Cardiology: A Case-Based Approach

Cardiology: A Case-Based Approach

Editor: Harrison Cox

FOSTER ACADEMICS
www.fosteracademics.com

www.fosteracademics.com

Cataloging-in-Publication Data

Cardiology : a case-based approach / edited by Harrison Cox.
p. cm.
Includes bibliographical references and index.
ISBN 978-1-63242-604-8
1. Cardiology. 2. Cardiology--Case studies. 3. Heart--Diseases. I. Cox, Harrison.
RC667 .C37 2019
616.1--dc23

Foster Academics,
118-35 Queens Blvd., Suite 400,
Forest Hills, NY 11375, USA

ISBN 978-1-63242-604-8 (Hardback)

Printed and bound in China.

Contents

1

A Rare Case of Complete Heart Block in a Young Patient

Zakaria Hindi,[1] **Yousef Hindi**,[2] **and Rami Batarseh**[1]

[1]*Internal Medicine Department, Texas Tech University Health Sciences Center, Permian Basin, Odessa, TX, USA*
[2]*Cardiology Department, University of Texas Health Science Center at San Antonio, San Antonio, TX, USA*

Correspondence should be addressed to Zakaria Hindi; dr.zhindi@hotmail.com

Academic Editor: Kjell Nikus

Introduction. Complete heart block (CHB) is considered as one of the dangerous rhythms since it can progress to lethal arrhythmias such as ventricular tachycardia. It can be congenital or acquired. Patients may present with frequent palpitations, presyncope, dyspnea, or chest pain but also may remain asymptomatic. Extensive work-up should be conducted to exclude secondary causes such as infections, cardiac ischemia or myopathies, autoimmune diseases, or endocrinological diseases. In our paper, we would like to present a case of CHB in the setting of aortic abdominal thrombus that nearly occluded both renal arteries. The CHB in this case is thought to be caused by hypertensive cardiomyopathy due to ongoing uncontrolled hypertension, which is caused by bilateral renal artery stenosis. *Case Presentation*. A 31-year-old male with history of active smoking was incidentally found to have high blood pressure, bradycardia, and CHB on electrocardiogram. The patient was admitted to a cardiology ward and extensive work-up revealed hypokinesia of the left ventricle with low ejection fraction and left ventricle concentric hypertrophy, large abdominal aortic thrombus with bilateral renal artery stenosis, and evidence of arterial collateral connections, which suggest chronicity. The patient then was placed on four antihypertensive medications but eventually, he underwent bilateral renal artery stenting and insertion of permanent pacemaker for his CHB. The patient's blood pressure then was under control with only one medication, and subsequent CT angiogram showed no evidence of stenosis of both renal arteries. *Conclusion*. Uncontrolled hypertension can lead to hypertensive cardiomyopathy, which in turn can cause conduction abnormalities such as CHB. Although hypertension can be secondary to a treatable underlying cause, permanent pacemaker is essential to treat CHB.

1. Introduction

Complete heart block (CHB) is considered as one of the dangerous rhythms since it can progress to lethal arrhythmias such as ventricular tachycardia. It can be congenital or secondary to infections, cardiac ischemia or myopathies, autoimmune diseases, or endocrinological diseases that require extensive work-up to be ruled out [1]. Out of secondary causes, hypertrophic obstructive cardiomyopathy and infiltrative myopathies such as sarcoidosis and amyloidosis are considered as potential causes for CHB [2].

Taking hypertensive heart disease into consideration, the condition is quite similar to hypertrophic cardiomyopathy. In that, both conditions have similar findings on physical exam and echocardiogram. They can be differentiated however on the basis of strain rate imaging [3]. Although the establishment of relation between hypertrophic cardiomyopathy and CHB has been reported before [4], yet the association between hypertensive cardiomyopathy and CHB has never been reported. Hence, we would like to report a case of CHB in a patient with bilateral renal artery stenosis, nonpreserved nonischemic hypertensive cardiomyopathy, and uncontrolled hypertension. We believe that this case would merit further investigation regarding the relation between hypertensive cardiomyopathy and CHB.

2. Case Presentation

A 30-year-old male with history of active smoking (1 pack per day for 10 years) and external hemorrhoids came to the preop anesthesia clinic for anesthesia evaluation fitness and was found to have high blood pressure (BP) (234/144). He was referred immediately to the emergency room (ER) for BP control. In the ER, BP was 221/125 and heart rate (HR) was 50 beats/minute. Routine electrocardiogram (EKG) showed 3rd-degree heart block (TDHB) and left ventricular

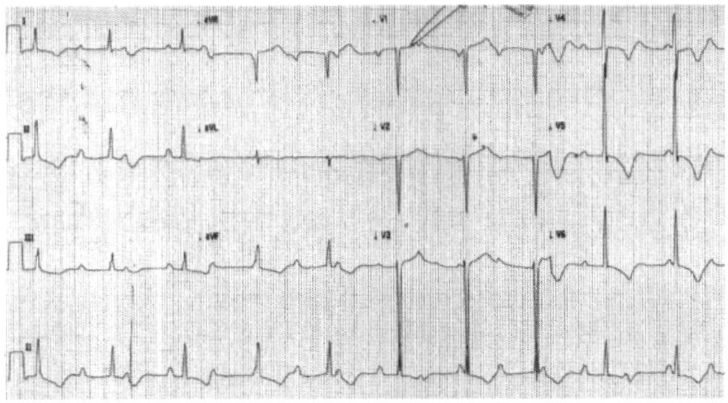

Figure 1: EKG showing complete heart block with T wave inversion in inferiolateral leads and LVH strain.

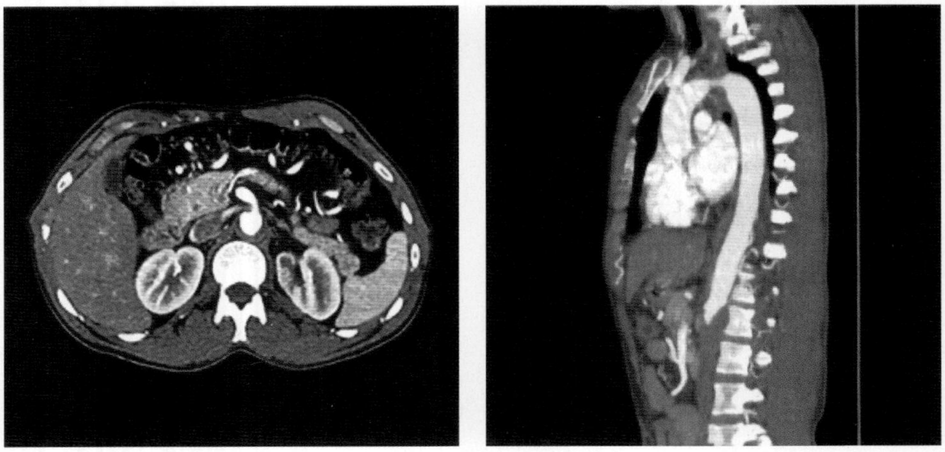

(a) (b)

Figure 2: CT angiogram of the abdomen. (a) Bilateral stenosis and near occlusion of renal arteries. (b) Abdominal aortic thrombus that extends to the level of renal arteries.

hypertrophy (LVH) with strain pattern (Figure 1). He denied chest pain, palpitation, dyspnea, dizziness, or syncope. The patient was started on antihypertensive medication for BP control and was admitted to the cardiology ward for evaluation and management of complete heart block. Further physical exam revealed absent arterial pulses except the left radial pulse which was weak. BP was significantly different between both upper limbs and between upper and lower limbs (right upper limb 126/86 and lower limb 85/54, left upper limb 145/85 and lower limb 75/50). His initial blood work showed mild renal impairment.

Computerized tomography (CT) thoracic aortogram was done to rule out coarctation of the aorta, which was normal; CT coronary angiogram showed no evidence of coronary artery disease (CAD). Magnetic resonance imaging (MRI) of the heart was normal as well. Transthoracic echocardiogram (TTE) showed moderate hypokinesia of the left ventricle (LV), ejection fraction (EF) 35–40%, grade 2/4 diastolic dysfunction, and moderate concentric LVH. Holter monitoring did not reveal any pauses. Ultrasound/Doppler of the kidneys showed increased parenchymal echogenicity with poorly defined corticomedullary junction impressive of renal parenchymal disease. CT abdominal aortogram showed large thrombus seen in the abdominal aorta starting at the level of renal arteries completely occluding the aorta and common iliac arteries with no blood flow seen beyond the renal artery level up to the aortic bifurcation; moderate to severe stenosis is noted at the origin of both renal arteries because of thrombus (Figures 2(a) and 2(b)). Multiple abdominal collaterals are seen with multiple collaterals in the anterior and lateral abdominal wall and paraspinal collaterals (Figure 3). Extensive blood work-up including thyroid function test and autoimmune and thrombophilia work-up was all unremarkable. No cause of aortic thrombosis and TDHB was identified.

Initial recommendation of the vascular surgeon was to follow up in the clinic with no intervention as it is a chronic process, and the patient was asymptomatic. Since the patient had uncontrolled hypertension despite being on maximum doses of four antihypertensive medications, eventually he underwent percutaneous stenting of bilateral renal arteries which was followed by an improvement in the BP and renal function and reduction in doses of antihypertensive medications. The patient also underwent permanent pacemaker insertion for TDHB. The patient was also placed on warfarin and was advised to see the vascular surgeon after 3 months. Unfortunately, the patient did not follow up.

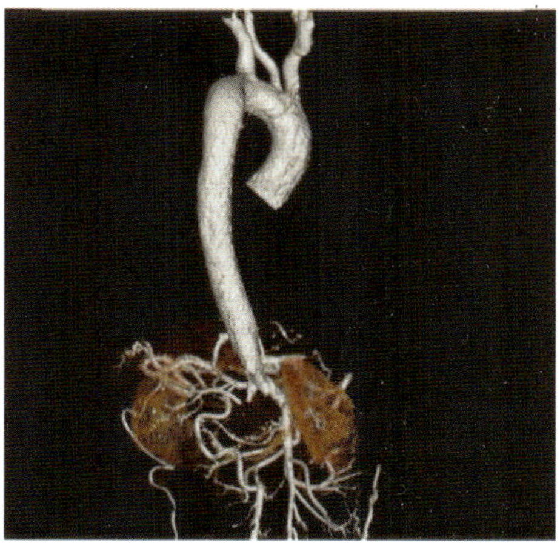

Figure 3: Aortogram extraction scan. It shows collateral arteries around renal arteries.

3. Discussion

This young patient had accidental findings of asymptomatic CHB, uncontrolled HTN with renal artery stenosis, and complete thrombosis of the abdominal aorta. After reviewing the literature, we could not find a unifying diagnosis for the patient's condition. The closest condition to our patient's presentation is Leriche's that is described as an aortoiliac disease, which partially explains the patient's thrombotic events [5]. Yet, Leriche's syndrome has no known association with CHB. We believe that the patient had initially bilateral renal artery stenosis which was a consequence of the chronic abdominal aortic thrombus as there were collateral arteries. The uncontrolled HTN which resulted from untreated bilateral renal artery stenosis led to hypertensive heart disease that was evident by EKG and echocardiogram findings.

Hypertensive heart disease (HHD) is a group of abnormalities that comprises LVH and systolic/diastolic dysfunction. HHD in general is considered as a risk factor for atrial and ventricular arrhythmias such as atrial fibrillation, supraventricular tachycardia, and ventricular tachycardia. Bradyarrhythmias, however, are mainly caused by drug side effects (such as beta blockers) when treating HTN [6–8]. The pathogenesis of arrhythmias in HHD arises mainly from LVH and left ventricular dysfunction [9]. Both may be associated with CHB if ischemic cardiomyopathy develops [10]. In our patient, ischemic cardiomyopathy was ruled out by coronary angiogram. This can indicate that HHD may cause atrioventricular block without developing ischemia.

The management of our patient was based on controlling HTN sufficiently. Our target blood pressure was below 130/80 mmHg. Despite medicating the patient with maximum doses of four different antihypertensive agents (which fits the definition of resistant HTN [11]), his blood pressure was not controlled. The stenting of both renal arteries was done as per American Heart Association recommendations [11]. As for CHB, the treatment of choice is permanent pacemaker regardless of the symptoms [12, 13].

4. Conclusion

It should be emphasized that CHB may be a rare consequence in HHD which requires permanent pacemaker regardless of cardiomyopathy stage or severity of symptoms. Moreover, the relation between CHB and HHD should be investigated.

References

[1] E. M. Kojic, T. Hardarson, N. Sigfusson, and H. Sigvaldason, "The prevalence and prognosis of third-degree atrioventricular conduction block: the Reykjavik study," *Journal of Internal Medicine*, vol. 246, no. 1, pp. 81–86, 1999.

[2] A. Harris, M. Davies, D. Redwood, A. Leatham, and H. Siddons, "Aetiology of chronic heart block. A clinico-pathological correlation in 65 cases," *British Heart Journal*, vol. 31, no. 2, pp. 206–218, 1969.

[3] T. S. Kato, A. Noda, H. Izawa et al., "Discrimination of nonobstructive hypertrophic cardiomyopathy from hypertensive left ventricular hypertrophy on the basis of strain rate imaging by tissue Doppler ultrasonography," *Circulation*, vol. 110, no. 25, pp. 3808–3814, 2004.

[4] M. Yesil, S. Bayata, I. Susam, H. Dinçkal, and N. Postaci, "Rare association of hypertrophic cardiomyopathy and complete atrioventricular block with prompt disappearance of outflow gradient after DDD pacing," *Europace*, vol. 1, no. 4, pp. 280–282, 1999.

[5] R. Leriche and A. Morel, "The syndrome of thrombotic obliteration of the aortic bifurcation," *Annals of Surgery*, vol. 127, no. 2, pp. 193–206, 1948.

[6] M. H. Drazner, "The progression of hypertensive heart disease," *Circulation*, vol. 123, no. 3, pp. 327–334, 2011.

[7] A. Aidietis, A. Laucevicius, and G. Marinskis, "Hypertension and cardiac arrhythmias," *Current Pharmaceutical Design*, vol. 13, no. 25, pp. 2545–2555, 2007.

[8] J. M. McLenachan, E. Henderson, K. I. Morris, and H. J. Dargie, "Ventricular arrhythmias in patients with hypertensive left ventricular hypertrophy," *New England Journal of Medicine*, vol. 317, no. 13, pp. 787–792, 1987.

[9] J.-P. Baguet, S. Erdine, and J.-M. Mallion, "European Society of Hypertension scientific newsletter: update on hypertension management: hypertension and dysrhythmias," *Journal of Hypertension*, vol. 24, no. 2, pp. 409–411, 2006.

[10] U. J. O. Gang, C. Jons, R. M. Jorgensen et al., "Risk markers of late high-degree atrioventricular block in patients with left ventricular dysfunction after an acute myocardial infarction: a CARISMA substudy," *Europace*, vol. 13, no. 10, pp. 1471–1477, 2011.

[11] J. L. Anderson, J. L. Halperin, N. Albert et al., "Management of patients with peripheral artery disease (compilation of 2005 and 2011 ACCF/AHA guideline recommendations): a report of the American College of Cardiology Foundation/American Heart Association Task Force on Practice Guidelines," *Journal of the American College of Cardiology*, vol. 61, no. 14, pp. 1555–1570, 2013.

[12] M. Brignole, A. Auricchio, G. Baron-Esquivias et al., "2013 ESC guidelines on cardiac pacing and cardiac resynchronization therapy: the task force on cardiac pacing and resynchronization therapy of the European Society of Cardiology (ESC). Developed in collaboration with the European Heart Rhythm

Association (EHRA)," *European Heart Journal*, vol. 34, no. 29, pp. 2281–2329, 2013.

[13] A. E. Epstein, J. P. DiMarco, K. A. Ellenbogen et al., "ACC/AHA/HRS 2008 guidelines for device-based therapy of cardiac rhythm abnormalities: a report of the American College of Cardiology/American Heart Association Task Force on Practice Guidelines (Writing Committee to Revise the ACC/AHA/NASPE 2002 Guideline Update for Implantation of Cardiac Pacemakers and Antiarrhythmia Devices) developed in collaboration with the American Association for Thoracic Surgery and Society of Thoracic Surgeons," *Journal of the American College of Cardiology*, vol. 51, no. 21, pp. e1–e62, 2008.

2

A Rare Case of Complete Fragmentation of Pacemaker Lead after a High-Velocity Theme Park Ride

Furqan Khattak, Muhammad Khalid, Sathvika Gaddam, Vijay Ramu, and Vipul Brahmbhatt

East Tennessee State University, Johnson City, TN, USA

Correspondence should be addressed to Furqan Khattak; Khattak@etsu.edu

Academic Editor: Domingo A. Pascual-Figal

Pacemaker lead fracture is one of the most common causes of pacemaker malfunction and is most frequently associated with weight lifting or chest trauma. These patients usually present with symptoms of dizziness, syncope, chest discomfort, and palpitations or less commonly with extracardiac symptoms. Diagnosis is made by ECG and careful review of chest imaging such as chest X-ray or fluoroscopy. Treatment involves placement of a new lead with or without extraction of the fractured lead. We present an interesting case of complete severance of the tip of a dual-chamber pacemaker's atrial lead after a high-velocity theme park ride. In our case, the fracture occurred during amusement park rides and went undiagnosed until the patient presented for routine pacemaker evaluation. This case indicates that extreme physical forces in the absence of direct trauma, such as during amusement park rides, may result in lead fractures and patients with pacemakers should be cautioned regarding such activities.

1. Introduction

Pacemaker lead fracture is one of the most common causes of pacemaker malfunction. Lead fractures are seen in approximately 0.1 to 4.2% of patients with pacemakers per year. Lead fractures are most commonly associated with physical exertion during weight lifting or chest trauma. Subclavian crush syndrome is one of the most commonly reported causes of traumatic pacemaker fractures. Stress or trauma due to physical exertion causes compression of a lead between the clavicle and first rib when implanted by subclavian approach. In our patient's case, fracture of a pacemaker lead occurred during accelerated rides in the absence of direct trauma.

2. Case Description

A 62-year-old male with history of hypertension, coronary artery disease, and sick sinus syndrome presented to outpatient device check clinic to establish care for a pacemaker device. He underwent implantation of a dual-chamber pacemaker device (St. Jude Accent generator with Medtronic CapSure SP Novus atrial and ventricular leads) in 2002 for sick sinus syndrome and had a generator changeout in 2011. The lead model was not implicated in a recall to our knowledge and search. The patient had his last device check performed in March 2017, and no problems with the device function were reported at that time. The patient denied any trauma to the chest or upper extremities, chest pain, shortness of breath, palpitations, presyncope, or syncopal episodes. He denied any device-related complications in the past. The patient reported a recent visit to a popular theme park in the 1st week of August, where he enjoyed multiple high thrill rides including high-velocity roller coaster rides. On physical examination, he was afebrile with normal pulse, blood pressure, and respiratory rate. His left pectoral pacemaker implant site showed no erythema, swelling, warmth, drainage, or signs of erosion. Labs showed normal blood counts and normal renal and liver function. A 12-lead ECG showed normal sinus rhythm with a heart rate of 60 beats per minute and atrial pacing spikes with loss of capture (Figure 1). Pacemaker device evaluation showed approximate remaining battery life of 9 years and programmed DDDR pacing mode. Heart rate histograms showed 54% atrial pacing and 15% ventricular pacing. The right

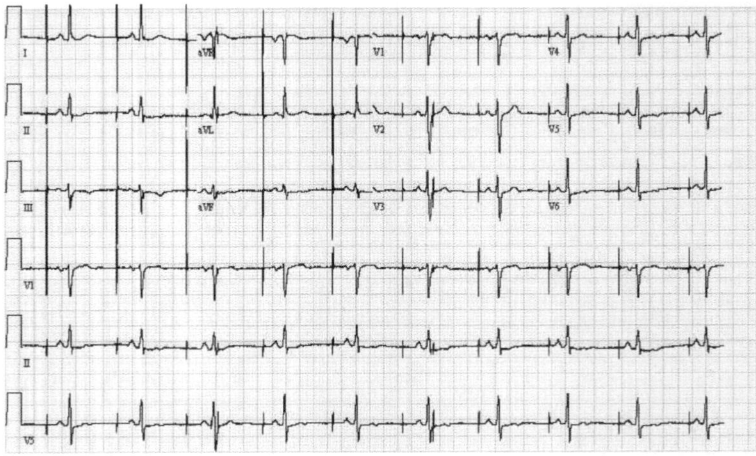

Figure 1: 12-lead ECG showed normal sinus rhythm with loss of capture of atrial lead.

ventricular lead showed normal sensing, impedance, and pacing threshold. The right atrial lead was noted to have unusually high impedance of 2175 ohms and no capture on testing at voltages as high as 7.5 mV. Lead impedance history clearly showed an abrupt increase in the atrial lead impedance in August, at the time patient had visited the theme park, from around 600 ohms to 1000 ohms and subsequently above 2000 ohms (Figure 2). EGM showed atrial lead noise. A chest X-ray (CXR) was obtained which revealed an intact right ventricular lead and complete severance of the right atrial lead tip (Figures 3 and 4). The pacemaker was reprogrammed from DDDR to VVIR mode. After discussion and review with the patient, it was decided not to retrieve the fractured lead or insert a new atrial lead, due to his intrinsic sinus rhythm having taken over, no evidence of atrioventricular (AV) block, and no current requirement for pacing. It was decided to follow the patient clinically to see if he will require insertion of an atrial lead in future.

3. Discussion

Pacemaker devices play an important role in the management of bradyarrhythmias, however, postimplantation complications can cause significant morbidity and mortality. Complications may occur during implant procedure, or, from pocket complications, generator malfunction, or lead failures. Pacemaker leads are considered the weakest link in this chain. Previous studies have reported lead-related complications such as lead dislodgement or lead damage during implantation, electrical failure, and lead fracture due to chest trauma or insulation defects in different pacemaker devices. Studies have also shown the benefit of postimplantation chest X-ray to look for immediate implantation-related complications, perforation, and malposition of leads. Early lead perforation is a rare complication of device implantation in the right atrium or right ventricle (0.1–0.8%) and occurs within one month of implantation. Delayed lead perforation occurs after the first month and is usually differentiated from early perforation by the absence of cardiac tamponade related to lead perforation. Lead fractures are seen with an incidence rate of 0.1 to 4.2% per patient year [1]. The most common site of lead fracture is at the site of entry (40%) followed by the area between the entry site and generator (28%) and lastly close to the generator site (23%). Only 7% are intravascular fractures [1]. Tricuspid valve has been reported as an unusual site of pacemaker lead fracture [2].

Most lead fractures occur in the pacemaker pocket or between clavicle and the first rib mainly due to compression of a lead lateral to the entry site between soft tissues muscles and ligaments. Pacemaker lead fracture due to physical exertion is an uncommon albeit recognized cause of lead malfunction. [3]. Few cases of traumatic lead fracture due to blunt chest trauma [4] and weight lifting due to crush injuries between clavicle and the first rib have been reported [5]. Subclavian crush syndrome is one of the most commonly reported causes of traumatic pacemaker fractures.

Studies have shown that fracture rate of multifilar coil leads is less than the single filar coil leads [6]. Lead fracture depends on factors such as coil diameter, radius of curvature, and approach used for implantation, with more fractures occurring with internal jugular vein approach than external jugular or cephalic vein approach. Usually, lead fracture is associated with high impedance, but there have been cases reported with normal impedance in multifilar coil lead fracture resulting from subclavian crush syndrome. The mechanism behind low impedance was a connection between inner and outer coil [7]. A case of lead fracture due to cardiac fibroma was also reported with low impedance [8]. Another case has been reported about loss of atrial pacing with possible atrial mode switch due to atrial oversensing in a patient with atrial arrhythmias [9].

Patients with a lead fracture may present with symptoms of dizziness, syncope, chest discomfort, and palpitations or less commonly extracardiac symptoms like hiccups or maybe completely asymptomatic as in our patient. Diagnosis is often made by ECG and careful review of chest imaging such as chest X-ray or fluoroscopy. Treatment involves placement of a new lead with or without extraction of the fractured lead. The decision regarding extraction of the old lead is individualized considering the age of the lead and expected fibrosis.

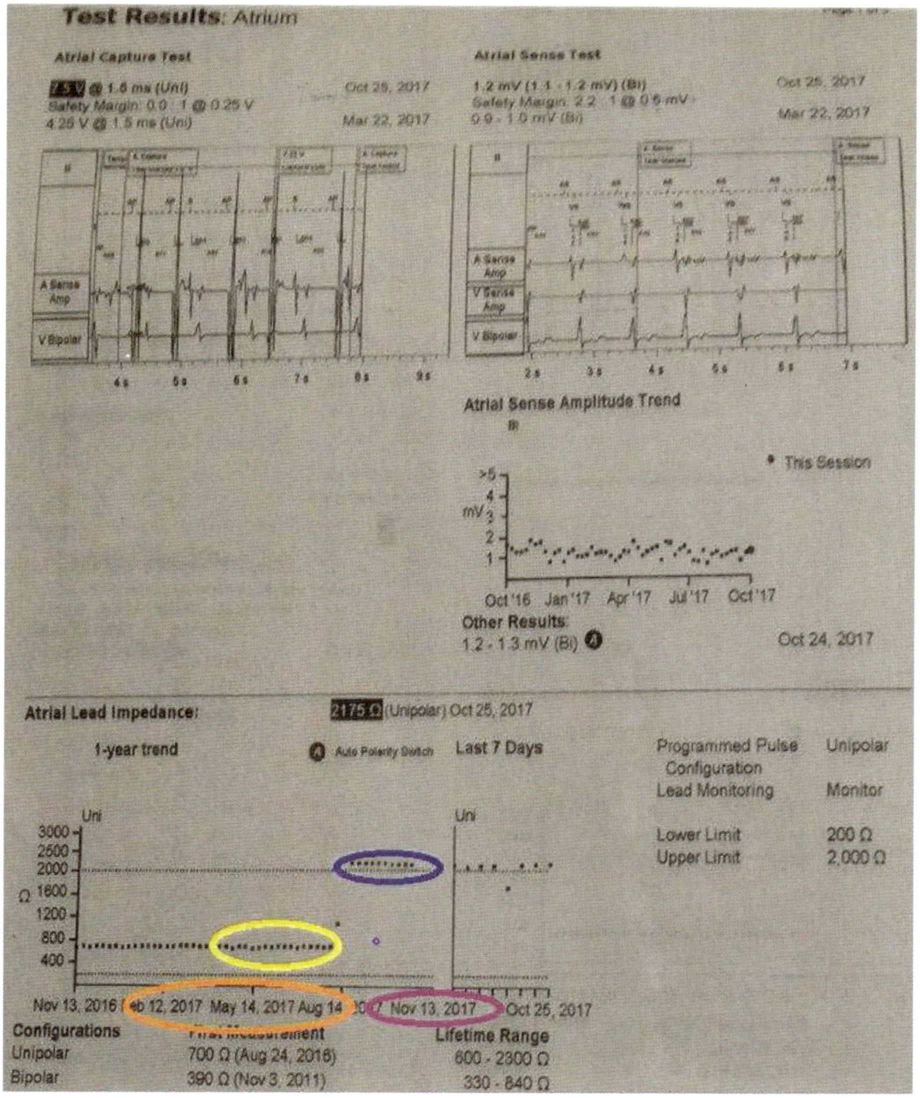

FIGURE 2: Device evaluation showed loss of atrial capture and sudden increase in lead impedance from normal in May 2017 (yellow circle) to 2000 ohms in August 2017 (blue circle).

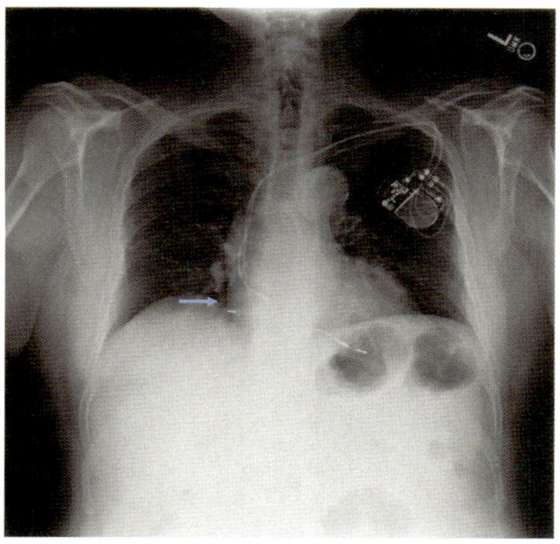

FIGURE 3: PA chest X-ray showed fractured right atrial lead (blue arrow).

Often, the old lead is capped and left alone to avoid complications of lead extraction such as arrhythmias and cardiac perforation.

Leadless pacemakers are now becoming available in the US market, and Micra, the first leadless pacemaker device, has been approved by FDA. Leadless devices implanted by transcatheter approach may theoretically reduce complications related to device implantation and those related to lead itself. This may be the future of pacing in suitable candidates who require only single chamber (right ventricle) pacing [10].

Our case is unusual to begin with as our patient had a dual-chamber pacemaker implanted for sick sinus syndrome at the age of 46 years; however, he did not show any progression to AV block after 16 years which is uncommon for molecular abnormalities of ion channel/cardiac proteins which usually undergo significant evolution to bradycardia/AV block with time. Second, to our knowledge, this is the first

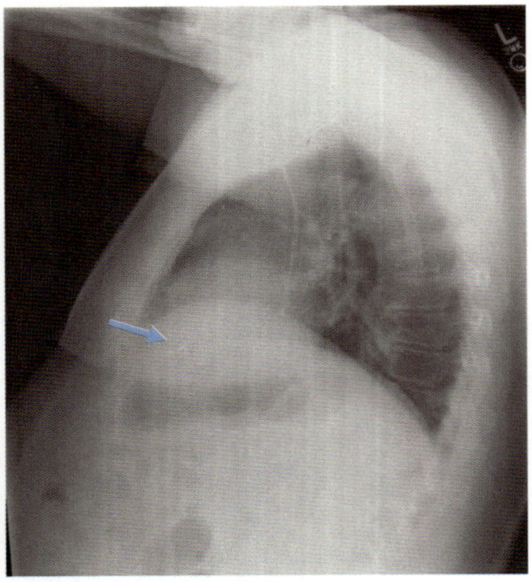

Figure 4: Lateral chest X-ray showed right atrial lead fracture (blue arrow).

case of a pacemaker lead fracture associated with a theme park ride and indicates that widely popular high-velocity theme park rides may pose risks to pacemaker leads. We hypothesize that the sheer stress generated by extreme acceleration and gravitational forces on a wire that is moving with cardiac cycle during the high-velocity rides may cause fracture even in the absence of direct physical trauma. The site of fracture in this case, which is a transition from ring to tip electrode of the atrial lead, rules out any possible role of surrounding skeletal structures, such as in cases of rib/clavicle/pocket fractures. The lack of previous chest X-ray in our center precluded the comparison between the current lead position and the position at implantation, which in fact could influence the fracture. Therefore, it cannot be inferred whether the lead tip was at the anterior-lateral location as the X-ray shows or if it migrated to this location after the lead body was snapped in two parts. This case may have important clinical implications such as the need for caution with theme park rides, and routine pacemaker interrogations after such visits especially in pacemaker-dependent patients. Luckily, our patient remained unharmed as he had intact intrinsic AV nodal conduction and required infrequent atrial pacing. Moreover, at the time of presentation, he had intrinsic sinus activity and intact AV nodal conduction and the failed atrial pacing programmed at 60 bpm was redundant.

References

[1] E. Alt, R. Völker, and H. Blömer, "Lead fracture in pacemaker patients," *The Thoracic and Cardiovascular Surgeon*, vol. 35, no. 2, pp. 101–104, 1987.

[2] B. Clarke, S. Jones, H. H. Gray, and E. Rowland, "The tricuspid valve: an unusual site of endocardial pacemaker lead fracture," *Pacing and Clinical Electrophysiology*, vol. 12, no. 7, pp. 1077–1079, 1989.

[3] O. J. Ohm, "Displacement and fracture of pacemaker electrode during physical exertion. Report on three cases," *Acta Medica Scandinavica*, vol. 192, no. 1-6, pp. 33–35, 1972.

[4] A. Bo"hm, G. Duray, and R. G. Kiss, "Traumatic pacemaker lead fracture," *Emergency Medicine Journal*, vol. 30, no. 8, p. 686, 2013.

[5] J. A. Deering and D. N. Pederson, "Pacemaker lead fracture associated with weightlifting: a report of two cases," *Military Medicine*, vol. 158, no. 12, pp. 833-834, 1993.

[6] J. Mugica and A. Ripart, "Twelve years' experience with cardiac pacing leads: clinical conclusions for 8,004 cases," *Clinical Progress in Pacing and Electrophysiology*, vol. 2, no. 6, pp. 513–532, 1984.

[7] E. De Maria, P. L. Fontana, L. Bonetti, and S. Cappelli, "An unusual presentation of complete pacing lead fracture with very low impedance values," *Journal of Cardiovascular Electrophysiology*, vol. 24, no. 12, pp. 1225–1425, 2013.

[8] D. Sato, H. Kitajima, H. Mani, C.-H. Park, and Y.-H. Chun, "Pacemaker lead fracture without an increase in lead impedance caused by cardiac fibroma," *Journal of Arrhythmia*, vol. 29, no. 6, pp. 357–359, 2013.

[9] E. E. Gul, U. Boles, F. S. Ali, and H. Abdollah, "Loss of atrial pacing in a patient with a dual-chamber permanent pacemaker: what is the mechanism?," *Journal of Arrhythmia*, vol. 33, no. 2, pp. 159-160, 2017.

[10] D. Reynolds, G. Z. Duray, R. Omar et al., "A leadless intracardiac transcatheter pacing system," *New England Journal of Medicine*, vol. 374, no. 6, pp. 533–541, 2016.

3

Successful Coronary Protection during TAVI in Heavily Calcified Aortic Leaflets in Patient with Short and Low Left Coronary System

Mohamad Kabach, Abdulah Alrifai, Lawrence Lovitz, Mark Rothenberg, Cristiano Faber, and Marcos Nores

JFK Medical Center, University of Miami School of Medicine, Atlantis, FL, USA

Correspondence should be addressed to Mohamad Kabach; mhd.kabach@gmail.com

Academic Editor: Man-Hong Jim

Transcatheter aortic valve replacement has been recently approved for patients who are high or intermediate risk for surgical aortic valve replacement. The procedure is associated with several known complications including coronary related complications. Coronary obstruction is rare but disastrous complication, and it is associated with a high mortality rate. Coronary protection technique has emerged as a preemptive technique to avoid this complication. We present a case of successful coronary protection during TAVR in severely calcified left cusp in patient with short and low left ostium.

1. Introduction

Surgical aortic valve replacement has been the mainstay of treatment of symptomatic severe aortic stenosis. The transcatheter approach comes to the rescue as a less invasive treatment in these high-risk patients [1] or old patients with intermediate risk [2] as well as inoperable patients [3]. TAVR has been associated with vascular, cerebrovascular, valvular, and conduction complications. A rare, life-threatening complication of TAVR is a coronary ostial obstruction. Several cases were reported in this field [4]. A systematic review of reported cases suggests that it occurs more often in women and in patients receiving a balloon-expandable valve. However, this complication has not been evaluated in comparative studies of CoreValve and SAPIEN transcatheter valve models [5]. Coronary protection during TAVI is a preemptive technique recommended in certain cases to avoid this complication. We report a case of successful coronary protection in patient with severely calcified aortic valve in patient with short and low left coronary system.

2. Case Presentation

An 86-year-old woman with known history of coronary artery disease and sick sinus syndrome was admitted to the hospital with dyspnea, orthopnea, and exertional dizziness. Physical exam revealed bibasilar crackles, a grade 5 crescendo-decrescendo murmur, elevated JVP, and lower extremity edema. Laboratory findings were pertinent for creatinine of 1.73, BUN of 45, and NT-pro-BNP of 10k. The rest of her physical exam and laboratory was normal. Electrocardiogram showed normal sinus rhythm with known left bundle branch block. 2D echocardiogram demonstrated severe aortic stenosis with mean aortic valve pressure gradient of 68.6 mmHg and peak velocity of 5.15 m/s with preserved systolic function. She received intravenous diuretics with some clinical improvement.

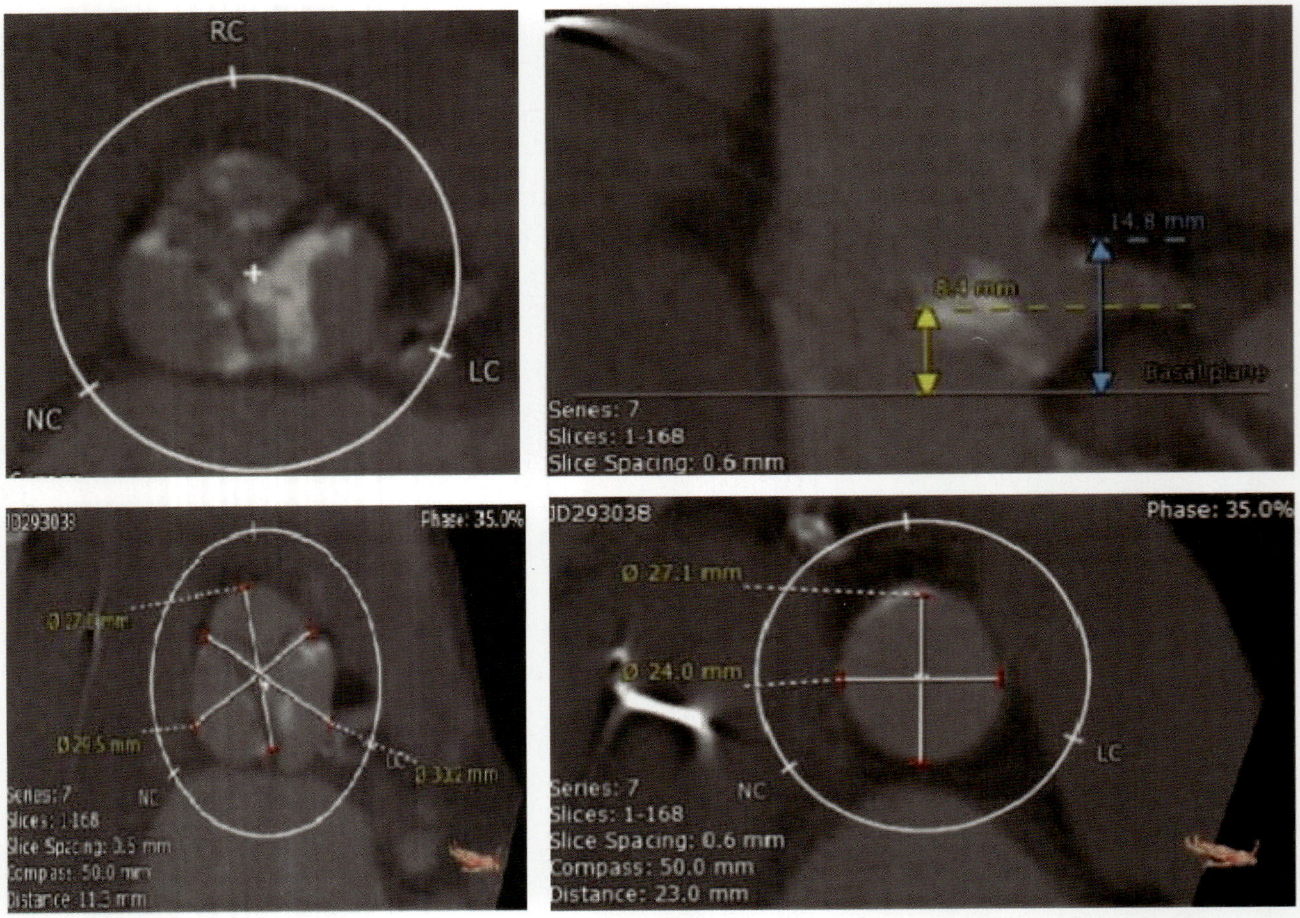

Figure 1: Cardiac computed tomography angiography showed severely calcified aortic leaflets with short and low left coronary system with coronary ostial height of 8.4 mm.

She was seen and evaluated by cardiothoracic surgeon for evaluation of aortic valve replacement but deemed high risk for surgical aortic valve replacement with an estimated surgical mortality by Society of Thoracic Surgeons score of 8.1%. Cardiac computed tomography angiography was done as part of transcatheter aortic valve replacement evaluation and showed severely calcified aortic leaflets with short and low left coronary system with coronary ostial height of 8.4 mm (Figure 1). Special attention was paid to the left coronary leaflet calcification and the short and low coronary ostium. Coronary angiography revealed 50% LAD stent restenosis, diffuse distal LCX disease, and 90% proximal RCA stenosis. A drug-eluting stent was implanted to the right coronary artery. The decision then was made to proceed with TAVI utilizing coronary protection technique during the procedure. TAVR was then undertaken from the right femoral artery through a 14F Edwards arterial sheath. Two 300 mm long Prowater wires were advanced to the LAD and LCX arteries. With rapid ventricular pacing over a long Amplatz extra stiff wire, balloon aortic valvuloplasty using an Edward 4×23 mm balloon with simultaneous root aortography to see how the left main flow was performed (Figure 2). There was flow compromise in the left main system to TIMI-2 flow; the wires were deformed and the large piece of calcium in the left cusp moved right over the left main coronary artery (Figure 2). We therefore made decision to place two 3.5×12 mm Robel bare-metal stents in the LAD and LCX. An Edward 23 mm SAPIEN 3 valve with rapid ventricular pacing was then deployed followed by deploying the two stents in a kissing fashion, and an excellent result was obtained (Figure 3). Position of the valve and function was confirmed by aortography and transesophageal echocardiography (TEE). The left main coronary flow was excellent. The patient tolerated the procedure well and recovered uneventfully and was discharged 2 days after the procedure without complications. At 30-day follow-up, she has notable improvement of her symptoms and physical activity with NYHA class I from class IV symptoms.

3. Discussion

TAVR is an acceptable and successful alternative to surgical aortic valve replacement in high-risk patients. A rare, life-threatening complication of TAVR is a coronary ostial obstruction. Scarce clinical data is available on this important complication as it has been reported in case reports

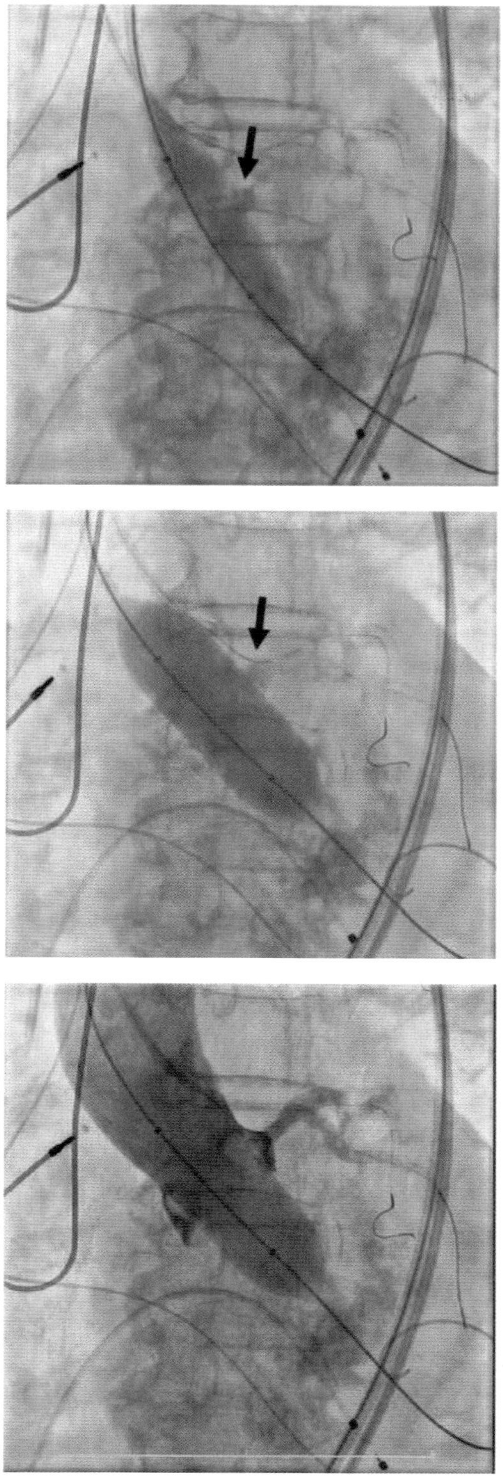

FIGURE 2: Balloon aortic valvuloplasty, notice the deformed wires and the large piece of calcium in the left cusp moved right over the left main coronary artery (arrows). Simultaneous aortic root injection showing decreased coronary flow TIMI-2. Echocardiogram demonstrated severe aortic stenosis with mean aortic valve pressure gradient of 68.6 mmHg and peak velocity of 5.15 m/s.

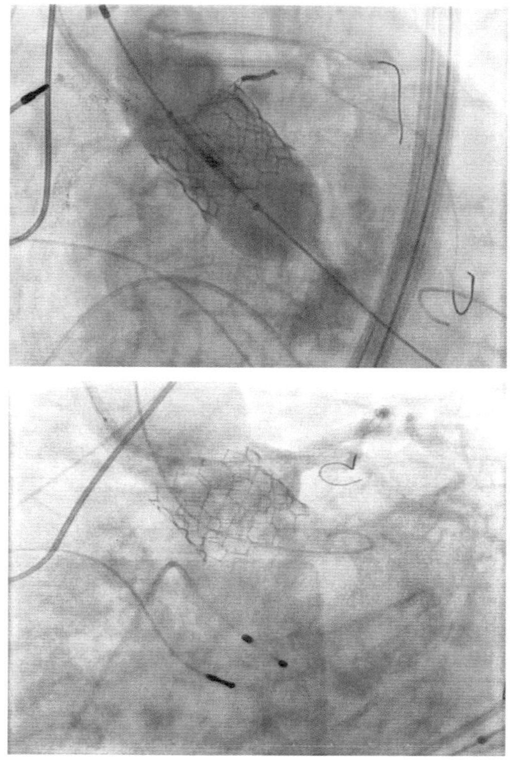

FIGURE 3: Final pictures demonstrating implantation of the Edward S3 valve with the kissing stents deflated prior and the final results after final implantation.

and small case series with an estimated incidence of <1% which carries a high mortality when it occurs (close to 40% at 30 days) [6]. A coronary ostial height cut-off of <10 mm increases the risk of coronary obstruction after TAVI [7, 8]. The LM protection technique should be considered in patients deemed to be at increased risk of LM compromise. It is mostly due to anatomical factors including low coronary ostia and shallow sinuses of Valsalva (SOV) and with valve in valve (VIV) for surgical bioprosthesis. LM protection should be considered in LM height of less than 9 mm, a difference of less than 2 mm between the SOV mean diameter, and the prosthesis diameter or severe aortic valve calcifications with the presence of left cusp large bulky calcium nodule(s). Preprocedural imaging and contingency planning must be utilized as it helps in the early diagnosis and treatment of coronary compromise following valve deployment. This involves preprocedural coronary angiography, EKG-gated, multislice CT angiography study with CT analysis that includes aortic annulus diameter and area, coronary height, SOV diameter, sinotubular junction (STJ) diameter, severity of aortic valve calcification, the presence of aortic valve calcium nodules (>10 mm), prosthesis size/annulus diameter ratio, and prosthesis area/annulus area ratio. Recent report of case series suggested a decision-making flow chart for the preprocedural evaluation of a patient believed to be at increased risk of LM compromise during TAVI (Figure 4) [9].

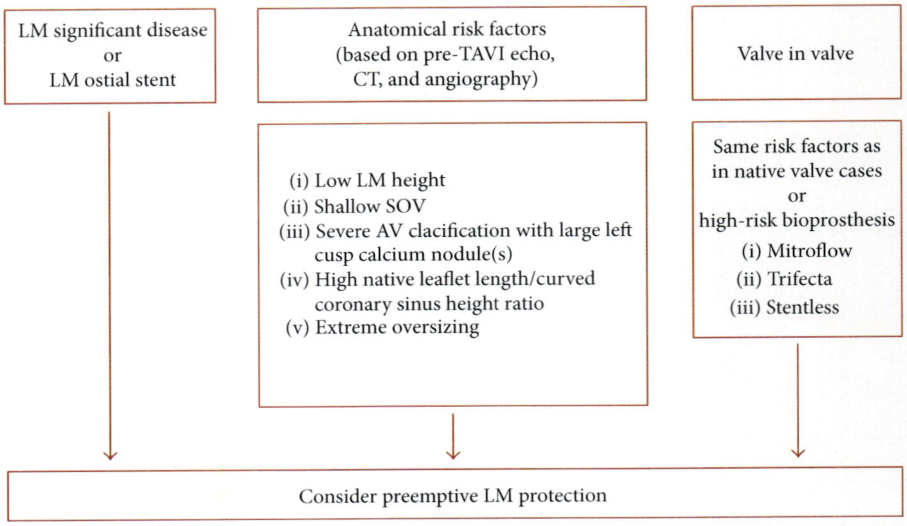

Figure 4: Suggested flow chart for preemptive LM protection based on pre-TAVR evaluation. AV: aortic valve; LM: left main; SOV: sinuses of Valsalva; TAVR: transcatheter aortic valve implantation.

4. Conclusion

The LM protection with preemptive technique is safe and feasible and should be considered in patients deemed to be at increased risk of LM compromise.

Disclosure

This case presentation was also presented at Cardiovascular Revascularization Therapies (CRT, 2017) [10].

References

[1] C. R. Smith, M. B. Leon, M. J. Mack et al., "Transcatheter versus surgical aortic-valve replacement in high-risk patients," *New England Journal*, vol. 364, no. 23, pp. 2187–2198, 2011.

[2] M. B. Leon, C. R. Smith, M. J. Mack et al., "Transcatheter or surgical aortic-valve replacement in intermediate-risk patients," *New England Journal*, vol. 374, no. 17, pp. 1609–1620, 2016.

[3] M. B. Leon, C. R. Smith, M. Mack et al., "Transcatheter aortic-valve implantation for aortic stenosis in patients who cannot undergo surgery," *New England Journal*, vol. 363, no. 17, pp. 1597–1607, 2010.

[4] M. Kabach, A. Alrifai, S. Furlan, and F. Alahdab, "Recurrent angina from chronic coronary obstruction following transcatheter aortic valve implantation," *Avicenna Journal of Medicine*, vol. 6, no. 3, pp. 86–88, 2016.

[5] H. B. Ribeiro, L. Nombela-Franco, M. Urena et al., "Coronary obstruction following transcatheter aortic valve implantation: a systematic review," *JACC: Cardiovascular Interventions*, vol. 6, no. 5, pp. 452–461, 2013.

[6] H. B. Ribeiro, J. G. Webb, R. R. Makkar et al., "Predictive factors, management, and clinical outcomes of coronary obstruction following transcatheter aortic valve implantation: insights from a large multicenter registry," *Journal of the American College of Cardiology*, vol. 62, no. 17, pp. 1552–1562, 2013.

[7] D. R. Holmes Jr., M. J. Mack, S. Kaul et al., "2012 ACCF/AATS/SCAI/STS expert consensus document on transcatheter aortic valve replacement," *Journal of the American College of Cardiology*, vol. 59, no. 13, pp. 1200–1254, 2012.

[8] J. B. Masson, J. Kovac, G. Schuler et al., "Transcatheter aortic valve implantation: review of the nature, management, and avoidance of procedural complications," *JACC: Cardiovascular Interventions*, vol. 2, no. 9, pp. 811–820, 2009.

[9] Y. Abramowitz, T. Chakravarty, H. Jilaihawi et al., "Clinical impact of coronary protection during transcatheter aortic valve implantation: first reported series of patients," *EuroIntervention*, vol. 11, no. 5, pp. 572–581, 2015.

[10] M. Kabach, "CRT," https://www.eventscribe.com/2017/CRT/aaSupperSessions.asp?day=2/19/2017&theday=Sunday&BCFO=&suppersession=Abstracts+%26+Interesting+Cases%3A+Session+5+-+Valve+Interesting+Cases, 2017.

Sick Sinus Syndrome and Takotsubo Cardiomyopathy

Ahmed S. Yassin[1], **Ahmed Subahi**,[1] **Hossam Abubakar**,[1] **Ahmed Rashed**,[2] **and Mohamed Shokr**[2]

[1]*Department of Internal Medicine, Wayne State University/Detroit Medical Center, Detroit, MI, USA*
[2]*Division of Cardiovascular Medicine, Department of Internal Medicine, Wayne State University/Detroit Medical Center, Detroit, MI, USA*

Correspondence should be addressed to Ahmed S. Yassin; gm0600@wayne.edu

Academic Editor: Gianluca Di Bella

Background. Takotsubo cardiomyopathy is associated with increased risk of ventricular arrhythmias, atrial fibrillation, and bradyarrhythmias. However, sinus node dysfunction is relatively infrequent in the setting of takotsubo cardiomyopathy. *Case Report.* We are reporting a case of a 73-year-old woman with a history of asymptomatic sinus bradycardia who developed sick sinus syndrome complicated by takotsubo cardiomyopathy. *Conclusion.* Acute symptomatic sick sinus syndrome in patients with preexisting silent sinus node dysfunction can trigger takotsubo cardiomyopathy. Understanding precipitating factors of takotsubo cardiomyopathy and identifying the patients at risk of life-threatening arrhythmia can help in refining risk stratification and therapy planning. Patients with sick sinus syndrome complicated by takotsubo cardiomyopathy may benefit from pacemaker implantation. However, evaluation on a case-by-case basis is mandatory.

1. Introduction

First described in Japan by Dote et al. in 1990, takotsubo cardiomyopathy (TC) became increasingly reported as a form of reversible focal myocardial hypokinesis following significant psychological or physical stress [1, 2]. Arrhythmias are common in patients with TC including atrial fibrillation (5–15% of the cases) and ventricular arrhythmias (4–9% of the cases) [2]. However, sinus node dysfunction (SND) is relatively infrequent in the setting of TC (1.3% of the cases) [3]. We describe the case of a 73-year-old woman with a history of asymptomatic sinus bradycardia who developed sick sinus syndrome (SSS) complicated by takotsubo cardiomyopathy.

2. Case Presentation

We present the case of a 73-year-old woman with a history of asymptomatic sinus bradycardia that presented to our facility with a chief complaint of acute chest pain. She was found to have elevated troponin I of 0.3 ng/ml (normal < 0.057). Chest X-ray was normal. Laboratory workup revealed normal complete blood count, bleeding profile, basic metabolic panel, thyroid-stimulating hormone, and random blood glucose. The 12-lead electrocardiogram (ECG) was suggestive of junctional escape rhythm with a heart rate (HR) of 37 beats/minute (Figure 1). Transthoracic echocardiography (TTE) showed reduced left ventricular function (ejection fraction (EF) of 30%), with apical ballooning suggestive of takotsubo cardiomyopathy versus acute coronary syndrome (Figure 2). Left ventriculogram also showed ventricular ballooning suggestive of takotsubo cardiomyopathy (Figure 3). Cardiac catheterization revealed normal coronary arteries. Thus, she was diagnosed with classical TC. Due to her symptomatic bradycardia, a temporary pacing wire was placed. Her diagnosis was suggestive of sick sinus syndrome as she had occasional P waves that were fine (Figure 4). Overnight, she went into an atrial flutter with a variable block (Figure 5). Although, no rate control agent was started, the HR was 83 beats/minute (Figure 5). Her atrial flutter continued over the next 24 hours. A dual-chamber pacemaker was recommended and placed without complications by the electrophysiology team. Her rhythm on discharge was rate-controlled

Vent. rate	37	BPM
PR interval	*	ms
QRS duration	88	ms
QT/QTc	510/400	ms
P-R-T axes	*86	79

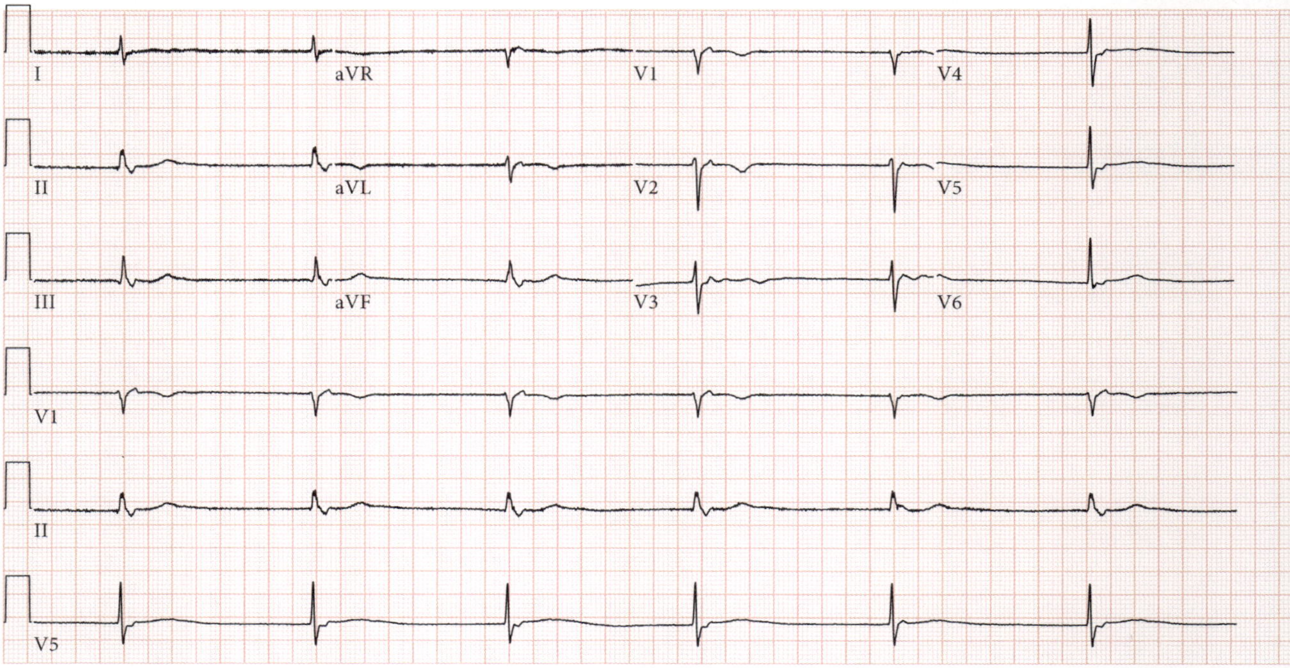

Figure 1: EKG shows junctional escape rhythm with a heart rate (HR) of 37 beats/minute.

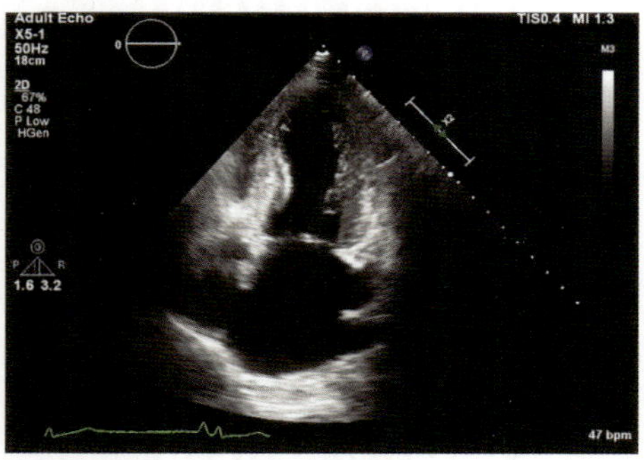

Figure 2: Echocardiogram (2-chamber long-axis view) showing the apical ballooning suggestive of takotsubo cardiomyopathy.

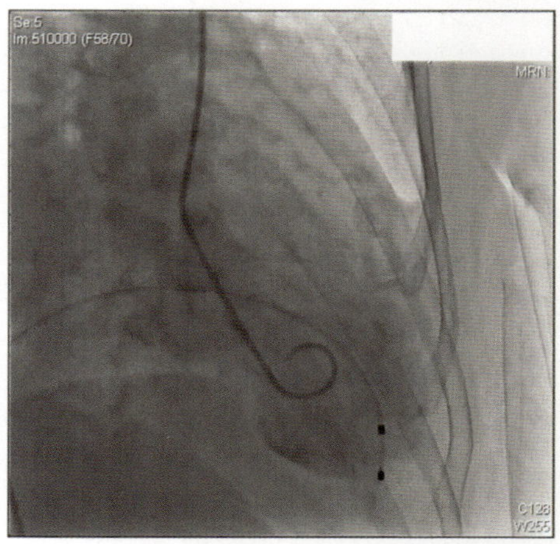

Figure 3: Left ventriculogram in the right anterior oblique projection showing the ventricular ballooning suggestive of takotsubo cardiomyopathy.

atrial flutter. She was discharged home on a beta-blocker, angiotensin-converting enzyme inhibitor, and anticoagulation. Her TTE findings were resolved on a follow-up visit two weeks later. However, pacemaker interrogation revealed frequent episodes of paroxysmal rate-controlled atrial fibrillation alternating with bradycardia requiring cardiac pacing. The patient is still under regular follow-up in the cardiology clinic.

3. Discussion

Takotsubo cardiomyopathy is characterized by reversible regional dyskinesia of the ventricular myocardium typically extending beyond a single coronary vascular bed [2]. TC can mimic acute heart failure or acute myocardial infarction in clinical presentation and be usually but not always triggered by medically or emotionally stressful events [2, 4]. The absence of significant coronary stenosis is a prerequisite for the diagnosis on almost all accepted diagnostic criteria [2, 4]. Arrhythmia is a common complication in patients with TC [2]. Also, TC can evolve after discrete episodes of arrhythmia [3]. However, SND in the setting of TC is

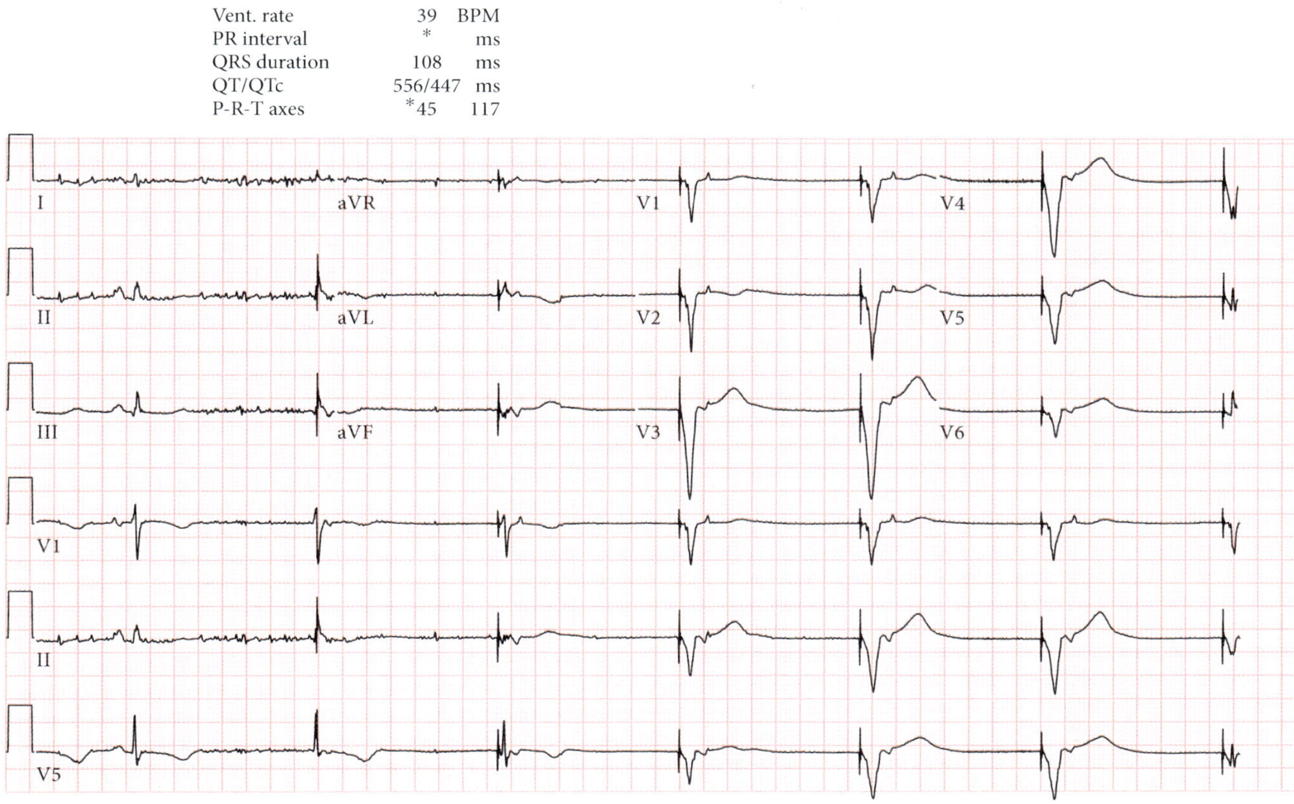

Figure 4: EKG shows one sinus beat followed by several ventricular paced beats.

relatively infrequent. In a review by Syed et al., new SND was observed in 11 of 816 TC patients (1.3%) [3]. Tsuchihashi et al. in a case series of 88 patients with TC reported sinus bradycardia in nine patients [5]. Dib et al. reported sinus pauses (up to 7.4 seconds) in one patient who eventually developed asystole mandating temporary pacemaker and inotropic support [6]. Hertting et al. reported one patient with symptomatic SSS requiring permanent pacemaker implantation [7]. Also, a case report by Kim described symptomatic SSS during the index episode requiring permanent pacemaker implantation [8]. However, in the previously reported cases, it is unclear whether TC is the cause or effect of SND. Theoretically, TC can cause SND through several mechanisms [3, 9]. Adrenergic compensative activation following bradycardia can induce transient myocardial dysfunction [10]. Ueyama et al. reported left ventriculography normalization in emotionally stressed rats with induced reversible LV apical ballooning, by pretreatment with adrenal receptor blockade [11, 12]. In time, catecholamine stress in TC can lead to a secondary increase in vagal tone with subsequent SND [3], and catecholamine-mediated myocardial stunning was considered crucial in the pathogenesis of TC. Therefore, reflex sympathetic stimulation to counteract severe SND may trigger TC. Age-related sinus node degeneration may also exacerbate that effect.

However, our patient had preexisting evidence of SND. She was seen in the cardiology outpatient clinic two months prior to admission for asymptomatic bradycardia. She was not on any negative chronotropic medication. Her EKG showed sinus bradycardia with no PR prolongation or conduction block. A 48 hr Holter monitor showed slow heart rate (HR) during sleep (30–40 beats/min) with an early morning pause of 3.5 seconds and an average HR of 61 beats/min. TTE showed EF 55–60%, with no regional wall motion abnormality. Thus, no intervention was necessary at that time. On admission emotional stress, medical stress and the intake of negative chronotropic drugs were ruled out during her focused history and examination. Therefore, reflex catecholamine surge to counteract bradycardia may have set the scene for TC evolution in this patient making SSS the most plausible trigger. Also, after the resolution of TC, our patient had episodes of bradycardia requiring cardiac pacing. Thus, TC is unlikely to be the cause of her SSS.

Pacemaker implantation was indicated in our patient due to the documented symptomatic bradycardia [13]. Dual-chamber pacemaker is recommended over single-chamber atrial pacing for all patients with sick sinus syndrome [14]. Also, in our patient, a concomitant atrioventricular nodal disease was expected. Furthermore, cardiac pacing allows adequate rate control (if needed) given that tachycardia-bradycardia syndrome persisted after TC resolution [13]. The patient also had prolongation of the QT interval during the acute phase of TC, which lowers her threshold for the development of torsades de pointes and ventricular

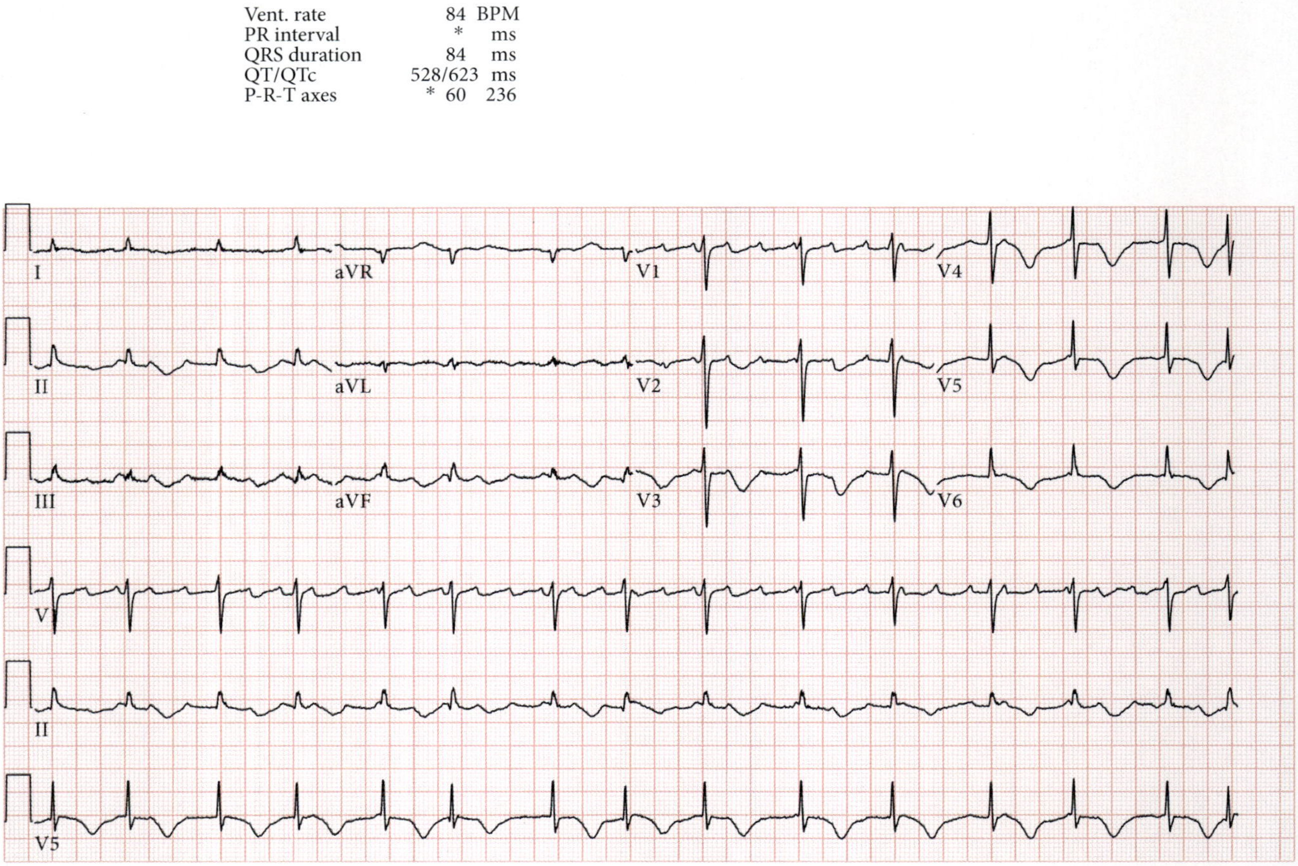

FIGURE 5: EKG shows atrial flutter with variable AV block.

fibrillation [2]. In addition, SND in patients with TC with QT prolongation can lead to significant rate variation and consequently higher risk torsades de pointes [3]. Thus, cardiac pacing may potentially reduce the risk of ventricular arrhythmias.

4. Conclusion

(i) Acute symptomatic sick sinus syndrome in patients with preexisting silent sinus node dysfunction can trigger takotsubo cardiomyopathy.

(ii) Understanding precipitating factors of takotsubo cardiomyopathy and identifying the patients at risk of life-threatening arrhythmia can help in refining risk stratification and therapy planning.

(iii) Patients with sick sinus syndrome complicated by takotsubo cardiomyopathy may benefit from pacemaker implantation. However, evaluation on a case-by-case basis is mandatory.

References

[1] K. Dote, H. Sato, H. Tateishi, T. Uchida, and M. Ishihara, "Myocardial stunning due to simultaneous multivessel coronary spasms: a review of 5 cases," *Journal of Cardiology*, vol. 21, no. 2, pp. 203–214, 1991.

[2] A. R. Lyon, E. Bossone, B. Schneider et al., "Current state of knowledge on takotsubo syndrome: a position statement from the taskforce on takotsubo syndrome of the heart failure Association of the European Society of Cardiology," *European Journal of Heart Failure*, vol. 18, no. 1, pp. 8–27, 2016.

[3] F. F. Syed, S. J. Asirvatham, and J. Francis, "Arrhythmia occurrence with takotsubo cardiomyopathy: a literature review," *Europace*, vol. 13, no. 6, pp. 780–788, 2011.

[4] S. W. Sharkey, "A clinical perspective of the takotsubo syndrome," *Heart Failure Clinics*, vol. 12, no. 4, pp. 507–520, 2016.

[5] K. Tsuchihashi, K. Ueshima, T. Uchida et al., "Transient left ventricular apical ballooning without coronary artery stenosis: a novel heart syndrome mimicking acute myocardial infarction. Angina pectoris-myocardial infarction investigations in Japan," *Journal of the American College of Cardiology*, vol. 38, no. 1, pp. 11–18, 2001.

[6] C. Dib, A. Prasad, P. A. Friedman et al., "Malignant arrhythmia in apical ballooning syndrome: risk factors and outcomes," *Indian Pacing Electrophysiol J.*, vol. 8, no. 3, pp. 182–192, 2008.

[7] K. Hertting, K. Krause, T. Harle, S. Boczor, J. Reimers, and K. H. Kuck, "Transient left ventricular apical ballooning in a community hospital in Germany," *International Journal of Cardiology*, vol. 112, no. 3, pp. 282–288, 2006.

[8] J. Kim, "Takotsubo cardiomyopathy complicating sick sinus syndrome," *International Journal of Arrhythmia*, vol. 14, no. 2, pp. 24–28, 2013.

[9] B. N. Limm, A. C. Hoo, and S. S. Azuma, "Variable conduction system disorders in takotsubo cardiomyopathy: a case series," *Hawai'i Journal of Medicine & Public Health*, vol. 73, no. 5, pp. 148–151, 2014.

[10] N. D. Brunetti, R. Ieva, M. Correale et al., "Combined exogenous and endogenous catecholamine release associated with Tako-Tsubo like syndrome in a patient with atrio-ventricular block undergoing pace-maker implantation," *Acute Cardiac Care*, vol. 13, no. 2, pp. 112–114, 2011.

[11] T. Ueyama, K. Kasamatsu, T. Hano, K. Yamamoto, Y. Tsuruo, and I. Nishio, "Emotional stress induces transient left ventricular hypocontraction in the rat via activation of cardiac adrenoceptors: a possible animal model of 'tako-tsubo' cardiomyopathy," *Circulation Journal*, vol. 66, no. 7, pp. 712-713, 2002.

[12] T. Ueyama, E. Senba, K. Kasamatsu, T. Hano, K. Yamamoto, and I. Nishio, "Molecular mechanism of emotional stress-induced and catecholamine-induced heart attack," *Journal of Cardiovascular Pharmacology*, vol. 41, pp. S115–S118, 2003.

[13] A. E. Epstein, J. P. DiMarco, K. A. Ellenbogen et al., "2012 ACCF/AHA/HRS focused update incorporated into the ACCF/AHA/HRS 2008 guidelines for device-based therapy of cardiac rhythm abnormalities: a report of the American College of Cardiology Foundation/American Heart Association Task Force on Practice Guidelines and the Heart Rhythm Society," *Circulation*, vol. 127, no. 3, pp. e283–e352, 2013.

[14] A. M. Gillis, A. M. Russo, K. A. Ellenbogen et al., "HRS/ACCF expert consensus statement on pacemaker device and mode selection," *Journal of the American College of Cardiology*, vol. 60, no. 7, pp. 682–703, 2012.

Dasatinib-Induced Pulmonary Arterial Hypertension Treated with Upfront Combination Therapy

Makoto Nishimori,[1] Tomoyuki Honjo,[1] Kenji Kaihotsu,[1] Naohiko Sone,[1] Sachiko Yoshikawa,[1] Junichi Imanishi,[1] Kazuhiko Nakayama,[2] Noriaki Emoto,[2,3] and Masanori Iwahashi[1]

[1]*Division of Cardiology, Department of Internal Medicine, Shinko Hospital, Kobe, Japan*
[2]*Division of Cardiovascular Medicine, Department of Internal Medicine, Kobe University Graduate School of Medicine, Kobe, Japan*
[3]*Department of Clinical Pharmacy, Kobe Pharmaceutical University, Kobe, Japan*

Correspondence should be addressed to Tomoyuki Honjo; honjo.tomoyuki@shinkohp.or.jp

Academic Editor: Aiden Abidov

Pulmonary arterial hypertension (PAH) is a rare complication of dasatinib that was approved as a first-line therapy for chronic myelocytic leukemia (CML). A 24-year-old man presenting dyspnea at rest and leg edema was admitted to our hospital. He had been diagnosed with CML and prescribed dasatinib for 4 years. Chest X-ray showed significant bilateral pleural effusion and heart enlargement. Echocardiography revealed interventricular septal compression and elevated peak tricuspid regurgitation pressure gradient of 66.7 mmHg indicating severe pulmonary hypertension. After the other specific diseases to provoke PAH were excluded, he was diagnosed with dasatinib-induced PAH. Despite discontinuation of dasatinib and intravenous administration of diuretic for two weeks, World Health Organization (WHO) functional class was still II and mean pulmonary arterial pressure (PAP) was high at 37 mmHg. Therefore, we administered sildenafil and bosentan together as an upfront combination therapy three weeks after dasatinib discontinuation. Six months later, his symptoms improved to WHO functional class I and mean PAP was decreased to 31 mmHg. Although PAH is a rare complication of dasatinib, symptomatic patients prescribed with dasatinib should have an echocardiogram for PAH screening. Moreover, the upfront combination therapy would be a useful option for symptomatic patients after discontinuation of dasatinib.

1. Introduction

Pulmonary hypertension (PH) is defined as an elevation in mean pulmonary arterial pressure (PAP) of 25 mmHg or more at rest. Pulmonary arterial hypertension (PAH) is a subgroup of PH and characterized by remodeling of pulmonary vasculature, resulting in increased pulmonary vascular resistance and PAP. It is reported that some drugs including dasatinib cause PAH [1].

Dasatinib, a second generated tyrosine kinase inhibitor (TKI), is widely used as a first-line therapy for chronic myelocytic leukemia (CML). Among the complications of dasatinib, PAH is a rare but severe complication. To treat dasatinib-induced PAH, some cases have demonstrated the effectiveness of pulmonary vasodilators [2]. However, data regarding the use of vasodilators are limited. Here, we present a case of dasatinib-induced PAH treated with an upfront combination therapy with vasodilators.

2. Case Presentation

A 24-year-old man with no past history of cardiopulmonary disease visited our hospital because of worsening of dyspnea at rest and leg edema. He had been diagnosed with CML seven years ago and initially treated with imatinib. Three years later, imatinib was switched to dasatinib (Sprycel®, Bristol-Myers; 100 mg/day) because of the incomplete molecular remission.

On admission, he developed increased nocturnal dyspnea, leg edema, and nausea. His blood pressure was 104/

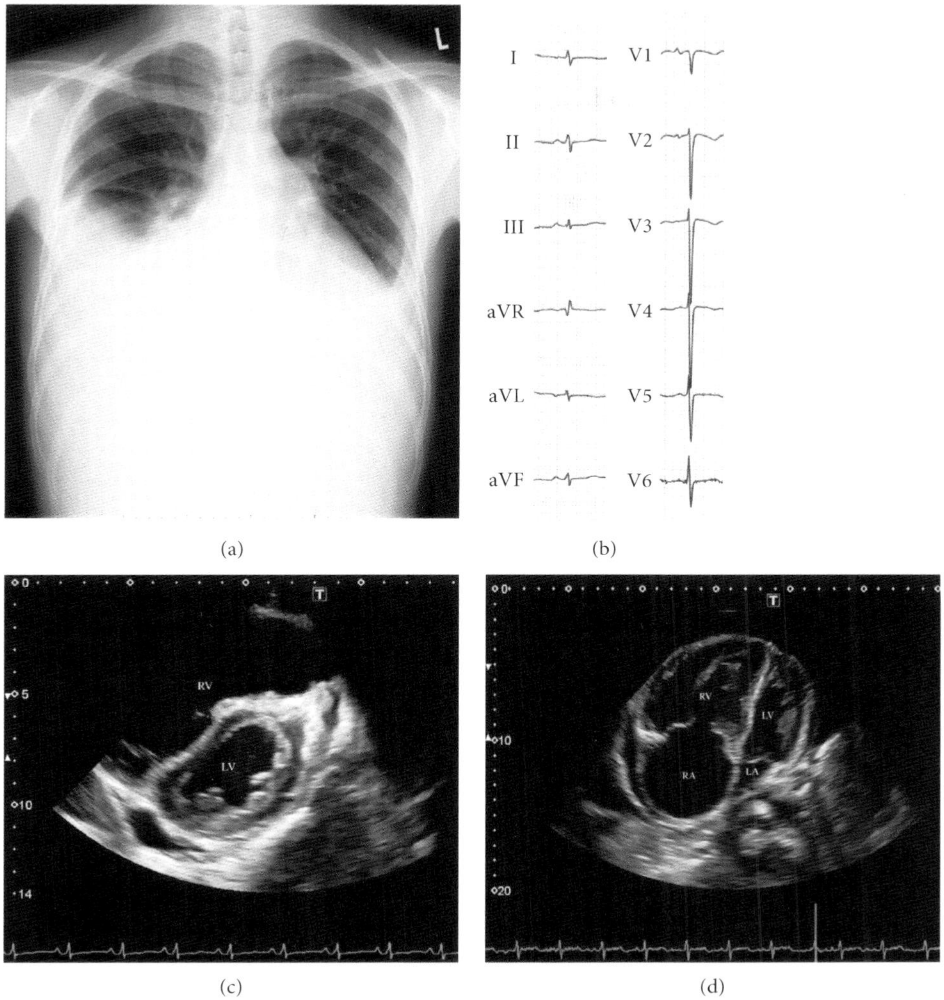

Figure 1: Clinical images on admission leading to diagnosis of pulmonary artery hypertension. (a) Chest X-ray on admission showed cardiac enlargement and severe bilateral plural effusion. (b) ECG suggested mild right ventricular overload and clockwise rotation. (c) Short axis view of the TTE showed flattening of the interventricular septum. (d) Apical four-chamber view of the TTE showed decreased left ventricular chamber size pressured by enlarged right ventricle. TTE: transthoracic echocardiography; LV: left ventricular; LA: left atrium; RV: right ventricular; RA: right atrium.

71 mmHg, heart rate was regular at 103 bpm, body temperature was 37.0°C, and oxygen saturation was 91% in room air. An X-ray examination found significant bilateral pleural effusion and heart enlargement (Figure 1(a)). An electrocardiogram showed low voltage in the limb lead, left axis deviation, clockwise rotation, and negative T waves in the V1-V2 lead indicating pleural effusion and right ventricular enlargement (Figure 1(b)). A transthoracic echocardiography revealed an enlarged right ventricle (D1 59 mm, D2 48 mm) with flattening of the interventricular septum during systolic and diastolic phases and severe tricuspid regurgitation with the elevated tricuspid regurgitation pressure gradient (TRPG) of 66 mmHg, indicating increased PAP and volume overload (Figures 1(c) and 1(d)). A chest contrast-enhanced computed tomography and a ventilation-perfusion lung scintigraphy showed no findings suggestive of thromboembolic disease. After the other specific diseases known to provoke PAH including human immunodeficiency virus infection, connective tissue disease, right-to-left shunt, and left heart disease were excluded, he was diagnosed with dasatinib-induced PAH in August 6, 2015.

After the admission as day 1, dasatinib was discontinued on day 2 and switched to bosutinib on day 14 which is another TKI used as a third choice for CML. In addition, bolus injection of loop diuretic (furosemide 20 mg daily from days 2 to 5) and oral diuretic (azosemide 60 mg qd from day 3) was started.

Two weeks after admission, his body weight decreased from 70.3 kg to 59.6 kg and pulmonary effusion disappeared. However, World Health Organization (WHO) functional class was still class II, and flattening of the interventricular septum and elevated TRPG (44 mmHg) was observed by the echocardiography. In right heart catheterization (RHC) on day 15, PAP was 55 (systolic)/26 (diastolic)/37 (mean) mmHg, pulmonary capillary wedge pressure was 8 mmHg, cardiac output was 6.55 l/min, cardiac index

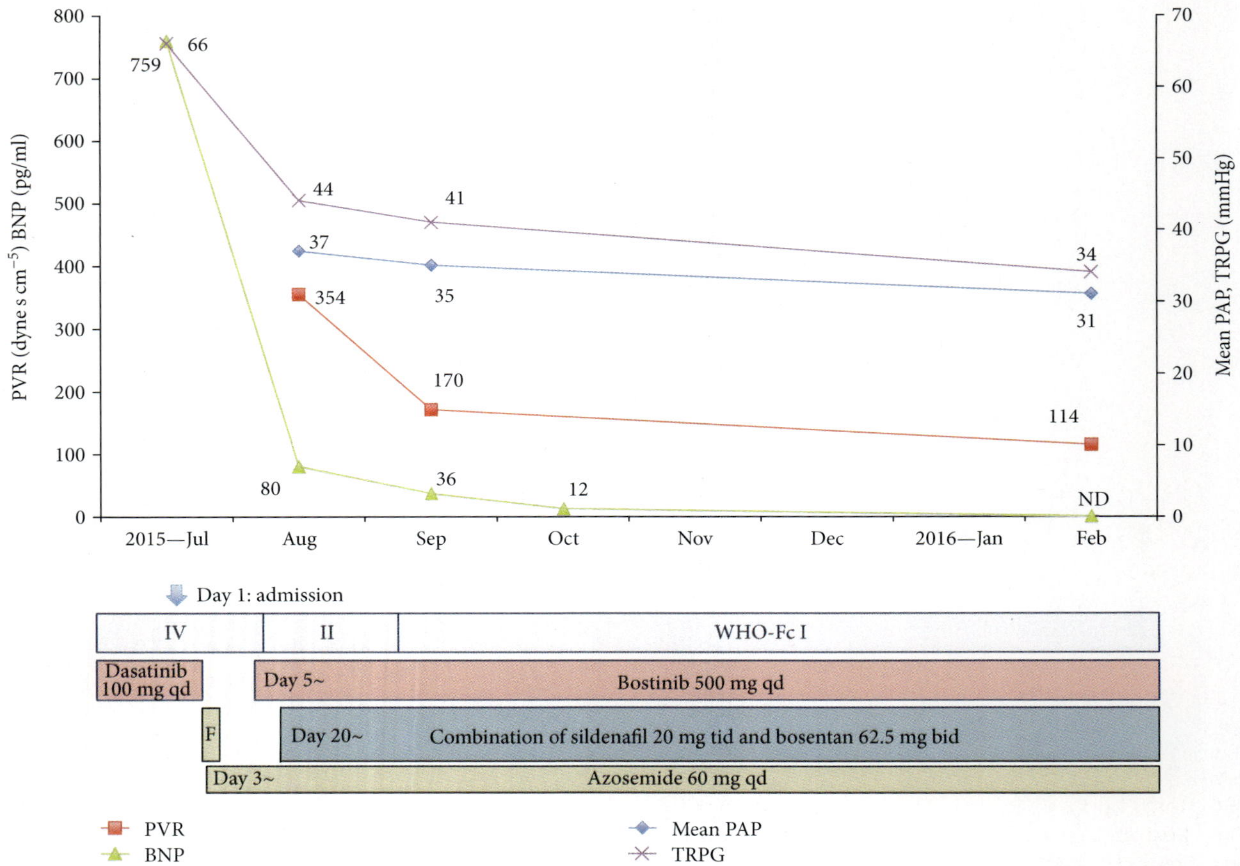

FIGURE 2: Clinical course of the case. BNP: B-type natriuretic peptide; PAP: pulmonary artery pressure; PVR: pulmonary vascular resistance; TRPG: tricuspid regurgitation peak gradient; WHO-Fc: World Health Organization functional class; F: furosemide 20 mg/day i.v. for three days; ND: not detected.

was 3.72 l/min/m^2, and pulmonary vascular resistance was 353 dyne s cm^{-5}, respectively (Figure 2).

Since discontinuation of dasatinib and diuretic administration had an insufficient therapeutic effect to decrease dyspnea and PAP, we started the upfront combination therapy with sildenafil, a phosphodiesterase-5 inhibitor, at 20 mg tid, and bosentan, an endothelin receptor antagonist, at 62.5 mg bid on day 20. One month later, his symptom was improved to WHO functional class I, mean PAP measured by RHC on day 15 was slightly reduced to 35 mmHg, and B-type natriuretic peptide level was decreased from 785 to 36 pg/ml. Six months later, mean PAP measured by RHC was decreased to 31 mmHg (Figure 2). The echocardiography also showed improvements in the right ventricular diameter (D1 48 mm, D2 40 mm) as shown in Figure 3. Finally, 12 months after the upfront combination therapy and dasatinib discontinuation, TRPG evaluated by the echocardiography was decreased to 24 mmHg.

3. Discussion

We encountered a case of severe dasatinib-induced PAH that was improved by the upfront combination therapy of vasodilators using a phosphodiesterase-5 inhibitor and an endothelin receptor antagonist.

Dasatinib is a second generated TKI that was recently approved as a first-line therapy for CML. Dasatinib inhibits not only the BCR-ABL oncogenic tyrosine kinase in Philadelphia chromosome-positive CML but also other tyrosine kinases. Bosutinib is also approved for salvage therapy in CML. Unlike other TKIs, bosutinib does not significantly inhibit Kit protein or platelet-derived growth factor receptor [3]. Among these tyrosine kinases, Src tyrosine kinase has been identified as likely the cause of PAH. The Src tyrosine kinase is abundantly expressed in vascular tissue. Activation of Src appears to play a critical role in proliferation of smooth muscle cells and vasoconstriction. Recently, Guignabert et al. demonstrated that chronic administration of dasatinib can cause pulmonary endothelial damage and PH in rats [4]. When monocrotaline and chronic hypoxic stress were given to the rats that were treated with dasatinib, imatinib, or a control vehicle, PH and pulmonary artery wall thickening occurred in only the dasatinib-treated rats in a dose-dependent manner. They highlighted that Src inhibitory profile of dasatinib exacerbated pulmonary hypertension, which was not observed in imatinib treatment. In addition, clinical report showed that

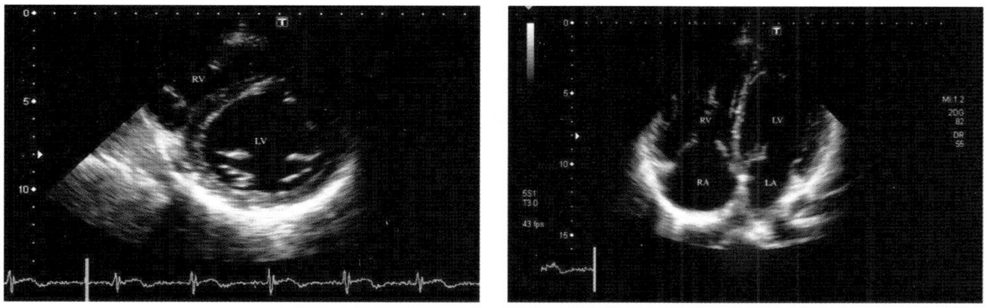

(a) (b)

Figure 3: Follow-up echocardiography, 6 months after the upfront combination therapy. (a) Short axis view of the TTE showed no compression of the interventricular septum. (b) Apical four chambers view the TTE showed improvement of the right ventricular size. TTE: transthoracic echocardiography; LV: left ventricular; LA: left atrium; RV: right ventricular; RA: right atrium.

imatinib improved exercise capacity and hemodynamics in advanced PAH patients [5]. Thus, it is important to know the character and kinase pathway when we choose TKIs for CML treatment. In this case, we changed dasatinib to bosutinib as a third-line therapy because there was no report of bosutinib-induced PAH at the time of the medication switch. However, recently, some case reports showed bosutinib occasionally provoked PAH [6], which has similar inhibitory profile on tyrosine kinases as dasatinib [3]. Given the patient's refractoriness to imatinib, an alternative TKI was used, which fortunately to date has not produced recurrent PH symptoms in the patient even though there are reported cases of bosutinib-associated PH and though the putative causative pathway may be invoked by both drugs.

A French group reported the incidence of dasatinib-induced PAH as 0.45% (13 out of 2900 patients) among symptomatic patients [1]. However, according to another report, increased right ventricular pressure was observed in 5 out of 38 patients (13.2%) assessed by echocardiography [7]. This incidence was higher than that in the previous report [1], suggesting the presence of asymptomatic dasatinib-induced PAH. Since pleural effusion and systemic edema are common side effects of dasatinib, it is quite difficult to distinguish PAH from common side effects by only symptoms. Therefore, early screening by echocardiography to detect the development of PAH is necessary in symptomatic patients.

It is reported that 34 out of 36 patients (94%) with dasatinib-induced PAH recovered by discontinuation of dasatinib, but 15 out of 36 patients (41.6%) did not show complete hemodynamic recovery [8]. Moreover, in another report on dasatinib-induced PAH, mean PAP did not decrease to less than 25 mmHg even with drug discontinuation or single vasodilator therapy [1]. Based on these findings, only drug discontinuation might not enough for complete remission of PH, suggesting the relevance of aggressive PH specific therapy. In fact, in our case, with the upfront combination therapy for 12 months, TRPG evaluated by the echocardiography was decreased to 24 mmHg.

The optimal timing and combination of the vasodilator intervention are still under debate. Since SUPER-2 trial showed that 12 weeks delay of the vasodilator made the prognosis of the patients worse [9], we decided to treat the patient with the upfront combination therapy after 4 weeks of dasatinib discontinuation aiming rapid and better outcome. Recently, AMBITION trial showed that initial combination therapy with ambrisentan and tadalafil resulted in a significantly lower risk of clinical failure events for the patients with PAH [10]. In this case, we chose bosentan and sildenafil because the AMBITION trial had not been published yet at the time of medication switch. Although the combination therapy with bosentan and sildenafil does not have evidence, initial use of these two drugs efficiently ameliorated the patient's symptoms. It could be another option for dasatinib-induced PAH treatment. Further accumulation of the cases is needed.

4. Conclusion

We experienced a case of dasatinib-induced PAH during the treatment of CML. We should consider the upfront combination therapy for symptomatic patients with PAH after discontinuation of dasatinib. Moreover, we strongly recommend routine screening of PAH by echocardiography during dasatinib or other TKI therapy in patients with edema or plural effusion.

References

[1] D. Montani, E. Bergot, S. Gunther et al., "Pulmonary arterial hypertension in patients treated by dasatinib," *Circulation*, vol. 125, no. 17, pp. 2128–2137, 2012.

[2] M. Sano, M. Saotome, T. Urushida et al., "Pulmonary arterial hypertension caused by treatment with dasatinib for chronic myeloid leukemia-critical alert," *Internal Medicine*, vol. 51, no. 17, pp. 2337–2340, 2012.

[3] J. J. Moslehi and M. Deininger, "Tyrosine kinase inhibitor-associated cardiovascular toxicity in chronic myeloid leukemia," *Journal of Clinical Oncology*, vol. 33, no. 35, pp. 4210–4218, 2015.

[4] C. Guignabert, C. Phan, A. Seferian et al., "Dasatinib induces lung vascular toxicity and predisposes to pulmonary hypertension," *Journal of Clinical Investigation*, vol. 126, no. 9, pp. 3207–3218, 2016.

[5] H. Mucke, "The role of imatinib in the treatment of pulmonary hypertension," *Drugs of Today*, vol. 49, no. 3, pp. 203–211, 2013.

[6] K. Seegobin, A. Babbar, J. Ferreira, B. Lyons, J. Cury, and V. Seeram, "A case of worsening pulmonary arterial hypertension and pleural effusions by bosutinib after prior treatment with dasatinib," *Pulmonary Circulation*, vol. 7, no. 4, pp. 808–812, 2017.

[7] M. Minami, T. Arita, H. Iwasaki et al., "Comparative analysis of pulmonary hypertension in patients treated with imatinib, nilotinib and dasatinib," *British Journal of Haematology*, vol. 177, no. 4, pp. 578–587, 2017.

[8] N. P. Shah, N. Wallis, H. W. Farber et al., "Clinical features of pulmonary arterial hypertension in patients receiving dasatinib," *American Journal of Hematology*, vol. 90, no. 11, pp. 1060–1064, 2015.

[9] L. J. Rubin, D. B. Badesch, T. R. Fleming et al., "Long-term treatment with sildenafil citrate in pulmonary arterial hypertension: the SUPER-2 study," *Chest*, vol. 140, no. 5, pp. 1274–1283, 2011.

[10] N. Galiè, J. A. Barberà, A. E. Frost et al., "Initial use of ambrisentan plus tadalafil in pulmonary arterial hypertension," *New England Journal of Medicine*, vol. 373, no. 9, pp. 834–844, 2015.

6

Catastrophic Prosthetic Valve Endocarditis Caused by Rare Black Fungi

Khurram Butt, Ranjeet Kumar, Jason D'Souza, Joseph Limback, Rajesh Shah, and Jeremy Burt

Florida Hospital, Orlando, USA

Correspondence should be addressed to Khurram Butt; khurram.butt.md@flhosp.org

Academic Editor: Aiden Abidov

Fungal infection of prosthetic heart valves is rare and can lead to severe complications including death. Dematiaceous mold, also known as "black fungi," are an extremely rare cause of endocarditis that usually affect immunocompromised hosts. The infection is usually chronic and can lead to heart failure and embolic complications. These fungi have limited antifungal treatment modalities. We present a rare case of prosthetic aortic valve, root, and graft infection in an immunocompetent host that revealed itself through renal, mesenteric, and cerebral embolic phenomenon. The patient underwent removal and replacement of the aortic graft followed by small bowel resection for mesenteric infarction. Patient had a successful postoperative course and underwent a long-term antifungal treatment with amphotericin B and voriconazole.

1. Introduction

Fungal infection of native and prosthetic cardiac valves in an immunocompetent patient is a rare occurrence and is a rather dreaded disease. Its estimated incidence can be as high as 2.9% [1] and mortality rate ranges from 23 to 46% [2–5]. The most common fungal agents affecting native heart valves are Candida, Aspergillus, and Histoplasma with Candida species being the most common amongst them [6, 7]. We hereby present a rare case of fungal prosthetic valve endocarditis (PVE) and ascending aortic root graft infection in an immunocompetent host caused by dematiaceous mold.

2. Case Presentation

A 68-year-old male with past medical history of coronary artery disease status post coronary artery bypass graft (CABG), aortic valve replacement along with replacement of the root of the ascending aorta 10 months prior to presentation and recent hemorrhagic cerebrovascular accident (CVA), came to the hospital with complains of acute onset of severe abdominal pain and melena for 1 day. He also attested to chronic abdominal pain and a 30-pound weight loss over the last 8 months prior to these acute symptoms. His physical exam on presentation was positive for severe bilateral lower abdominal tenderness. Apart from a hemoglobin of 10 mg/dl and a positive stool occult blood test, the rest of his basic lab work up was unremarkable (white blood cell/platelet count, comprehensive metabolic panel, and PT/INR included). Hepatitis B, hepatitis C, and human immunodeficiency virus (HIV) testing were negative. The electrocardiogram (EKG) showed sinus rhythm and left ventricular hypertrophy (Figure 1). An emergent computerized tomography (CT) scan of the abdomen revealed features suggestive of an embolic infarct in the left kidney (Figures 2(a) and 2(b)) and within the mid-one-third of the superior mesenteric artery causing luminal narrowing and also suspected to be extending to the takeoff of small bowel branches. Segmental mural thickening of at least one small bowel loop was noted which strongly favored acute bowel ischemia as a cause of his abdominal pain (Figure 2(c)). Incidental findings on CT of the abdomen were also strongly suspicious for large eccentric thrombus in the ascending aortic graft and the aortic root which were further investigated and confirmed with a CT scan of the chest (Figure 3). Cardiology and cardiothoracic surgery were consulted. A CT scan of the

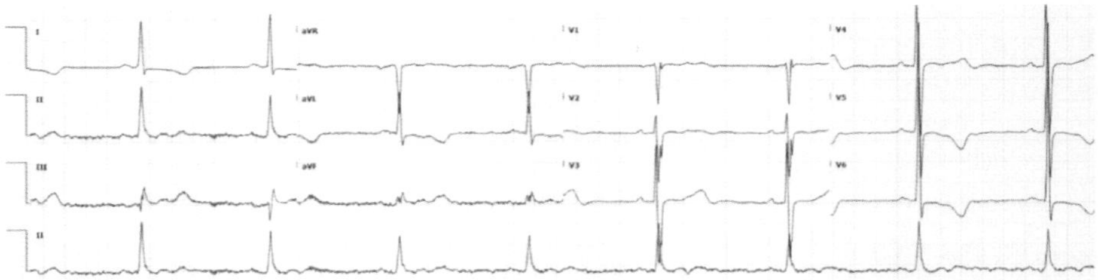

Figure 1: Electrocardiogram showing sinus bradycardia and left ventricular hypertrophy.

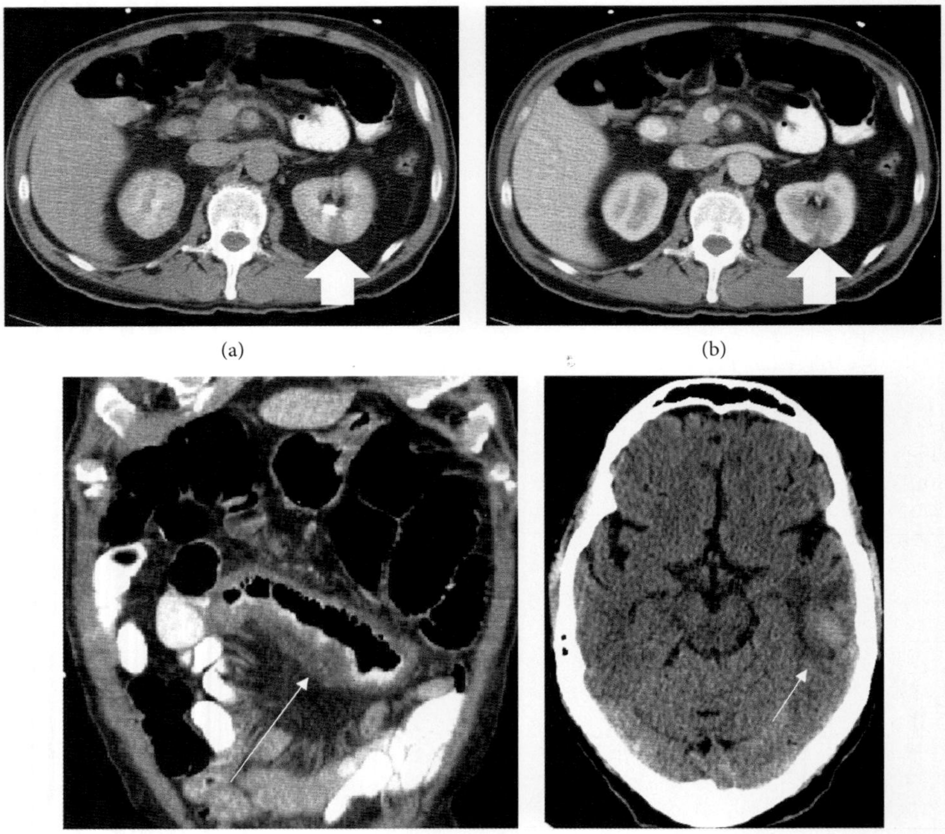

(a) (b) (c) (d)

Figure 2: (a, b) Axial contrast-enhanced abdominal CT demonstrates a segmental infarct in the posterior aspect of the left kidney (short thick arrow). (c) Coronal reformatted CT showing infarcted small bowel (long thin arrow). (d) Noncontrast head CT showing a subacute hemorrhagic infarct in the left temporal lobe (short thin arrow).

head was performed to assess the recent CVA and showed a subacute hemorrhage along the left-sided temporal parenchyma (Figure 2(d)). CT head imaging was obtained from the facility where the patient presented 3 months prior for cerebral hemorrhage and in comparison, to the most recent CT scan of the head, the hemorrhage appeared stable. The hemorrhage was suspected to be secondary to thromboembolism. After a review of the risks and benefits of anticoagulation to prevent extension of this suspected thrombus, heparin was initiated. An echocardiogram revealed dilatation of the ascending aorta and mild paravalvular leak around the bioprosthetic aortic valve. Gastroenterology was consulted and an emergent esophagogastroduodenoscopy was performed which was negative for any causes of upper gastrointestinal bleed. A hypercoagulable workup was performed which did not reveal any apparent cause of a prothrombotic state. Anticoagulation was held and subsequently, the patient underwent a redo sternotomy under cardiopulmonary bypass with extensive lysis of adhesions, removal of the thrombosed aortic valve and graft, ascending and proximal aortic arch replacement utilizing a 30 mm Dacron graft, and aortic valve replacement with a 25 mm Edwards Magna Ease bovine pericardial valve. The patient also underwent an explorative laparotomy as a part of a staged procedure

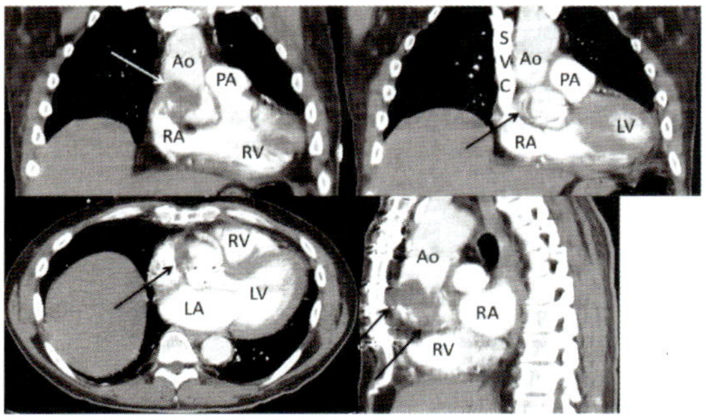

FIGURE 3: Axial, sagittal, and coronal contrast-enhanced CT images of the chest showing a fungal ball in the aortic root adherent to the prosthetic valve (arrows). Ao = aorta; PA = main pulmonary artery; RA = right atrium; LA = left atrium; RV = right ventricle; LV = left ventricle; SVC = superior vena cava.

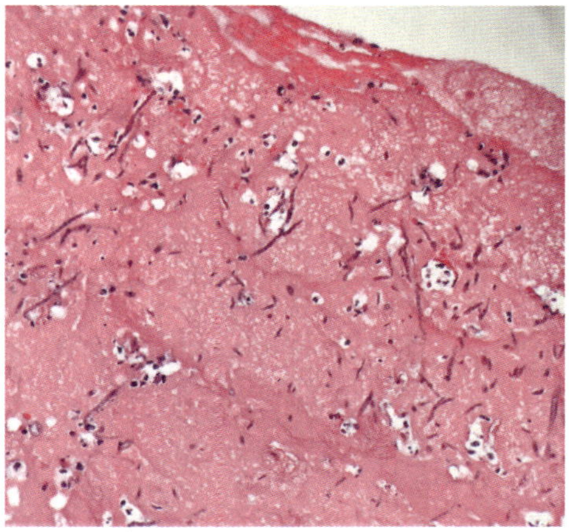

FIGURE 4: Histopathological sample of the aortic graft shows chronic inflammation and fungus with acute angle branching hyphae.

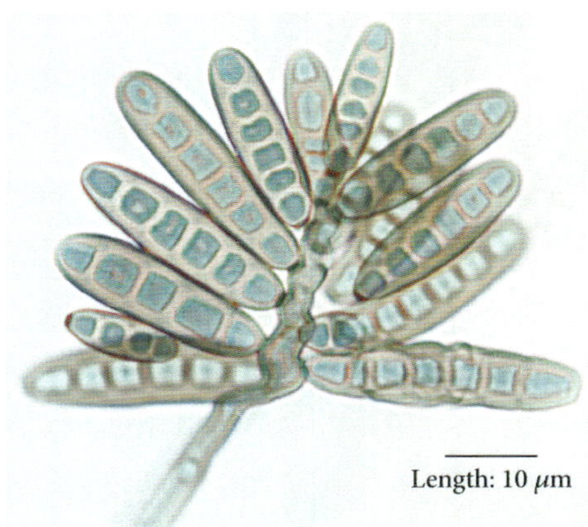

FIGURE 5: Image demonstrating conidia of Bipolaris hawaiiensis [16].

to address the ischemic bowel caused by the presumed septic emboli. Intraoperatively, the patient was found to have a portion of small bowel that had become necrotic. The necrotic bowel was excised and an end to end anastomosis was performed.

The aortic graft and thrombus were sent for culture and pathology. Histopathological examination of the aortic graft and cusps of the aortic valve revealed chronic inflammation and was also notable for abundant acute angle branching septate fungal hyphae (Figure 4). The patient was immediately started on amphotericin B and voriconazole pending finalization of cultures and sensitivities. On postoperative day four, three culture reports from the graft came back positive for dematiaceous mold, suggestive of Bipolaris species. The minimum inhibitory concentration (MIC) was 0.25 ug/dl for voriconazole and 0.03 ug/ml for amphotericin B. A decision was made to continue the same antifungal regimen on the basis of sensitivities and further speciation was not performed. Patient had a good postoperative course and was later discharged on amphotericin B and voriconazole for at least 1 month with continued follow-up with an infectious disease specialist.

3. Discussion

Dematiaceous mold, also known as "black fungi" owing to the presence of melanin like pigments, are a heterogeneous group of filamentous molds. These saprophytic and plant pathogenic fungi are now increasingly being recognized as causes of human infection, particularly in immunocompromised persons, such as diabetics, transplant recipients, and patients with human immunodeficiency virus (HIV) infection [8]. Dematiaceous molds are often found in soil and thus have a worldwide distribution. These molds cause a heterogeneous group of infections referred to as phaeohyphomycosis which include local infections, pneumonia, brain abscesses, and disseminated infections. Phaeohyphomycosis is characterized by the presence of black-pigmented hyphae or pseudohyphae.

Bipolaris genus belongs to the group of dematiaceous molds and has more than 100 species. These organisms are mostly pathogens of plants; however, a few saprobic species are potentially able to infect humans and animals. Morphologically, Bipolaris species are differentiated by their rapidly growing dark colonies, large conidia with transverse distosepta (Figure 5), and bipolar method of germination. Bipolaris species are an extremely rare cause of endocarditis and aortic root infection, especially in an immunocompetent host. These infections evolve chronically and predispose to thromboembolic phenomenon which can be the primary manifestation of infection as evidenced by our case.

Vallabhaneni et al. [9] identified 21 cases of surgical site infection caused by Bipolaris species in over ten hospitals located in Texas, Arkansas, and Florida out of which 6 cases involved valve replacement. Pauzner et al. [10] reported a case of homograft aortic valve infected with Bipolaris spicifera now termed as "Curuvularia spicifera" which was treated with surgical valve replacement and antifungal medications. The patient had a good long-term outcome. Ogden et al. [11] also reported fungal endarteritis of the ascending aorta by Bipolaris species following replacement of the aortic valve with a porcine valve which ultimately resulted in the patient's death. Our case represents a rare success story with a successful treatment outcome in endocarditis/endarteritis caused by dematiaceous mold in an immunocompetent patient managed aggressively with surgical and antifungal treatments.

The European Society of Clinical Microbiology and Infectious Diseases (ESCMID) and European Confederation of Medical Mycology (ECMM) guidelines recommend using voriconazole, posaconazole, itraconazole, or in some cases amphotericin B to target infections caused by dematiaceous molds [12]. However, the current antifungal treatment modalities for patients infected with dematiaceous mold are limited, and the outcome of antifungal treatment appears dismal. In one survey, it was shown that only 23% of the patients treated with amphotericin B survived [13]. Itraconazole has been shown to be active against many species of the dematiaceous molds and there are case reports of successful treatment of some patients with systemic forms of phaeohyphomycosis, such as arthritis and osteomyelitis, including those refractory to other agents [14]. Treatment with newer agents, such as voriconazole, or treatment with combinations of antifungal agents may prove to be encouraging in the management of these infections [15]. Due to limited data on sensitivities and treatment response, usually, a two or more drug combination is employed and treatment continued under supervision of an infectious disease specialist after discharge from the hospital.

References

[1] M. G. Threlkeld and C. G. Cobbs, "Infectious disorders of prosthetic valves and intravascular devices," in *Principles and Practice of. Infectious Diseases*, G. L. Mandell, J. E. Bennett, and R. Dolin, Eds., pp. 783–793, Churchill-Livingstone, New York, NY, USA, 4th edition, 1995.

[2] S. B. Calderwood, L. A. Swinski, A. W. Karchmer, C. M. Waternaux, and M. J. Buckley, "Prosthetic valve endocarditis. Analysis of factors affecting outcome of therapy," *The Journal of Thoracic and Cardiovascular Surgery*, vol. 92, no. 4, pp. 776–783, 1986.

[3] G. Fang, T. F. Keys, L. O. Gentry et al., "Prosthetic valve endocarditis resulting from nosocomial bacteremia. A prospective, multicenter study," *Annals of Internal Medicine*, vol. 119, no. 7, Part 1, pp. 560–567, 1993.

[4] F. L. Grover, D. J. Cohen, C. Oprian, W. G. Henderson, G. Sethi, and K. E. Hammermeister, "Determinants of the occurrence of and survival from prosthetic valve endocarditis. Experience of the veterans affairs cooperative study on valvular heart disease," *The Journal of Thoracic and Cardiovascular Surgery*, vol. 108, no. 2, pp. 207–214, 1994.

[5] S. S. Sett, M. P. Hudon, W. R. Jamieson, and A. W. Chow, "Prosthetic valve endocarditis. Experience with porcine bioprostheses," *The Journal of Thoracic and Cardiovascular Surgery*, vol. 105, no. 3, pp. 428–434, 1993.

[6] M. E. Ellis, H. Al-Abdely, A. Sandridge, W. Greer, and W. Ventura, "Fungal endocarditis: evidence in the world literature, 1965–1995," *Clinical Infectious Diseases*, vol. 32, no. 1, pp. 50–62, 2001.

[7] G. R. Melgar, R. M. Nasser, S. M. Gordon, B. W. Lytle, T. F. Keys, and D. L. Longworth, "Fungal prosthetic valve endocarditis in 16 patients. An 11-year experience in a tertiary care hospital," *Medicine*, vol. 76, no. 2, pp. 94–103, 1997.

[8] M. E. Brandt and D. W. Warnock, "Epidemiology, clinical manifestations, and therapy of infections caused by dematiaceous fungi," *Journal of Chemotherapy*, vol. 15, pp. 36–S47, 2013.

[9] S. Vallabhaneni, A. E. Purfield, K. Benedict et al., "Cardiothoracic surgical site phaeohyphomycosis caused by *Bipolaris* mould, multiple US states, 2008-2013: a clinical description," *Medical Mycology*, vol. 54, no. 3, pp. 318–321, 2016.

[10] R. Pauzner, A. Goldschmied-Reouven, I. Hay et al., "Phaeohyphomycosis following cardiac surgery: case report and review of serious infection due to Bipolaris and Exserohilum species," *Clinical Infectious Diseases*, vol. 25, no. 4, pp. 921–923, 1997.

[11] P. E. Ogden, D. L. Hurley, and P. T. Cain, "Fatal fungal endarteritis caused by Bipolaris spicifera following replacement of the aortic valve," *Clinical Infectious Diseases*, vol. 14, no. 2, pp. 596–598, 1992.

[12] A. Chowdhary, J. F. Meis, J. Guarro et al., "ESCMID and ECMM joint clinical guidelines for the diagnosis and management of systemic phaeohyphomycosis: diseases caused by black fungi," *Clinical Microbiology and Infection*, vol. 20, pp. 47–75, 2014.

[13] S. G. Revankar, J. E. Patterson, D. A. Sutton, R. Pullen, and M. G. Rinaldi, "Disseminated phaeohyphomycosis: review of an emerging mycosis," *Clinical Infectious Diseases*, vol. 34, no. 4, pp. 467–476, 2002.

[14] E. M. Johnson, A. Szekely, and D. W. Warnock, "In-vitro activity of voriconazole, itraconazole and amphotericin B against filamentous fungi," *The Journal of Antimicrobial Chemotherapy*, vol. 42, no. 6, pp. 741–745, 1998.

[15] J. R. Perfect, K. A. Marr, T. J. Walsh et al., "Voriconazole treatment for less-common, emerging, or refractory fungal infections," *Clinical Infectious Diseases*, vol. 36, no. 9, pp. 1122–1131, 2003.

[16] S. G. Revankar and D. A. Sutton, "Melanized fungi in human disease," *Clinical Microbiology Reviews*, vol. 23, no. 4, pp. 884–928, 2010.

7

Advanced Biventricular Heart Failure due to Left Ventricular Noncompaction Cardiomyopathy Leading to the Formation of a Gastric Bezoar: The Implications of Heart Failure on the Gastrointestinal Tract

Daria Yunina,[1] **Dikshya Sharma**,[1] **Richard Fazio**,[2] **Hossam Amin**,[1] **Yuriy Tsirlin**,[2] **and Vijay Shetty**[3,4]

[1]*Department of Medicine, Maimonides Medical Center, Brooklyn, NY, USA*
[2]*Division of Gastroenterology, Department of Medicine, Maimonides Medical Center, Brooklyn, NY, USA*
[3]*Department of Cardiology, Department of Medicine, Maimonides Medical Center, Brooklyn, NY, USA*
[4]*Department of Medicine, SUNY Downstate School of Medicine, Brooklyn, NY, USA*

Correspondence should be addressed to Daria Yunina; dyunina@maimonidesmed.org

Academic Editor: Nurten Sayar

Congestive heart failure (CHF) is a chronic disease process affecting multiple organ systems and is associated with significant morbidity and mortality. We report a case of a 43-year-old male with a history of unspecified cardiomyopathy who presented to the hospital with abdominal pain, distention, and nausea for 4 months. He was diagnosed with left ventricular noncompaction and gastroparesis. While symptoms of dyspnea, orthopnea, or increasing peripheral edema are the first that come to mind when thinking of a CHF exacerbation, we must broaden our scope to include such things as nausea, vomiting, abdominal pain, and bloating which can also indicate worsening cardiac function. This case report highlights the significant yet often forgotten gastrointestinal (GI) symptoms that result from advanced biventricular heart failure, with emphasis on impaired gastric and intestinal motility.

1. Introduction

Congestive heart failure (CHF) is a chronic disease process affecting multiple organ systems and is associated with significant morbidity and mortality. In the United States (U.S.) alone, its prevalence is close to 6 million, with a yearly incidence of over 550,000 and a death rate of 300,000 per year [1]. This case report will highlight the significant yet often forgotten gastrointestinal (GI) symptoms that result from advanced biventricular heart failure, with emphasis on impaired gastric and intestinal motility.

2. Case Presentation

A 43-year-old male with past medical history of hypertension, depression, and an unspecified cardiomyopathy presented to the hospital with complaints of abdominal pain, distention, and nausea for 4 months, worse in recent weeks. The patient had multiple episodes of vomiting with inability to tolerate anything by mouth. His primary care doctor prescribed metoclopramide and famotidine, which provided minimal relief. In parallel to his GI symptoms, the patient also described symptoms of fatigue and worsening shortness of breath on exertion. He denied chest pain, palpitations, diarrhea, constipation, or increased swelling of the legs. The patient was a former cigarette smoker and drank alcohol socially.

On physical examination, there was jugular venous distention and trace peripheral edema. Auscultation of the lungs was significant for mildly diminished breath sounds in bilateral lower lobes with bibasilar crepitations. Cardiac auscultation was significant for a 2/6 holosystolic murmur of mitral

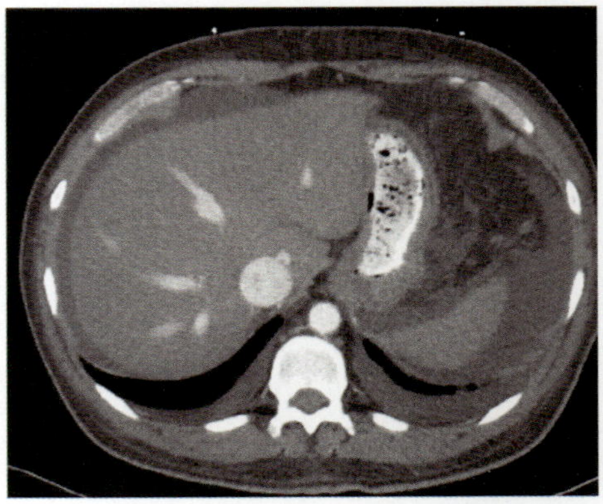

Figure 1: CT scan of the abdomen.

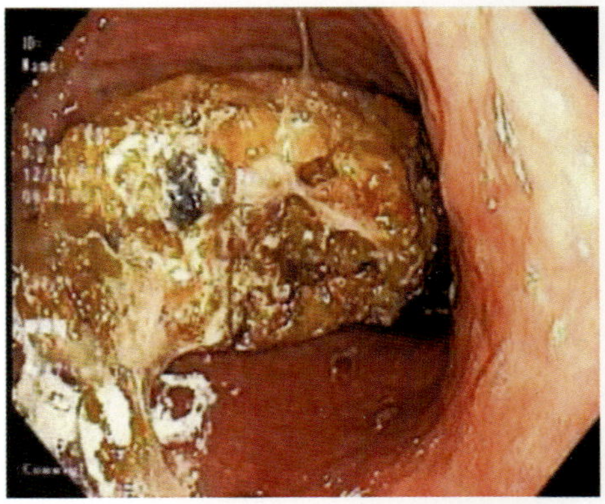

Figure 2: Gastric bezoar.

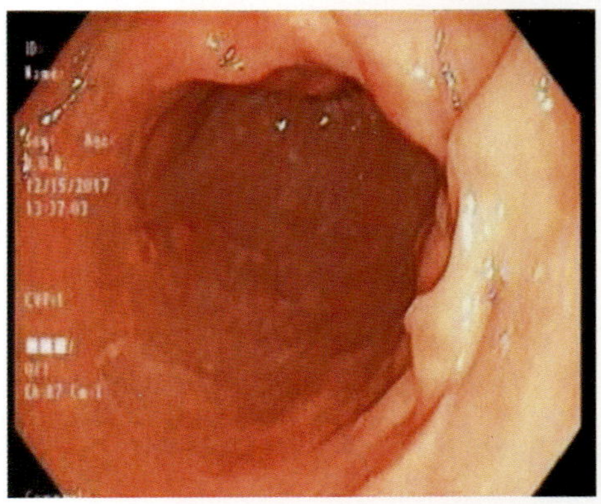

Figure 3: Body of the stomach.

and tricuspid regurgitation. Bowel sounds were normal. The abdomen was soft but mildly distended with diffuse tenderness. There was no guarding or rigidity.

Initial laboratory findings showed a B-type natriuretic peptide (BNP) of 1374 pg/ml consistent with volume overload. The basic metabolic panel was normal. Venous blood gas showed an elevated lactic acid level of 3.2 mmol/l suggesting tissue hypoperfusion. Complete blood count (CBC) and coagulation panel showed a platelet count of 66 K/Ul and an international normalized ratio (INR) of 2.3 (the patient was not taking anticoagulants prior to admission). These findings indicated some degree of liver dysfunction which was confirmed by abnormal liver function tests (LFTs) that showed an albumin of 3 g/dl, direct bilirubin of 1.9 mg/dl, total bilirubin of 4.0 mg/dl, aspartate aminotransferase of 98 IU/l, alanine aminotransferase of 121 IU/l, and an alkaline phosphatase of 87 IU/l. Chest radiograph showed cardiac enlargement. The patient was admitted for further workup of abdominal pain and management of acute decompensated heart failure.

Computerized tomography (CT) of the abdomen and pelvis with oral and intravenous (IV) contrast was performed showing wall thickening of the cardia of the stomach, a moderate amount of abdominal ascites, and diffuse anasarca and thickening within the proximal sigmoid colon (Figure 1). Abdominal ultrasound (US) showed fatty infiltration of the liver and distention of the intrahepatic inferior vena cava (IVC) and hepatic veins. Echocardiogram (ECHO) showed a severely decreased left ventricular (LV) systolic function with ejection fraction (EF) of 21–25%. There was global cardiomyopathy, moderate LV diastolic dysfunction, and severe mitral and tricuspid valve regurgitation. The right ventricle (RV) was moderately dilated and hypokinetic. The patient's last known EF was reported to be 40% a year ago.

Cardiology evaluated the patient and recommended medical optimization and diuresis with plans for eventual right and left heart catheterization once he was euvolemic. Gastroenterology evaluated the patient for his abdominal pain, nausea, vomiting, and elevated LFTs. The patient's liver function was suggestive of cirrhosis. Viral hepatitis panel, iron studies, serum ceruloplasmin, alpha-1-antitrypsin, anti-mitochondrial antibodies, anti-smooth muscle antibodies, and anti-nuclear antibodies were unremarkable, ruling out infectious and autoimmune causes, making the etiology of his cirrhosis and abdominal complaints likely cardiogenic in origin.

Upper endoscopy was performed on hospital day 2 to rule out peptic ulcer disease as a cause of his nausea and vomiting, revealing desquamation of the esophageal mucosa in linear streaks and a large gastric bezoar obstructing the view of the underlying mucosa (Figure 2).

After the endoscopy, the patient was given one can of Pepsi Cola and otherwise kept nil per os (NPO) for repeat endoscopy the following day with plans of possible bezoar removal. Repeat esophagogastroduodenoscopy (EGD) showed no evidence of the bezoar (Figure 3).

Despite resolution of the bezoar, the patient continued to have complaints of intermittent nausea. Right and left heart catheterization was performed on hospital day 8, showing normal coronaries, reduced cardiac output, and mild pulmonary hypertension. It was suspected that the reason pulmonary pressures were noted to be lower than expected was because the patient had received aggressive dieresis in the days leading up to the catheterization and was relatively euvolemic.

His medications were optimized and he was fitted for a LifeVest prior to discharge from the hospital. After discharge, he underwent cardiac magnetic resonance imaging (CMR) which revealed a diagnosis of left ventricular noncompaction cardiomyopathy (LVNC) (Figure 4). Cardiac output of the

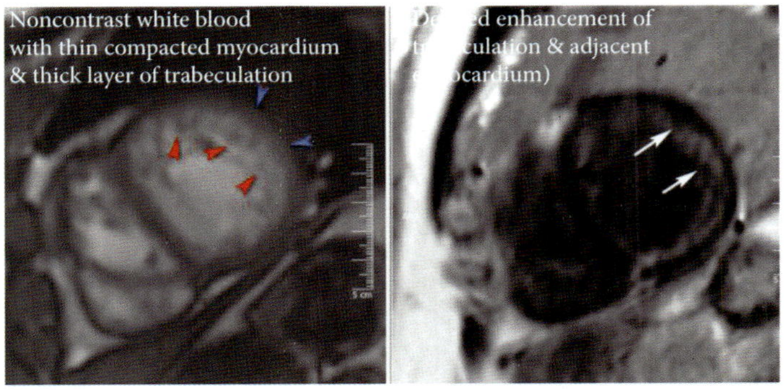

FIGURE 4: CMR showing compacted myocardium and trabeculated layer.

LV in cardiac MRI was measured to be 4.08 l/min with and EF of 28%. The RV was moderately dilated and noted to have an EF of 27%.

He also underwent a nuclear medicine gastric emptying study, which showed 24% gastric emptying at 90 minutes with the majority of the radioactive meal remaining in the proximal stomach. This study confirmed gastroparesis in our patient, presumably secondary to worsening cardiac function in the presence of biventricular failure due to noncompaction cardiomyopathy.

3. Discussion

As the prevalence of heart failure increases, so does the number of organ systems we see being affected by the disease. While symptoms of dyspnea, orthopnea, or increasing peripheral edema are the first that come to mind when thinking of a CHF exacerbation, we must broaden our scope to include such things as nausea, vomiting, abdominal pain, and bloating which can also indicate worsening cardiac function. Here, we look into the pathophysiology of the failing heart and its effect on the structure and function of the gastrointestinal system.

In the stomach, there can be notable thickening of the mucosa and areas of vascular ectasias [2]. The small intestine and the colon may display sonographic evidence of bowel wall edema with increased intestinal wall thickness. Increased distance between the basal membrane of the intestinal cells and the capillary blood flow leads to impaired nutrition of the enterocytes resulting in decreased absorptive function of the bowel wall [2]. The sigmoid colon is of particular importance as increased thickness positively correlates with an increase in blood concentrations of C-reactive protein and leukocytes [2].

Naturally, changes in the structure of the GI tract affect its function. The intestine is one of the most perfused organs at rest, receiving approximately 25% of the cardiac output [2]. At maximal exercise intensity, gut perfusion drops to 4% of the cardiac output [3]. The sympathetic nervous system innervates the splanchnic circulation, thus at a time of increased sympathetic stimulation, there is constriction of the blood vessels leading to decreased intestinal perfusion [2]. Thus, even minimal changes in cardiac output (i.e., ejection fraction) can lead to significant intestinal ischemia [2]. Ischemia results in a decrease in intestinal motility and absorption and an increase in bowel wall permeability [3]. Bowel wall edema and decreased perfusion cause the gut wall to lose its integrity, becoming more permeable to bacteria, increasing rates of bacterial colonization. Food and nutrients are absorbed into enterocytes and later the capillaries via transcellular and paracellular transport. Sugar absorption studies show an increased absorption of transfer proteins in the small and large bowel, suggesting disruption of the intestinal membrane [2].

There is a phenomenon that occurs in end-stage CHF patients in which there is impaired absorption of fats and proteins resulting in severe unintentional weight loss. Cardiac cachexia is found in 16–42% of heart failure patients [2]. This finding is most pronounced in patients with functional class III and IV heart failure. These patients were measured to have an increased amount of protein and fat in their feces in comparison to patients without CHF [2]. Cardiac muscle wasting causes further decline of cardiac function. Cardiac cachexia is a predictive factor of increased mortality in patients with heart failure [2].

In heart failure, there is overactivity of the sympathetic system and a blunted parasympathetic response [4]. Although the sympathetic activity can be regulated pharmacologically with beta blockers and renin-angiotensin-aldosterone inhibitors, this is not the case for the parasympathetic system [4]. The parasympathetic vagus nerve innervates multiple organs including the heart and the GI tract [4]. Trials and studies have analyzed the use of vagal nerve stimulation (VNS) in advanced heart failure. Results show improvements in NYHA class, quality of life and end-systolic volumes measured via ECHO [4]. VNS has also been studied in patients with drug refractory gastroparesis, a chronic impairment in gastric motility and delayed emptying. Noninvasive cervical vagus nerve stimulation (nVNS) similar to implanted gastric electric stimulation (GES) shows reduction in symptoms of nausea, vomiting, early satiety, and abdominal bloating [5].

Cardiogenic cirrhosis, also known as congestive hepatopathy, occurs as a result of right-sided heart failure or in the case of our patient, biventricular heart failure [6]. The backup of blood from the right ventricle into the liver results in hepatic congestion and subsequent damage. Interestingly, the changes on the GI tract that occur with advanced heart failure are very similar to the ones that occur as a result of liver cirrhosis. These include delayed gastric emptying, slowed gut motility, increased bowel permeability, and bacterial translocation [6].

CMR revealed that our patient had LVNC, a structural abnormality in which the left ventricle has a thinner than normal compacted layer and trabeculae [7]. This defect occurs during embryonic development with the premature cessation of endomyocardial compaction within the left ventricle, resulting in the formation of trabeculations and deep intratrabecular recesses [8]. This can lead to cardiomyopathy; however, it is a rare incidental finding in healthy individuals with preserved LV function, which accounts for approximately 35% of LVNC cases [8]. In adults, the prevalence of LVNC is about 0.05% [8]. 3-4% of heart failure patients sent for ECHO are found to have LVNC [8]. LVNC is more commonly found in African Americans and in males, with average age of diagnosis being 40–50 years old [8]. Overall, about 8 forms of LVNC exist with varying heterogeneity [8]. The diagnosis is made with ECHO or CMR by measuring the ratio of noncompacted to compacted layers of the LV muscle wall, with a ratio of $\geq 2:1$ meeting the criteria for LVNC [8]. Although the etiology of LVNC is uncertain, it is thought to be genetic in origin [8]. Research has shown links between abnormalities in certain genes, metabolic, mitochondrial, and chromosomal diseases, with the occurrence of LVNC [7]. The genetic defects most commonly associated with LVNC are of the sarcomere genes which are also involved with both dilated and hypertrophic cardiomyopathies [8].

Mitochondrial disorders also known as mitochondriopathies (MCPs) can be either syndromic or nonsyndromic and can present at any age, affect any organ, and have broad symptomatology [9]. The heart is one of the most commonly affected organs in MCPs [9]. Cardiac manifestations can include cardiomyopathies, LVNC, and arrhythmias [9]. Gastrointestinal manifestations of MCPs include dysphagia, gastroparesis, vomiting, malabsorption, diarrhea, pseudoobstruction, pancreatitis, and hepatopathy [10]. Over 50% of MCPs show some GI involvement although this is often underdiagnosed [10]. Episodic vomiting is a common manifestation and often first presenting symptom of mitochondrial encephalomyopathy, lactic acidosis, and stroke-like episode syndrome (MELAS) [10]. Gastroparesis is a less frequent manifestation of nonsyndromic MCPs and occurs due to a metabolic defect in the smooth muscle cells or from decreased parasympathetic innervation [10]. Hepatopathy in MCPs although more commonly seen in children may result in elevated liver enzymes and hepatic steatosis [10]. Involvement of the liver can be seen in up to 20% of patients with mitochondrial disorders [10].

4. Conclusion

Advanced stage heart failure is not a typical or well-studied cause of gastroparesis. Although gastric emptying studies demonstrated that our patient did indeed have gastroparesis, it is possible that he had components of both bowel wall edema and vagal nerve dysfunction from his enlarged heart, leading to delayed gastric emptying, abdominal discomfort, and formation of a gastric bezoar. The ultimate culprit was his failing heart. Better control of the patient's heart failure with recovery of function and improvement in ejection fraction may give some symptom relief. This can only be monitored by close patient follow-up. It will also be interesting to conduct more research in the future to investigate mitochondriopathies to understand the link between LVNC and gastroparesis.

References

[1] A. L. Bui, T. B. Horwich, and G. C. Fonarow, "Epidemiology and risk profile of heart failure," *Nature Reviews Cardiology*, vol. 8, no. 1, pp. 30–41, 2011.

[2] F. G. Romeiro, K. Okoshi, L. A. Zornoff, and M. P. Okoshi, "Gastrointestinal changes associated to heart failure," *Arquivos Brasileiros de Cardiologia*, vol. 98, no. 3, article 22527026, pp. 273–277, 2011.

[3] A. Krack, R. Sharma, H. R. Figulla, and S. D. Anker, "The importance of the gastrointestinal system in the pathogenesis of heart failure," *European Heart Journal*, vol. 26, no. 22, pp. 2368–2374, 2005.

[4] A. J. Camm and I. Savelieva, "Vagal nerve stimulation in heart failure," *European Heart Journal*, vol. 36, no. 7, pp. 404–406, 2015.

[5] E. Paulon, D. Nastou, F. Jaboli, J. Marin, E. Liebler, and O. Epstein, "Proof of concept: short-term non-invasive cervical vagus nerve stimulation in patients with drug-refractory gastroparesis," *Neurogastroenterology*, vol. 8, no. 4, pp. 325–330, 2018.

[6] E. Kalaitzakis, "Gastrointestinal dysfunction in liver cirrhosis," *World Journal of Gastroenterology*, vol. 20, no. 40, pp. 14686–14695, 2014.

[7] E. Arbustini, V. Favalli, N. Narula, A. Serio, and M. Grasso, "Left ventricular noncompaction: a distinct genetic cardiomyopathy," *Journal of the American College of Cardiology*, vol. 68, no. 9, pp. 949–966, 2016.

[8] J. A. Towbin and J. L. Jefferies, "Cardiomyopathies due to left ventricular noncompaction, mitochondrial and storage diseases, and inborn errors of metabolism," *Circulation Research*, vol. 121, no. 7, pp. 838–854, 2017.

[9] J. Finsterer, "Overview on visceral manifestations of mitochondrial disorders," *The Netherlands Journal of Medicine*, vol. 64, no. 3, pp. 61–71, 2006.

[10] J. Finsterer and M. Frank, "Gastrointestinal manifestations of mitochondrial disorders: a systematic review," *Therapeutic Advances in Gastroenterology*, vol. 10, no. 1, pp. 142–154, 2017.

8

Late Diagnosis of Anomalous Aortic Origin of a Coronary Artery from the Inappropriate Sinus of Valsalva during Investigation of Chest Pain

Brunna Priscylla Américo Carvalho,[1] Marcio Antônio Dos Santos,[2] Wilson Pedro Guimarães Neto,[2] Júlio César Queiroz De França,[2] Márcio Rogério de Souza Braite,[2] Rodrigo Bottura De Araújo,[2] Isabella Gomes Carvalho,[2] and Moacir Fernandes de Godoy[1,2]

[1]*Cardiology and Cardiovascular Surgery Department, São José do Rio Preto Medical School, São José do Rio Preto, SP, Brazil*
[2]*Hemodynamic and Interventional Cardiology Service, Hospital de Base, São José do Rio Preto, SP, Brazil*

Correspondence should be addressed to Wilson Pedro Guimarães Neto; wguimaraesn@hotmail.com

Academic Editor: Kjell Nikus

In this work are reported two cases of anomalous aortic origin of a coronary artery (AAOCA), with the left main coronary artery (LMCA) arising at the right sinus of Valsalva in a 77-year-old woman and in a 79-year-old man submitted to angiography after positive ischemic tests. The origin of the LMCA or the left descendant artery (LDA) from the right sinus of Valsalva has a prevalence of 0.2%, the origin of the circumflex artery (CXA) from the right sinus 0.5%, and the origin of the right coronary artery (RCA) from the left sinus of Valsalva has a prevalence of 0.3%. It is the subgroup of the coronary anomalies that has the greatest potential for clinical repercussions, especially the sudden cardiac death (SCD). We discuss the diagnostic methods and treatment options for this kind of coronary anomaly in symptomatic cases.

1. Introduction

The anomalous aortic origin of a coronary artery (AAOCA) is a rare disease with a range in prevalence from 0.3% to 1.5%, and it can be fatal depending on its anatomy [1, 2]. The symptoms may appear in childhood or only in adult life when the diagnosis is, most of the times, late due to normal ischemic tests. With the advancement of image methods, we may have a better understanding of the coronary anatomy and an early confirmation of this anatomical variant.

The objective of this report is to show the image diagnosis of two cases of anatomical variation of the left main coronary artery that arises at the right semilunar leaflet of the aortic valve in patients evaluated in the emergency room for precordial pain and treatment options for the symptomatic cases.

2. Case Reports

2.1. Case 1. A 77-year-old woman, with high blood pressure, in use of atenolol and losartan, presented to the emergency room with a complaint of chest pain that began during rest, tightness-like, without irradiation, of great intensity, associated with nausea, becoming worse during inspiration, and getting better at rest. The initial electrocardiogram showed atrial fibrillation, and the dosages of troponins were negative. A scintigraphy was performed with sestamibi that showed myocardial ischemia of small-to-moderate extension in the anteroseptal and inferoapical regions of the left ventricle (LV). Invasive stratification performed with coronary angiography showed an anomalous aortic origin of the left main coronary artery at the right semilunar cusp of the aortic valve, with a prepulmonic course and sharing a common ostium with the RCA (Figure 1).

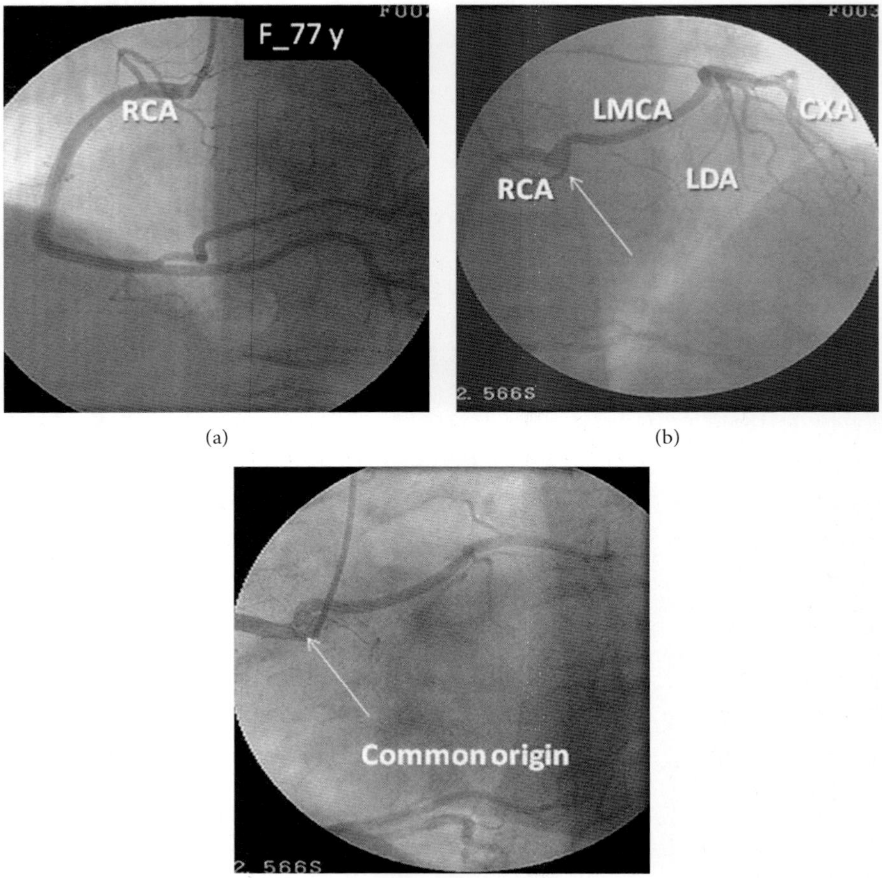

(a) (b) (c)

Figure 1: Coronary angiography showing the right coronary artery and the left main coronary artery arising from the same ostium, with a prepulmonic course of the LMCA.

There were no significant coronary obstructions. Synchronized scintigraphy of cardiac chambers showed enlarged left ventricle with global contractile performance depressed in mild-to-moderate grades and a left ventricular ejection fraction (LVEF) of 0.36. As the coronary anomaly was a fortuitous discovery and not related to the myocardial perfusion imaging abnormalities, the patient was discharged for clinical treatment using furosemide 40 mg once a day, carvedilol 25 mg twice a day, losartan 50 mg twice a day, and simvastatin 40 mg per day.

2.2. Case 2. A 79-year-old man, farmer, with no history of medication intake, presented to the emergency room with chest pain, started at physical stress, tightness-like, of moderate intensity, without irradiation, without associated factors, and getting better at rest. The electrocardiogram showed sinus rhythm, without suggestive signals of myocardial ischemia, and dosages of troponins were negative. The scintigraphy with sestamibi showed myocardial ischemia of a small-to-moderate area, involving parts of the apical region and inferoapical and inferior regions of the left ventricle. Invasive stratification performed with coronary angiography showed the anomalous aortic origin of the left main coronary artery at the right semilunar cusp of the aortic valve. The CT angiography showed a long and trifurcated left main coronary artery, with a prepulmonic course (Figure 2). Once again, this AAOCA pattern was not recognized as potentially serious, and the patient was discharged asymptomatic.

3. Discussion

Coronary anomaly can be defined as any change in the anatomical pattern, such as the number of ostium, proximal course, distal bed, and it is rarely found in the general population [3].

The anomalous aortic origin of the left main coronary artery from the right aortic sinus may be related to SCD, usually during or after exhausting exercise. It is currently the second most common cause of SCD in athletes [2]. The anatomical variation can follow five different paths: interarterial, subpulmonic (intraconal or intraseptal), prepulmonic, retroaortic, or retrocardiac. The interarterial variation is the pattern that has stronger relationship with SCD [2, 4, 5].

In most cases of AAOCA, there are no symptoms, and the only clinical manifestation of the interarterial course

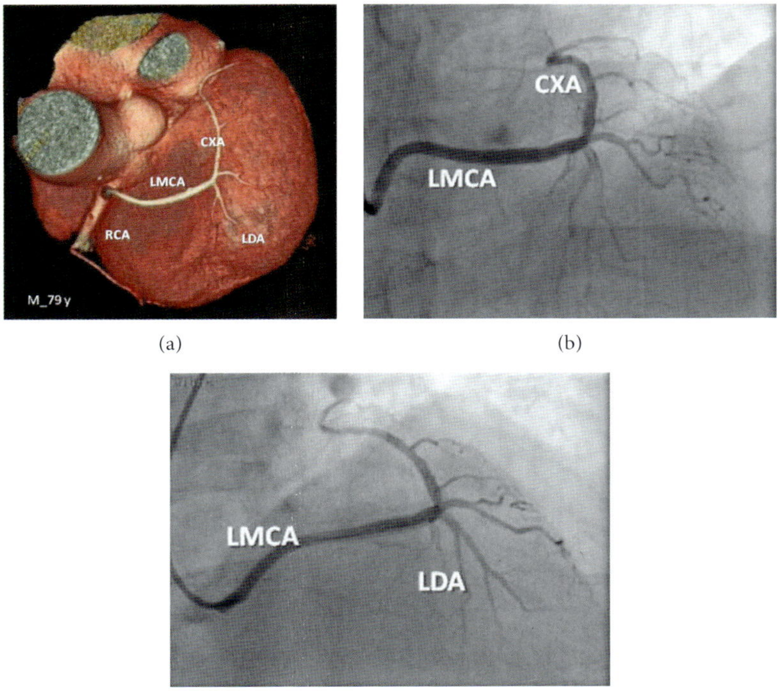

(a) (b) (c)

Figure 2: CT angiography and coronary angiography showing a long and trifurcated left main coronary artery with a prepulmonic course.

may be SCD. When symptomatic, the patients may complain of syncope, chest pain, and palpitations. The lack of symptoms difficults the diagnosis. In symptomatic patients, the initial investigation should follow with electrocardiogram, stress testing, and echocardiography [5].

The coronary angiography is traditionally the gold standard for the diagnosis of these anomalies, with the disadvantage of being an invasive test that uses potentially nephrotoxic contrast and ionizing radiation. Besides that, the usual two-dimensional images may generate failures in interpretation [6].

On the other hand, computed tomography of coronary arteries has had a fast evolution as the coronary evaluation method. This method has shown excellent accuracy in evaluating the origin and proximal course of the coronary anomalies, being superior to coronary angiography. The middle and distal segments have also been better visualized. Some comparative studies with coronary angiography have shown superior efficiency, suggesting that multislice computed tomography is the ideal test for coronary anomaly diagnosis [3, 6].

Transthoracic echocardiogram is the most useful method for children because it is not invasive and does not use radiation, contrast, or sedation. It also allows visualization of the origin of the coronary vessels [7].

In asymptomatic patients, there is no consensus on treatment management. However, in symptomatic individuals, with interarterial course, surgical treatment should be the first option, but there are no data that define which is the best surgical technique to be used. Coronary artery bypass grafting should be avoided, unless there is concomitant obstructive coronary artery disease [4]. Surgical techniques are beyond the scope of this work and will not be discussed. In some symptomatic individuals or in cases with reversible myocardial ischemia, beta-blockers and calcium channel blockers can be used in order to reduce ischemic symptoms [6, 7].

4. Conclusion

The two cases presented above show patients with suspected acute coronary artery syndromes, in which the clinical investigation with invasive strategy diagnosed anomalous aortic origin of the left main coronary artery without atherosclerotic obstructions and no relationship with the myocardial ischemic changes. These case reports highlight this rare diagnostic possibility in patients undergoing angiography.

References

[1] O. Yamanaka and R. E. Hobbs, "Coronary artery anomalies in 126,595 patients undergoing coronary arteriography," *Catheterization and Cardiovascular Diagnosis*, vol. 21, no. 1, pp. 28–40, 1990.

[2] C. Tuncer, T. Batyraliev, R. Yilmaz, M. Gokce, B. Ervonuku, and S. Koroglu, "Origin and distribution anomalies of the left anterior descending artery in 70,850 adult patients: multicenter data collection," *Catheterization and Cardiovascular Interventions*, vol. 68, no. 4, pp. 574–585, 2006.

[3] D. R. Rabelo, M. V. Barros, M. C. Nunes, C. C. Oliveira, and M. H. Siqueira, "Multislice coronary angiotomography in the assessment of coronary artery anomalous origin," *Arquivos Brasileiros de Cardiologia*, vol. 98, no. 3, pp. 266–272, 2012.

[4] M. K. Cheezum, R. R. Liberthson, N. R. Shah et al., "Anomalous aortic origin of a coronary artery from the inappropriate sinus of Valsalva," *Journal of the American College of Cardiology*, vol. 69, no. 12, pp. 1592–1608, 2017.

[5] J. S. Ho and N. E. Strickman, "Anomalous origin of the right coronary artery from the left coronary sinus: case report and literature review," *Texas Heart Institute Journal*, vol. 29, no. 1, pp. 37–39, 2002.

[6] A. T. Marler, J. A. Malik, and A. M. Slim, "Anomalous left main coronary artery: case series of different courses and literature review," *Case Reports in Vascular Medicine*, vol. 2013, Article ID 380952, 5 pages, 2013.

[7] J. M. Peñalver, R. S. Mosca, D. Weitz, and C. K. L. Phoon, "Anomalous aortic origin of coronary arteries from the opposite sinus: a critical appraisal of risk," *BMC Cardiovascular Disorders*, vol. 12, p. 83, 2012.

9

Takotsubo Cardiomyopathy Associated with Polycythemia Vera

Sijan Basnet,[1] **Priya Rajagopalan**,[2] **Rashmi Dhital**,[1] **and Biswaraj Tharu**[3]

[1]*Department of Medicine, Reading Hospital, 420 S Fifth Avenue, West Reading, PA 19611, USA*
[2]*Jefferson Medical College, 1025 Walnut Street, Philadelphia, PA 19107, USA*
[3]*Maharajgunj Medical Campus, Tribhuvan University, Kathmandu, Nepal*

Correspondence should be addressed to Sijan Basnet; sijan.basnet@towerhealth.org

Academic Editor: Nurten Sayar

Takotsubo cardiomyopathy is characterized by transient apical ballooning with preserved basal ventricular function triggered by physical or emotional stressors. We present a case of a 75-year-old man referred to our facility for the management of acute myocardial infarction later diagnosed as takotsubo cardiomyopathy. We believe platelet-mediated adrenaline release from massive thrombocytosis might have been the precipitating factor for the pathogenesis of takotsubo cardiomyopathy.

1. Introduction

Takotsubo cardiomyopathy (TTC) was first reported by Sato et al. in 1990 [1]. TTC, named after a semblance of the left ventricle in systole with an octopus trap, is characterized by transient, reversible, apical ballooning with preservation of basal ventricular function, commonly seen in postmenopausal women after emotional or physical stressors [1, 2]. We present a case of TTC which developed during a hospital stay for pneumonia suspected secondary to rapidly increasing platelet count in an elderly gentleman with a history of polycythemia vera (PV).

2. Case Description

The patient is a 75-year-old man referred to our facility for the further management of ST-elevation myocardial infarction (STEMI). He had presented 3 days earlier to an outside hospital with shortness of breath and productive cough of one-day duration. The evaluation was positive for right-sided pneumonia and was started on intravenous ceftriaxone and oral azithromycin. He was gradually improving but on day 3 of admission developed worsening shortness of breath with tachypnea and oxygen desaturation. He denied any precordial pain. His electrocardiogram (EKG) showed ST-segment elevation in anterolateral precordial leads with QT/QTc interval prolongation (Figure 1). Troponin T then was 0.01 ng/mL (reference range: <0.01 ng/mL). Chest X-ray (CXR) showed diffuse pulmonary edema. He was started on intravenous (IV) furosemide and intubated for hypoxic respiratory failure. He was then transferred to our facility for expectant cardiac catheterization.

On presentation, the patient was intubated, and history was obtained from the patient's family. According to them, the patient was functionally active at baseline prior to presentation. He ambulated with a cane but was able to go up a flight of stairs without anginal symptoms. His past medical history was significant for heart failure with reduced ejection fraction, polycythemia vera, obstructive sleep apnea, hypertension, hyperlipidemia, aortic stenosis, anemia, chronic kidney disease stage IV, and stroke. He had undergone cardiac catheterization 2 years ago which had shown 40–50% stenosis of ostial left anterior descending (LAD) artery and 50% stenosis of the first diagonal branch. The patient was diagnosed with JAK2 V617F mutation-positive polycythemia vera 22 years ago and was maintained on hydroxyurea and darbepoetin alfa. Hydroxyurea was discontinued 2 weeks prior to presentation for anemia (hemoglobin 7 g/dL; reference range: 14–17 g/dL) requiring a blood transfusion and was started on ruxolitinib. Hydroxyurea was restarted 2 days prior at the referring hospital for worsening thrombocytosis.

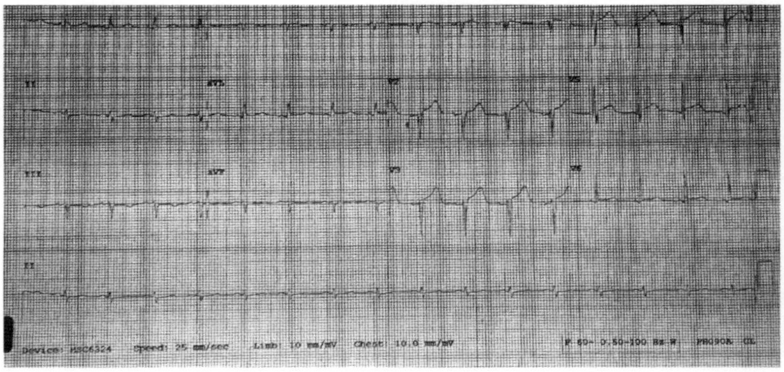

Figure 1: 12-lead electrocardiogram showing ST-segment elevation in the anterolateral precordial leads with QT/QTc interval prolongation.

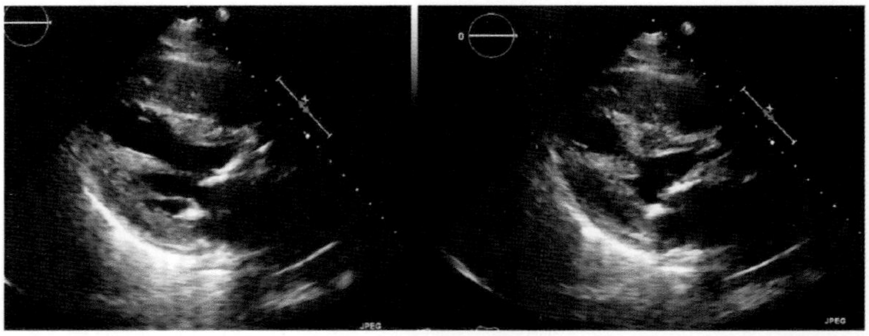

Figure 2: Transthoracic echocardiography with akinetic distal half of both left and right ventricles with resulting left ventricle outflow tract obstruction from the hyperkinetic basal myocardium.

On examination, the patient was afebrile with a pulse of 80 beats per minute (bpm), blood pressure of 98/56 mmHg, respiratory rate of 28/min, and 99% saturation on FiO2 of 70% intubated on assist control mode of ventilation. Chest examination revealed diffuse crackles and aortic stenosis murmur. He did not have pedal edema. His platelet count was 3,321,000/μL (reference range: 140,000–400,000/μL) and was described as giant platelets on peripheral smear. During the stay, his platelet count peaked at 4,145,000/μL. His white cell count was 13,100/μL (reference range: 4000–11,000/μL), and hemoglobin was 7.5 g/dL. Creatinine was elevated at 3.1 mg/dL (reference range: 0.7–1.4 mg/dL; baseline: 2.3–2.5 mg/dL) His probrain natriuretic peptide (pro-BNP) was 12,885 pg/mL (reference range: <450 pg/mL). Troponin T was 0.99 ng/mL. As EKG in the outside hospital showed ST elevation, he received 2 units packed red cells to reach goal hemoglobin between 9–10 g/dl. Repeat hemoglobin was 9.3 g/dL. He was continued on dual antiplatelet therapy and metoprolol tartrate 50 mg twice daily. He was started on heparin infusion. Transthoracic echocardiography showed an ejection fraction of 35% and moderately decreased left ventricular systolic function with dyskinetic to akinetic distal half of both ventricles consistent with takotsubo cardiomyopathy (Figure 2). Cardiac catheterization revealed nonobstructive coronary artery disease (Figure 3). Heparin infusion was discontinued. Post catheterization, his hospital stay was uneventful. He was successfully extubated and discharged a week later (hydroxyurea 1000 mg and ruxolitinib 5 mg both twice daily).

3. Discussion

Several theories have been postulated to explain the pathogenesis of TTC. The leading mechanism is direct myocardial damage from increased catecholamine release [1]. Acute stressors activate central and peripheral adrenergic sympathetic nervous system stimulating massive amounts of catecholamine secretion [1, 3]. This leads to increased cardiac workload with coronary microvascular spasm, consequent demand ischemia, and postischemic stunning [3]. This effect is profound in the apical myocardium where negatively inotropic β-adrenergic receptors are abundant. This differential distribution leads to the characteristic takotsubo-like appearance on echocardiography. In postmenopausal women, the loss of the effect of estrogen exaggerates the responses of central neurons and cardiac cells and possibly attenuates the production of cardioprotective substances. Abnormalities in glucose or fatty acid metabolism and excessive coronary vasoconstriction from defect in endothelial relaxation are other proposed mechanisms for the development of TTC [1].

4. Polycythemia Vera

TTC has previously been reported in association with esophageal carcinoma [4]. It has not been described in association with PV. Polycythemia vera (PV) is a myeloproliferative disorder with an increased risk of both arterial and venous thromboembolism including acute myocardial infarction through increased risk for clot formation [5]. In most

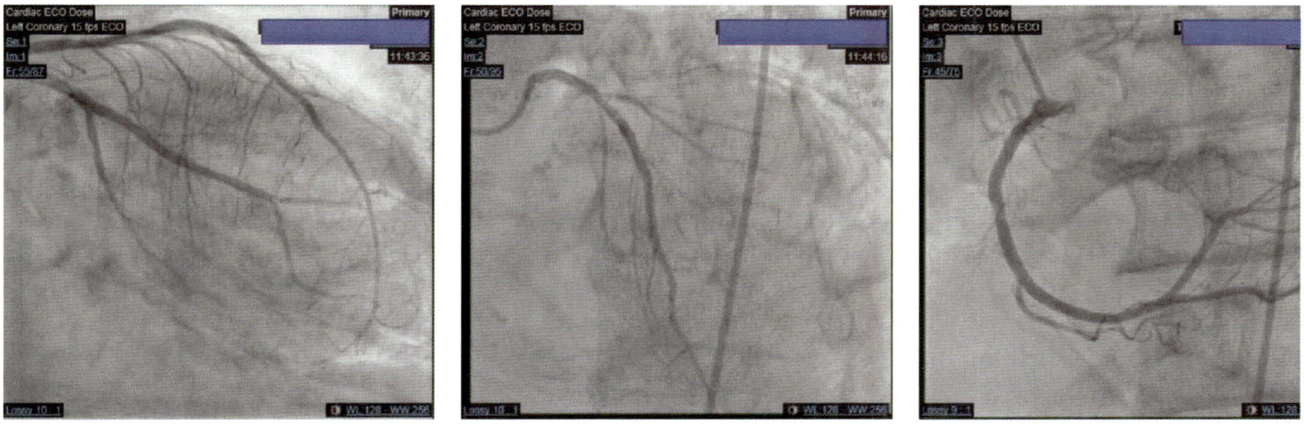

(a) (b) (c)

FIGURE 3: Cardiac catheterization with nonobstructive coronary artery disease of (a) left anterior descending and left circumflex arteries, (b) left main and left anterior descending, and (c) right coronary artery.

patients with PV, elevated hemoglobin > 18.5 g/dL is associated with thrombocytosis (platelet count > 450,000/μL in 53%) [6]. Contrastingly, our patient was anemic and had nonobstructive coronary artery disease on cardiac catheterization. His platelet counts were rapidly increasing prior to presentation possibly due to discontinuation of hydroxyurea. Platelets are one of the earliest responders at the site of injury. Their antimicrobial properties come from releasing cytokines and internalizing microorganisms [7]. They also have stores of adrenaline which are released at the same time [8]. We suspect an exaggerated adrenaline release from an abnormally elevated number of platelets might have acted as a stressor and triggered TTC.

5. Clinical Presentation

TTC is estimated to account for 1% to 2% of cases among patients presenting with acute coronary syndrome [1]. Deshmukh et al. reported that it was exceedingly common in women than in men, more so in women > 55 years of age [9]. There is usually an identifiable physical (36.0%) trigger like surgery, trauma, infection, and exacerbation of lung disease or emotional trigger (27.7%) [1, 10]. Common presenting complaints include chest pain, shortness of breath, and syncope. On rare occasions, cardiac arrest, cardiogenic shock, and life-threatening ventricular arrhythmias may occur [1]. Cardiogenic shock is commonly seen in the setting of left ventricular outflow tract (LVOT) obstruction from basal hypercontractility [11]. Our patient had demonstrated LVOT obstruction but was not in cardiogenic shock.

6. Diagnosis

Mayo Clinic criteria proposed for the diagnosis of TTC requires fulfillment of 4 conditions [12]:

1. Transient hypokinesis, akinesis, or dyskinesis of the left ventricular mid segments with or without apical involvement; the regional wall motion abnormalities extending beyond a single epicardial vascular distribution; a stressful trigger often but not always present
2. The absence of obstructive coronary disease or angiographic evidence of acute plaque rupture
3. New electrocardiographic abnormalities (either ST-segment elevation and/or T-wave inversion) or modest elevation in cardiac troponin
4. The absence of pheochromocytoma and myocarditis

We did not work up our patient for pheochromocytoma or myocarditis during his hospital stay. However, he had an old imaging of his abdomen which was negative for any adrenal mass. Clinical history did not co-relate with the presentation of pheochromocytoma or myocarditis. Wall motion abnormality on echocardiography with characteristic apical ballooning and basal hypercontractility makes TTC more likely. Our patient had ST-segment elevation and QT/QTc interval prolongation on EKG which is characteristic for TTC [1, 10]. Regarding cardiac biomarkers, troponin is only modestly elevated in TTC in comparison to STEMI [1] whereas brain natriuretic peptide (BNP) levels are usually higher in TTC than in STEMI [3, 10]. Although levels of both cardiac biomarkers may have been confounded by his stage IV chronic kidney disease, our patient had manifold elevation in pro-BNP than troponin T. Coronary angiography typically shows normal coronary arteries or nonobstructive coronary artery disease with wall motion abnormalities that extend beyond the distribution of a single coronary artery [1, 3, 10]. Thus, coronary atherosclerosis does not exclude a diagnosis of TTC [10].

7. Treatment

TTC is initially managed as acute myocardial infarction with oxygen, aspirin, intravenous heparin, and beta blockers [1, 11]. Cardiac catheterization should not be delayed with suspicion for TTC [10]. Once confirmed, aspirin can be discontinued in the absence of coronary artery disease [1, 11].

Intravenous heparin should be continued in the absence of contraindications to prevent left ventricular apical thrombus formation. This should be bridged to warfarin which should be continued until documented resolution of regional wall motion abnormalities. In the presence of an LVOT obstruction, nitroglycerin or inotropes should be avoided as it can worsen obstruction [11]. TTC usually resolves in a few days to weeks [3, 11]. The prognosis is favorable with in-hospital mortality ranging from 0 to 8% [11].

8. Conclusion

This is the first case to relate excess adrenaline release from platelets as a physical stressor in a patient with PV leading to TTC. We hope this case will bring forward other similar observations and help in better understanding the underlying pathogenetic mechanism.

References

[1] R. Ono and L. M. Falcão, "Takotsubo cardiomyopathy systematic review: pathophysiologic process, clinical presentation and diagnostic approach to takotsubo cardiomyopathy," *International Journal of Cardiology*, vol. 209, pp. 196–205, 2016.

[2] W. Chen and V. Dilsizian, "Exploring the pathophysiology of takotsubo cardiomyopathy," *Current Cardiology Reports*, vol. 19, no. 6, p. 53, 2017.

[3] F. Pelliccia, J. C. Kaski, F. Crea, and P. G. Camici, "Pathophysiology of takotsubo syndrome," *Circulation*, vol. 135, no. 24, pp. 2426–2441, 2017.

[4] T. C. Gangadhar, E. Von der Lohe, S. G. Sawada, and P. R. Helft, "Takotsubo cardiomyopathy in a patient with esophageal cancer: a case report," *Journal of Medical Case Reports*, vol. 2, no. 1, article 379, 2008.

[5] M. H. Kroll, L. C. Michaelis, and S. Verstovsek, "Mechanisms of thrombogenesis in polycythemia vera," *Blood Reviews*, vol. 29, no. 4, pp. 215–221, 2015.

[6] A. Tefferi, E. Rumi, G. Finazzi et al., "Survival and prognosis among 1545 patients with contemporary polycythemia vera: an international study," *Leukemia*, vol. 27, no. 9, pp. 1874–1881, 2013.

[7] E. M. Golebiewska and A. W. Poole, "Platelet secretion: from haemostasis to wound healing and beyond," *Blood Reviews*, vol. 29, no. 3, pp. 153–162, 2015.

[8] G. V. R. Born, "The uptake of adrenaline by human blood platelets," *Naunyn-Schmiedebergs Archiv für Experimentelle Pathologie und Pharmakologie*, vol. 259, no. 2, pp. 155-156, 1968.

[9] A. Deshmukh, G. Kumar, S. Pant, C. Rihal, K. Murugiah, and J. L. Mehta, "Prevalence of takotsubo cardiomyopathy in the United States," *American Heart Journal*, vol. 164, no. 1, pp. 66–71.e1, 2012.

[10] D. C. Scantlebury and A. Prasad, "Diagnosis of takotsubo cardiomyopathy," *Circulation Journal*, vol. 78, no. 9, pp. 2129–2139, 2014.

[11] S. Kurisu and Y. Kihara, "Clinical management of takotsubo cardiomyopathy," *Circulation Journal*, vol. 78, no. 7, pp. 1559–1566, 2014.

[12] M. Madhavan and A. Prasad, "Proposed Mayo Clinic criteria for the diagnosis of Tako-Tsubo cardiomyopathy and long-term prognosis," *Herz*, vol. 35, no. 4, pp. 240–244, 2010.

Carney Complex: A Rare Case of Multicentric Cardiac Myxoma Associated with Endocrinopathy

Yehia Saleh,[1,2] Basma Hammad,[2,3] Abdallah Almaghraby,[2] Ola Abdelkarim,[2] Mohamed Seleem,[2] Mahmoud Abdelnaby,[3] Hoda Shehata,[2] Mahmoud Hammad,[2] Bassem Ramadan,[2] Mohamed Elshafei,[2] Eman Elsharkawy,[2] and Mohamed Ayman Abdel-hay[2]

[1]*Michigan State University, East Lansing, MI, USA*
[2]*Faculty of Medicine, Alexandria University, Alexandria, Egypt*
[3]*Massachusetts General Hospital and Harvard Medical School, Boston, MA, USA*

Correspondence should be addressed to Yehia Saleh; yehia.saleh@hc.msu.edu

Academic Editor: Kuan-Rau Chiou

Carney complex is a rare autosomal dominant disorder characterized by multiple tumors, including cardiac and extracardiac myxomas, skin lesions, and various endocrine disorders. We are reporting a 21-year-old female patient with past surgical history significant for excision of a cutaneous myxoma who presented with multicentric cardiac myxomas involving the four cardiac chambers. She also presented with endocrinal disorders in the form of an enlarged right lobe of the thyroid, hyperthyroid state, and an incidentally noted adrenal cyst; hence, she was diagnosed with carney complex syndrome.

1. Introduction

Cardiac myxoma is the most common benign cardiac tumor. It usually presents as a sporadic isolated condition in the left atrium of middle-aged women [1]. A condition of multiple cardiac myxomas was reported in the familial forms. Carney complex (CNC) is one of those familial forms characterized by multiple cardiac myxomas, skin lesions, and various endocrine disorders [2].

2. Case Presentation

A 21-year-old female patient presented with progressive exertional dyspnea and irregular palpitations for 3 months. She had past surgical history significant for excision of a cutaneous myxoma in her left arm. Physical examination revealed a high jugular venous pressure and a diastolic murmur. An electrocardiogram showed atrial fibrillation. Laboratory investigations were within normal limits except for a low TSH and elevated free T3 and T4. Transthoracic echocardiography (TTE) showed a large echogenic mobile mass with central constriction attached to the interventricular septum (IVS), occupying the entire right atrium and right ventricle (RV) and obstructing the flow of the tricuspid valve. There were two other masses of the same echogenicity: one was occupying the left ventricle (LV) and the other was in the left atrium attached to the interatrial septum at the site of fossa ovalis (Figure 1, Videos 1–5). The left ventricular dimensions and function were normal. Cardiac magnetic resonance showed similar findings with no septal invasion and tissue characterization suggestive of multiple myxomas (Figure 2). Computed tomography of the chest, abdomen, and pelvis revealed the same findings (Figure 3) in addition to an enlarged thyroid nodule and a left adrenal cyst that measures 65×57 mm (Figure 4). Ultrasonography of the thyroid gland revealed a markedly enlarged right lobe of the thyroid with normal vascularity. Serum aldosterone, dexamethasone suppression test, dehydroepiandrosterone sulfate, and 24-hour urine metanephrines were within normal limits.

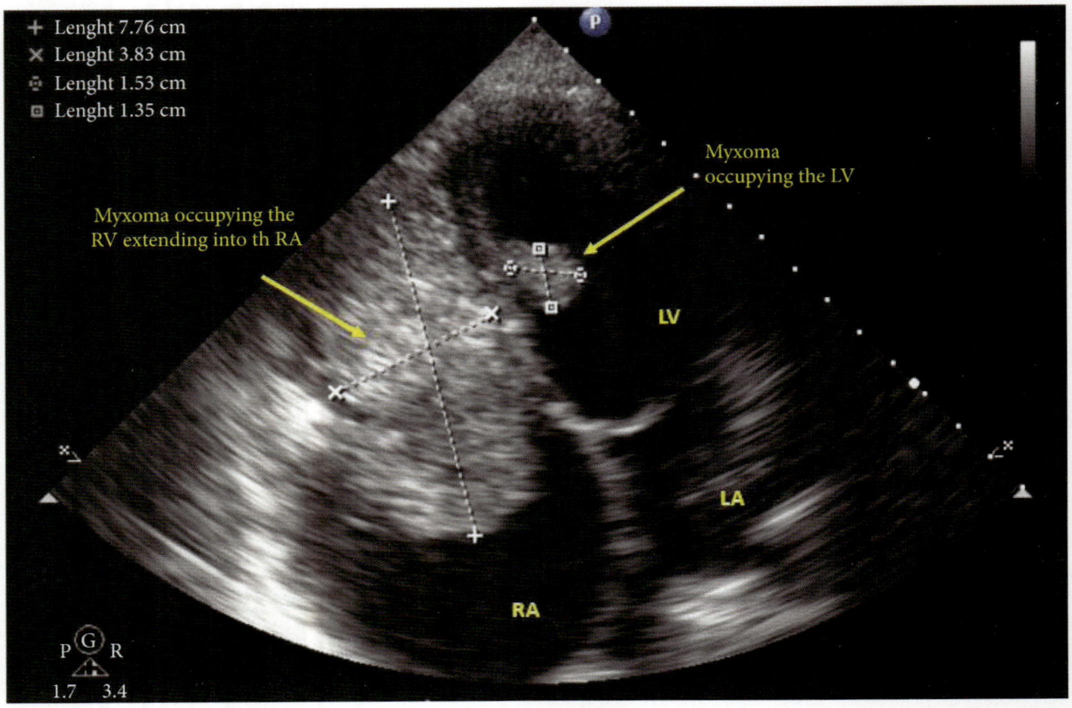

Figure 1: Transthoracic echocardiogram modified apical 4-chamber view showing a large mass in the right ventricle and atrium measuring 7.7 × 3.8 cm and another mass in the left ventricle attached to interventricular septum measuring 1.5 × 1.3 cm.

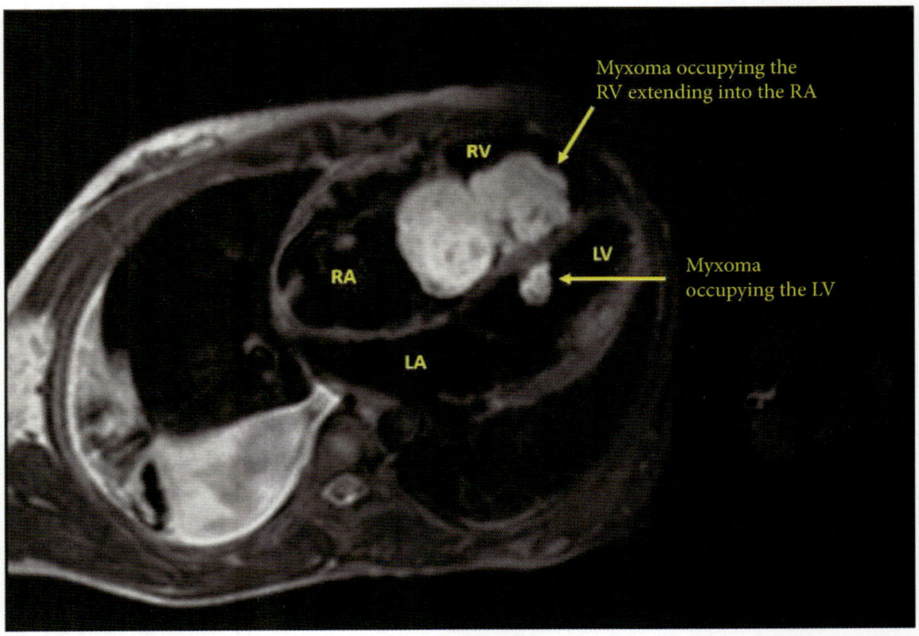

Figure 2: Cardiac magnetic resonance showing a myxoma occupying the right ventricle and atrium and another myxoma in the left ventricle attached to the interventricular septum.

The patient underwent surgery where all three masses were excised. However, the tricuspid valve was inseparable from the RV mass; hence, it was replaced with a tissue prosthesis. The masses were grossly reddish grey in color, fleshy, and gelatinous in consistency (Figure 5). The histopathological examination of the excised masses revealed myxomatous cellular proliferations with sparse collagen fibers consistent with multiple myxomas (Figures 6(a) and 6(b)). The patient was followed up on 6-month intervals. After 2 years of follow-up, the adrenal cyst was stable in size; however, TTE showed a mass in the left ventricular outflow tract (Figures 7 and 8, Videos 6–10). The newly developed mass

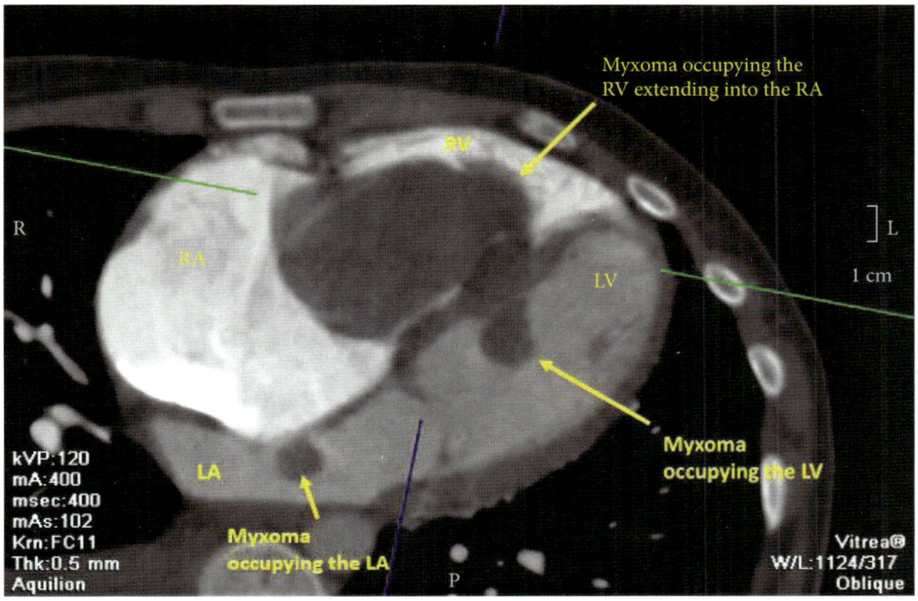

FIGURE 3: Computed tomography showing a large myxoma occupying the right ventricle and atrium, another myxoma occupying the left atrium, and a third myxoma occupying the left ventricle.

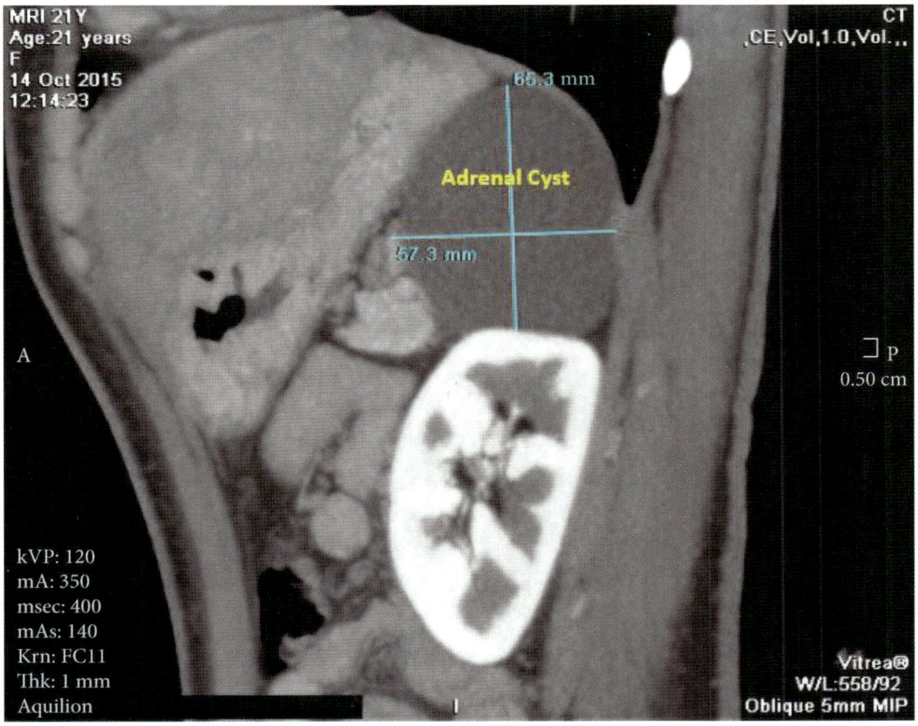

FIGURE 4: Computed tomography showing a large adrenal cyst measuring 65 × 57 mm.

was surgically excised, and histopathology revealed myxomatous tissue.

3. Discussion

Primary intracardiac tumors are extremely rare in comparison to secondary tumors. However, myxoma is the most common primary cardiac neoplasm [1]. Cardiac myxoma usually presents as a sporadic mass; it can occur in any chamber of the heart but mainly occurs in the left atrium, and it affects women more than men with a mean age of 56. If myxoma presents as multiple masses, which rarely occurs, it is usually a familial form [2].

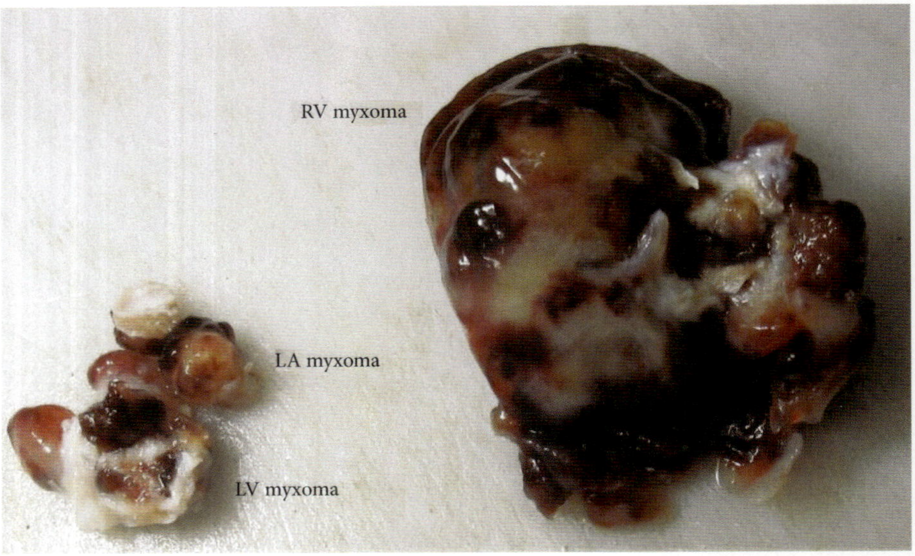

FIGURE 5: Gross specimen of the myxomas.

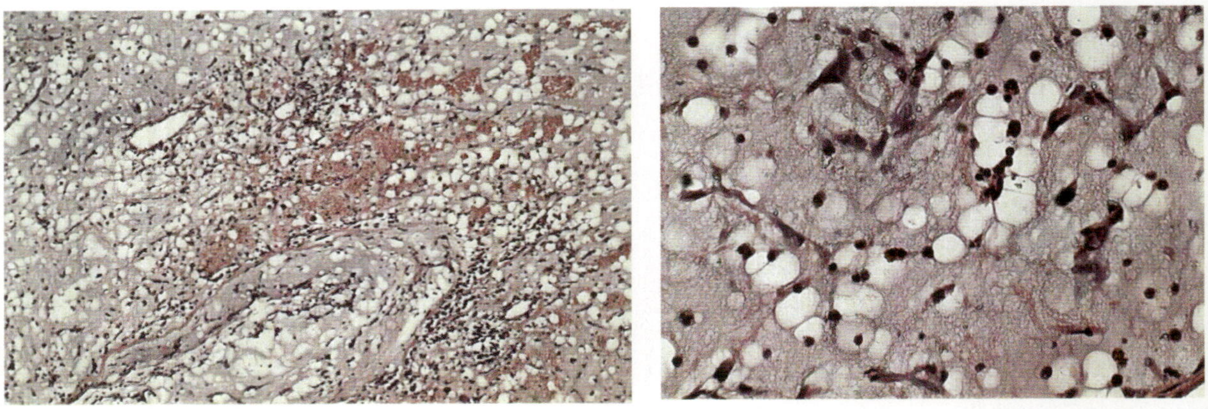

(a) (b)

FIGURE 6: (a, b) Histopathology of mass showing myxomatous cellular proliferations with sparse collagen fibers consistent with myxoma.

Carney complex (CNC) is one of the familial forms inherited in an autosomal dominant fashion. CNC is most frequently associated with mutations in the protein kinase A type I-alpha regulatory subunit gene (*PRKAR1A*). However, twenty-five percent of the cases occur sporadically secondary to de novo mutation [3]. CNC is characterized by multiple tumors, including cardiac and extracardiac myxomas, skin lesions, and various endocrine disorders [2].

Cardiac myxomas associated with CNC are characterized by the following: occurring at a younger age, multicentric, and a higher tendency of recurrence after resection in comparison to solitary ones [2, 4]. Our patient presented with three myxomas initially and had a recurrence after 2 years in a different location.

CNC-associated skin lesions can present as a spotty skin pigmentation which occurs in more than 80% of patients [5] or a cutaneous myxoma which is a benign dermal tumor present in less than 50% of patients. Cutaneous myxoma is a well-demarcated subcutaneous nodule that can reach 15 mm in diameter and most commonly affects the head, neck, and trunk. When nodules are confirmed to be myxomas histologically, the diagnosis of CNC is highly suggested [5, 6]. Hence, we would suggest screening any patient who present with cutaneous myxomas for other features of CNC. Our patient did not develop any skin pigmentation. However, she had history of a surgically removed cutaneous myxoma.

Endocrine abnormalities due to tumors of the adrenal and pituitary glands or testicular tumors are the most frequent systemic manifestations of CNC. Cushing's syndrome can occur in up to 45% of patients diagnosed with CNC [7]. Our patient had no symptoms that would suggest Cushing's syndrome, and the adrenal gland laboratory work-up was within normal limits. However, an adrenal cyst was detected on computed tomography and was followed up for 2 years without any change in size.

Thyroid disease is also common; almost 75% of patients with CNC will develop thyroid nodules typically early in life,

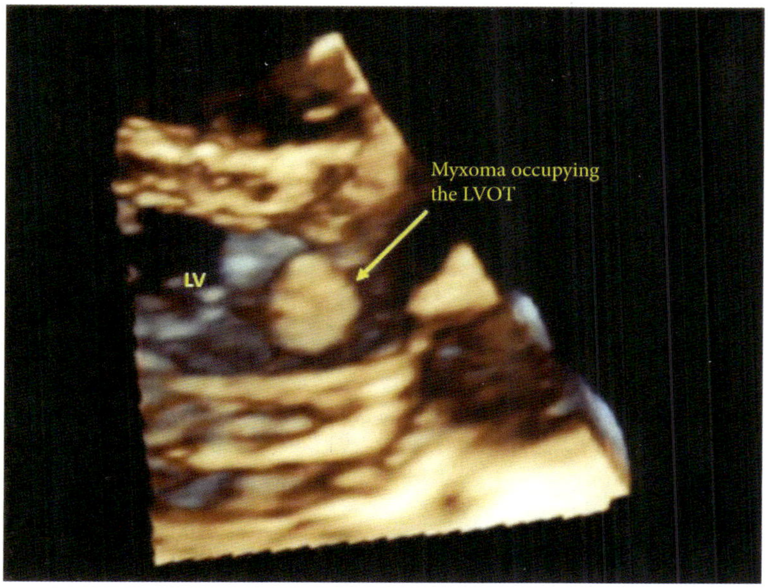

FIGURE 7: Transthoracic echocardiogram parasternal long-axis view 3-dimensional reconstruction showing a myxoma in the left ventricular outflow tract.

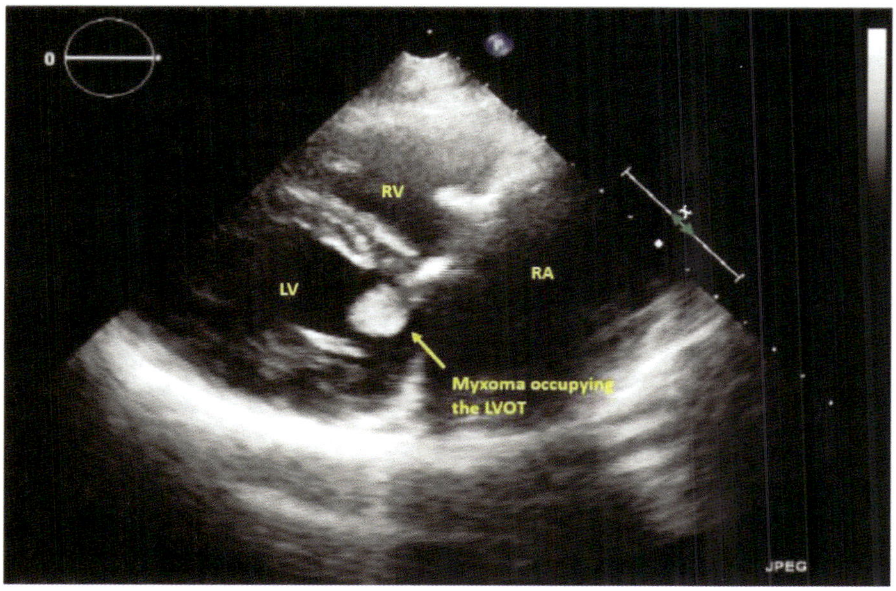

FIGURE 8: Transthoracic echocardiogram modified parasternal long-axis view showing a myxoma in the left ventricular outflow tract.

and 25% will develop adenomatous disease. Less than 10% will develop thyroid cancer. Hence, fine-needle aspiration is indicated for patients with thyroid nodules. Regardless of the previous pathologies, most CNC patients are euthyroid [8]. Our patient presented with a nodule and was diagnosed with hyperthyroidism which is uncommon.

In order to diagnose CNC, Stratakis et al. defined the diagnostic criteria (Table 1). Diagnosis is established if the patient has two or more major criteria, or, alternatively, one major criterion in addition to either an inactivating mutation of the *PRKAR1A* gene or a first-degree relative has CNC [9, 10].

Although the clinical diagnostic criteria are reliable, nowadays genetic testing for mutations in the *PRKAR1A* gene is more commonly used for diagnostic certainty. In addition, genetic screening of potentially affected family members of patients with CNC could be useful especially in younger family members. However, clinical surveillance is still advisable for family members even when a *PRKAR1A* pathogenic variant is not identified.

In cases of cardiac myxomas, surgical resection is the treatment of choice with a 6-month follow-up via TTE afterwards due to the high incidence of recurrence. In addition, a multidisciplinary approach is recommended in

Table 1: Diagnostic criteria for carney complex.

(1) Spotty skin pigmentation with a typical distribution (lips, conjunctiva and inner or outer canthi, vaginal and penile mucosa)
(2) Myxoma (cutaneous and mucosal)[a]
(3) Cardiac myxoma[a]
(4) Breast myxomatosis[a] or fat-suppressed magnetic resonance imaging findings suggestive of this diagnosis
(5) PPNAD[a] or paradoxical positive response of urinary glucocorticosteroids to dexamethasone administration during Liddle's test
(6) Acromegaly due to GH-producing adenoma[a]
(7) LCCSCT[a] or characteristic calcification on testicular ultrasonography
(8) Thyroid carcinoma[a] or multiple, hypoechoic nodules on thyroid ultrasonography, in a young patient
(9) Psammomatous melanotic schwannoma[a]
(10) Blue nevus, epithelioid blue nevus (multiple)[a]
(11) Breast ductal adenoma (multiple)[a]
(12) Osteochondromyxoma[a]
Supplemental criteria
(1) Affected first-degree relative
(2) Inactivating mutation of the *PRKARIA* gene

To make a diagnostic of CNC, a patient must either (1) exhibit two of the manifestations of the diseases listed or (2) exhibit one of these manifestations and meet one of the supplemental criteria (an affected first-degree relative or an inactivating mutation of the PRKARIA gene). [a]With histologic information.

order to screen for endocrinopathies and malignancies. Clinical surveillance is advisable for family members and possibly genetic testing. In our patient, clinical screening of the family was not significant; hence, we concluded she developed a de novo mutation.

4. Conclusion

Multiple intracardiac myxomas account for less than 5% of all cases of myxoma. Its presence should warrant screening for endocrinal disorders and should be treated by complete surgical excision with a generous safety margin in addition to close follow-up as it carries high risk of recurrence.

Disclosure

Yehia Saleh and Basma Hammad are co-first authors.

Authors' Contributions

Yehia Saleh and Basma Hammad contributed equally to the development of this manuscript.

References

[1] O. Azevedo, J. Almeida, T. Nolasco et al., "Massive right atrial myxoma presenting as syncope and exertional dyspnea: case report," *Cardiovascular Ultrasound*, vol. 8, no. 1, p. 23, 2010.

[2] H. J. Vidaillet, J. B. Seward, F. E. Fyke, W. P. Su, and A. J. Tajik, ""Syndrome myxoma": a subset of patients with cardiac myxoma associated with pigmented skin lesions and peripheral and endocrine neoplasms," *Heart*, vol. 57, no. 3, pp. 247–255, 1987.

[3] L. S. Kirschner, J. A. Carney, S. D. Pack et al., "Mutations of the gene encoding the protein kinase A type I-alpha regulatory subunit in patients with the carney complex," *Nature Genetics*, vol. 26, no. 1, pp. 89–92, 2000.

[4] A. D. Irani, A. L. Estrera, L. M. Buja, and H. J. Safi, "Biatrial myxoma: a case report and review of the literature," *Journal of Cardiac Surgery*, vol. 23, no. 4, pp. 385–390, 2008.

[5] A. Horvath and C. A. Stratakis, "Carney complex and lentiginosis," *Pigment Cell & Melanoma Research*, vol. 22, no. 5, pp. 580–587, 2009.

[6] C. Mateus, A. Palangié, N. Franck et al., "Heterogeneity of skin manifestations in patients with carney complex," *Journal of the American Academy of Dermatology*, vol. 59, no. 5, pp. 801–810, 2008.

[7] K. Reynen, "Frequency of primary tumors of the heart," *The American Journal of Cardiology*, vol. 77, no. 1, p. 107, 1996.

[8] C. A. Stratakis, "Hereditary syndromes predisposing to endocrine tumors and their skin manifestations," *Reviews in Endocrine and Metabolic Disorders*, vol. 17, no. 3, pp. 381–388, 2016.

[9] M. Q. Almeida and C. A. Stratakis, "Carney complex and other conditions associated with micronodular adrenal hyperplasias," *Best Practice & Research Clinical Endocrinology & Metabolism*, vol. 24, no. 6, pp. 907–914, 2010.

[10] C. A. Stratakis, L. S. Kirschner, and J. A. Carney, "Clinical and molecular features of the carney complex: diagnostic criteria and recommendations for patient evaluation," *The Journal of Clinical Endocrinology & Metabolism*, vol. 86, no. 9, pp. 4041–4046, 2001.

A Rare Case of Spontaneous Cardiac Tamponade Induced by Concomitant Use of Rivaroxaban and Amiodarone

Oreoluwa Oladiran,[1] Jared Segal,[1] Ifeanyi Nwosu,[2] and Salik Nazir[1]

[1] *Reading Hospital, Tower Health System, Reading, PA, USA*
[2] *Benenden Hospitals Trust, Kent, UK*

Correspondence should be addressed to Oreoluwa Oladiran; oreoluwa.oladiran@towerhealth.org

Academic Editor: Assad Movahed

Rivaroxaban is a direct oral anticoagulant (DOAC) approved as an important alternative to warfarin in patients with nonvalvular atrial fibrillation. We report the case of an 87-year-old man with past medical history of nonvalvular atrial fibrillation on rivaroxaban and recently started amiodarone for pulseless ventricular tachycardia who presented to our hospital with intermittent chest pain and was diagnosed with spontaneous hemopericardium causing cardiac tamponade. The culprit drugs were discontinued, and the patient was treated with emergent pericardiocentesis. Both rivaroxaban and amiodarone are substrates for the CYP3A4 hepatic pathway, and concomitant use can result in increased plasma rivaroxaban levels causing an increased propensity to bleeding. While most physicians are cognizant of the need for renal dosing of rivaroxaban, this article aims to increase awareness of its interactions with drugs that are also metabolized through the same hepatic CYP450 pathway.

1. Background

Rivaroxaban is a direct oral anticoagulant approved by the United States Food and Drug Administration (FDA) for stroke prevention in nonvalvular atrial fibrillation [1]. Amiodarone is an antiarrhythmic agent indicated for the prevention of recurrent life-threatening ventricular arrhythmias [2]. All anticoagulants including rivaroxaban are associated with increased risk of bleeding. The risk of bleeding with rivaroxaban can be accentuated by the concomitant use of medications such as amiodarone [3] which compete for metabolism via the CYP3A4 hepatic pathway [4]. The incidence of spontaneous hemopericardium due to rivaroxaban is unknown, likely due to its rarity as only few cases have been documented so far [5–7]. However, with increasing use of this medication, rare side effects like this will be encountered more often. Clinicians must be aware of this rare catastrophic possibility that could result from the lethal combination of rivaroxaban and amiodarone. We suggest that rivaroxaban package insert should include more information on medications considered to be inhibitors of CYP3A4 and P-glycoprotein system.

2. Case Presentation

An 87-year-old male with medical history of paroxysmal atrial fibrillation on 20 mg of rivaroxaban daily, recent pulseless ventricular tachycardia with implantable cardiac defibrillator in situ, and nonischemic cardiomyopathy (ejection fraction 35%) presented to the emergency room (ER) with intermittent chest pain and light headedness of 2 days duration. Chest pain was exertional, left sided, and pleuritic. He also reported shortness of breath but denied cough, fever, or any other infectious. Of note, he was commenced on 200 mg amiodarone daily four months prior to presentation following an episode of syncope due to pulseless ventricular tachycardia.

Initial vital signs showed blood pressure of 89/60 mmHg with pulse rate of 59/min, temperature of 98.2°F, and respiratory rate of 14 breaths/min with normal oxygen saturation of

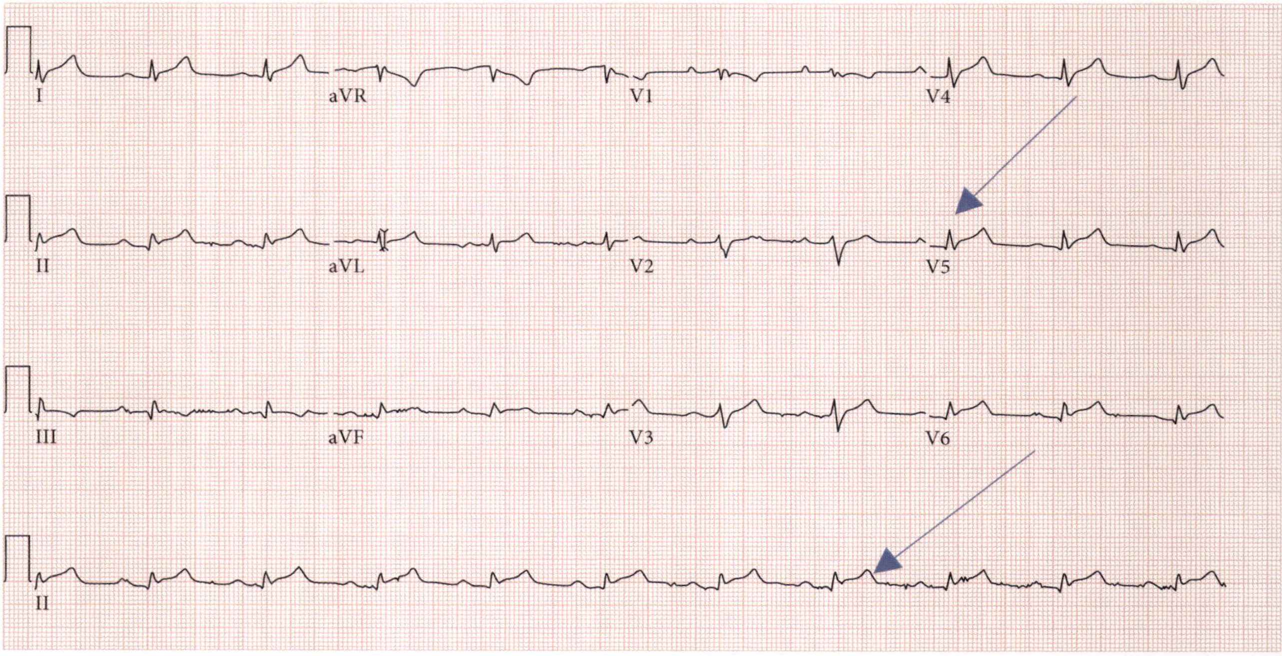

FIGURE 1: Electrocardiogram showing diffuse ST segment elevation with low voltage QRS complexes.

100% on ambient air. On physical examination, he was in no acute distress and was alert and oriented to time, place, and person. Jugular venous distention was noted on neck examination. Heart sounds were muffled, but lung fields were clear to auscultation. Peripheral pulses were also weak but palpable.

3. Investigations

His EKG on arrival to the emergency room showed new widespread ST segment elevation (Figure 1). His troponin was trended and remained <0.03 ng/mL (normal <0.05 ng/mL). Complete blood count showed hemoglobin of 11.2 g/dL (normal 14–17.5 g/dL), white blood cell count of 11.7/microliter (normal 4.8–10.8/microliter), and normal platelet count of 211/microliter (normal 130–400/microliter). Basic metabolic panel revealed creatinine of 3.4 mg/dL from baseline of <0.8 mg/dL (normal 0.6–1.3 mg/dL) with BUN of 58 mg/dL (normal 7–25 mg/dL). His liver function test showed AST of 90 U/L (normal 13–39 U/L), ALT of 126 U/L (normal 7–52 U/L), and total bilirubin of 1.2 mg/dL (0.3–1.0 mg/dL). INR was also elevated at 2.2 (normal 0.9–1.1) with prothrombin time of 24.7 seconds (normal 12.3–14.6 seconds). Initial lactate was also elevated at 3.2 meq/L (normal 0.6–1.4 meq/L).

Chest X-ray revealed enlargement of the cardiomedistinal silhouette. CT chest revealed new moderate-sized pericardial effusion (Figure 2).

Transthoracic echocardiogram (TTE) revealed large circumferential pericardial effusion and evidence for tamponade physiology with multichamber collapse and significant respirophasic variation to the mitral inflow pattern (Figure 3). Please see Supplementary Material (available here).

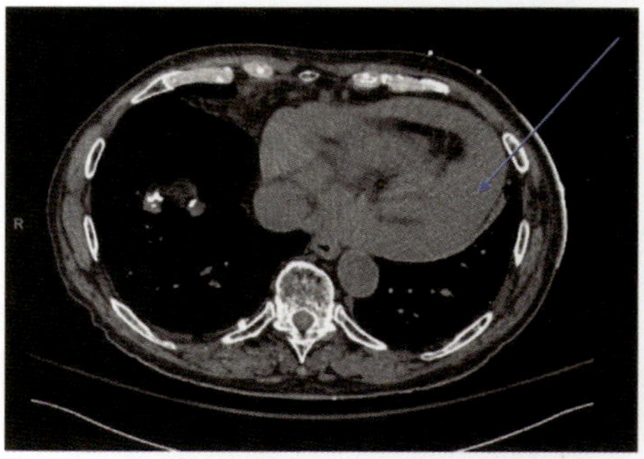

FIGURE 2: Chest CT scan (transverse view) showing fluid in the pericardial space.

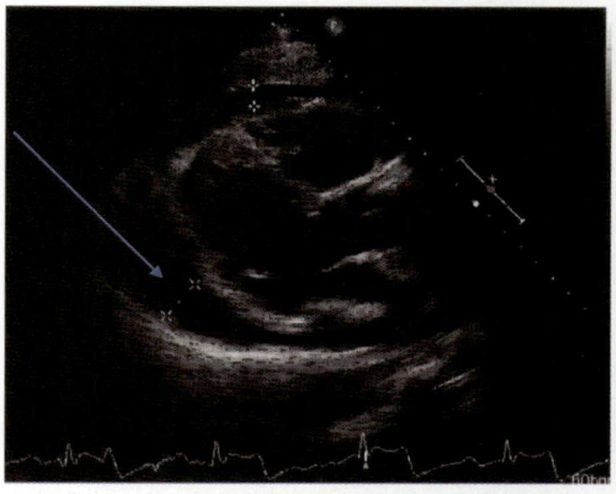

FIGURE 3: Parasternal long axis view of transthoracic echocardiogram showing fluid within the pericardial space.

4. Differential Diagnosis

Given the patient's history of intermittent chest pain and presence of ST segment elevation on EKG, our initial suspicion was an ST segment elevation myocardial infarction. However, at the time of evaluation by the cardiologist, the patient had no chest pain and serial troponin levels remained normal. Notably, patient had coronary angiography done 9 months prior to index presentation revealed minimal plaquing of the coronary arteries. We now know that the hypotension, muffled heart sounds, and jugular venous distention were part of the Beck's triad of cardiac tamponade. The lactic acidosis, acute kidney injury, and elevated liver enzymes were likely the result of tissue hypoperfusion from hypotension while the leucocytosis was likely reactive.

5. Treatment

Based on the initial finding of ST segment elevation on EKG, he received a loading dose of 324 mg of ASA by EMS. Amiodarone was discontinued due to deranged liver and renal functions. We also held his rivaroxaban due to abnormal clotting profile and finding of hemopericardium on imaging studies. He had urgent pericardiocentesis in the catheterization laboratory with initial drainage of 825 mLs of sanguinous fluid, and postprocedural TTE showed evidence of resolution of tamponade. The pericardiocentesis catheter was left in place to drain any residual collections, and patient was transferred to the intensive care unit. He had daily TTE at the bedside, and his pericardial drainage volume progressively reduced from 160 cc on day 1 to 100 cc on day 2 to 80 cc on day 3 postpericardiocentesis when the drain was removed. Pericardial fluid analysis was negative for organisms or malignancy.

6. Outcome and Follow-Up

Our patient experienced significant improvement of his symptoms following pericardiocentesis. His blood pressure normalized, and IV dopamine was discontinued immediately after pericardiocentesis. His renal function also improved significantly evidenced by a reduction in creatinine to normal at the time of discharge. He went home 5 days after admission and was instructed to stop his amiodarone and rivaroxaban in the mean time until his office appointment with his cardiologist.

7. Discussion

Based on the Naranjo causality assessment scale [8], there is probable relationship between our patient's spontaneous hemopericardium and rivaroxaban use.

Serious bleeding events have been reported with rivaroxaban, mainly intracranial and gastrointestinal [9], but only a few case reports of nontraumatic hemopericardium exist.

Altered hepatic metabolism resulting from coadministration with amiodarone and transient renal impairment synergistically resulted in supratherapeutic serum levels of rivaroxaban in our patient resulting in nontraumatic hemopericardium and eventual cardiac tamponade.

Elimination of rivaroxaban occurs through a dual pathway—hepatic metabolism occurs via the CYP450 pathway (mainly by CYP3A4 and CYP2J2) while renal excretion via P-glycoprotein-mediated secretion [4]. Amiodarone and its main metabolite N-desethylamiodarone (NDEA) inhibit CYP3A4 and P-glycoprotein resulting in supratherapeutic concentrations of rivaroxaban when used simultaneously.

When used for stroke prophylaxis in patients with nonvalvular atrial fibrillation, clinical trials evaluating the safety and efficacy of rivaroxaban using the cockroft-gault formula recommend that for creatinine clearance greater than 50 mL/minute as was the case in our patient prior to this admission, a standard dose of 20 mg once daily is adequate. However, for CrCl between 15 and 50 mL/minute, a dose adjustment to 15 mg once daily may be considered. Most clinicians recommend discontinuing rivaroxaban in acute kidney injury or CrCl less than 15 mL/minute [9]. No guidelines exist for dose adjustment when used with other medications undergoing CYP450 metabolism.

Andexanet alfa, a recombinant modified human factor Xa protein, is an antidote recently approved by the United States Food and Drug Administration (FDA) [10] for patients treated with rivaroxaban and apixaban when reversal of anticoagulation is needed for life-threatening bleeding [11].

However, there are neither routinely available laboratory tests to measure the anticoagulant effect of rivaroxaban nor consensus guidelines on the use of prothrombin complex concentrates, recombinant factor VIIa, and the newly approved reversal agents in patients on direct oral anticoagulants.

This article aims to alert clinicians to this rare but increasingly reported side effect of rivaroxaban. A high index of suspicion is needed for recognition and diagnosis of spontaneous hemopericardium. Caution should be observed especially in elderly patients with declining renal function and increased likelihood of polypharmacy. With increasing use of rivaroxaban and other novel anticoagulants and the recent approval of a new reversal agent, more research is needed to develop monitoring laboratory parameters to determine and monitor their therapeutic range.

References

[1] M. R. Patel, K. W. Mahaffey, J. Garg et al., "Rivaroxaban versus warfarin in nonvalvular atrial fibrillation," *New England Journal of Medicine*, vol. 365, no. 10, pp. 883–891, 2011.

[2] S. M. Al-Khatib, W. G. Stevenson, M. J. Ackerman et al., "2017 AHA/ACC/HRS guideline for management of patients with ventricular arrhythmias and the prevention of sudden cardiac death: a report of the American College of Cardiology/American Heart Association Task Force on Clinical Practice Guidelines and the Heart Rhythm Society," *Heart Rhythm*, 2017.

[3] R. Latini, G. Tognoni, and R. E. Kates, "Clinical pharmacokinetics of amiodarone," *Clinical Pharmacokinetics*, vol. 9, no. 2, pp. 136–156, 1984.

[4] C. Weinz, T. Schwarz, D. Kubitza, W. Mueck, and D. Lang, "Metabolism and excretion of rivaroxaban, an oral, direct factor Xa inhibitor, in rats, dogs, and humans," *Drug Metabolism*

and Disposition, vol. 37, no. 5, pp. 1056–1064, 2009.

[5] N. M. Kham and M. Song, "Spontaneous, life-threatening hemorrhagic cardiac tamponade secondary to rivaroxaban," *American Journal of Therapeutics*, vol. 23, no. 4, pp. e1128–e1131, 2016.

[6] S. Boone, "Cardiac tamponade associated with rivaroxaban," *Delaware Medical Journal*, vol. 87, no. 7, pp. 206-207, 2015.

[7] D. Menendez and J. Michel, "Hemopericardium with tamponade following rivaroxaban administration and its attenuation by CYP3A4 inhibitors," *Baylor University Medical Center Proceedings*, vol. 29, no. 4, pp. 414-415, 2016.

[8] Naranjo algorithm, "A method for estimating the probability of adverse drug reactions | pmidCALC online calculators," May 2018, http://www.pmidcalc.org/?sid=7249508&newtest=Y.

[9] W. Mueck, J. Stampfuss, D. Kubitza, and M. Becka, "Clinical pharmacokinetic and pharmacodynamic profile of rivaroxaban," *Clinical Pharmacokinetics*, vol. 53, no. 1, pp. s–16, 2014.

[10] A. Alfa, "First reversal agent for factor Xa inhibitors, finally gains FDA approval," May 2018, http://TCTMD.com, http://www.tctmd.com/news/andexanet-alfa-first-reversal-agent-factor-xa-inhibitors-finally-gains-fda-approval..

[11] *Andexanet Alfa for Acute Major Bleeding Associated with Factor Xa Inhibitors* | *NEJM*May 2018, https://www.nejm.org/doi/full/10.1056/NEJMoa1607887.

12

An Interesting Case and Literature Review of a Coronary Stent Fracture in a Current Generation Platinum Chromium Everolimus-Eluting Stent

Sammy San Myint Aung,[1] **Htun Latt**,[2] **Kyaw Kyaw**,[1] **and Chanwit Roongsritong**[1]

[1]*Institute for Heart and Vascular Health, Renown Regional Medical Center, 1500 E 2nd St No. 302, Reno, NV 89502, USA*
[2]*Department of Internal Medicine, School of Medicine, University of Nevada-Reno, 1155 Mill St No. W11, Reno, NV 89502, USA*

Correspondence should be addressed to Sammy San Myint Aung; aung.sammy@gmail.com

Academic Editor: Aiden Abidov

Coronary interventions are the mainstay of treatment for stenotic coronary vascular lesions. New stent designs are constantly being evaluated to improve stent performances and clinical outcomes. Coronary stent fracture is uncommon; however, it is associated with potential major consequences including acute coronary syndrome and the need for repeated target vessel revascularization due to in-stent restenosis or stent thrombosis. We report a case of a 66-year-old man with an extensive cardiac disease history, who presented with intractable angina and was found to have a fracture of a current generation, platinum chromium everolimus-eluting stent (Synergy, Boston Scientific Inc.).

1. Introduction

Coronary stent fracture is defined as a discontinuation of any part of the stent structure seen on angiogram. Stent fracture (SF) was first described with bare-metal stents in 2002 [1]. In 2004, it was subsequently reported with drug-eluting stents [2]. Newer designs, materials, and eluting drugs are being developed to improve the performance, safety, and long-term patency of drug-eluting stents (DES). Synergy stent (Boston Scientific Inc.) is one of the commonly used, current generation of platinum chromium everolimus-eluting stents (EES). To the best of our knowledge, there has been no previously reported case of a stent fracture involving this particular stent.

2. Case Presentation

The following case is of a 66-year-old man with a complicated cardiac history, who for some time has been experiencing limiting angina despite being on maximally titrated medical therapy of aspirin, prasugrel, carvedilol, ranolazine, isosorbidemononitrate (sustained release), atorvastatin, lisinopril, nitroglycerin patch, and as needed sublingual nitroglycerin. His cardiac history includes extensive coronary artery disease (CAD).

(i) Status post coronary artery bypass graft 15 years ago (CABG: reverse saphenous vein graft to first and second obtuse marginal arteries in a sequential fashion and reverse saphenous vein graft to posterior descending artery and posterolateral artery in a sequential fashion)

(ii) Status post redo CABG 2 years ago (CABG: left internal mammary artery [LIMA] to the left anterior descending artery [LAD])

(iii) Status post multiple stents

He also has a history of hypertension, diabetes (on metformin), dyslipidemia, and prior bilateral carotid endarterectomy. He was evaluated by cardiothoracic surgery 8 months prior, and they recommended against reoperation.

About 4 months prior, he underwent another coronary angiography. This angiogram showed a relatively long 95%

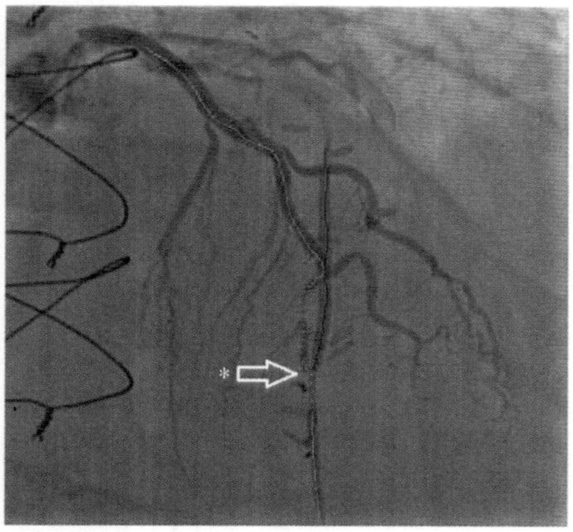

FIGURE 1: Coronary angiogram showing a long mid-LAD stenosis of 95%, extending from the mid-LAD (dotted blue line) to an area just below the anastomosis with LIMA (white asterisk), with retrograde filling into LIMA (red line).

stenosis in the mid-LAD. The stenosis extended from the mid-LAD to a bit passed the LIMA anastomosis, with retrograde flow into the LIMA (Figure 1). Some tenting of the LAD at the anastomotic site was also noted. Several predilations were performed at 8 and 10 atmospheres with no significant improvement to the stenosis. A 2.25 × 28 mm Synergy drug-eluting stent (Boston Scientific) was then deployed at 12 atmospheres and postdilated with 2.25 × 20 mm noncompliant balloon at 14 atmospheres. The stent was successfully deployed in the mid-LAD with no residual stenosis. A slight kink in the distal one-third of the stent at the LIMA insertion point was noted (Figure 2). Figure 3 further demonstrates the movement of the intact stent during diastole and systole. The patient's symptoms temporarily improved.

A short time after, he presented again with rest pain. His vital signs were stable. Physical examinations, including cardiac exams, were unimpressive. Electrocardiogram (EKG) showed normal sinus rhythm without significant ST/T changes. Two troponin levels drawn 12-hour apart were both normal. Repeat coronary angiography was performed. It revealed a mid-LAD stent fracture with 70% in-stent restenosis (fractional flow reserve of 0.78) (Figure 4). Coronary intervention was performed and a Xience Alpine DES was deployed inside the fractured Synergy DES with TIMI III flow and no residual stenosis (Figure 5). The patient tolerated the procedure and was discharged in stable condition.

3. Discussion

A coronary stent fracture is a discontinuation of any part of the stent structure seen on angiogram [3]. Depending on the study and type of stent, the incidences of SF lie between 0.5% and 19% [4–7]. In a pathological study, the incidence rose as high as 29% [8]. SF rates in sirolimus-eluting stent (SES) were mainly used in these studies. One study by Kuramitsu et al. had shown the incidence of SF in everolimus-eluting stent (EES) to be 2.9% [3]. However, with regard to SF rates, no study has included the Synergy PtCr EES, as yet. Synergy is an EES with a platinum chromium (PtCr) platform. It is a modification from the Promus Element PtCr platform and has thinner struts with a bioabsorbable polymer on the abluminal side [9]. In a randomized trial comparing safety and efficacy, Synergy was shown to be as effective, and slightly better trending, as the Promus element in their clinical endpoints [10].

Coronary SF is thought to be due to a combination of unfortunate factors. These factors are all related to abnormal forces placed on the stent, creating metal fatigue and eventual fracture. Vessel tortuosity (especially in the right coronary artery), vessel calcification, ostial stent location, hinge motion, overlapping stents, increased stent length, smaller stent diameter, coronary aneurysm, and balloon overdilation are some of the known risk factors for SF [3, 4, 6, 7, 11]. The design of the Synergy due to its thin-strut and platinum chromium platform is said to incur flexibility and strength to prevent SF [3, 9]. However, a mechanism for SF in thin-strut DES is longitudinal stent deformation (LSD) [3]. LSD can be caused by balloon overexpansion and abnormalities in the vessel wall such as calcifications [6].

Our patient had experienced intractable chest pain believed to be caused by the in-stent restenosis precipitated by the stent fracture. Clinically concerning complications of coronary stent fractures are acute coronary syndromes (ACS), in-stent restenosis (ISR), stent thrombosis (ST), and the possible need for target vessel revascularization (TVR) [3, 4, 11–13]. These manifestations are related to the disruption of the stent structure and the malapposition of the stent struts to the intimal surface of the vessel. Normally, a DES will provide sufficient amounts of antiproliferative drugs in the vicinity of smooth muscle cells on the vessel intima. However, during a SF, the struts that usually elute the drug are no longer adequately pressed against the vessel walls, thus allowing smooth muscle cells to proliferate. The fractured strut can also mechanically irritate the vessel wall and stimulate smooth muscle cell division, as well as become foci for thrombogenesis [3, 6, 7, 14, 15]. This can lead to a series of cascading events that ultimately disrupts the surrounding hemodynamic environment and lead to the abovementioned complications.

In our case, the SF occurred at the mid-LAD, in the vicinity of the LIMA anastomosis (Figure 4). We believe that the Synergy EES came under a lot of external mechanical strain due to the vessel curvature, as well as the additional tenting force generated by the anastomosis with the LIMA. With each cardiac cycle, the hinge motion (Figure 3), created by the vessel's tortuosity, lead to the eventual metal fatigue and fracture.

The reported incidences of coronary SF may actually be underestimated. Considering the higher incidence reported by Nakazawa et al.'s pathological analysis and the varying incidences of 0.5% to 19% in other studies [4, 6–8], we can infer that a large number of SF are going undetected and are possibly asymptomatic. Like our case, most studies identify SF through angiography [4, 7]. The disadvantage, however, is the lower spatial resolution of angiography compared with other imaging techniques (intravascular ultrasound and optical coherence tomography). Recent technological advancements have introduced the use of stent

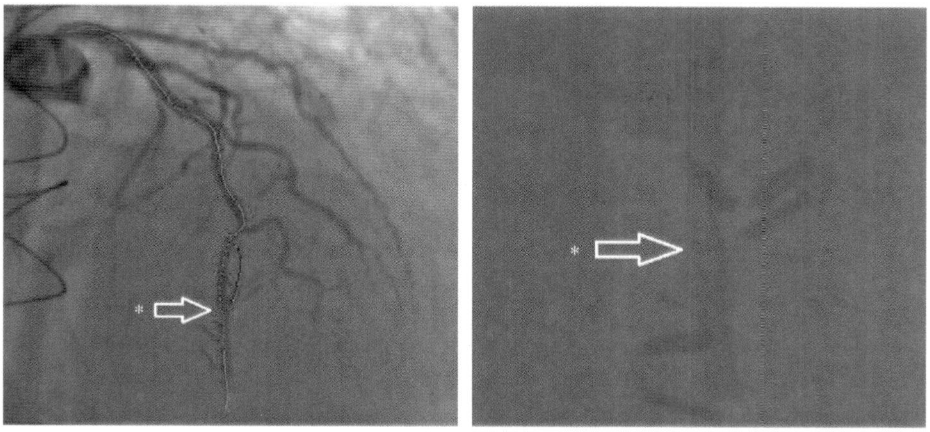

FIGURE 2: Coronary angiogram showing TIMI III flow over mid-LAD (dotted blue line) and the point of anastomosis (asterisk) after the deployment of Synergy PtCr EES. Note that there is a mild deformity of the stent, which conforms to the coronary anatomy and anastomotic site.

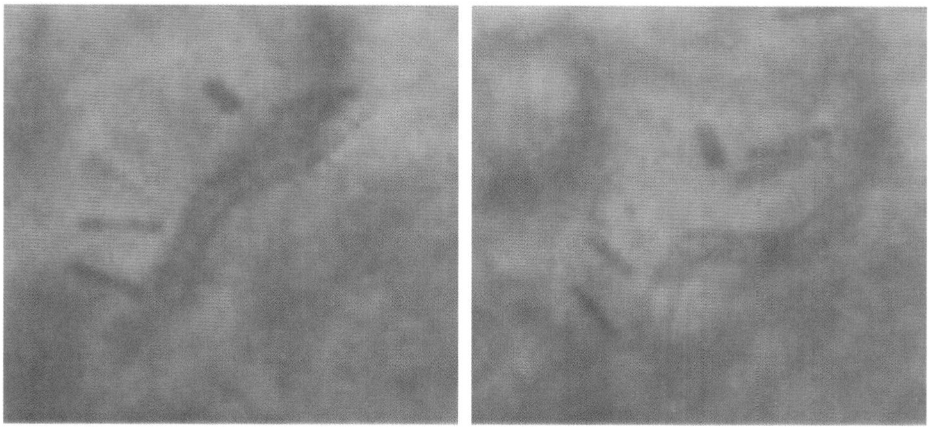

FIGURE 3: Coronary angiogram showing conformational changes of intact stent during the cardiac cycle (diastole on the left, systole on the right). It can be inferred that various forces are creating a hinge-type motion on the intact stent.

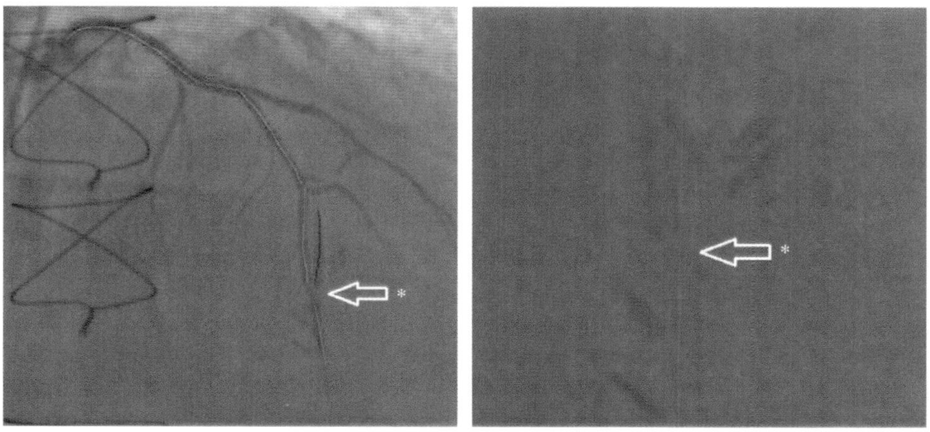

FIGURE 4: Repeat coronary angiogram showing mid-LAD stent fracture with 70% in-stent restenosis at the site of anastomosis between LAD and LIMA (asterisk).

boost with angiography, a high resolution cine-angiography, that allows easier SF identification [7]. Optical frequency domain imaging has also demonstrated a good ability to detect coronary SFs, in addition to other vessel wall details [16]. Once a SF is identified, classification of the lesion becomes important, for both communication and future

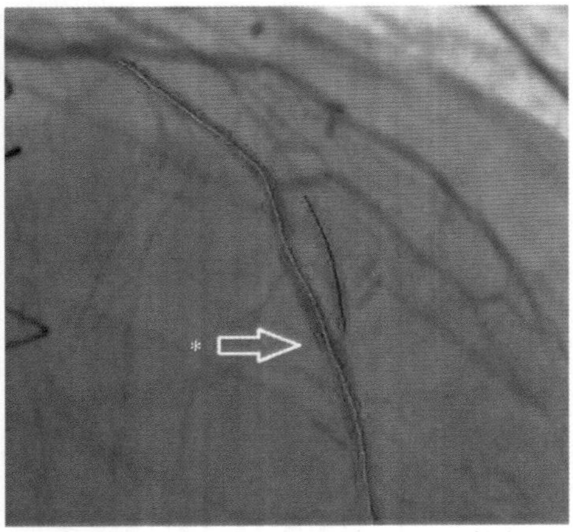

FIGURE 5: Repeat coronary angiogram showing TIMI III flow in mid-LAD at the point of anastomosis with LIMA (asterisk) after Xience Alpine DES was deployed inside the fractured Synergy DES.

management. Lee et al. had used the following classification in their study [15].

(i) Type I: single strut fracture

(ii) Type II: multiple strut fractures

(iii) Type III: complete transverse fracture with no displacement

(iv) Type IV: complete transverse fracture with displacement

Based on this, our case would be considered a type IV fracture, the most severe form. There is no formal management guideline for treating coronary SF. In a single-center study by Lee et al., they proposed to treat SF with no signs of ISR with dual or triple antiplatelet therapy for an unknown duration of time. Significant ISR with severe SF (type II to type IV) warranted coronary intervention [15]. DES use in the treatment of SF was shown to have lower rates of target vessel revascularization than plain old balloon angioplasty [17]. Our patient was managed in a way consistent with the recommendations above. We treated our patient with a repeated coronary intervention using the Xience Alpine EES. Although overlapping stents are known to be a risk factor for further SF, it was important that such a severe stent fracture and in-stent restenosis be amended in an attempt to return maximal perfusion to distal tissues.

4. Conclusion

Regardless of stent type and design, stent fractures are a complication that should always be considered. Vessel anatomy, hinge motions, overlapping stents, calcifications, and stent types are a few of the risk factors mentioned that should be incorporated in the decision process prior to performing coronary intervention. Having a simple yet accurate description of stent fractures based on image modality will help in standardizing appropriate treatment guidelines of coronary SF. Further studies on the clinical outcomes in patients who received stent-within-a-stent treatment, as our patient, would help in determining if this is the best treatment option for coronary SF.

References

[1] P. S. Chowdhury and R. G. Ramos, "Images in clinical medicine: coronary-stent fracture," *The New England Journal of Medicine*, vol. 347, no. 8, p. 581, 2002.

[2] G. Sianos, S. Hofma, J. M. R. Ligthart et al., "Stent fracture and restenosis in the drug-eluting stent era," *Catheterization and Cardiovascular Interventions*, vol. 61, no. 1, pp. 111–116, 2004.

[3] S. Kuramitsu, M. Iwabuchi, T. Haraguchi et al., "Incidence and clinical impact of stent fracture after everolimus-eluting stent implantation," *Circulation: Cardiovascular Interventions*, vol. 5, no. 5, pp. 663–671, 2012.

[4] M. Chinikar and P. Sadeghipour, "Coronary stent fracture: a recently appreciated phenomenon with clinical relevance," *Current Cardiology Reviews*, vol. 10, no. 4, pp. 349–354, 2014.

[5] H. S. Kim, Y. H. Kim, S. W. Lee et al., "Incidence and predictors of drug-eluting stent fractures in long coronary disease," *International Journal of Cardiology*, vol. 133, no. 3, pp. 354–358, 2009.

[6] D. M. Wiktor, S. W. Waldo, and E. J. Armstrong, "Coronary stent failure: fracture, compression, recoil, and prolapse," *Interventional Cardiology Clinics*, vol. 5, no. 3, pp. 405–414, 2016.

[7] A. Omar, L. K. Pendyala, J. A. Ormiston, and R. Waksman, "Review: stent fracture in the drug-eluting stent era," *Cardiovascular Revascularization Medicine*, vol. 17, no. 6, pp. 404–411, 2016.

[8] G. Nakazawa, A. V. Finn, M. Vorpahl et al., "Incidence and predictors of drug-eluting stent fracture in human coronary artery: a pathologic analysis," *Journal of the American College of Cardiology*, vol. 54, no. 21, pp. 1924–1931, 2009.

[9] J. Bennett and C. Dubois, "A novel platinum chromium everolimus-eluting stent for the treatment of coronary artery disease," *Biologics: Targets and Therapy*, vol. 7, pp. 149–159, 2013.

[10] I. T. Meredith, S. Verheye, C. Dubois et al., "Final five-year clinical outcomes in the EVOLVE trial: a randomised evaluation of a novel bioabsorbable polymer-coated, everolimus-eluting stent," *EuroIntervention*, vol. 13, no. 17, pp. 2047–2050, 2018.

[11] F. Amico, S. Geraci, and C. Tamburino, "Acute coronary syndrome due to early multiple and complete fractures in sirolimus-eluting stent: a case report and brief literature review," *Catheterization and Cardiovascular Interventions*, vol. 81, no. 1, pp. 52–56, 2013.

[12] A. A. Rafighdust and A. Eshraghi, "Acute ST-elevation myocardial infarction after coronary stent fracture," *The Journal of Tehran University Heart Center*, vol. 10, no. 4, pp. 205–207, 2015.

[13] T. Chakravarty, A. J. White, M. Buch et al., "Meta-analysis of incidence, clinical characteristics and implications of stent fracture," *The American Journal of Cardiology*, vol. 106, no. 8, pp. 1075–1080, 2010.

[14] S. Biscaglia, M. Tebaldi, C. Tumscitz et al., "Prospective identification of stent fracture by enhanced stent visualization system during percutaneous coronary intervention," *Circulation Journal*, vol. 81, no. 1, pp. 82–89, 2017.

[15] S. E. Lee, M. H. Jeong, I. S. Kim et al., "Clinical outcomes and optimal treatment for stent fracture after drug-eluting stent implantation," *Journal of Cardiology*, vol. 53, no. 3, pp. 422–428, 2009.

[16] M. Nakano, M. Vorpahl, F. Otsuka, and R. Virmani, "Optical frequency domain imaging of stent fracture and coronary dissection associated with intraplaque hemorrhage," *JACC: Cardiovascular Interventions*, vol. 4, no. 9, pp. 1047-1048, 2011.

[17] S. Mitomo, T. Naganuma, K. Takagi et al., "Comparison between plain old balloon angioplasty and drug-eluting stent implantation for the treatment of stent fracture," *Journal of Interventional Cardiology*, vol. 28, no. 4, pp. 365–373, 2015.

13

Streptococcus pyogenes Pericarditis with Resultant Pulmonary Trunk Compression Secondary to Mycotic Pseudoaneurysm

E. Fry, J. Urbanczyk, J. Price, R. Digiovanni, M. Jepson, and D. Gantt

Baylor Scott and White Medical Center, Temple, TX, USA

Correspondence should be addressed to D. Gantt; david.gantt@bswhealth.org

Academic Editor: Kuan-Rau Chiou

Purulent pericarditis is a rare disease in the era of antibiotics, with *Streptococcus pyogenes* being a possible, though uncommon etiology. Even more uncommon are mycotic aneurysms secondary to group A strep purulent pericarditis and bacteremia. We report a case of an 18-year-old female with a history of strep pharyngitis develop *Streptococcus pyogenes* purulent pericarditis with subsequent ventricular fibrillation (VF). Following initial stabilization, she ultimately developed a 4.8 cm mycotic aneurysm of the ascending aorta, with resultant compression of the pulmonary trunk and right pulmonary arteries.

1. Introduction

Purulent pericarditis is a rare but rapidly progressing and in some cases deadly event. Rapid detection via imaging and high clinical suspicion are paramount. Purulent pericarditis can, in limited cases, complicate clinical course by instigating mycotic pseudoaneurysm formation in the aorta. Proper imaging and prompt treatment with antibiotic therapy and either endovascular or open surgical repair are vital. We present a case of group A strep purulent pericarditis that resulted in formation of a mycotic pseudoaneurysm in an otherwise healthy 18-year-old female. She underwent subsequent urgent surgical repair with complete recovery. To our knowledge, this is the second reported case of purulent pericarditis complicated by mycotic pseudoaneurysm.

2. Case Description

An 18-year-old female with an allergy to penicillin and a past medical history of migraines presented to the emergency department with pleuritic chest pain and dyspnea on exertion. Three months prior she had an upper respiratory infection. Her initial workup was unrevealing, including negative troponin and normal complete blood count. Her electrocardiogram (ECG) revealed normal sinus rhythm. A computed tomography angiogram (CTA) chest had no significant findings. She was diagnosed with atypical chest pain and discharged home.

She returned three days later with worsening chest pain. ECG (Figure 1(a)) was significant for sinus tachycardia, PR depressions, and diffuse ST elevations, consistent with pericarditis. Significant findings at that time included a Troponin-I of 0.28 ng/ml and white blood cell count (WBC) of 16.2 (16,200). Shortly after admission, she was transferred to the intensive care unit (ICU) for hypotension and tachycardia in the 150's. Echocardiography demonstrated a moderate pericardial effusion with evidence of tamponade. Pericardiocentesis yielded 300 ml of serous fluid and established hemodynamic stability. She was initiated on empiric antibiotic therapy with vancomycin and meropenem. Later that same day, she underwent emergent intubation and vasopressor support after two separate episodes of ventricular fibrillation and pulseless electrical activity, requiring multiple rounds of advanced cardiac life support. After stabilization, fluid aspiration from the pericardial drain revealed 130 ml of purulent fluid. Her final pericardial fluid cultures and blood cultures grew *Streptococcus pyogenes*. Antibiotic coverage was weaned to intravenous cefazolin monotherapy. She continued to drain 240–360 milliliters of purulent pericardial fluid daily and was on norepinephrine for pressure support. Post resuscitation, she developed acute renal failure that required intermittent renal replacement

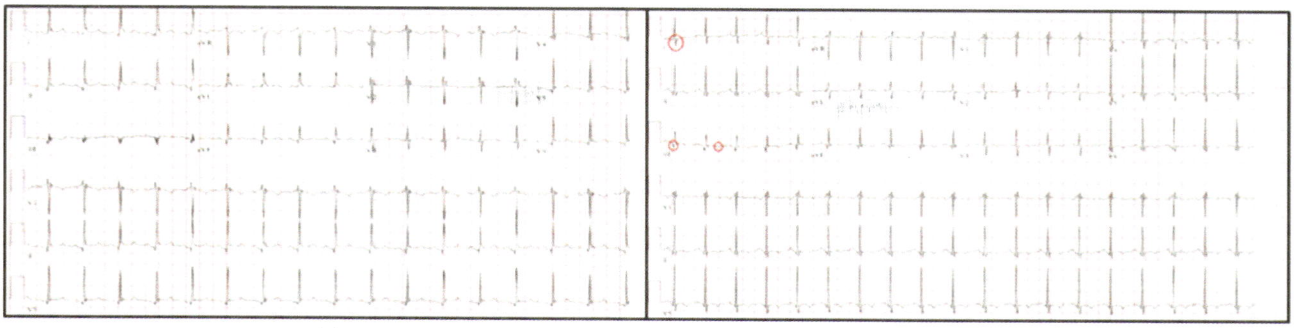

(a) (b)

FIGURE 1: Significant ECGs. (a) Diffuse ST elevation and PR depressions indicating pericarditis. (b) S1Q3T3 phenomenon.

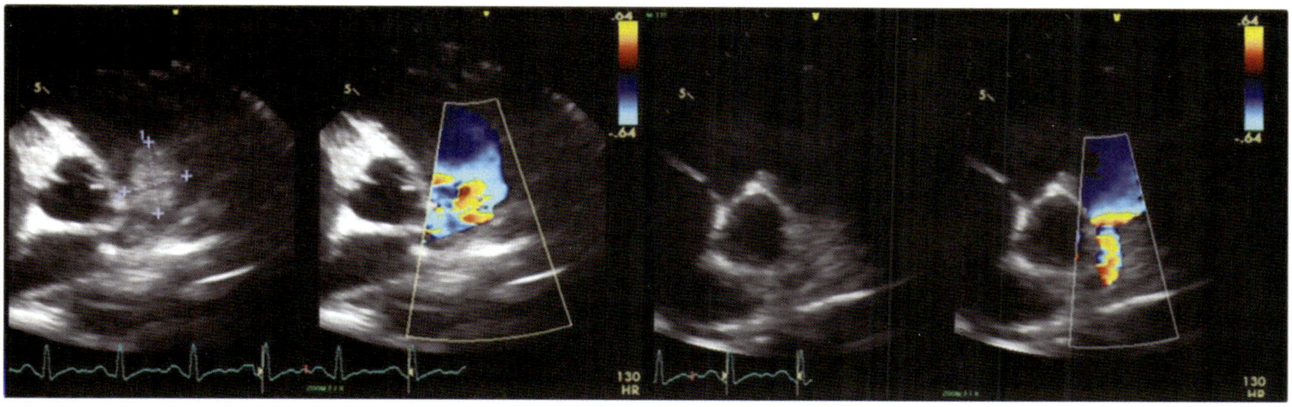

FIGURE 2: Transthoracic 2D echocardiography images. Echo images concerning for compression of the pulmonary vasculature.

therapy secondary to acute tubular necrosis. Antibiotic coverage was broadened to vancomycin and cefepime after the development of acute respiratory distress syndrome (ARDS) secondary to multifocal pneumonia. She was gradually weaned from the ventilator and subsequently extubated. The remaining hospital course was uneventful, and she was discharged home on oral levofloxacin for completion of her antibiotic course.

The patient returned to the ED several days later with shortness of breath and worsening back pain that radiated to her chest. The ECG (Figure 1(b)) at that time was significant for sinus tachycardia and an S1Q3T3 phenomenon. She was admitted for severe sepsis and started on ceftriaxone for concern of recurrent bacteremia. Repeat transthoracic echocardiography demonstrated right ventricular strain and what appeared to be a near to total occlusion of her pulmonary trunk (Figure 2). Computed tomography (CT) angiography was significant for a 4.8 cm small-necked pseudoaneurysm arising off the anterolateral aspect of the aorta and was found to be compressing the pulmonary trunk and right pulmonary artery (Figure 3).

Our patient was again transferred to the ICU. A subsequent CT chest with contrast demonstrated pseudoaneurysm expansion to 5.3 cm. Emergent cardiothoracic surgery with circulatory arrest was performed. The operation revealed a 2 cm × 1 cm wall defect in the distal ascending aorta, extending into the arch of the aorta. Intraoperative transesophageal echocardiography revealed right ventricular remodeling resulting in a severely strained D-shaped ventricle and severely dilated RVOT of 4 cm (Figure 4). Additionally, there was significant clot burden in the anterior mediastinum encasing the ascending aorta and the pulmonary artery. A CorMatrix patch was used to close the defect, and a specimen of the anterior mediastinal mass was sent for pathological analysis, confirming our diagnosis of a mycotic pseudoaneurysm. The patient tolerated the surgical procedure well and did not require additional operations during her inpatient hospital recovery.

3. Discussion

Purulent pericardial effusions are a relatively uncommon occurrence, particularly in the post antibiotic era. A retrospective study in Spain, done between 1972 and 1991, indicated an incidence of 33 in a population of 593,600 [1]. It is most often caused by gram positive cocci (40–45%) with *Staphylococcus aureus* comprising the majority of cases. Other commonly reported organisms include *Streptococcus pneumoniae*, *Haemophilus influenzae*, viridans streptococci, and anaerobic bacteria [2, 3]. There is a scarcity of reported group A streptococcal purulent pericardial effusions in current publications. Literature review yielded 11 previously

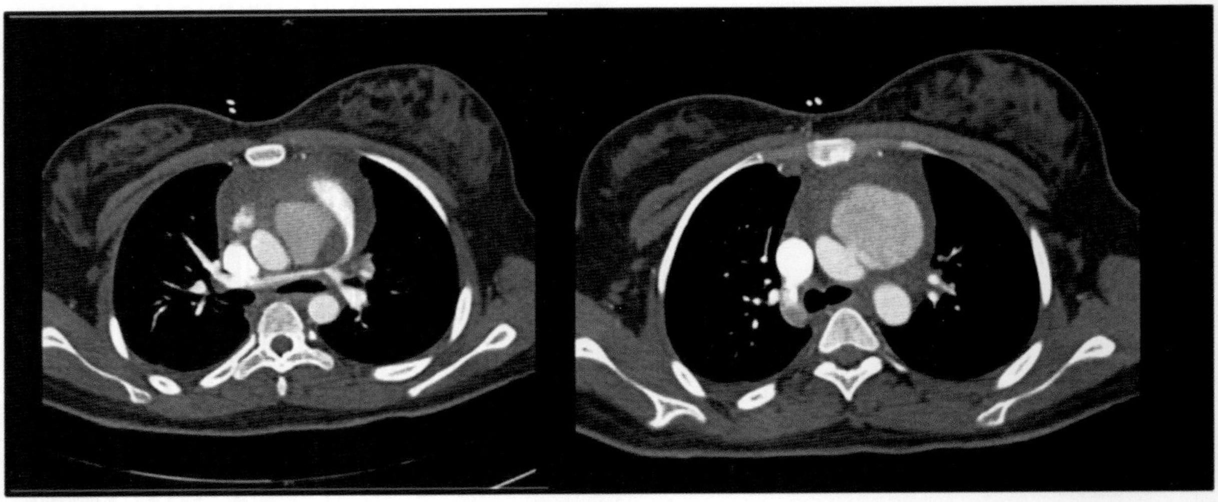

(a) (b)

Figure 3: CT scans identifying pseudoaneurysm. Pseudoaneurysm compressing on the pulmonary trunk and right main stem (a) and 4.8 cm aortic pseudoaneurysm (b).

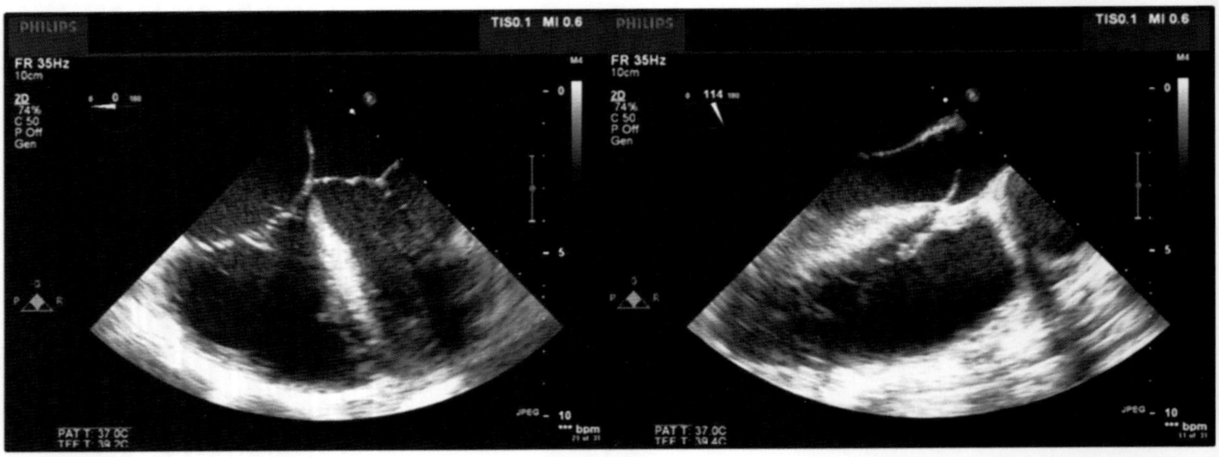

Figure 4: Intraoperative transesophageal echocardiogram. D-shaped ventricle indicating right heart strain seen in multiple frames.

reported cases of which only one formed a mycotic pseudoaneurysm [4]. Patients' age ranged from 4 months to 14 years old [4–12]. Dissemination of the bacteria to the pericardium typically occurs via 4 major mechanisms: (1) direct pulmonary extension such as streptococcal pneumonia/pharyngitis infection 20–25%; (2) hematogenous spread 22–29%; (3) perforating injury or surgery 24–29%; and (4) myocardial abscess and/or endocarditis in 14–22% [2, 3]. Certain factors can predispose towards their occurrence, such as transplant recipients, immunocompromised state, or chronic comorbidities. Common complications from purulent pericarditis can include constrictive pericardial disease due to thickening and scarring of the pericardium or pericardial empyema [13]. Despite treatment, up to 40% of patients die from tamponade, constriction, or toxicity [14]. Previously described successful treatments include a 2-to-4-week duration of intravenous antibiotic monotherapy with β-lactam agents or combination therapy with a β-lactam and aminoglycoside [7].

Mycotic pseudoaneurysms are rarely described following purulent pericardial effusions and only comprise a small minority of all aneurysms (0.7%) [15]. Hematogenous seeding of a damaged atherosclerotic wall is the most frequently described pathogenesis for infected aortic aneurysms [16], with staphylococcal and salmonella spp. being the most common [17]. Other predisposing factors include impaired immunity, arterial injury, or preexisting aneurysm [15, 18, 19]. Foroulis et al. and Sorensen et al. previously describe aortic aneurysms involving pulmonary artery compression, though neither was mycotic in origin [20, 21]. Management of pseudoaneurysm typically consists of antibiotic therapy and either endovascular or open repair. An endovascular approach is preferred in high-risk patient, patients with significant comorbidities, or as a bridge to future surgical repair [19, 22]. Inherently, endovascular repair carries an increased risk of secondary infections and graft failure. Open surgical repair has been shown to have an initial higher mortality rate compared with endovascular repair but displays improved long-term bacterial clearance and mortality benefit [19, 22].

4. Conclusion

Purulent pericarditis is a rare and serious condition with a high chance of complications and mortality. We describe a rare case of group A streptococcal purulent pericarditis with multiple complications, including mycotic pseudoaneurysm formation and resultant compression on the pulmonary vasculature. While unusual, mycotic aortic pseudoaneurysms are a reported complication following purulent pericardial infection. Appropriate and early antibiotic therapy was key in our patient's recovery as well as swift pseudoaneurysm identification and surgical intervention.

Disclosure

This case was previously presented at the American College of Cardiology 2018 in the clinical decision-making section of poster presentations.

References

[1] J. Sagristà-Sauleda, J. A. Barrabés, G. Permanyer-Miralda, and J. Soler-Soler, "Purulent pericarditis: review of a 20-year experience in a general hospital," *Journal of the American College of Cardiology*, vol. 22, no. 6, pp. 1661–1665, 1993.

[2] R. H. Rubin and R. C. Moellering Jr., "Clinical, microbiologic and therapeutic aspects of purulent pericarditis," *The American Journal of Medicine*, vol. 59, no. 1, pp. 68–78, 1975.

[3] P. G. Klacsmann, B. H. Bulkley, and G. M. Hutchins, "The changed spectrum of purulent pericarditis: an 86 year autopsy experience in 200 patients," *The American Journal of Medicine*, vol. 63, no. 5, pp. 666–673, 1977.

[4] H. Barth, R. Moosdorf, J. Bauer, D. Schranz, and H. Akintürk, "Mycotic pseudoaneurysm of the aorta in children," *Pediatric Cardiology*, vol. 21, no. 3, pp. 263–266, 2000.

[5] M. C. Schwartz, M. J. Gillespie, P. Stephens, and B. Fisher, "Cardiac tamponade due to group A streptococcal pericarditis in a 10-month-old boy and a review of the literature," *Open Journal of Pediatrics*, vol. 1, no. 4, pp. 87–89, 2011.

[6] F. Angoulvant, H. Bellanger, S. Magnier, P. Bidet, C. Saizou, and S. Dauger, "Acute purulent pericarditis in childhood: don't forget β-haemolytic group-A *Streptococcus*," *Intensive Care Medicine*, vol. 37, no. 10, pp. 1709-1710, 2011.

[7] S. Bhaduri-McIntosh, M. Prasad, J. Moltedo, and M. Vázquez, "Purulent pericarditis caused by group A streptococcus," *Texas Heart Institute Journal*, vol. 33, no. 4, pp. 519–522, 2006.

[8] W. M. Gersony and G. H. McCracken Jr., "Purulent pericarditis in infancy," *Pediatrics*, vol. 40, no. 2, pp. 224–232, 1967.

[9] J. L. Pruitt, "Group A streptococcal pericarditis in a previously well child," *The Pediatric Infectious Disease Journal*, vol. 8, no. 5, p. 338, 1989.

[10] B. Thébaud, D. Sidi, and J. Kachaner, "Purulent pericarditis in children: a 15 year-experience," *Archives de Pédiatrie*, vol. 3, no. 11, pp. 1084–1090, 1996.

[11] W. T. Vigneswaran, R. Hardie, J. C. Ferguson, and A. Faichney, "Cardiac tamponade due to Lancefield group A beta haemolytic streptococcal pericarditis," *Thorax*, vol. 40, no. 7, pp. 549-550, 1985.

[12] B. Al-Waili, S. Zacharias, and E. Aslem, "Group A streptococcal pericarditis in a four-month-old infant: case report," *Sultan Qaboos University Medical Journal*, vol. 17, no. 2, pp. e241–e243, 2017.

[13] I. P. Hall, "Purulent pericarditis," *Postgraduate Medical Journal*, vol. 65, no. 765, pp. 444–448, 1989.

[14] B. Maisch and A. D. Ristic, "Practical aspects of the management of pericardial disease," *Heart*, vol. 89, no. 9, pp. 1096–1103, 2003.

[15] G. S. Oderich, J. M. Panneton, T. C. Bower et al., "Infected aortic aneurysms: aggressive presentation, complicated early outcome, but durable results," *Journal of Vascular Surgery*, vol. 34, no. 5, pp. 900–908, 2001.

[16] K. Chandrikakumari, J. B. Giot, L. de Leval et al., "Report of a case of *Streptococcus agalactiae* mycotic aneurysm and review of the literature," *International Journal of Surgical Pathology*, vol. 16, no. 3, pp. 314–319, 2008.

[17] R. Marques da Silva, D. A. Caugant, E. R. K. Eribe et al., "Bacterial diversity in aortic aneurysms determined by 16S ribosomal RNA gene analysis," *Journal of Vascular Surgery*, vol. 44, no. 5, pp. 1055–1060, 2006.

[18] M. H. Samore, M. A. Wessolossky, S. M. Lewis, S. J. Shubrooks Jr., and A. W. Karchmer, "Frequency, risk factors, and outcome for bacteremia after percutaneous transluminal coronary angioplasty," *The American Journal of Cardiology*, vol. 79, no. 7, pp. 873–877, 1997.

[19] B. J. Gardiner, J. Wong, M. Yii, T. Buckenham, and T. M. Korman, "*Streptococcus pyogenes* aortic aneurysm infection: forgotten but not gone," *Infectious Disease Reports*, vol. 5, no. 2, article e11, 2013.

[20] C. N. Foroulis, N. A. Desimonas, and N. B. Tsilimingas, "Large ascending aorta aneurysm compressing and thrombosing the right pulmonary artery," *European Journal of Cardio-Thoracic Surgery*, vol. 29, no. 5, p. 841, 2006.

[21] B. Sorensen, C. Moyal, O. Marlois, B. Vaisse, J. R. Montiès, and L. Poggi, "Compression of the right pulmonary artery by a dissecting aneurysm of the ascending aorta. Apropos of a case occurring long after aortic valve replacement," *Archives des Maladies du Coeur et des Vaisseaux*, vol. 79, no. 7, pp. 1111–1115, 1986.

[22] C. Setacci, G. de Donato, and F. Setacci, "Endografts for the treatment of aortic infection," *Seminars in Vascular Surgery*, vol. 24, no. 4, pp. 242–249, 2011.

14

Left Ventricle Outflow Obstruction by Reverse-Oriented Tricuspid Semilunar Valve-Like Endocardial Duplicatures

Kristína Mikuš-Kuracinová, Pavel Babál, and Eliška Kubíková

Department of Pathology and Institute of Anatomy, Comenius University Faculty of Medicine Bratislava, Sasinkova 4, 81372 Bratislava, Slovakia

Correspondence should be addressed to Pavel Babál; pavel.babal@fmed.uniba.sk

Academic Editor: Ramazan Akdemir

A 57-year-old female had a history of hypertension disease, and one year before her death, her ECG showed signs of left ventricle hypertrophy. She died with signs of heart failure with pulmonary edema development. At autopsy, there was left ventricle hypertrophy (wall thickness: 21 mm). In the left ventricle outflow channel, 15 mm below the aortic valve on the muscular wall, there were three white 1–1.5 mm thick membranous semilunar valve-like structures with the sizes of 9, 7, and 5 mm, with concavities opened into the left ventricle, reducing the outflow area by 21.5%. These structures were hanging on the regular muscular ventricular wall, without any visible fibrous anchoring structure and without formation of commissures, and were composed of fine collagen and elastic fibers. Gross anatomy as well as histological structure was different from the subaortic membrane. The reported accessory reverse-oriented tricuspid semilunar valve-like structure is an unusual finding of a structure in the left ventricular outflow tract, to which we could not find an analogy in the available literature.

1. Introduction

The heart is a three-dimensional organ with complicated configuration including the four heart valves pushing the blood to flow in a unidirectional way [1]. Defects of the heart valves represent the most frequent congenital pathological condition in the heart [2–5].

Subvalvar aortic stenosis corresponds to about 1% of congenital heart diseases. A rare cause of this congenital condition is the obstruction by an accessory mitral valve tissue, approximately half of these corresponding to an accessory mitral leaflet [6, 7]. Discrete subvalvar aortic stenosis represents a unique cardiac lesion. As compared to most other congenital heart defects, the last mentioned is virtually never recognized in early infancy but appears to be an "acquired" lesion, although with anatomic precursors [8]. The stenosis is caused by a fibrous ridge in the left ventricular outflow tract just proximal to the aortic valve [9]. Here, we report an unusual bizarre finding of an accessory reverse-oriented tricuspid semilunar valve-like structure in the left ventricular outflow, found postmortem.

2. Case

A 57-year-old woman was admitted to hospital for ileus status and metabolic disturbance. She had a history of paranoid schizophrenia, thyroid gland hypofunction, and hypertensive disease. No records of positive heart auscultation finding were found. Her ECG 1 year before death showed signs of left ventricular hypertrophy; echocardiography was not performed. The patient died with symptoms of heart failure and was indicated for autopsy. At autopsy, the main findings were distended intestines with numerous *skybala* in the colon and pulmonary edema.

3. The Heart Gross Finding

The heart was $10 \times 12 \times 7$ cm; the ventricles were in diastolic position, left ventricle wall 21 mm, right ventricle 4 mm thick,

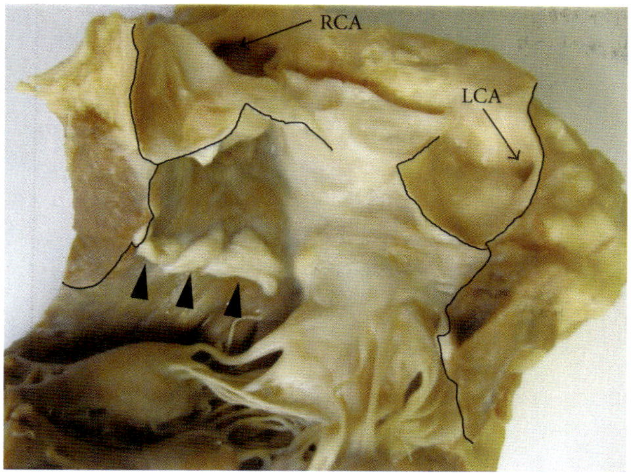

FIGURE 1: Left ventricle outflow channel opened with the cut delineated by the black line. On the ventricular septum wall, there are three membranous semilunar valve-like structures with concavities opened into the ventricle (arrowheads). Coronary arteries' ostia—left: LCA; right: RCA.

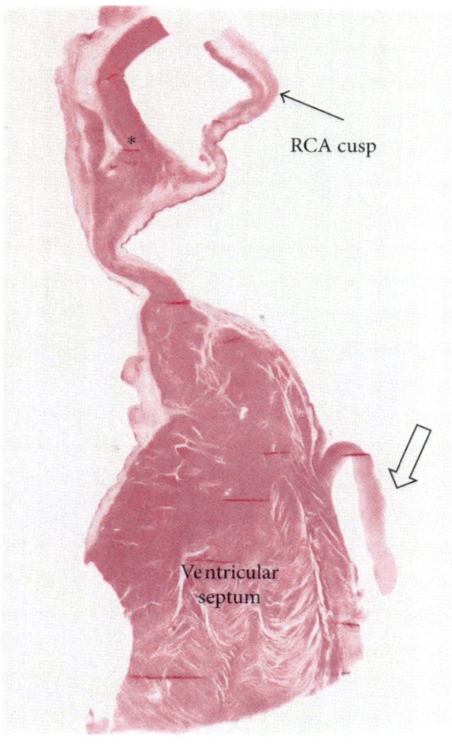

FIGURE 2: Section through the muscular wall of the left ventricular outflow and the aortic root. Membranous valve-like structure (large arrow) on the ventricular septum, aortic wall (asterisk), and the right coronary artery cusp (RCA cusp) of the aortic valve.

myocardium on cross-section was brown, with a white hard elastic focal lesion of 10 mm in diameter in the middle of the anterior wall of the left ventricle; circumference of the tricuspid valve was 13 cm, mitral valve 10 cm, pulmonary valve 8 cm, aortic valve 7 cm; the valves were anatomically correct, leaflets were elastic, without thickening. The coronary arteries were without significant narrowing, with fibrous plaques covering 10% of the intima.

In the left ventricle outflow channel, 15 mm below the aortic valve on the muscular wall, there were three white 1–1.5 mm thick membranous semilunar valve-like structures with the sizes of 9, 7, and 5 mm, with concavities opened into the left ventricle. These structures were hanging on regular muscular ventricular wall, without any visible fibrous anchoring structure, and without formation of commissures (Figure 1). The internal area of the left ventricle outflow was reduced 21.5% by the valve-like structures.

3.1. The Heart Histology. In the myocardium, there was diffuse interstitial fibrosis and myocytes were enlarged, with large hyperchromic nuclei. The endocardium was without any significant thickening. Direct projection of the histological slide shows the valve-like structure hanging on the ventricular wall with normal myocardium appearance, without fibrous anchoring structure unlike the normal aortic valve (Figure 2).

The valve-like structures were composed of fibrillary material with staining properties of collagen with scattered very fine elastic fibers, only lightly more condensed on both surfaces. There was no evident continuation or anchorage of fiber fascicles of the leaflets into the left ventricle wall. The only finding was thickening of the adjacent endocardium with a coarse compact layer of elastic fibers (Figure 3). This was different from the normal aortic valve leaflet, which was underlayed on the ventricular aspect by a continuous thick layer of elastic fibers that had a tendency to separate into thinner subunits towards the edge of the leaflet (Figure 3(f)). The normal aortic valve leaflet was outgoing from structures of the annulus fibrosus formed by dense meshwork of fine collagen fibers (Figure 2).

4. Discussion

Most frequent pathologies affecting the left ventricular outflow are inborn defects of the aortic valve. Embryologically, the semilunar valves are derived from mesenchymal swelling in the aortic and pulmonary trunk after they have been separated. Abnormal cusp formation results either from aberrant fusion of the aorticopulmonary septum or from abnormal mesenchymal proliferation in the common trunk, clinically leading to a severe regurgitation [4, 10]. The abovementioned inborn defects of aortic valve development encompass the tissues of the valve.

The substantial difference of the valve-like structures found in our case differed from normal aortic valve cusps in their histological structure. No collagen accumulation in the left ventricular outflow wall was observed that could be considered an analogy of the annulus fibrosus [1]. In the area of attachment of the valve cusp-like structure to the ventricular wall, there was a markedly thickened layer of elastic fibers but without their continuation into the cusp body, which was different from the normal aortic valve with characteristic thick layer of elastic fibers at the ventricular side

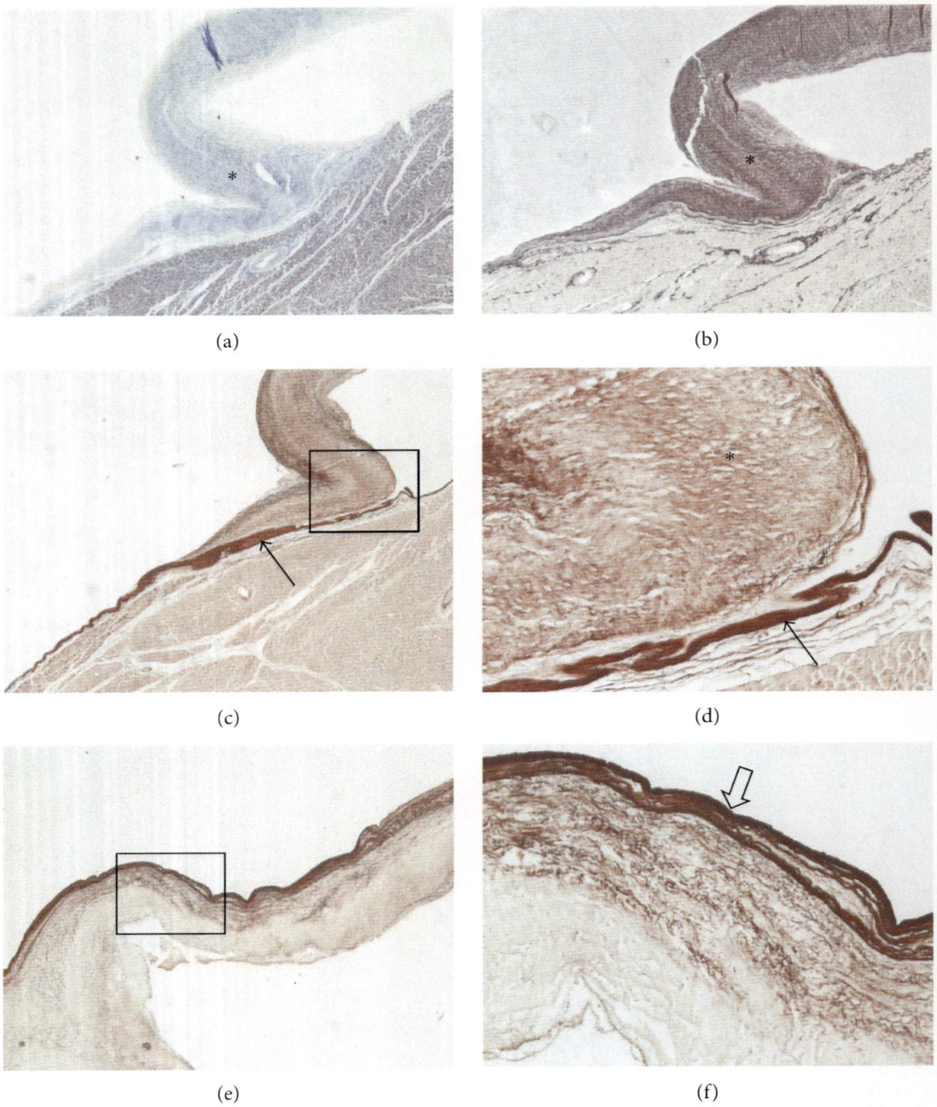

FIGURE 3: The valve-like structure was composed of fibrillary material with staining properties of fine fibrillary collagen (asterisk) stained with trichrome (a) and methenamine silver impregnation (b), with scattered very fine elastic fibers stained with orcein (c, d); the anchorage of the valve-like structure was on a thickening of the adjacent endocardium with a coarse compact layer of elastic fibers (arrow, c, d). Normal aortic valve leaflet is underlayed on the ventricular aspect by a continuous thick layer of elastic fibers (e, f, large arrow) separating into thinner subunits (orcein). 25x (a, b, c, e). 100x (d, f).

of the valve cusps wall that extend from the thick elastic layer in the endocardium above the annulus fibrosus [11].

The abnormal accessory reverse-oriented tricuspid semilunar valve-like structure described in our case could remotely suggest subaortic membrane. This condition causes circumferential subaortic stenosis that ranges from a discrete subaortic membrane to a tunnel-type narrowing of the entire left ventricular outflow tract to stenosis associated with multilevel obstruction in Shone's complex [12]. Subaortic membrane is usually diagnosed early in childhood with clinical manifestation of aortic stenosis, although this lesion may be diagnosed also late in adulthood [13]. The histological structure of subaortic membranes is characterized by stack-like layers of fibroelastic tissue with underlying bundles of smooth muscle cells towards the subendocardial region [14], which is different from the observed histological composition of the above-described valve-like structures.

Accessory mitral valve leaflet is another lesion in the left ventricular outflow tract to be considered. This lesion leads to subvalvular aortic stenosis and usually also to severe aortic incompetence. In our case, semilunar valve-like structures were positioned on the muscular part of the outflow channel, which differed from the accessory mitral valve leaflet that outgoes from the membranous structure—the anterior mitral valve leaflet, and is connected to the anterolateral papillary muscle via a strand of chordal tissue [15]. Other pathologies that could produce left ventricular outflow obstruction account tumors, that is, myxoma [16] or a dynamic left ventricular outflow obstruction induced by other preexisting pathological conditions [17, 18].

In conclusion, the above-reported accessory reverse-oriented tricuspid semilunar valve-like structure is an unusual finding of an obstruction in the left ventricular outflow tract, to which we could not find an analogy in the available literature. The patient's history does not elucidate the pathogenesis of the lesion, whether it was a congenital or an acquired-during-life structure. Since no inflammatory cells, nor structures that could be considered remains of a reparatory process in the area were recorded, the second option is not likely.

Acknowledgments

This article was created with the support of the OP Research and Development for the project: Completion of the Multidisciplinary Center for Biomedical Research—BIOMEDIRES, ITMS 26210120041, cofinanced by the European Regional Development Fund.

References

[1] M. Misfeld and H. H. Sievers, "Heart valve macro- and microstructure," *Philosophical Transactions of the Royal Society B: Biological Sciences*, vol. 362, no. 1484, pp. 1421–1436, 2007.

[2] I. Mordi and N. Tzemos, "Bicuspid aortic valve disease: a comprehensive review," *Cardiology Research and Practice*, vol. 2012, Article ID 196037, 7 pages, 2012.

[3] S. C. Siu and C. K. Silversides, "Bicuspid aortic valve disease," *Journal of the American College of Cardiology*, vol. 55, no. 25, pp. 2789–2800, 2010.

[4] A. D'Aloia, E. Vizzardi, S. Bugatti et al., "A quadricuspid aortic valve associated with severe aortic regurgitation and left ventricular systolic dysfunction," *European Heart Journal - Cardiovascular Imaging*, vol. 10, no. 5, pp. 724-725, 2009.

[5] E. O. Abreu Silva, A. G. Iglesias, and A. Silva Ede, "Quadricuspid aortic valve by transthoracic echocardiography," *Arquivos Brasileiros de Cardiologia*, vol. 91, no. 2, pp. e22–e24, 2008.

[6] A. Gaspar, J. Almeida, B. Marinho, V. Monteiro, A. Abreu, and P. Pinho, "Images in cardiovascular medicine. Accessory mitral valve with cordal attachments to mitral and aortic valves: an unusual cause of left ventricular outflow tract obstruction and both mitral and aortic insufficiencies," *Circulation*, vol. 124, no. 17, pp. e434–e436, 2011.

[7] M. A. Pavione, J. T. Mendonça, I. S. Souza, and M. A. Russo, "Accessory mitral leaflet: an uncommon form of subaortic stenosis," *Revista Brasileira de Cirurgia Cardiovascular*, vol. 27, no. 3, pp. 477–480, 2012.

[8] J. Y. Choi and I. D. Sullivan, "Fixed subaortic stenosis: anatomical spectrum and nature of progression," *British Heart Journal*, vol. 65, no. 5, pp. 280–286, 1991.

[9] W. M. Gersony, "Natural history of discrete subvalvar aortic stenosis: management implications," *Journal of the American College of Cardiology*, vol. 38, no. 3, pp. 843–845, 2001.

[10] L. E. Hurwitz and W. C. Roberts, "Quadricuspid semilunar valve," *The American Journal of Cardiology*, vol. 31, no. 5, pp. 623–626, 1973.

[11] M. G. Bateman, A. J. Hill, J. L. Quill, and P. A. Iaizzo, "The clinical anatomy and pathology of the human arterial valves: implications for repair or replacement," *Journal of Cardiovascular Translational Research*, vol. 6, no. 2, pp. 166–175, 2013.

[12] R. G. Ohye, E. J. Devaney, and E. L. Bove, "Resection of discrete subaortic membranes," *Operative Techniques in Thoracic and Cardiovascular Surgery*, vol. 7, no. 4, pp. 172–175, 2002.

[13] J. A. Carr, L. Sugeng, L. Weinert, V. Jeevanandam, and R. M. Lang, "Images in cardiovascular medicine. Subaortic membrane in the adult," *Circulation*, vol. 112, no. 23, article e347, 2005.

[14] J. Butany, P. Vaideeswar, and T. E. David, "Discrete subaortic membranes in adults—a clinicopathological analysis," *Cardiovascular Pathology*, vol. 18, no. 4, pp. 236–242, 2009.

[15] S. S. Tamin, J. Dillon, K. Aizan, S. Kadiman, and H. A. Latiff, "An accessory mitral valve leaflet causing left ventricular outflow tract obstruction and associated with severe aortic incompetence," *Echocardiography*, vol. 29, no. 2, pp. E34–E38, 2012.

[16] S. H. Baek, H. Y. Kim, H. J. Kim et al., "Left ventricular outflow tract obstruction due to a left ventricular myxoma that was misidentified as an accessory mitral valve tissue," *Journal of Thoracic Disease*, vol. 9, no. 3, pp. E258–E263, 2017.

[17] S. Kim, S. J. Kim, J. Kim, P. Yoon, J. Park, and J. Moon, "Dynamic obstruction induced by systolic anterior motion of the mitral valve in a volume-depleted left ventricle: an unexpected cause of acute heart failure in a patient with chronic obstructive pulmonary disease," *Journal of Thoracic Disease*, vol. 7, no. 9, pp. E365–E369, 2015.

[18] J. S. Evans, S. J. Huang, A. S. McLean, and M. Nalos, "Left ventricular outflow tract obstruction-be prepared!," *Anaesthesia & Intensive Care*, vol. 45, no. 1, pp. 12–20, 2017.

Decitabine Induced Delayed Cardiomyopathy in Hematologic Malignancy

Pradyumna Agasthi,[1] Hemalatha Narayanasamy,[1] Dan Sorajja,[1] James Slack,[2,3] and Farouk Mookadam[1,2]

[1]*Department of Cardiovascular Diseases, Mayo Clinic, Arizona 85259, USA*
[2]*Department of Cardio-Oncology, Mayo Clinic, Arizona 85259, USA*
[3]*Department of Internal Medicine, Mayo Clinic, Arizona 85259, USA*

Correspondence should be addressed to Pradyumna Agasthi; pradyumna_agasthi@hotmail.com

Academic Editor: Hiroaki Kitaoka

Decitabine is a pyrimidine analogue of nucleoside cytidine, used for the treatment of myelodysplastic syndromes, chronic myelogenous leukemia, and acute myelogenous leukemia. We present a case of cardiomyopathy associated with decitabine used for secondary acute myelogenous leukemia. The patient presented with new heart failure symptoms and an ejection fraction decline.

1. Introduction

Decitabine is a pyrimidine analogue of the nucleoside cytidine [1]. It inhibits DNA methylation and plays a role in reversing epigenetic silencing in malignant cells. Decitabine is currently indicated in the treatment of myelodysplastic syndromes (MDS) [2–4]. To our knowledge, one case of myocarditis [5] and one case of reversible nonischemic cardiomyopathy [6] from decitabine have been reported, this being the 3rd case.

2. Case Report

A 71-year-old female with a history significant for hypertension, hepatitis B, and hypothyroidism, underwent bone marrow biopsy which showed a hypercellular bone marrow with >90% cellularity and 81% myeloblasts expressing CD 34 and CD 117 markers, confirming a diagnosis of acute myeloid leukemia (AML). Molecular testing showed no evidence for FMS-like tyrosine kinase 3 internal tandem duplication, absence of nucleophosmin1 and KIT exon 8, and 17 mutations, suggesting a lower risk of relapse after chemotherapy. Based on cytogenetic studies, secondary AML was diagnosed. Given her advanced age, decitabine therapy was commenced. A baseline 2-D transthoracic echocardiogram (TTE) showed normal function with an ejection fraction (EF) of 55–60%. After completing 10 cycles of decitabine, she was noted to have a tachycardia and dyspnea by self-report. She was therefore referred to cardiology with these symptoms in preparation for allogeneic stem cell transplant.

The heart rate was 110/min, and a 2/6 ejection systolic murmur and a loud P2 with an S3 and S4 gallop were heard. Lungs were clear. No jugular venous distension or pedal edema was noted.

Laboratory data is significant for a serum creatinine level of 0.8 mg/dl, estimated glomerular filtration rate of 80 ml/min per 1.73 m^2, and N-terminal pro-b-type natriuretic peptide level of 517 pg/ml. Her complete blood count showed a white blood cell count of 12.6×10^9/l with greater than 50% blasts, low hemoglobin at 7.8 g/dl, hematocrit value of 25%, large platelet count of 212×10^9/l, and lactate dehydrogenase level of 588 U/l. Serum troponin or creatinine phosphokinase levels were not performed due to a lack of discernibility in patients undergoing chemotherapy for cancer. Echocardiogram showed severe left ventricular systolic dysfunction (EF 28%), mildly abnormal end systolic

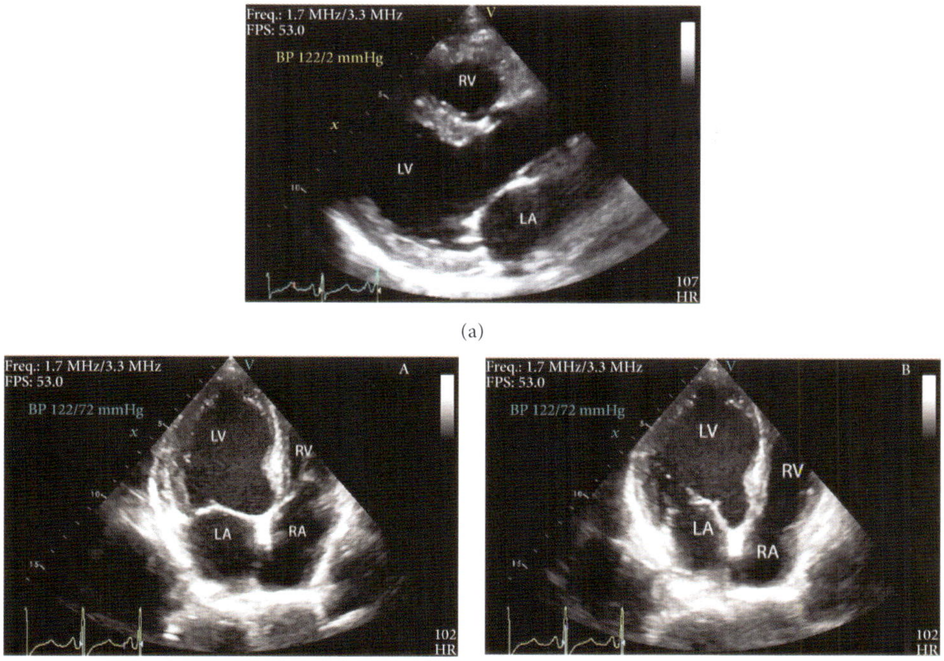

(a)

(b) (c)

FIGURE 1: Transthoracic echocardiogram of the patient in parasternal long axis view (a) demonstrating an enlarged left ventricular cavity, in apical (four-chamber) view demonstrating a mildly abnormal end systolic (b) and normal end diastolic (c) left ventricular dimension (RV: right ventricle; LV: left ventricle; LA: left atrium; RA: right atrium).

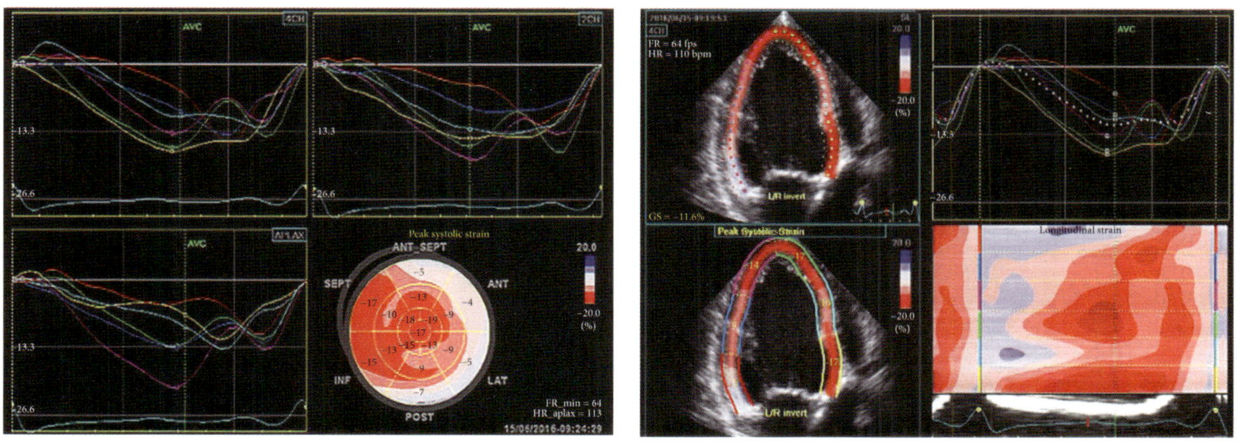

(a) (b)

FIGURE 2: Peak systolic strain pattern in cross-sectional view (a) and longitudinal view (b) demonstrates decrease in left ventricular strain pattern.

dimension (Figure 1), and a mild reduction in right ventricular systolic function. Global averaged left ventricular longitudinal peak systolic strain was abnormal at −12% (normal more negative than −18%) (Figure 2). Nuclear stress test showed no evidence of coronary disease. Patient was euthyroid at the time of diagnosis.

The patient was diagnosed with New York Heart Association class II and American Heart Association stage B heart failure with reduced ejection fraction. In the absence of any viral illness, toxins, or coronary disease, or concomitant cardiotoxic medication use and known recent normal ejection fraction, the etiology was attributed to decitabine use. The patient was subsequently started on metoprolol succinate 50 mg twice a day and furosemide 20 mg daily. Follow-up echocardiogram 4 weeks later showed no change in the ejection fraction of 28%, but there was mild improvement in the global left ventricular longitudinal peak systolic strain at −15% (improved from −12%).

Table 1: Baseline characteristics of patients.

	Age/sex	Comorbid conditions	Decitabine	EF 1[a]	Biomarker	Test[b]	EF 2[c]	EF Δ[d]
De et al. [6] (2012)	75 yrs/M	DM type II, DVT	2 cycles	35%	BNP: 259	Coronary angiogram	50% (after 7 days)	Yes
Our patient	71 yrs/F	HTN, Hep B, hypothyroidism	10 cycles	28%	Pro-BNP: 517	Nuclear stress test	28% (after 4 weeks) but with improvement in strain	No

[a]Baseline left ventricular ejection fraction. [b]Test to rule out coronary artery disease. [c]Repeat left ventricular ejection fraction. [d]Reversibility of ejection fraction. Note: both patients received decitabine as part of treatment for acute myeloid leukemia. Abbreviations: BNP: brain natriuretic peptide; DM: diabetes mellitus; DVT: deep vein thrombosis; EF: ejection fraction; HTN: hypertension; Hep B: hepatitis B; BNP units: pg/ml.

3. Discussion

3.1. Decitabine. Decitabine is an azanucleoside (AZN), a pyrimidine analogue of cytidine. Cancer cells often exhibit severely altered chromatin structure and methylation patterns leading to promoter hypermethylation and silencing of key tumor suppressor genes. The inactivation of tumor suppressor genes and other critical genes leads to unopposed proliferation of cancer cells [7–9].

Low dose AZNs have shown optimal inhibition of DNA methylation leading to subsequent cellular differentiation [10]. Decitabine inhibits the action of DNA methyltransferase and restores the normal growth and differentiation of cells [11]. Decitabine was approved in 2006 for high-risk myelodysplastic syndromes of all French-American-British subtypes, chronic myelogenous leukemia, acute myelogenous leukemia, and sickle cell anemia [3, 6, 12]. The common cardiovascular adverse effects ascribed to decitabine include peripheral edema (25%), cardiac murmurs (16%), chest discomfort (7%), and hypotension (6%) [4, 6].

Reports of decitabine-related cardiotoxicity in the literature are scant with a case of myocarditis in a 50-year-old female treated with azacitidine and decitabine for MDS [5]. A reversible nonischemic cardiomyopathy from decitabine in a 75-year-old patient treated with decitabine for AML, presented with heart failure and an EF of 35%. Left heart catheterization showed no obstructive coronary artery disease. With guideline-based heart failure therapy, EF normalised [6].

We present a 71-year-old female treated with AML for 10 cycles presenting with symptoms of EF decline. Table 1 [6] shows the comparison of the previously reported reversible cardiomyopathy.

Approval for the use of decitabine in the treatment of myelodysplastic syndromes are based on two clinical trials [3, 13]. The number of patients in the clinical trials were 170 and 66, respectively. Mean ages of the patients were 68 yrs and 70 yrs. None of the patients participating in the clinical trials developed cardiomyopathy or heart failure. However, no routine echocardiograms or biomarkers were used during the study. The literature suggests that the mechanism for cardiomyopathy is likely myocarditis based on patent coronaries on coronary angiogram and biomarker elevation [6]. The current package insert mentions cardiomyopathy as a potential side effect without the suggestion that it may be attributable to myocarditis [14]. A recent retrospective study of 111 patients with AML treated with decitabine showed a higher incidence of cardiotoxic side effects in patients with renal dysfunction. New onset heart failure was noted only in patients with renal dysfunction [15]. Our patient developed cardiac dysfunction despite normal kidney function. Contrary to prior reports, our patient had a delayed onset of cardiac dysfunction, which is unique. Clearly, the etiology for cardiac dysfunction with decitabine therapy may be bimodal (early onset versus delayed) and may be due either to hypersensitivity to hypomethylating agents causing myocarditis or to cardiac cell injury. This has yet to be elucidated. We hypothesize that the reason for the lack of cardiac function recovery in our patient might be directly related to the extent or duration of cardiomyocyte injury endured over the prolonged course of decitabine therapy.

The prevalence of chemotherapy-induced cardiomyopathy is increasing because of longer cancer survivorship and multiple new chemotherapeutic regimens where cardiac side effects are understudied. Early detection and prompt treatment is the best strategy. Many of the chemotherapeutic agents have not been studied a priori for cardiotoxicity and are symptom driven. Cardiac dysfunction symptoms may mimic the side effects attributable to the chemotherapy and no standard screening guidelines exist, especially for newer drugs.

Lessons learned from the monoclonal antibody, trastuzumab, which was shown to have a much higher incidence of cardiotoxicity post marketing, need to be applied to newer agents. Well-designed clinical trials involving chemotherapeutic agents or registries for chemotherapeutic agents should be studied for the potential for cardiotoxicity.

4. Conclusion

We present a third case of cardiomyopathy with decitabine used for secondary AML. Since older populations are more prone to chemotherapy-associated cardiomyopathy, screening these vulnerable groups may be helpful for early diagnosis and early treatment.

References

[1] F. Sorm, A. Piskala, A. Cihak, and J. Vesely, "5-Azacytidine, a new, highly effective cancerostatic," *Experientia*, vol. 20, no. 4, pp. 202-203, 1964.

[2] P. Fenaux, G. J. Mufti, E. Hellstrom-Lindberg et al., "Efficacy of azacitidine compared with that of conventional care regimens in the treatment of higher-risk myelodysplastic syndromes: a randomised, open-label, phase III study," *The Lancet Oncology*, vol. 10, no. 3, pp. 223–232, 2009.

[3] H. Kantarjian, J. P. J. Issa, C. S. Rosenfeld et al., "Decitabine improves patient outcomes in myelodysplastic syndromes: results of a phase III randomized study," *Cancer*, vol. 106, no. 8, pp. 1794–1803, 2006.

[4] M. Nieto, P. Demolis, E. Béhanzin et al., "The European Medicines Agency review of decitabine (Dacogen) for the treatment of adult patients with acute myeloid leukemia: summary of the scientific assessment of the Committee for Medicinal Products for Human Use," *The Oncologist*, vol. 21, no. 6, pp. 692–700, 2016.

[5] J. E. Bibault, N. Cambier, J. M. Lemahieu, B. Quesnel, M. Auffret, and C. Rose, "Acute myocarditis induced by hypomethylating agents," *Journal of Clinical Oncology: Official Journal of the American Society of Clinical Oncology*, vol. 29, no. 14, pp. e411–e412, 2011.

[6] C. De, J. Phookan, V. Parikh et al., "Decitabine induced transient cardiomyopathy: a case report," *Clinical Medicine Insights: Oncology*, vol. 6, 2012.

[7] D. D. von Hoff, M. Slavik, and F. M. Muggia, "5-Azacytidine: a new anticancer drug with effectiveness in acute myelogenous leukemia," *Annals of Internal Medicine*, vol. 85, no. 2, pp. 237–245, 1976.

[8] P. A. Jones and D. Takai, "The role of DNA methylation in mammalian epigenetics," *Science*, vol. 293, no. 5532, pp. 1068–1070, 2001.

[9] P. A. Jones and S. M. Taylor, "Cellular differentiation, cytidine analogs and DNA methylation," *Cell*, vol. 20, no. 1, pp. 85–93, 1980.

[10] P. A. Jones and S. M. Taylor, "Hemimethylated duplex DNAs prepared from 5-azacytidine-treated cells," *Nucleic Acids Research*, vol. 9, no. 12, pp. 2933–2947, 1981.

[11] J. Diesch, A. Zwick, A. K. Garz, A. Palau, M. Buschbeck, and K. S. Gotze, "A clinical-molecular update on azanucleoside-based therapy for the treatment of hematologic cancers," *Clinical Epigenetics*, vol. 8, no. 1, p. 71, 2016.

[12] H. M. Kantarjian, X. G. Thomas, A. Dmoszynska et al., "Multicenter, randomized, open-label, phase III trial of decitabine versus patient choice, with physician advice, of either supportive care or low-dose cytarabine for the treatment of older patients with newly diagnosed acute myeloid leukemia," *Journal of Clinical Oncology: Official Journal of the American Society of Clinical Oncology*, vol. 30, no. 21, pp. 2670–2677, 2012.

[13] P. Wijermans, M. Lübbert, G. Verhoef et al., "Low-dose 5-aza-2′-deoxycytidine, a DNA hypomethylating agent, for the treatment of high-risk myelodysplastic syndrome: a multicenter phase II study in elderly patients," *Journal of Clinical Oncology: Official Journal of the American Society of Clinical Oncology*, vol. 18, no. 5, pp. 956–962, 2000.

[14] *Decitabine [Package Insert]*, MGI PHARMA, INC., Bloomington, MN, 2006.

[15] L. B. Levine, J. V. F. Roddy, M. Kim, J. Li, G. Phillips, and A. R. Walker, "A comparison of toxicities in acute myeloid leukemia patients with and without renal impairment treated with decitabine," *Journal of Oncology Pharmacy Practice*, vol. 24, no. 4, pp. 290–298, 2018.

16

Cardiac Dedifferentiated Liposarcoma Requiring a Mitral Valve Replacement Complicated by Severe Paravalvular Leak: A Rare Case Report with Literature Review

Anju Adhikari[1,2] **Adam Hafeez**[1,2] **and Alexandra Halalau**[1,2]

[1]Internal Medicine Department, Beaumont Hospital, Royal Oak, MI, USA
[2]Oakland University William Beaumont School of Medicine, Rochester, MI, USA

Correspondence should be addressed to Anju Adhikari; anju.adhikari@beaumont.org

Academic Editor: Ertugrul Ercan

Cardiac sarcomas have a high infiltrative and metastatic potential and are often associated with poor prognosis. These tumors are often identified incidentally by thoracic and cardiac imaging. However, when symptomatic, their presentation can differ based on the localized structural effects on the endocardium, myocardium, pericardium, and valves as well as on dynamic effects on the cardiac function. We report a case of a 61-year-old female who presented to the emergency room with recurrent chest pain, fatigue, and chronic anemia. A transthoracic echocardiogram demonstrated a left atrial mass attached to the septal wall and anterior leaflet of the mitral valve. The mass was further characterized by a transesophageal echocardiogram and cardiac MRI. The patient underwent a resection of the left atrial mass with mitral valve replacement (MVR) and atrial septal defect repair. MVR was later complicated by paravalvular leak leading to acute congestive heart failure. Tissue immune histology was consistent with dedifferentiated liposarcoma. Cardiac dedifferentiated liposarcoma is extremely rare with only few cases reported in literature. We attempt to review the clinical features, diagnosis, and management of cardiac sarcoma with great emphasis.

1. Background

Cardiac tumors in general are relatively rare and can be either primary or secondary. Secondary cardiac involvement from metastasis and local extension are slightly more common, although still relatively rare when compared with other organ systems. Secondary metastatic tumors are commonly known to arise from the malignancies originating in the lungs, breast, kidney, skin, or lymphatic tissue (lymphoma) [1]. On the other hand, primary cardiac tumors are known to be extremely rare with some studies reporting less than 0.1 percent incidence [2].

Primary cardiac tumors are commonly benign while malignant primary cardiac tumors remain very rare with autopsy series reporting a prevalence of 0.001% [3]. The Japanese Association of Thoracic Surgery (JATS) along with the Japanese Circulation Society (JCS) compiled a compendium of cardiac tumors from 1999 to 2010 [4]. They found that the most common benign cardiac tumor was myxoma (34.0–43.1%), followed by papillary fibroelastoma (11.4–17.7%). This was followed by lipoma and hemangioma in this order. On the other hand, they found that malignant cardiac tumors were most commonly angiosarcoma (8.2–9.5%), followed by fibrous histiocytoma and leiomyosarcoma. Cardiac dedifferentiated liposarcoma is extremely rare with less than 10 cases reported in the literature. It is a type of liposarcoma with an infiltrative and metastatic potential. We report a case of a female presenting with cardiac liposarcoma of primary cardiac origin.

2. Case

A 61-year-old female with past medical history significant for type 2 diabetes mellitus, hypertension, and dyslipidemia and family history of breast cancer in her brother and maternal aunt presented to the emergency room for recurrent chest pain. She also reported fatigue for the past few months and was being evaluated for worsening anemia by her primary care physician. Her hemoglobin was 6 gm/dl with iron panel consistent with anemia of chronic disease. Her electrocardiogram (ECG) at arrival showed an "RSR pattern" in V1 and V2 leads but was otherwise normal. She underwent a stress myocardial perfusion imaging (MPI) which was negative for cardiac ischemia. A transthoracic echocardiogram revealed a 1.6 cm × 1.5 cm atrial mass attached to the anterior wall of the left atrium, which appeared to cross the mitral valve in ventricular diastole. The left atrial mass was further characterized by a transesophageal echocardiogram (TEE) as a solid, irregularly shaped, partly mobile mass attached to the atrial septum and extending to the anterior mitral valve leaflet (Figure 1). The segment attached to the septum measured 2.6 cm × 1.43 cm, and the segment attached to the valve measured 1.4 cm × 2.22 cm. In addition, MRI of the heart with gadolinium was done preoperatively which confirmed the circumscribed hypodense mass with speckled appearance which originated at the atrial septum and extended along the anterior mitral valve leaflet (Figure 2). The mitral valve flow was normal with no evidence of obstruction, stenosis, or regurgitation. The patient underwent a minimal incision valve surgery for resection of the mass which was presumed to be myxoma due to its location. Intraoperatively, on open examination of the left atrium, it was noted that the mass originated from the fossa ovalis region of the interatrial septum and infiltrated the atrial wall down onto the entire anterior leaflet of the mitral valve. A fibrotic density that surrounded the tumor was also noted. The mass along with a portion of the interatrial septum and the mitral valve was resected. The mitral valve was replaced using a 27 mm Hancock II bioprosthetic valve. The atrial septal defect caused by the resection was repaired with a bovine pericardial patch. A postoperative TEE was performed which confirmed the successful placement of the bioprosthetic valve with no paravalvular leak. The patient had an otherwise unremarkable postoperative recovery and was discharged home after fourteen days of hospital stay.

Two weeks following discharge, the patient presented to the emergency with cough, diaphoresis, and palpitations. She was noted to have jugular venous distention and bibasilar crackles on auscultation of the lungs and was found to be in acute heart failure. An urgent transesophageal echocardiography demonstrated severe mitral regurgitation with paravalvular leak (Figures 3, 4, 5, and 6). At the same time, the histopathologic examination of the atrial mass showed a high-grade sarcoma consistent with dedifferentiated liposarcoma. The tissue exhibited spindle cells with pleomorphism, multinucleated giant cells, and inflammatory cells. Immunohistochemical stains demonstrated that the neoplastic cells were positive for vimentin, focally positive for S-100, and weakly positive for CDK4 and negative for p53 (Figure 7). FISH studies performed showed an MDM-2 gene amplification in 95–200 nuclei examined. The patient was aggressively treated with intravenous diuretics and afterload reduction using furosemide and nicardipine infusion. Blood cultures were obtained with suspicion of postsurgical infective endocarditis causing valvular dehiscence. However, cultures did not grow any bacteria. The patient clinically deteriorated due to new-onset atrial fibrillation and worsening heart

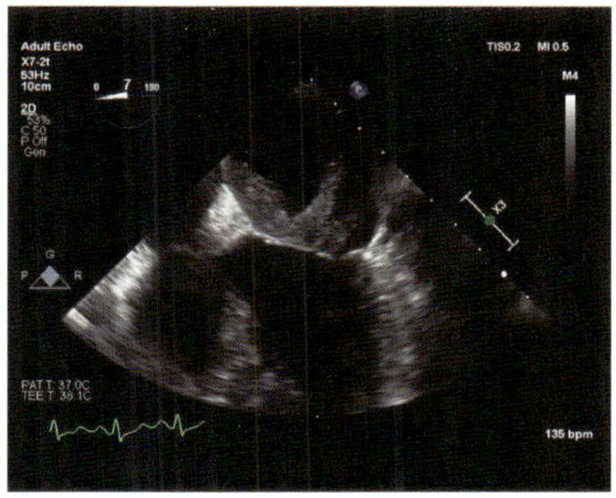

Figure 1: Preoperative midesophageal TEE 4-chamber view showing a large echo-dense atrial mass; one segment is attached to the atrial septum (2.67 cm × 1.43 cm) and another segment is attached to the anterior mitral leaflet (1.43 cm × 2.22 cm).

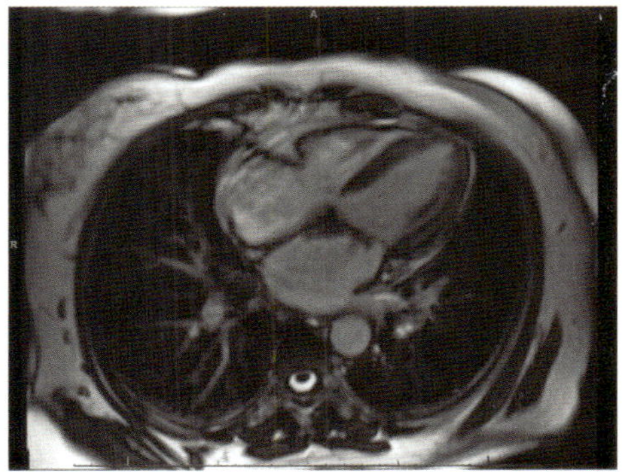

Figure 2: Cardiac MRI first-pass perfusion imaging showing mass originating on the atrial septum and extending along the atrial aspect of the anterior mitral valve leaflet.

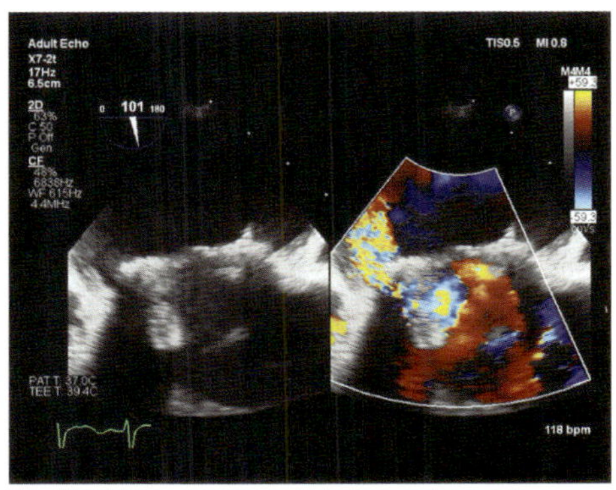

Figure 3: TEE 2-chamber view at hospital readmission showing severe paravalvular leak of the bioprosthetic mitral valve. 180° rotation showed leak extending along the medial aspect of the valve from the posterior to the anterior.

failure despite medical treatment in CCU. CT chest obtained showed a 1.3 cm lytic iliac bone lesion and 3.1 cm × 2.5 cm right upper mediastinal soft tissue density. Due to high suspicion of metastatic disease, MVR and cardiac transplant were not offered until further evaluation for metastasis.

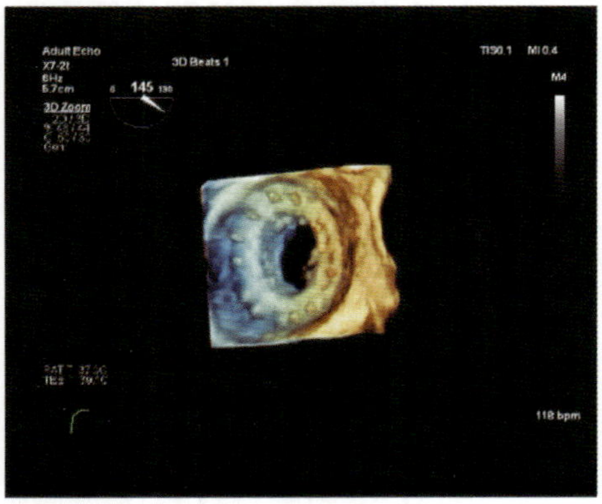

FIGURE 4: TEE 3D reconstruction showing bioprosthetic mitral valve in the short axis with paravalvular dehiscence that extends along the medial aspect of the valve from the posterior to the anterior.

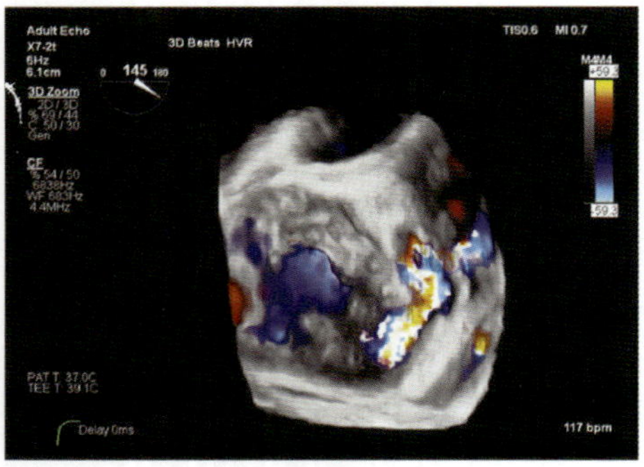

FIGURE 5: TEE 3D reconstruction with color Doppler showing a bioprosthetic mitral valve with paravalvular leak on the short axis.

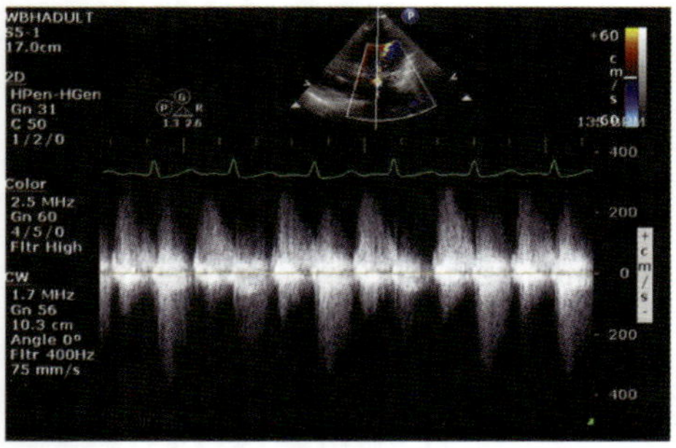

FIGURE 6: TEE continuous wave showing severe mitral regurgitation.

Unfortunately, due to rapid clinical decline with a new diagnosis of high-grade cardiac tumor with possible metastases, the patient opted for hospice care. PET study was not obtained.

3. Discussion

Among malignant cardiac tumors, cardiac sarcomas appear to be the most common. In a retrospective study done in Germany from 1989 to 2012 that looked at 181 diagnosed cardiac tumors, cardiac sarcoma represented 75% of all malignant cardiac tumors [5]. Histologically, soft tissue sarcomas in general have been classified by the World Health Organization (WHO) to include more than 100 different histologic subtypes on the basis of the morphologic pattern most often noted on immunohistochemical staging (IHC) [6]. The most common soft tissue sarcoma subtypes in adults include undifferentiated/unclassified soft tissue sarcoma, undifferentiated pleomorphic sarcoma, liposarcoma, leiomyosarcoma, and gastrointestinal stromal tumors (GIST). Liposarcoma constitutes only 13% of all cardiac sarcomas, arises from adipocytes, and has three main morphologic subgroups that vary in their metastatic potential according to 2013 WHO classification of soft tissue sarcoma: (1) myxoid, (2) dedifferentiated, and (3) pleomorphic liposarcoma [7]. Myxoid liposarcoma are low-grade tumors while dedifferentiated and pleomorphic liposarcomas are highly aggressive tumors. Dedifferentiated liposarcoma, as seen in our patient, is extremely rare with less than 10 reported cases in PubMed and Embase together (Table 1). However, dedifferentiated liposarcomas of the mediastinum, retroperitoneum, and extremities were more commonly reported.

Common clinical symptoms of cardiac tumors include dyspnea, orthopnea, paroxysmal nocturnal dyspnea, hemoptysis, edema, and nonspecific constitutional symptoms such as fevers, chills, or fatigue, arthralgias, and myalgias [8]. Laboratory studies are inconsistent and may show anemia due to chronic disease, mildly elevated white blood cell count, and elevated erythrocyte sedimentation rate. Tumors can cause direct obstruction, valvular dysfunction, coronary artery spasm, changes in the electrical conduction of the heart with arrhythmias, and production of a malignant pericardial effusion. Cardiac tumors may metastasize or embolize causing distant complications with brain infarction being a feared complication. One study on atrial myxomas reported as high as 12% incidence of central nervous system complications from left atrial tumors [9].

Left atrial tumors are commonly presumed to be benign myxomas. Although left atrial tumors are commonly benign, the possibility of malignancy should always be considered given that 50% of cardiac sarcomas occur in the left atrium [10]. As shown in Table 1, most reported cases of dedifferentiated liposarcoma arose in the left atrium. These tumors are known to impede blood flow and cause mitral valve obstruction. Clinically, patients often present with symptoms of heart failure or pulmonary hypertension (Table 1). Although not commonly reported, physical exam maneuvers may produce a tumor plop in early diastole.

Evaluation for cardiac tumors rests heavily on imaging modalities. There are three major imaging modalities that aid with the diagnosis of cardiac tumors. Transthoracic echocardiography remains at the heart of diagnosing and screening of cardiac neoplasms as it has a high sensitivity and specificity (90% and 95%, respectively) for detecting intracavitary and endocardial lesions [1, 11]. TEE can be utilized for a more accurate evaluation as it provides superior spatial resolution and is optimal for tumors where areas such as the atria, interatrial septum, superior vena cava, and atrioventricular valves are difficult to visualize. In our patient, TEE provided a more accurate view of the tumor size, extent, and

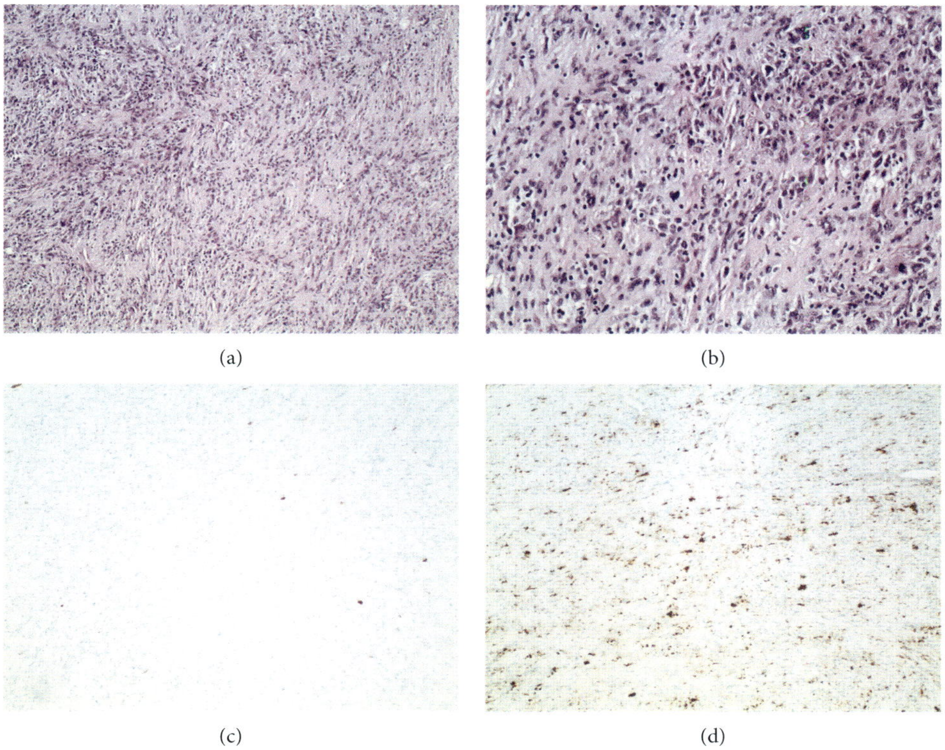

Figure 7: (a) 10x H&E, (b) 20x H&E, (c) tumor negative for p53, and (d) tumor focally positive for S100.

Table 1: Case reports of cardiac dedifferentiated liposarcoma indexed in PubMed and Embase.

Number	Publication	Year	Primary/Metastatic	Location of tumor	Presentation
1	Seaweed floating in the pericardium: a rare case of primary dedifferentiated liposarcoma [14]	2016	Primary	Pericardium	Dyspnea
2	Primary cardiac dedifferentiated liposarcoma with homologous and heterologous differentiation: a case report [15]	2015	Primary	Left atrium	Dyspnea on exertion, fatigue, palpitation
3	Large left ventricular metastasis in patient with liposarcoma [16]	2016	Metastasis from pleura	Left ventricle	Not mentioned
4	Synchronous primary heart liposarcoma and papillary renal carcinoma–a case report (abstract only) [17]	2003	Not available	Not available	Not available
5	Metastatic cardiac liposarcoma of the small intestine causing enteroenteric intussusception: a case report and a review of the literature [18]	2015	Primary with metastasis to the small intestine	Left atrium	Dyspnea on exertion
6	A case of dedifferentiated liposarcoma of the heart and stomach [19]	2017	Unknown	Left atrium	Anorexia and weight loss
7	Mitral stenosis secondary to high-grade liposarcoma in a young pregnant [20]	2015	Primary	Left atrium and right pulmonary vein	Acute dyspnea
8	Multiple skeletal muscle metastases revealing a cardiac intimal sarcoma [21]	2018	Primary cardiac with skeletal muscle metastasis	Left atrium	Thigh swelling

attachment than the initial TTE. MRI is currently the modality of choice to evaluate tissue infiltration, pericardial image, and extracardiac extension whenever a malignant lesion is suspected. Multidetector CT is a relatively new modality which produces images with higher spatial resolution in a shorter exposure span and also better demonstrates calcifications, fatty lesions, and cardiac valves [12]. Clinical signs and symptoms along with imaging can help formulate a presumed diagnosis of a cardiac tumor but, as seen in our patient, cannot be relied on to help differentiate between benign or metastatic diseases. The tumor stage and grade can only be made with histological confirmation. Minimally invasive techniques can be used if the malignancy is in pericardial fluid or if an imaging-guided percutaneous biopsy can be performed. However, in endocardial tumors, the risk of embolization often outweighs the benefits of biopsy of the tumor, given that the tumor will eventually be resected anyways. Of note, percutaneous needle biopsy is not adequate for the diagnosis and grade determination of lipomatous tumors. These tumors require larger tissue specimens obtained by incisional or excisional biopsy which further complicates and delays their diagnosis [5].

Surgical resection with or without chemotherapy or radiotherapy remains the treatment of choice for cardiac malignancies including liposarcoma. Management begins by assessing the extent and size of tumor as that determines the approach to excise such tumors. Positron emission tomography (PET) as well as coronary angiography is important as mapping the blood supply of tumors helps cardiac surgeons know where to also resect or graft involved arteries. Simple tumor resection is selected for benign tumors with no infiltration while complex tumor resection and ex situ resection are utilized for malignant tumors. Implantation of an artificial heart and heart transplantation are reserved for young patients with no evidence of distant metastasis [5].

Unfortunately, sarcomas in general, regardless of the morphologic type, are known to rapidly proliferate. They are known to infiltrate the myocardium, obstruct blood flow through the heart, and cause metastasis. In a study of 181 patients with cardiac tumors, among which 25% were malignant, the 5-year survival rates for malignant tumors following treatment was 30% [5]. The study also reported that complete tumor resection and adjuvant radiation therapy contributed to the reduced risk of local recurrence and metastasis. Specifically with liposarcoma, recurrence was seen in approximately 40% of the cases and was reported to be up to 14 years after the initial surgical resection [7].

Our patient developed paraprosthetic leak following mitral valve replacement (MVR). Mild paravalvular leak (PVL) is a fairly common complication occurring in almost 20% post-MVR. Of note, however, clinically significant PVL occurs in only 1–5% [13]. Calcification and fibrosis of the annulus are known to increase the risk of PVL. On the other hand, it is well known that malignant tissue often displays fibrosis or calcification. Our patient had fibrotic changes around the atrial cancer which was easily noticed during resection. Hence, it is possible that the remnant friable malignant tissue or its sclerotic surrounding tissue might have contributed to the PVL in our patient leading to poor clinical outcome. Keeping in mind the limitations of echocardiogram, cardiac MRI, and CT in diagnosing a malignant tumor, we suggest the utilization of PET scan whenever malignancy is suspected. Presurgical diagnosis of malignant tumors would not only help surgeons plan a complete tumor resection and anticipate complications but would also allow neoadjuvant radiation or chemotherapy. At present, the prognosis of cardiac malignancy remains poor with high mortality and tumor recurrence. The advent of new modalities to diagnose cardiac malignancy before curative surgery could potentially decrease the mortality in the future.

Acknowledgments

The authors would like to thank Kausar Jabbar, MD, Department of Clinical and Laboratory Pathology at Oakland University William Beaumont Hospital for the assistance with immunohistopathology images and description. We also express our gratitude to Richard J. Bloomingdale, MD, Department of Cardiology, for the assistance with cardiac images and description.

References

[1] I. A. Paraskevaidis, C. A. Michalakeas, C. H. Papadopoulos, and M. Anastasiou-Nana, "Cardiac tumors," *ISRN Oncology*, vol. 2011, Article ID 208929, 5 pages, 2011.

[2] K. Y. Lam, P. Dickens, and A. C. Chan, "Tumors of the heart. a 20-year experience with a review of 12,485 consecutive autopsies," *Archives of Pathology & Laboratory Medicine*, vol. 117, no. 10, pp. 1027–1031, 1993.

[3] G. Sütsch, R. Jenni, L. von Segesser, and J. Schneider, "Heart tumors: incidence, distribution, diagnosis. Exemplified by 20,305 echocardiographies," *Schweizerische Medizinische Wochenschrift*, vol. 121, no. 17, pp. 621–629, 1991.

[4] J. Amano and J. Nakayama, *Epidemiology and Frequency of Cardiac Tumors. Textbook of Cardiac Tumors*, Nanzando, Tokyo, 2011.

[5] A. Hoffmeier, J. R. Sindermann, H. H. Scheld, and S. Martens, "Cardiac tumors— diagnosis and surgical treatment," *Deutsches Ärzteblatt International*, vol. 111, no. 12, pp. 205–211, 2014.

[6] C. D. M. Fletcher, J. A. Bridge, P. C. W. Hogendoorn, and F. Mertens, *World Health Organization Classification of Tumours of Soft Tissue and Bone*, IARC Press, Lyon, 4th edition, 2013.

[7] C. M. Steger, "Primary liposarcoma of the heart," *BMJ Case Reports*, vol. 2011, article bcr0320114013, 2011.

[8] L. M. Shapiro, "Cardiac tumours: diagnosis and management," *Heart*, vol. 85, no. 2, pp. 218–222, 2001.

[9] V. H. Lee, H. M. Connolly, and R. D. Brown, "Central nervous system manifestations of cardiac myxoma," *Archives of Neurology*, vol. 64, no. 8, pp. 1115–1120, 2007.

[10] A. Burke and F. Tavora, "The 2015 WHO classification of tumors of the heart and pericardium," *Journal of Thoracic Oncology*, vol. 11, no. 4, pp. 441–452, 2016.

[11] E. E. Salcedo, G. I. Cohen, R. D. White, and M. B. Davison, "Cardiac tumors: diagnosis and management," *Current Problems in Cardiology*, vol. 17, no. 2, pp. 73–137, 1992.

[12] P. J. Sparrow, J. B. Kurian, T. R. Jones, and M. U. Sivananthan, "MR imaging of cardiac tumors," *Radiographics*, vol. 25, no. 5, pp. 1255–1276, 2005.

[13] G. Smolka, "Paravalvular leak – important complication after implantation of prosthetic valve," 2010, February 2018, https://www.escardio.org/Journals/E-Journal-of-Cardiology-Practice/Volume-9/Paravalvular-leak-important-complication-after-implantation-of-prosthetic-valve.

[14] G. Zanini, E. Gorga, F. Pasini et al., "Seaweed floating in the pericardium: a rare case of primary dedifferentiated liposarcoma," *Cardiovascular Pathology*, vol. 25, no. 4, pp. 333–335, 2016.

[15] D. He, M. Chen, H. Chen et al., "Primary cardiac dedifferentiated liposarcoma with homologous and heterologous differentiation: a case report," *International Journal of Clinical and Experimental Pathology*, vol. 8, no. 8, pp. 9662–9666, 2015.

[16] G. Dendramis, D. Di Lisi, C. Paleologo, G. Novo, and S. Novo, "Large left ventricular metastasis in patient with liposarcoma," *Journal of Cardiovascular Medicine*, vol. 17, pp. e166–e168, 2016.

[17] K. Gałazka, M. Ciezarek, J. Soja et al., "Synchronous primary heart liposarcoma and papillary renal carcinoma - a case report," *Polish Journal of Pathology*, vol. 54, no. 2, pp. 153–159, 2003.

[18] G. Gomez, M. Bilal, P. Klepchick, and K. Clarke, "Rare case of entero-enteric intussusception caused by small bowel metastasis from a cardiac liposarcoma," *World Journal of Gastrointestinal Oncology*, vol. 8, no. 3, pp. 326–329, 2016.

[19] Y. Hisata, Y. Tasaki, S. Kozaki, and T. Yamada, "A case of dedifferentiated liposarcoma of the heart and stomach," *International Journal of Surgery Case Reports*, vol. 41, pp. 36–38, 2017.

[20] C. Morgan, M. Shah, S. Bailey, and J. Nunez, "Mitral stenosis secondary to high-grade liposarcoma in a young pregnant female," *Journal of the American College of Cardiology*, vol. 65, no. 10, article A719, 2015.

[21] A. Crombé, P.-F. Lintingre, F. le Loarer, D. Lachatre, and B. Dallaudière, "Multiple skeletal muscle metastases revealing a cardiac intimal sarcoma," *Skeletal Radiology*, vol. 47, no. 1, pp. 125–130, 2017.

17

His-Bundle Pacing in a Patient with Transcatheter Aortic Valve Implantation-Induced Left Bundle Branch Block

Jonathan Sen, Michael Mok, and Mark Perrin

University Hospital Geelong, Barwon Health, PO Box 281, Geelong, VIC 3220, Australia

Correspondence should be addressed to Jonathan Sen; research@jonathansen.com

Academic Editor: Hajime Kataoka

Transcatheter aortic valve implantation (TAVI) is an effective intervention for severe aortic stenosis in patients at intermediate or high surgical risk, but damage to the native conduction system such as left bundle branch block (LBBB) may offset its benefits. New onset LBBB is associated with a higher risk of cardiovascular morbidity and mortality. His-bundle pacing (HBP) may be useful to treat TAVI-induced LBBB but has yet to be reported. We present the case of a 76-year-old man with severe symptomatic aortic stenosis treated with TAVI. His preoperative electrocardiogram showed sinus rhythm with a narrow QRS complex. Insertion of a CoreValve Evolut R transcatheter aortic valve was uneventful apart from the development of LBBB with a long PR interval. A dual-lead DDD pacemaker was implanted via the left cephalic vein on the following day. HV was mildly prolonged at 60 ms. Capture of the proximal His restored AV synchrony without correction of LBBB. Repositioning of the lead with capture of the left bundle branch enabled complete ventricular resynchronisation with a single lead. Our case demonstrates that LBBB in the setting of TAVI may be corrected by HBP.

1. Introduction

Transcatheter aortic valve implantation (TAVI) is an effective treatment for severe aortic stenosis in patients at intermediate or high surgical risk [1, 2]. However, damage to the native conduction system including complete atrioventricular (AV) block (6–25%) and new left bundle branch block (LBBB) (4–65%) may occur and offset the benefit of the intervention [3–5]. New-onset LBBB causes a delay in depolarisation of the left ventricle and predicts higher cardiovascular morbidity and mortality and high rates of pacemaker implantation [2, 6].

Pacing at the distal His bundle may correct LBBB. Case reports support the concept of longitudinal dissociation in the His bundle [7], that is, fibres within the His bundle are predestined for the left or right bundle branch. Pacing at the His bundle may capture fibres of a bundle branch distal to the site of intra-Hisian block [6]. However, to our knowledge, the correction of TAVI-induced LBBB via HBP has not been reported [7, 8]. This is likely due to more distal block and the relative inaccessibility of the left bundle branch conduction fibres to the pacing lead helix. Here, we describe HBP as a therapeutic intervention for patients with TAVI-induced LBBB.

2. Case Presentation

A 76-year-old man was electively admitted for intervention and management of severe symptomatic aortic stenosis resulting in worsening New York Heart Association Class III cardiac failure. His medical history included stage III chronic kidney disease, type 2 diabetes mellitus, hypertension, and prior coronary artery bypass grafting. Coronary angiography demonstrated a patent left internal mammary artery graft to the left anterior descending coronary artery and a saphenous vein graft to the dominant distal left circumflex artery with a severe stenosis distal to the surgical anastomosis.

Transthoracic echocardiography was performed and showed a thickened and calcified aortic valve with reduced cusp excursion, mild concentric left ventricular hypertrophy with normal left ventricular cavity size, and systolic function.

The left atrium was severely dilated. Left ventricular ejection fraction was above 55%. Valve area was estimated at 0.8 cm^2, with a measured mean gradient of 44 mmHg.

A cardiac conference was held to discuss intervention for his severe aortic stenosis. TAVI was chosen in preference to a redo sternotomy in the setting of the Society of Thoracic Surgeons score of 5.8% (intermediate risk cardiac surgery), stable coronary artery disease, and in accordance with the patient's preference.

The preoperative electrocardiogram (ECG) showed sinus rhythm with a narrow QRS complex (Figure 1(a)). Using a right femoral approach, a CoreValve Evolut R 29 mm (Medtronic, Minneapolis, Minnesota) transcatheter aortic valve was deployed after balloon aortic valvuloplasty with an 18 mm Cristal balloon. TAVI was uneventful. Postdilatation was performed using a 23 mm Cristal balloon due to moderate paravalvular aortic regurgitation around the left coronary cusp seen on a postprocedure transoesophageal echocardiogram. At the time of TAVI, the patient developed LBBB (average QRS duration of 180 ms) with a prolonged PR interval of 240 ms (Figure 1(b)). Within the first 24 hours post-TAVI, he also had episodes of high-grade AV block.

A dual-lead Boston Scientific Accolade™ Extended Life DR Pacemaker was implanted via the left cephalic vein (Figure 2). The HV interval was mildly prolonged at 60 ms. Proximal His capture (selective) threshold was less than 1 V without recruitment of the left bundle branch; RV myocardial capture threshold was 1.5 V at 1 ms; correction of LBBB—due to the presumed capture of distal His bundle and recruitment of the left bundle branch—occurred at 4.5-5 V at 1 ms. A Medtronic 5076 lead was then placed in the right atrial appendage with a threshold less than 1 V. The device was programmed DDD 50. The paced QRS duration on 12 lead ECG was 125 ms consistent with nonselective HBP (para-Hisian morphology) (Figure 1(c)). At 1 month, 12 lead electrocardiogram tracing showed continued correction of LBBB at 5 V @ 1 ms.

3. Discussion

TAVI is an increasingly common intervention for patients with severe symptomatic aortic stenosis at intermediate or high risk with standard surgery. The multinational randomized Surgical Replacement and Transcatheter Aortic Valve Implantation trial (SURTAVI) demonstrated that TAVI was noninferior to surgical replacement based on a composite of all-cause mortality or disabling stroke at 2 years; however, TAVI had markedly higher rates of pacemaker implantation [9].

The risk of heart block and the need for permanent pacing is higher with CoreValve (25%) than other TAVI models [10, 11]. The CoreValve's self-expanding frame and deeper implantation into the left ventricular outflow tract may result in mechanical injury of the His bundle and/or left bundle branch accounting for this higher risk [11].

LBBB is the most common TAVI-induced conduction abnormality reported in 29–65% of patients implanted with CoreValve [11, 12]. LBBB causes rhythmic and haemodynamic complications, is associated with worse outcomes, and can lead to heart failure [13]. The effect of new-onset LBBB on mortality is uncertain, but some studies found a significantly higher mortality rate in patients who develop LBBB post-TAVI [11, 14]. Even though the incidence of new-onset LBBB is higher in patients implanted with CoreValve compared to Edwards SAPIEN valve, no difference in mortality was observed [14].

There is no published guideline on the management of LBBB post-TAVI. In our case, we elected to place a pacemaker due to the presence of a long PR interval, new-onset LBBB, and an expanding valve. The His bundle contains fibres predestined to form the right and left bundle branches, a theory confirmed by correction of bundle branch block by pacing at the His bundle presumably due to the recruitment of fibres distal to the site of block [15]. In our case, these fibres were found by mapping for the His bundle potential, with small movements of the lead tip until a suitable pacing site where correction of the underlying LBBB was achieved, albeit at high pacing output.

A standard dual-chamber device would resynchronise the atrial and ventricular chambers, but leave the ventricular chambers dyssynchronous. We placed a dual-chamber His bundle device to allow resynchronisation of all chambers. In the largest series to date of HBP in patients with heart block postprosthetic valve replacement, Sharma and colleagues included four patients post-TAVI—all Edward SAPIEN valves: in two cases, HBP was unsuccessful and a standard right ventricular lead was placed—in the remaining two patients, HBP was employed successfully to correct RBBB in one case and to retain a narrow QRS complex in the other [8]. In our case, we were able to obtain selective HBP at a low threshold, but true correction of LBBB—presumably due to more distal disease—was only possible at higher output.

The tools for HBP are rudimentary. The Medtronic SelectSecure lead has an exposed helix screw with no inner lumen and must be delivered through a fixed sheath (Medtronic 315His) delivered through a 7 French introducer sheath, or a deflectable sheath (Medtronic SelectSite C304) delivered through a 9Fr introducer sheath. Implantation is therefore limited by anatomy. It may be that improved delivery tools allow more precise placement of the lead with lower subsequent thresholds. To some extent, the higher output required in our case may be mitigated through device programming by increased pulse width, pacing with output marginally (0.5-1 V) above the left bundle branch threshold, and the use of a pacemaker with an extended-life battery.

4. Conclusion

Our case demonstrates that LBBB in the setting of TAVI may be corrected by pacing at the His bundle. To our knowledge, this is the first report of HBP with a self-expanding valve and the first report for left bundle branch recruitment in this setting. HBP allows complete AV and ventricular resynchronisation with two leads. Longer-term follow-up will be needed to determine the chronic threshold of LBBB correction.

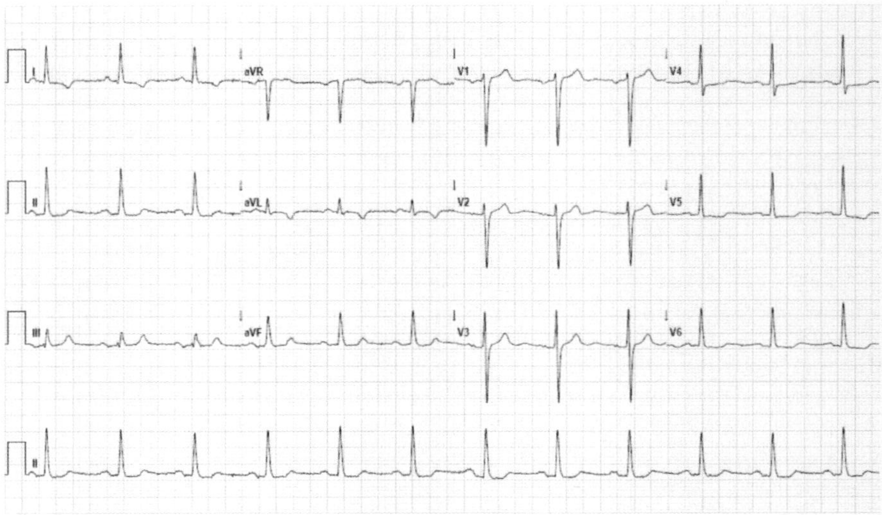

(a)

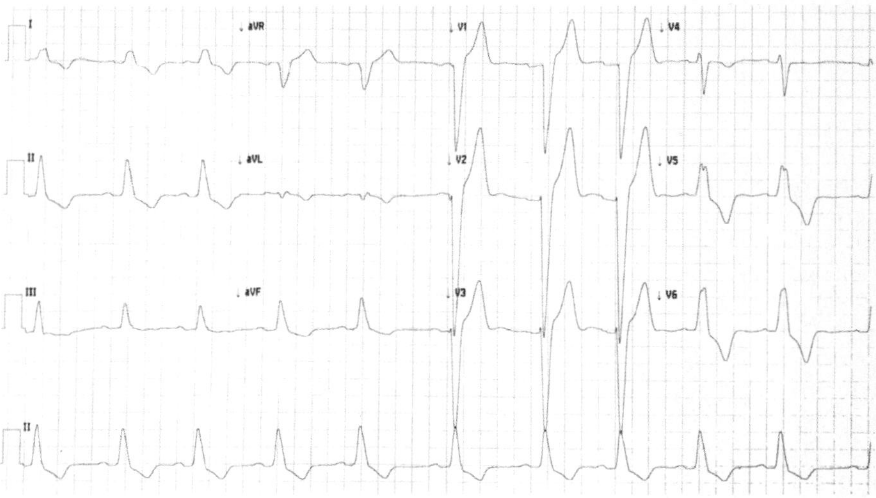

(b)

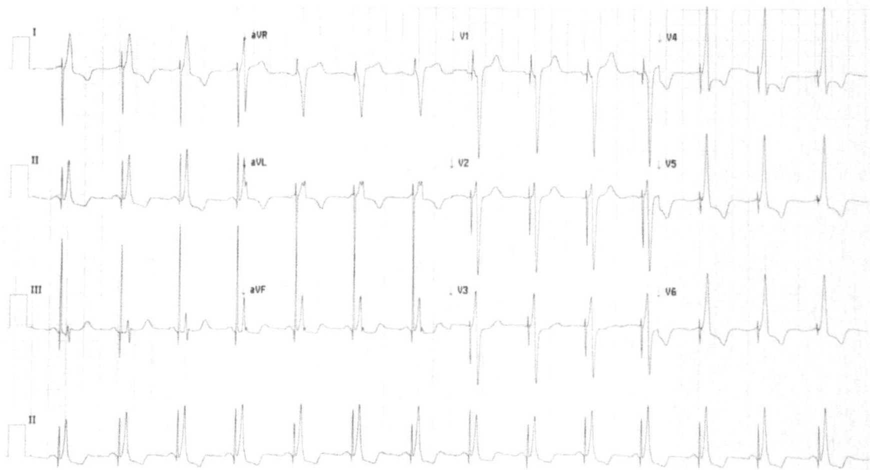

(c)

FIGURE 1: Electrocardiogram tracings at different time points. (a) Pre-transcatheter aortic valve implantation; (b) prolonged PR interval with left bundle branch block post-transcatheter aortic valve implantation; (c) post-His-bundle pacing with correction of the left bundle branch block.

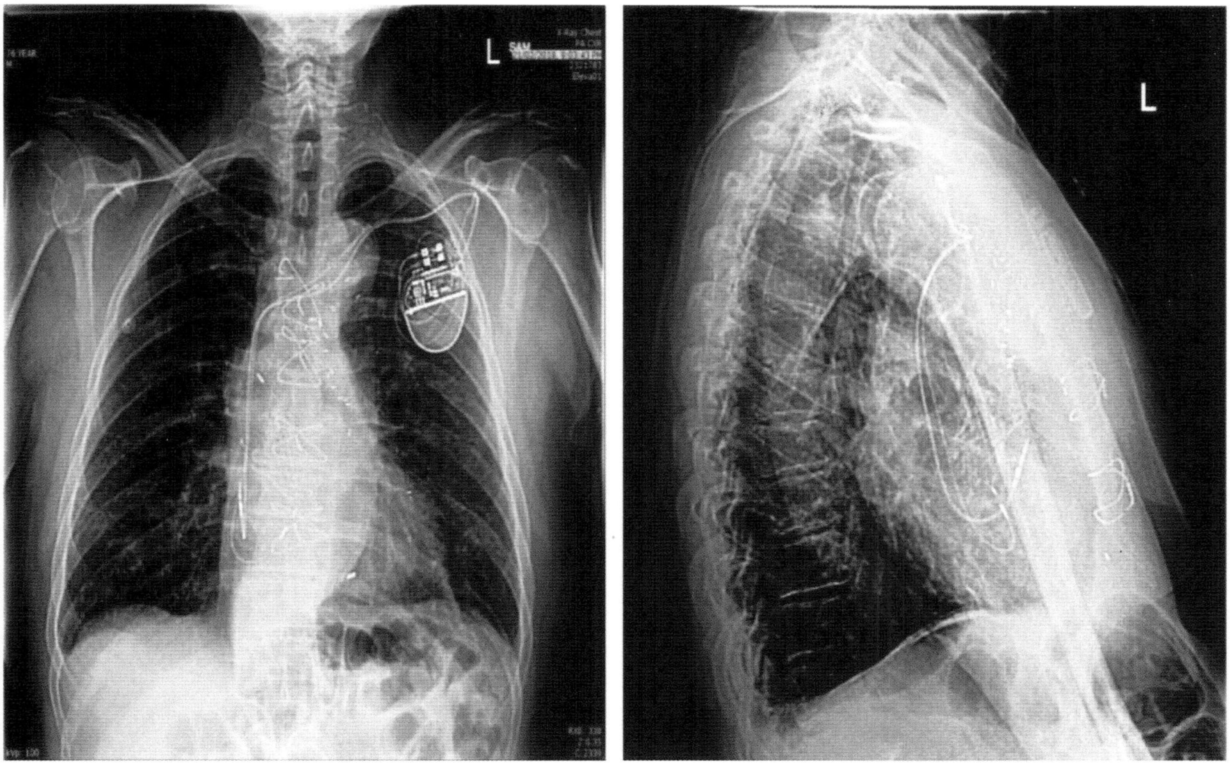

FIGURE 2: Chest X-rays (posterior-anterior and lateral views) after transcatheter aortic valve implantation and His-bundle pacemaker insertion.

Authors' Contributions

All three authors (Jonathan Sen, Michael Mok, and Mark Perrin) made significant contributions to the manuscript, which included a review of patient charts, data collection, and interpretation. Jonathan Sen was responsible for drafting the initial case report, which was subsequently reviewed by Michael Mok and Mark Perrin. All authors reviewed the final and full manuscript and approved the manuscript for submission.

References

[1] M. Pighi, R. Serdoz, I. D. Kilic, S. A. Sherif, A. Lindsay, and C. di Mario, "TAVI: new trials and registries offer further welcome evidence - U.S. CoreValve, CHOICE, and GARY," *Global Cardiology Science and Practice*, vol. 2014, no. 1, pp. 78–87, 2014.

[2] V. Calvi and G. P. Pruiti, "Pacemaker implantation and need for ventricular pacing during follow-up after transcatheter aortic valve implantation," *Pacing and Clinical Electrophysiology*, vol. 37, no. 12, pp. 1589–1591, 2014.

[3] A. Kostopoulou, P. Karyofillis, E. Livanis et al., "Permanent pacing after transcatheter aortic valve implantation of a CoreValve prosthesis as determined by electrocardiographic and electrophysiological predictors: a single-centre experience," *Europace*, vol. 18, no. 1, pp. 131 137, 2016.

[4] E. B. Engels, T. T. Poels, P. Houthuizen et al., "Electrical remodelling in patients with iatrogenic left bundle branch block," *Europace*, vol. 18, Supplement_4, pp. iv44–iv52, 2016.

[5] F. Sundh and M. Ugander, "Impact of left bundle branch block after transcatheter aortic valve replacement," *Journal of Electrocardiology*, vol. 47, no. 5, pp. 608–611, 2014.

[6] A. E. Teng, D. L. Lustgarten, P. Vijayaraman et al., "Usefulness of His bundle pacing to achieve electrical resynchronization in patients with complete left bundle branch block and the relation between native QRS Axis, duration, and normalization," *The American Journal of Cardiology*, vol. 118, no. 4, pp. 527–534, 2016.

[7] P. S. Sharma, K. Ellison, H. N. Patel, and R. G. Trohman, "Overcoming left bundle branch block by permanent His bundle pacing: evidence of longitudinal dissociation in the His via recordings from a permanent pacing lead," *HeartRhythm Case Reports*, vol. 3, no. 11, pp. 499–502, 2017.

[8] P. S. Sharma, F. A. Subzposh, K. A. Ellenbogen, and P. Vijayaraman, "Permanent His-bundle pacing in patients with prosthetic cardiac valves," *Heart Rhythm*, vol. 14, no. 1, pp. 59–64, 2017.

[9] M. J. Reardon, N. van Mieghem, J. J. Popma et al., "Surgical or Transcatheter aortic-valve replacement in intermediate-risk patients," *New England Journal of Medicine*, vol. 376, no. 14, pp. 1321–1331, 2017.

[10] T. M. Nazif, J. M. Dizon, R. T. Hahn et al., "Predictors and clinical outcomes of permanent pacemaker implantation after transcatheter aortic valve replacement: the PARTNER (Placement of AoRtic TraNscathetER Valves) trial and registry," *JACC: Cardiovascular Interventions*, vol. 8, no. 1, Part A, pp. 60–69, 2015.

[11] M. Young Lee, S. Chilakamarri Yeshwant, S. Chava, and D. Lawrence Lustgarten, "Mechanisms of heart block after

Transcatheter aortic valve replacement – cardiac anatomy, clinical predictors and mechanical factors that contribute to permanent pacemaker implantation," *Arrhythmia & Electrophysiology Review*, vol. 4, no. 2, pp. 81–85, 2015.

[12] R. M. van der Boon, R. J. Nuis, N. M. van Mieghem et al., "New conduction abnormalities after TAVI–frequency and causes," *Nature Reviews Cardiology*, vol. 9, no. 8, pp. 454–463, 2012.

[13] G. Massoullié, P. Bordachar, D. Irles et al., "Prognosis assessment of persistent left bundle branch block after TAVI by an electrophysiological and remote monitoring risk-adapted algorithm: rationale and design of the multicentre LBBB–TAVI study," *BMJ Open*, vol. 6, no. 10, article e010485, 2016.

[14] G. Schymik, P. Tzamalis, P. Bramlage et al., "Clinical impact of a new left bundle branch block following TAVI implantation: 1-year results of the TAVIK cohort," *Clinical Research in Cardiology*, vol. 104, no. 4, pp. 351–362, 2015.

[15] O. S. Narula, "Longitudinal dissociation in the His bundle. Bundle branch block due to asynchronous conduction within the His bundle in man," *Circulation*, vol. 56, no. 6, pp. 996–1006, 1977.

Percutaneous Coronary Intervention in a Patient with Right-Sided Heart: Invert the Views?

Miguel López Hidalgo [1] and Risshi D. Rampersad [2]

[1] *Interventional Cardiology Unit, Hospital Metropolitano Del Norte, Valencia, Venezuela*
[2] *Caribbean Heart Care, Medcorp Ltd., St Clair Medical Centre, Port of Spain, Trinidad and Tobago*

Correspondence should be addressed to Miguel López Hidalgo; lopezh900@hotmail.com

Academic Editor: Filippo M. Sarullo

Situs inversus totalis considered a malposition syndrome is a very rare condition, occurring in 1 : 8000 births, usually without associated structural congenital heart disease. The diagnosis is often incidental as in this case, which presented with an acute coronary syndrome as a manifestationof multivessel coronary artery disease. Here, we present the challenges encountered during the diagnosis and management of this entity via percutaneous intervention.

1. Introduction

Right-sided heart is a rare congenital anomaly that is related to malposition of the internal organs, and it can be found usually with all the organs changed in the opposite direction, known as situs inversus totalis (mirror-image dextrocardia) or less commonly as isolated dextrocardia in situs solitus (dextroversion) [1]. Mirror-image dextrocardia (situs inversus) has an incidence of associated congenital heart disease same as normal population, usually does not affect survival, and can be incidentally found in the presence of a cardiothoracic pathology such as coronary artery disease [2]. This situation offers a technical challenge to interventional cardiologists. Here, we describe a patient with postinfarction unstable angina having situs inversus with coronary artery disease, treated with percutaneous coronary intervention (PCI). The challenges in the diagnosis and treatment by an endovascular approach imposed by the anatomical changes of the usual topography of the heart and the presence of multivessel coronary artery disease as a very unusual presentation are shown and discussed.

2. Case Presentation

A 69-year-old Afro-American man was admitted in the emergency department of a public institution in Port of Spain, Trinidad, in February 2015 with EKG findings consistent of an acute coronary syndrome: an inferior wall ST elevation myocardial infarction (inferior STEMI). The symptoms of chest pain initiated 5 hours before admission, he was in Killip-Kimball class I, and he received thrombolytic therapy with Tenecteplase, with clinical, ECG, and biomarkers criteria of successful reperfusion and good clinical in-hospital outcome; primary PCI was not performed because there was not a catheterization laboratory available in that public hospital.

The patient's prior history is that he smokes 10 to 15 cigarettes a day for the last 15 years and had no previous heart disease, hypertension, diabetes, and dyslipidemia nor family history of early coronary artery disease. He was discharged with medical treatment since he had an uncomplicated inferior myocardial infarction (MI) that was stratified for noninvasive evaluation, but due to the presence of postmyocardial infarction effort angina 5 days after discharge, he was admitted to Caribbean Heart Care Medcorp (CHCM) at St. Clair Medical Centre Hospital for diagnostic catheterization. The EKG revealed sinus rhythm with an inverted p wave in DI, aVL, and aVR, with right axis deviation, positive QRS complex in aVR, and poor progression of r waves in precordial leads and signs consistent of a prior inferior MI with q waves at DII, DIII, and aVF.

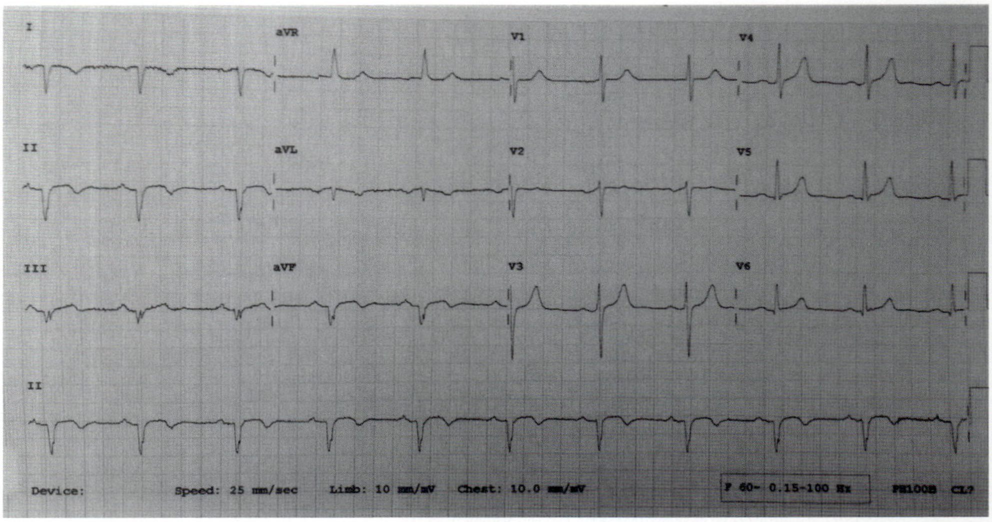

Figure 1: EKG shows the classical elements found in dextrocardia: right axis deviation of p wave with an inverted QRS axis of aVR. Signs of previous inferior MI: q waves in inferior leads.

The TIMI risk score was 2 (8% risk of event at 30 days). The EKG findings made us suspicious of a malposition syndrome (Figure 1).

The physical exam with right-sided heart sounds, including a 4th heart sound and a right-sided apex with a palpable liver in the left side, and the radiogram findings with right-sided cardiac apex and gastric chamber Figure 2 confirmed our suspicion of situs inversus totalis, which was an incidental diagnosis.

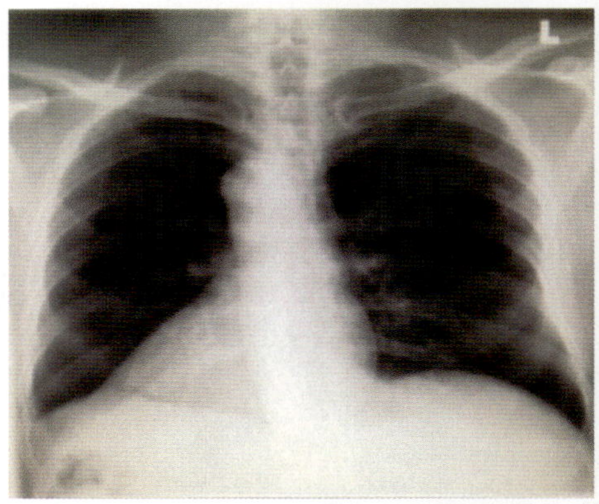

Figure 2: Chest radiogram shows the right-sided heart (apex to the right) and gastric chamber to the right, which adds to the diagnosis of situs inversus.

Coronary angiography was performed via femoral access using the standard Judkins technique [3] with 6 French catheters (Judkins left: JL 4.0 and Judkins right: JR 3.5), which showed right-sided aortic arch and mirror image of coronary circulation. Horizontal axis mirror-image inversion of the angiographic views was used. A two-vessel coronary artery disease was diagnosed. There were a significant 70% stenosis at the proximal segment of the left anterior descending artery (LAD) and a right coronary artery (RCA) 90% stenosis in the distal segment.

On May 25, 2015, percutaneous coronary intervention (PCI) was performed with an extra-backup support EBU 3.5, 6 French guiding catheter with the standard Judkins technique, using inverted horizontal axis angiographic views of the left coronary artery, to mimic a left anterior oblique (LAO) with a cranial view for the left anterior descending artery (LAD), an inverted view; that is, to the other side, a right anterior oblique (RAO) view was used, to proceed with a direct stenting of the proximal segment stenosis of the LAD, implanting a 2.5 × 16 mm drug-eluting (everolimus) stent (Promus Premier, Boston Scientific) successfully (Figures 3(a) and 3(b)). Then, we proceeded to treat the right coronary artery 90% distal segment stenosis; for this, we used a right Judkins 3.5, 6F guiding catheter with horizontal mirror imaging, using a RAO view to mimic the LAO view; the anatomical right coronary artery was engaged easily using an opposite maneuver to the usual, with the tip of the catheter pointing leftward and rotated counterclockwise (instead of rotating clockwise), and then, we passed a Whisper 0.014 angioplasty guidewire and crossed the distal stenosis; predilatation was done with a 1.5 × 10 mm balloon (Apex, Boston Scientific), and then, a 2.5 × 12 mm zotarolimus-eluting stent (Resolute Integrity, Medtronic) was successfully implanted, obtaining excellent angiographic results and final TIMI grade 3 flow (Figures 4(a) and 4(b)).

The patient had an excellent in-hospital follow-up, without any symptoms and complications; there was no rise in cardiac biomarkers and was discharged after 48 hrs. With life style modification and receiving coated aspirin 81 mg/d, clopidogrel 75 mg/d, and atorvastatin 80 mg/d, a 3-month follow-up showed no recurrent ischemia, and a treadmill stress test (positioning electrodes to the right side) was performed which was negative.

3. Discussion

Dextrocardia is a rare cardiac anomaly of development, characterized by an opposite orientation of the apex to the

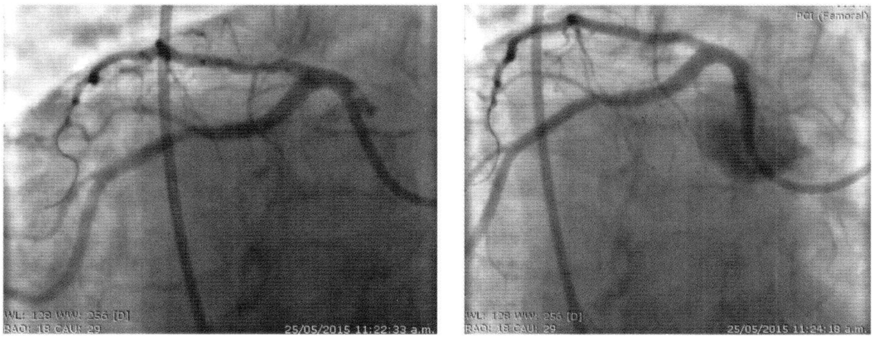

(a) (b)

Figure 3: Sequence of percutaneous intervention with drug-eluting stent implantation in the proximal segment of the LAD. (a) Pre-PCI: shows a 70% stenosis at the proximal segment of LAD (stent in posistion, preimplantation). (b) Post-PCI: DES implantation.

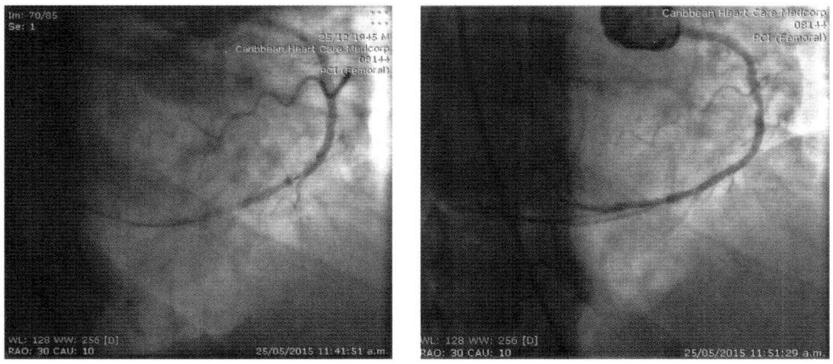

(a) (b)

Figure 4: (a, b) Sequence of stent implantation in the distal segment stenosis of the right coronary artery with previous balloon predilatation.

usual one; it is in the right hemithorax, with its axis directed to the right and caudally. This can occur with situs solitus or more frequently in association with situs viscerum inversus totalis (all the organs inverted); it can also be found as situs ambiguous. With situs solitus and situs inversus, the atrial situs always corresponds to the visceral situs; with situs ambiguous, the arrangement of the organs is not as ordered, and the relation between the atria and the viscera is inconsistent [1, 2, 4]. Dextrocardia with situs inversus is an infrequent condition occurring with an estimated range of 1 : 8000 to 1 : 10,000. In situs inversus totalis, the incidence of structural congenital heart disease is low, estimated to be near 3%. It is known that dextrocardia with situs inversus has a 15% association of another rare disease that affects primarily the respiratory tract and the epithelia of the sexual organs, the Kartagener syndrome (immotile cilia syndrome characterized by bronchitis, chronic sinusitis, and infertility in men). It is believed that these patients share the same risk as the general population to develop ischemic heart disease because of the high prevalence of atherosclerosis [4]. The majority of patients with dextrocardia and situs inversus totalis are ignorant of their variant anatomy until they are forced to seek medical attention, most frequently for cardiothoracic pathology [1, 4]. Our patient was not aware of his malposition syndrome until this admission, when he presented for the first time with acute coronary syndrome. The presence of coronary artery disease (CAD) in this population presents several challenges to the interventional cardiologists due to the abnormal anatomic position of the heart, usually right position of the aortic arch and unfamiliar coronary anatomy especially at their origin. Once the diagnosis of dextrocardia is made in the context of an acute coronary syndrome, a reversed or right-sided ECG should be done; this will show the exact localization of the infarct in an ST elevation myocardial infarction, particularly if it is in the anterior and/or lateral wall [5].

The first report of diagnostic cardiac catheterization in a patient with dextrocardia was done in 1973 by Hynes. Fourteen years later, Moreyra and coworkers in 1987 in the USA performed the first balloon angioplasty in a patient with dextrocardia and single-vessel CAD [6], and PCI with balloon angioplasty in a dextrocardia patient with multivessel CAD has been reported from Japan by Yoshimasa Yabe since 1995 [7, 8]. The first stent deployment in a patient with dextrocardia in situs inversus was performed in Italy by Patti et al. in 1999 [9].

This is the first case of diagnostic and therapeutic catheterization of dextrocardia in situs inversus totalis documented in Trinidad. It was our first encounter with this rare scenario, so we had to search and review the literature to understand and approach this variety of presentation. We learned that, with the inversion technique of mirror-image views, it was easier to approach the lesions and that, with the RCA, the inverted maneuver of counterclockwise rotation as suggested by Gaglani et al. in 1989 [10] made the difference in engaging it. Note that with the image inversion technique, one gets a partly normalized intended view in the horizontal axis, but the apex is always pointing to the opposite side of the conventional angiogram; that is, to the right, to correct this, the double inversion technique was developed.

Although we only used the inversion technique to facilitate the viewing, this does not normalize completely the views. There have been some advances applied to the newer fluoroscopy equipment such as the "horizontal sweep reverse" feature used in the method of double-inversion technique for coronary angiogram viewing in dextrocardia, developed by Goel. With this, the unfamiliar angulated coronary angiograms seen in dextrocardia are digitally corrected into a conventionally normal angiogram [11–12].

In dextrocardia patients, there are several considerations that should be taken into account: (1) image acquisition, a mirror image between LAO and RAO; using an image reversal technology will give an advantage to the operator for the intervention; (2) the technique of torque of the catheter, a reverse maneuver of the usual between clockwise and counterclockwise rotation for the RCA; (3) transfemoral access gives a better access, even though some reports of transradial approach are also good for dextrocardia cases; and (4) anatomical variation in dextrocardia, variable position of the aortic arch (left/right), will require different catheter selection, that is, in the presence of a right aortic arch, as in this case, but in a case with an isolated right aortic arch, a left Judkins catheter can be used to selectively cannulate the left coronary artery and is also able to cannulate a right-sided right coronary artery [9–12].

Acknowledgments

The authors thank Iván Machado H., MD, Professor of Cardiology, Pediatric Cardiology Section, Head Cardiology Department, Universidad Central de Venezuela, for his observations and corrections made, as a pediatric interventional cardiologist point of view.

References

[1] T. S. Dhanjal, P. Davison, and J. M. Cotton, "Primary percutaneous coronary intervention for acute myocardial infarction in a patient with dextrocardia," *Cardiology Journal*, vol. 16, no. 2, pp. 168–171, 2009.

[2] R. Vijayvergiya and A. Grover, "Percutaneous coronary intervention for acute myocardial infarction in a patient with dextrocardia," *World Journal of Cardiology*, vol. 2, no. 4, pp. 104–106, 2010.

[3] C. Pepine, J. A. Hill, and C. A. Lambert, *Diagnostic and Therapeutic Cardiac Catheterization*, Williams & Wilkins, Baltimore, USA, 3rd edition, 1998.

[4] D. Kawecki, W. Wojakowski, R. Wyderka et al., "Acute myocardial infarction in a patient with situs inversus totalis," *American Journal of Case Reports*, vol. 11, pp. 113–115, 2010.

[5] C. Johnson and E. Nicol, "Getting the right diagnosis: ST-elevation myocardial infarction in situs inversus," *Europa Heart Journal*, vol. 34, no. 7, p. 485, 2012.

[6] A. E. Moreyra, G. J. Saviano, and J. B. Kostis, "Percutaneous transluminal coronary angioplasty in situs inversus," *Catheterization and Cardiovascular Diagnosis*, vol. 13, no. 2, pp. 114–116, 1987.

[7] R. P. Sinha, D. Agarwal, A. M. Sarang et al., "Successful transradial percutaneous coronary intervention in a patient with dextrocardia and situs inversus," *Journal of Clinical and Diagnostic Research*, vol. 9, no. 1, pp. 4-5, 2015.

[8] Y. Yabe and R. Tsukahara, "Percutaneous transluminal coronary angioplasty for culprit lesions in patients with post myocardial infarction angina based on dextrocardia and anomalous coronary arteries," *Angiology*, vol. 46, pp. 431–440, 1995.

[9] G. Patti, A. D'Ambrosio, and G. Di Sciacio, "Coronary stenting in patients with situs viscerum inversus," *Giornale Italiano di Cardiologia*, vol. 29, pp. 304–307, 1999.

[10] R. Gaglani, D. K. Gabos, B. H. Sangani et al., "Coronary angioplasty in a patient with dextrocardia," *Catheter and Cardiovascular Diagnostics*, vol. 17, no. 1, pp. 45–47, 1989.

[11] M. Munawar, B. Hartono, K. Iskandarsyah, and T. N. Nguyen, "Successful percutaneous coronary intervention for chronic total occlusion of right coronary artery in patient with dextrocardia," *Cardiovascular Interventions and Therapeutics*, vol. 28, no. 3, pp. 303–306, 2013.

[12] K. T. Koh, S. Asri, Y. Y. Oon et al., "ST-elevation myocardial infarction in situs inversus dextrocardia: a case report," *Asean Heart Journal*, vol. 24, no. 1, pp. 122–124, 2016.

19

A Case of Lyme Carditis Presenting with Atrial Fibrillation

Peter J. Kennel,[1] Melvin Parasram,[2] Daniel Lu,[3] Diane Zisa,[1] Samuel Chung,[1] Samuel Freedman,[1] Katherine Knorr,[1] Timothy Donahoe,[1] Steven M. Markowitz,[3] and Hadi Halazun[3]

[1]*Department of Medicine, Weill Cornell Medicine, New York, NY, USA*
[2]*Department of Neurology, Weill Cornell Medicine, New York, NY, USA*
[3]*Department of Cardiology, Weill Cornell Medicine, New York, NY, USA*

Correspondence should be addressed to Hadi Halazun; hjh7001@med.cornell.edu

Academic Editor: Kjell Nikus

We report a case of a 20-year-old man who presented to our institution with a new arrhythmia on a routine EKG. Serial EKG tracings revealed various abnormal rhythms such as episodes of atrial fibrillation, profound first degree AV block, and type I second degree AV block. He was found to have positive serologies for *Borrelia burgdorferi*. After initiation of antibiotic therapy, the atrial arrhythmias and AV block resolved. Here, we present a case of Lyme carditis presenting with atrial fibrillation, a highly unusual presentation of Lyme carditis.

1. Background

Lyme disease is the most commonly reported vector-borne illness in the United States [1]. In 2016, 26,203 confirmed diagnoses of Lyme disease were reported [2]. The incidence of Lyme disease has been consistent over the last decade at approximately 8 cases per 100,000 persons in the US with 95% of confirmed Lyme disease cases reported from only 14 states, mostly in the Northeast region of the US. The most common clinical presentation of Lyme disease is erythema migrans (70%), followed by arthritis (30%), Bell's palsy (9%), radiculoneuropathy (4%), and meningitis/encephalitis (2%). Only 1% present with cardiac manifestations [3]. Cardiac manifestations of Lyme disease are rare but well described. Lyme carditis (LC) occurs in 0.3–4% of untreated adults with Lyme disease in Europe and in 1.5–10% of untreated adult patients in the United States [4]. For reasons yet to be determined, there is a male predominance of 3 to 1 in LC [5]. Cardiac involvement occurs during the early, disseminated phase of the disease [5], and cardiac symptoms can develop between the 7th day and the 7th month (median 21 days) after the onset of erythema migrans [4, 6]. Pathophysiologically, myocardial biopsy specimens usually show transmural inflammatory infiltrates with characteristic endocardial lymphocytic infiltrates and occasionally spirochetes [7]. Most cases of LC appear to be clinically asymptomatic. If symptomatic, typical presentations may be complaints of fatigue, dyspnea, palpitations, lightheadedness, syncope, and chest pain [8]. LC usually has a benign clinical course with complete resolution of symptoms. However, serious and even fatal cardiac complications have been reported, including fatal cardiac arrhythmias, myocarditis, cardiac tamponade, heart failure, and sudden cardiac death [4]. The typical cardiac presentations are various degrees of atrioventricular block [8, 9]. Rarely, LC has been reported to cause isolated bundle branch blocks or other conduction abnormalities [4, 8, 10]. There are rare reports of ventricular and supraventricular arrhythmias associated with LC. A recent case reported by Frank et al. describes a new-onset junctional tachycardia in a pediatric case of LC [11]. In another recent publication, Wenger et al. report a case of an adult man presenting with atrial fibrillation, complete atrioventricular block, and escape rhythm attributed to LC [12]. Here, we report a case of a young adult man with Lyme

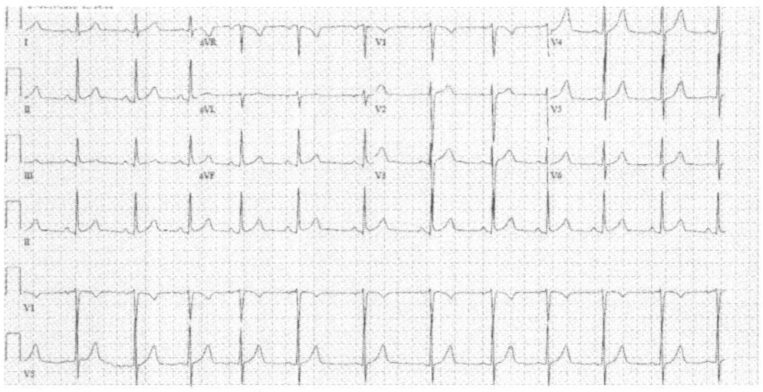

FIGURE 1: Baseline EKG. Normal sinus rhythm with a short PR interval.

disease presenting with atrial fibrillation, profound first degree AV block, and type I second degree AV block.

2. Case Presentation

A 20-year-old man was referred to our institution from an oncological clinic where he was undergoing maintenance chemotherapy for metastatic alveolar rhabdomyosarcoma. In routine EKG, there was concerning new EKG abnormalities with a possible new AV block. Prior EKGs had been without abnormal findings (Figure 1). Given the new EKG changes, the patient was admitted to an outside hospital for observation. Prior to his admission, the patient had been asymptomatic and had unlimited exercise capacity. He denied any tick bites or rashes in the recent past but reported that he had been hiking over the summer in Orange County, NY.

The patient had a medical history of left forearm alveolar rhabdomyosarcoma, diagnosed 16 months prior to this presentation for which he had undergone radiation therapy to his arm and chemotherapy including irinotecan, carboplatin, vincristine, doxorubicin (cumulative dose 300 mg/m^2; initial regimen, which had been completed), and a combination of cyclophosphamide, vinorelbine, and temsirolimus (maintenance chemotherapy regimen). Recent imaging including PET had shown no evidence of disease, and the patient was deemed to be in remission at the time of presentation. The patient's baseline EKG prior to his presentation showed a normal sinus rhythm with a PR interval of 152 msec (Figure 1).

The patient's home medications were sulfamethoxazole and trimethoprim prophylaxis, cyclophosphamide, and zolpidem. He was a lifetime nonsmoker, did not consume alcohol or illicit drugs, and lived with his family with no cardiac family history.

On arrival to our institution, the patient was asymptomatic. His blood pressure was 108/63 mmHg, heart rate was regular and between 80 and 115 bpm, he was afebrile at 36.4°C, and his oxygen saturation was 100% on room air. His physical exam was unremarkable, with no cardiopulmonary findings, no focal neurological deficits, and no abnormal skin findings. The initial EKG on admission revealed coarse atrial fibrillation with a ventricular rate of 60 beats per minute (Figure 2).

Initial laboratory results were only notable for a hemoglobin of 10.0 mg/dl, a mild relative lymphocytopenia with

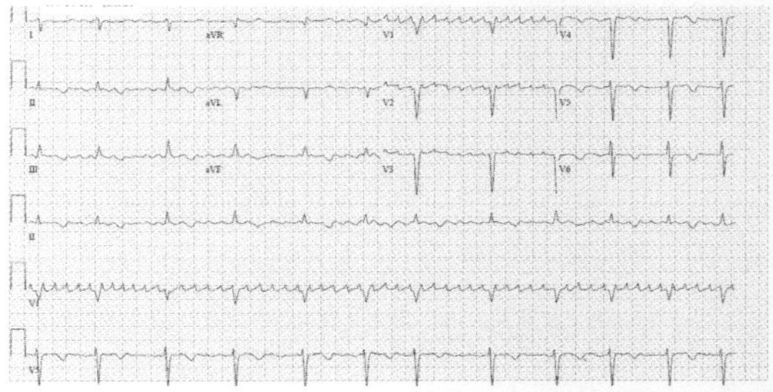

FIGURE 2: EKG on admission shows coarse atrial fibrillation with a slow ventricular response. Whereas the tracings in the precordial leads to appear organized, the tracing in lead II suggests coarse atrial fibrillation.

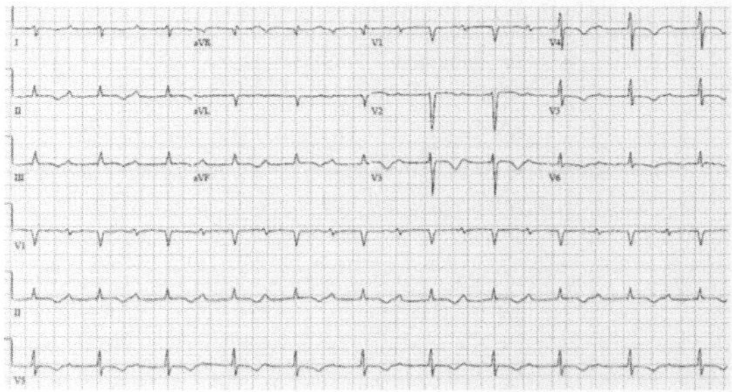

FIGURE 3: Profound PR prolongation.

a normal white blood cell count. TSH and troponin I levels were within normal limits. Echocardiogram showed normal left and right heart function with no wall motion abnormalities, mild tricuspid valve regurgitation, and no pericardial effusion.

A cardiac MRI, performed 2 days after presentation, showed mild right atrial dilatation and no other abnormalities. In particular, no signs of inflammation or masses were found. Additionally, on hospital day 2, telemetry monitoring and EKG revealed spontaneous conversion to normal sinus rhythm with a profoundly prolonged PR interval of 460 msec (Figure 3).

Further workup during the hospital course revealed a twice positive *B. burgdorferi* IgG and IgM immunoblot (performed at ARUP Laboratories; IgG: bands present: 66, 45, 41, 39, 23, and 18 kDa, IgM: bands present: 41 and 39 kDa).

3. Treatment

Given the positive Lyme serology in the setting of a new AV block and atrial fibrillation, antibiotic therapy with intravenous ceftriaxone (2 grams every 24 h) was initiated. The patient was monitored with daily EKGs and continued telemetry monitoring. Telemetry showed intermittent episodes of abrupt changes from relatively short to long PR intervals. Figure 4 shows an abrupt spontaneous shift from short to long PR. Abrupt shortening of the PR interval occurred following a late-coupled spontaneous premature ventricular complex (PVC) consistent with retrograde

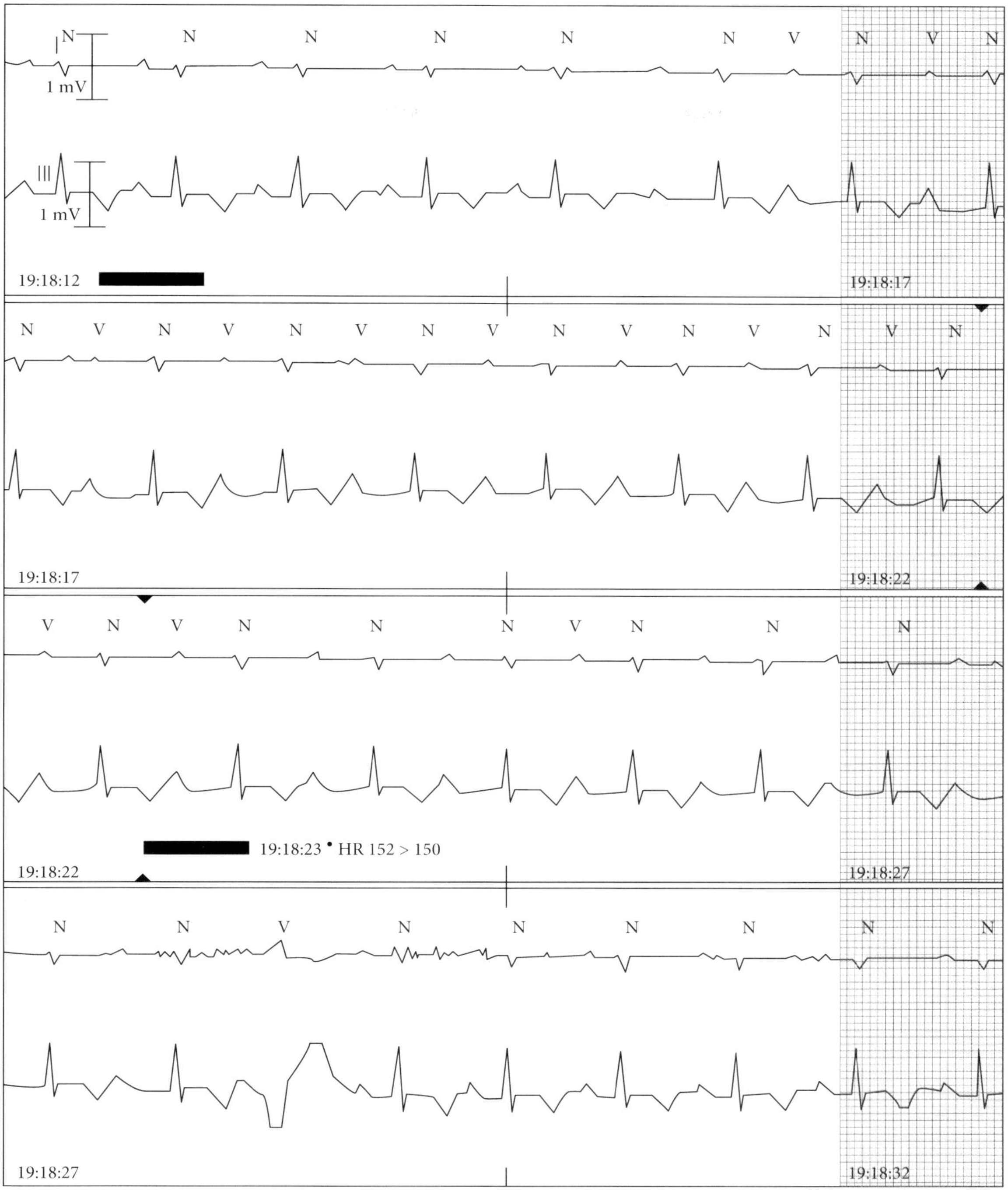

Figure 4: Abrupt change of PR intervals. Abrupt shift from relatively short PR to long PR (first line) and recurrent shift from long PR to shorter PR (last line). This second shift occurs after a PVC, which is a known phenomenon in which the PVC resets conduction to allow the fast pathway to conduct on the next beat.

concealed conduction into the AV node facilitating antegrade fast pathway conduction on the subsequent beats.

On continued antibiotic therapy, the patient remained in sinus rhythm with shortening PR intervals to 390 msec on the day of discharge. The patient was discharged with a 21-day course of home IV ceftriaxone, a home telemetry monitor, and close follow-up with our electrophysiology clinic.

4. Outcome

At home, an event monitor for 1 week showed no advanced AV block or profound bradycardia. Recorded events were a HR 53 to 137 bpm, average 85 bpm, 147 supraventricular runs up to 33 beats; no advanced AV blocks were recorded. Over the course of his antibiotic therapy, the PR interval on

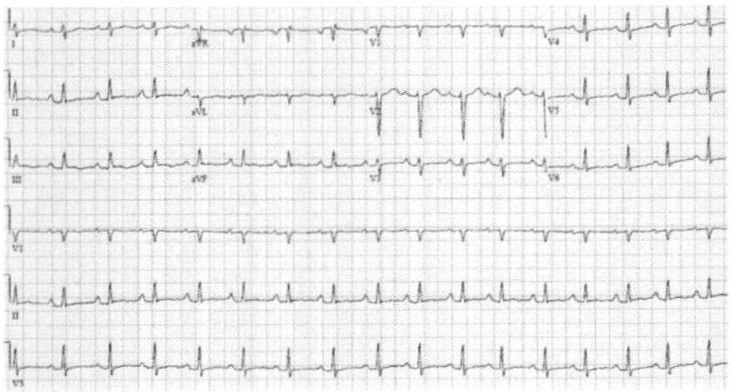

Figure 5: After antibiotic therapy, resolution of AV block.

serial EKG recordings shortened from 460 msec on admission to 184 msec after 3 weeks of intravenous ceftriaxone, without any evidence of episodes of higher degree AV blocks (Figure 5). At the end of his treatment, the PR intervals were consistently short.

5. Discussion

Here, we report a case of a young adult man with Lyme disease presenting with atrial fibrillation, profound first degree AV block, and type I second degree AV block. This is an unusual presentation of LC, in which AV block is a known entity; however, atrial fibrillation is highly unusual. Lyme disease is an overall rare disease with only around 26,000 cases reported in the US per year. Only around 4% of these cases will develop LC. Among these patients, the vast majority experiences some degree of AV block. To our knowledge, there are only anecdotal reports of LC presenting with supraventricular arrhythmias as we describe in the case at hand. Of note, the patient also had alterations in his PR interval, sometimes occurring from one beat to the next. This pattern suggests the presence of dual AV nodal physiology whereby abrupt PR prolongation occurs following antegrade block in the fast pathway. Dual atrial inputs are likely to be an intrinsic property of the AV node, but this manifestation of abrupt PR changes is rarely seen in normal individuals. Interestingly, this phenomenon has been reported as a manifestation of Lyme disease in another case report [13]. Decremental physiology of the fast pathway is favored by gradual PR prolongation until block occurs in the fast pathway and conduction proceeds down a slow AV nodal pathway. It is possible that Lyme carditis preferentially affected particular components of the AV node associated with the fast pathway.

While the patient was diagnosed with LC, a rare presentation of a rare disease, his past medical history was also notable for ARMS, a rare pediatric malignancy, which has an incidence of around 1 per 1 million. Notably, the patient was diagnosed with stage 4 disease with an overall poor prognosis, but underwent an experimental radiochemotherapeutic protocol and was deemed free of disease after completion of the treatment. Given his prior exposure to chemotherapeutic drugs, cardiotoxic effects of these agents needed to be reviewed as possible causes for his new-onset arrhythmias: the experimental chemotherapeutic regimen consisted of irinotecan, carboplatin, vincristine, cyclophosphamide and vinorelbine, and doxorubicin (Clinical Trials Identifier NCT00077285). While the aforementioned drugs are not associated with cardiotoxic effects, doxorubicin is known to be cardiotoxic and can cause atrial fibrillation [14]. However, atrial fibrillation would usually present as an acute cardiotoxic effect and unlikely as delayed cardiotoxicity. The patient had completed the chemotherapeutic regimen containing doxorubicin (cumulative dose 300 mg/m^2) around a year prior to the onset of atrial arrhythmias, and MRI and echocardiogram did not show signs of myocarditis or heart failure. Furthermore, the patient was exposed to a low cumulative dose of doxorubicine. Cardiac complications at comparable doses have been found to be as low as 0–2.8% [15]. Hence, it appears unlikely that the chemotherapeutic agents contributed to the cardiac findings.

Other rare differential diagnoses to consider in this case may be other causes for myocarditis or cardiomyopathies, familial syndromes such as Lenegre disease, cardiac tumors given his history of rhabdomyosarcoma, or syndromes in the rheumatologic realm. However, an extensive workup including cardiac MRI showing no evidence of structural abnormalities, signs of inflammation, or heart failure, repeat echocardiogram, and serologic studies including troponin, RPR, and toxoplasmosis remained unrevealing.

Our case report is limited in that we are unable to conclusively identify the cause of the new-onset atrial fibrillation in this patient as, even though serologies and response to antibiotic treatment hint towards LC being the cause for the arrhythmia, other causes cannot be excluded. Of note, given the finding of mild atrial dilation on cardiac MRI, it is possible that LC could have been a "second hit" in the setting of a preexisting abnormal substrate.

In summary, LC needs to be considered as a differential diagnosis in patients presenting with new-onset supraventricular arrhythmias if they may have been exposed to vectors of borrelia or live in endemic areas.

Acknowledgments

We thank Dr. Viktor Gamarnik and Donavan White for their contribution.

References

[1] https://www.cdc.gov/lyme/stats/index.html.

[2] https://www.cdc.gov/lyme/stats/tables.html.

[3] https://www.cdc.gov/lyme/stats/graphs.html.

[4] P. Rostoff, G. Gajos, E. Konduracka, A. Gackowski, J. Nessler, and W. Piwowarska, "Lyme carditis: epidemiology, pathophysiology, and clinical features in endemic areas," *International Journal of Cardiology*, vol. 144, no. 2, pp. 328–333, 2010.

[5] P. S. Munk, S. Ørn, and A. I. Larsen, "Lyme carditis: persistent local delayed enhancement by cardiac magnetic resonance imaging," *International Journal of Cardiology*, vol. 115, no. 3, pp. e108–e110, 2007.

[6] J. Cox and M. Krajden, "Cardiovascular manifestations of lyme disease," *American Heart Journal*, vol. 122, no. 5, pp. 1449–1455, 1991.

[7] N. Scheffold, B. Herkommer, R. Kandolf, and A. E. May, "Lyme carditis–diagnosis, treatment and prognosis," *Deutsches Arzteblatt International*, vol. 112, no. 12, pp. 202–208, 2015.

[8] T. Kostić, S. Momčilović, Z. D. Perišić et al., "Manifestations of Lyme carditis," *International Journal of Cardiology*, vol. 232, pp. 24–32, 2017.

[9] M. R. van der Linde, "Lyme carditis: clinical characteristics of 105 cases," *Scandinavian Journal of Infectious Diseases*, vol. 77, pp. 81–84, 1991.

[10] P. Lelovas, I. Dontas, E. Bassiakou, and T. Xanthos, "Cardiac implications of Lyme disease, diagnosis and therapeutic approach," *International Journal of Cardiology*, vol. 129, no. 1, pp. 15–21, 2008.

[11] D. B. Frank, A. R. Patel, G. R. Sanchez, M. J. Shah, and W. J. Bonney, "Junctional tachycardia in a child with Lyme carditis," *Pediatric Cardiology*, vol. 32, no. 5, pp. 689–691, 2011.

[12] N. Wenger, C. Pellaton, P. Bruchez, and J. Schläpfer, "Atrial fibrillation, complete atrioventricular block and escape rhythm with bundle-branch block morphologies: an exceptional presentation of Lyme carditis," *International Journal of Cardiology*, vol. 160, no. 1, pp. e12–e14, 2012.

[13] U. Rastogi and N. Kumars, "Lyme arrhythmia in an avid golfer: a diagnostic challenge and a therapeutic dilemma," *Journal of Atrial Fibrillation*, vol. 8, no. 5, p. 1378, 2016.

[14] Y. Kaakeh, B. R. Overholser, J. C. Lopshire, and J. E. Tisdale, "Drug-induced atrial fibrillation," *Drugs*, vol. 72, no. 12, pp. 1617–1630, 2012.

[15] A. M. Rahman, S. W. Yusuf, and M. S. Ewer, "Anthracycline-induced cardiotoxicity and the cardiac-sparing effect of liposomal formulation," *International Journal of Nanomedicine*, vol. 2, no. 4, pp. 567–583, 2007.

20

A Young Male with Severe Myocarditis and Skeletal Muscle Myositis

Abdalla Ibrahim,[1] **Eoghan Meagher**,[1] **Alexander Fraser**,[2] **and Thomas J. Kiernan**[1]

[1]*Cardiology Department, University Hospital Limerick, St. Nessan's Road, Dooradoyle, Limerick, Ireland*
[2]*Rheumatology Department, University Hospital Limerick, St Nessan's Road, Dooradoyle, Limerick, Ireland*

Correspondence should be addressed to Abdalla Ibrahim; abdalla.ibrahimmd@gmail.com

Academic Editor: Domingo A. Pascual-Figal

A 34-year-old male presented with retrosternal chest pain, fatigue, shortness of breath, and a history of a previous episode of myocarditis four years prior. He had elevated troponin T, normal skeletal muscle enzymes, and negative inflammatory markers. Cardiac magnetic resonance imaging (MRI) confirmed active myocarditis with extensive myocardial fibrosis and normal left ventricular ejection fraction (LVEF). His myocarditis symptoms resolved with steroids and anti-inflammatory treatment, but on closer questioning, he reported a vague history of long-standing calf discomfort associated with episodes of stiffness, fatigue, and flu-like symptoms. MRI of the lower legs consequently demonstrated active myositis in the calf muscles. Immunomodulatory therapy was commenced with good effect. The patient is undergoing regular follow-up in both cardiology and rheumatology outpatient departments. Repeated MRI of the legs showed significant interval improvement in his skeletal muscle myositis, and repeat cardiac MRI demonstrated the resolution of myocarditis along with persistent stable extensive myocardial fibrosis and preserved LVEF. The patient has returned to full-time work.

1. Introduction

The diagnosis of myocarditis remains challenging given the diverse nature of clinical presentations [1]. The exact incidence is difficult to determine since endomyocardial biopsy, the gold standard diagnostic test, is used infrequently [2]. It has been reported that as few as 10% of people with polymyositis present with a cardiac involvement as the initial feature of the disease compared to 70% of patients with known polymyositis who experience some cardiac involvement as their disease progresses [3]. Clinically significant cardiac involvement has rarely been reported in myositis patients [4], while subclinical manifestations more commonly present as conduction abnormalities and arrhythmias detected on electrocardiography (ECG) [5].

2. Case Presentation

A 34-year-old male was admitted to the hospital with recurrent episodes of retrosternal chest pain, fatigue, and shortness of breath with an elevated troponin T. He had suffered an acute episode of myocarditis four years previously requiring hospital admission. He had no other relevant medical history and no family history of cardiac disease. He is a nonsmoker and consumed alcohol occasionally. Clinical examination was unremarkable and did not show any evidence of heart failure or systemic disease. ECG showed normal sinus rhythm without any ischemic changes, and chest X-ray showed no evidence of infection or heart failure. Routine blood tests including antinuclear antibody, creatinine kinase (CK), rheumatoid factor, and C-reactive protein were all within normal limits apart from an elevated cardiac troponin T with a peak value of 2700 ng/l (<14 ng/l). Further extensive inflammatory, viral, and autoimmune screening was carried out and found to be negative. Subsequent coronary angiogram showed normal coronary arteries, and transthoracic echocardiography demonstrated left ventricular ejection fraction (LVEF) >55% with trace mitral regurgitation. Cardiac magnetic resonance imaging (MRI) demonstrated extensive subepicardial and midwall

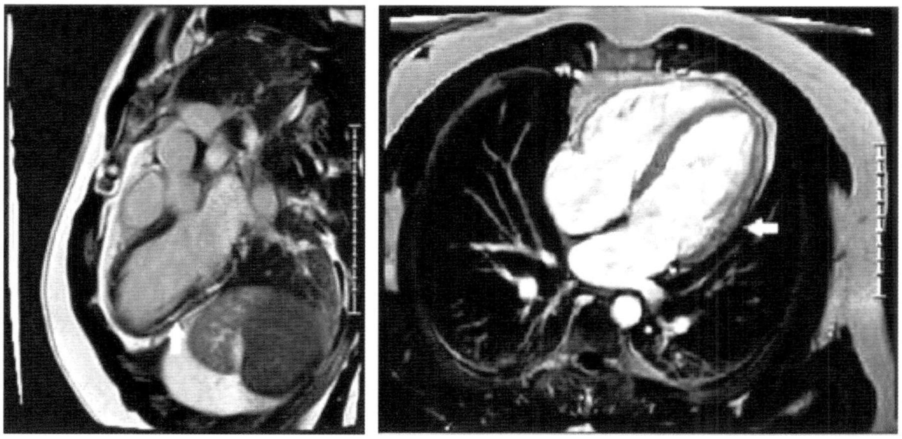

FIGURE 1: Cardiac MRI showing extensive subepicardial and midwall late enhancement typical of myocarditis in the anterior, lateral, and inferior walls.

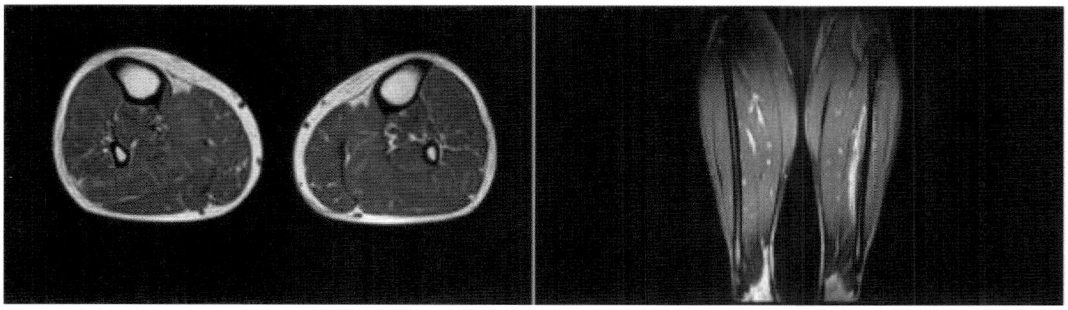

FIGURE 2: MRI of the left leg showing patchy increased STIR signal in the muscles but predominately involving the gastrocnemius muscles.

late enhancement typical of myocarditis in the anterior, lateral, and inferior walls along with extensive fibrosis with normal LVEF (Figure 1).

A short course of steroids and anti-inflammatory medication as an inpatient resulted in the resolution of his myocarditis symptoms. The troponin T level normalized and the patient was discharged with a plan to repeat cardiac MRI in six months. On follow-up as an outpatient, it was decided to refer the patient to rheumatology for an opinion regarding ongoing immunomodulatory therapy. At this juncture, the patient stated that he also had symptoms of stiffness and aching in his calf muscles for quite some time but he did not consider it to be relevant. Despite persistently normal skeletal muscle enzyme levels, an MRI of the lower legs was performed and this showed active myositis involving the gastrocnemius muscles bilaterally (Figure 2). As the patient was demonstrated to have ongoing myositis despite minimal symptoms, and as he had accrued significant myocardial scarring from previous episodes of myocarditis, it was decided to commence long-term immunomodulatory therapy in the form of methotrexate and prednisolone. Clinically, the patient reported a significant improvement in his symptoms and a repeat of the lower limb MRI demonstrated a significant interval improvement in his skeletal muscle myositis. Six months later, a repeat of the cardiac MRI demonstrated resolution of myocarditis along with persistent, stable, and extensive myocardial fibrosis and preserved LVEF (Figure 3). The patient is tolerating the immunomodulatory therapy well without major side effects, and he has returned to full-time work.

3. Discussion

We describe an elusive case of a young male with recurrent episodes of acute myocarditis presenting with chest pain and elevated troponin T. All biochemical, immune, and autoimmune tests were within normal limits. However, he described a long-standing and persistent history of calf aching and discomfort. Consequently, lower limb MRI revealed that the patient had active myositis of his gastrocnemius muscles. This unexpected finding demonstrated that this inflammatory myositis was not isolated to cardiac muscle and by definition was still active despite initial treatment. As this patient had already accrued significant myocardial scarring, the finding of active myositis demonstrated the need for more effective long-term immunomodulatory therapy in order to preserve cardiac function. Cardiac involvement in patients with skeletal myositis was first reported in 1899 [6]. Subclinical conduction abnormalities and arrhythmias discovered by ECG are considered to be more frequent

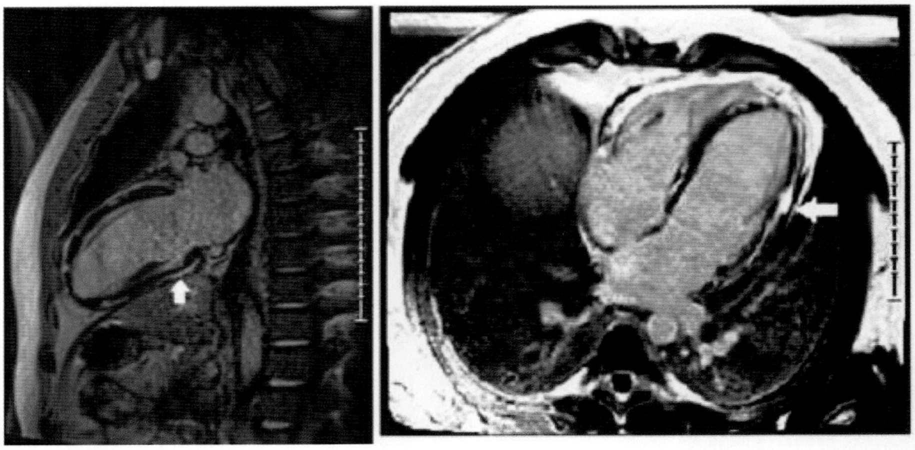

Figure 3: Cardiac MRI showing extensive epicardial and midwall fibrosis in the anterolateral, lateral, inferolateral, and inferior walls from base to apex.

than clinically manifest heart involvement [5]. The number of reported cases of clinically overt cardiac involvement in patients with myositis has increased recently, largely due to the increased use of noninvasive sensitive tests such as troponin [5]. The overall incidence of heart involvement in myositis patients ranges from 6% to 75% depending on the type (clinical or subclinical), definition of cardiac involvement, and tests used to confirm the diagnosis [3, 7]. Cardiovascular involvement is considered to be one of the major causes of mortality in patients with myositis [8, 9]. Mortality due to myocardial infarction in patients with myositis was reported to be increased by 16 times, especially among female patients [10]. Despite the lack of large epidemiological studies, cardiac involvement has been reported as a cause of death in 10–20% of patients with polymyositis [11, 12]. A number of cases of cardiac and skeletal myositis have been reported in the literature in which an underlying cause was identified. Kerr and Spiera reported six cases of myocarditis as a complication in scleroderma patients with myositis. In contrast to our patient, all of the six patients had an elevated CK, and five of them had reduced LVEF [13]. Infectious agents such as influenza virus and toxoplasma have been reported to cause polymyositis and myocarditis in a 4-year-old and a 13-year-old immunocompetent patient, respectively [14, 15]. Greaves et al. investigated the prevalence of myocarditis and skeletal myositis using CK, CK-MB, and troponin I/T in 152 adults with acute viral infection. The study showed that skeletal muscle injury was far more common than cardiac muscle injury in that cohort of patients [16]. Further literature review revealed a recently reported case of myocarditis and skeletal myositis in a 65-year-old following a seasonal influenza vaccination. Similar to our case, his myocarditis was diagnosed with cardiac MRI and an elevated troponin I, but in contrast to our case, his CK level was markedly elevated [17].

Our case is unique as there was no evidence from the history, clinical examination, or extensive laboratory investigations to indicate a specific aetiology of this man's myositis. Endomyocardial biopsy is the gold standard test for myocarditis; however, the clinical presentation in conjunction with the raised troponin level and a cardiac MRI demonstrating myocardial muscle oedema in keeping with myocarditis was considered sufficient to make a diagnosis without a myocardial biopsy, since such a procedure would be invasive and not without significant side effects. Consequently, the patient was noted to have calf muscle symptoms and MRI demonstrated skeletal muscle oedema in a distribution in keeping with skeletal muscle myositis. At this juncture, a skeletal muscle biopsy was proposed but the patient was not happy to consent to this procedure. However, in light of the history and clinical and MRI findings, it was considered reasonable to make a diagnosis of skeletal muscle myositis on a background of myocarditis and to treat the patient accordingly.

The first-line treatment of idiopathic inflammatory myositis is a high dose of corticosteroids (60–100 mg), which should be tapered after 4–6 weeks according to response [18]. Most patients require an additional immunosuppressive agent such as methotrexate, azathioprine, or mycophenolate mofetil [18]. There are very few studies comparing immunosuppressant regimes (azathioprine with methotrexate, cyclosporine with methotrexate, and intramuscular methotrexate with oral methotrexate plus azathioprine). They showed no statistically significant difference in efficacy between the treatment regimes [19]. We chose methotrexate due to our extensive experience with the drug and the fact that no trials have shown the superiority of one agent over the other. Other treatment options such as intravenous immunoglobulins, cyclophosphamide, and rituximab can be used but are reserved for severe or refractory cases [18].

In conclusion, we report a rare case of clinically significant cardiac and skeletal myositis whose cause is unclear. In patients with acute myocarditis, it is important to consider the possibility of an associated skeletal myositis when suggestive symptoms are present. MRI can be useful to establish the diagnosis particularly if laboratory tests are not conclusive. Further trials are needed to determine whether cardiac involvement is associated with certain types and subtypes of myositis or not.

References

[1] P. Richardson, W. McKenna, M. Bristow et al., "Report of the 1995 World Health Organization/International Society and Federation of Cardiology Task Force on the Definition and Classification of Cardiomyopathies," *Circulation*, vol. 93, no. 5, pp. 841-842, 1996.

[2] O. Leone, J. P. Veinot, A. Angelini et al., "2011 consensus statement on endomyocardial biopsy from the Association for European Cardiovascular Pathology and the Society for Cardiovascular Pathology," *Cardiovascular Pathology*, vol. 21, no. 4, pp. 245–274, 2012.

[3] J. S. Gottdiener, H. S. Sherber, R. J. Hawley, and W. K. Engel, "Cardiac manifestations in polymyositis," *The American Journal of Cardiology*, vol. 41, no. 7, pp. 1141–1149, 1978.

[4] I. E. Lundberg, "Cardiac involvement in autoimmune myositis and mixed connective tissue disease," *Lupus*, vol. 14, no. 9, pp. 708–712, 2005.

[5] I. E. Lundberg, "The heart in dermatomyositis and polymyositis," *Rheumatology*, vol. 45, Supplement_4, pp. iv18–iv21, 2006.

[6] H. Oppenheim, "Zur dermatomyositis," *Berliner Klinische Wochenschrift*, vol. 36, pp. 805–807, 1899.

[7] L. Gonzalez-Lopez, J. I. Gamez-Nava, L. Sanchez et al., "Cardiac manifestations in dermato-polymyositis," *Clinical and Experimental Rheumatology*, vol. 14, no. 4, pp. 373–379, 1996.

[8] K. Danko, A. Ponyi, T. Constantin, G. Borgulya, and G. Szegedi, "Long-term survival of patients with idiopathic inflammatory myopathies according to clinical features: a longitudinal study of 162 cases," *Medicine*, vol. 83, no. 1, pp. 35–42, 2004.

[9] A. Bohan, J. B. Peter, R. L. Bowman, and C. M. Pearson, "Computer-assisted analysis of 153 patients with polymyositis and dermatomyositis," *Medicine*, vol. 56, no. 4, pp. 255–286, 1977.

[10] R. Devere and W. G. Bradley, "Polymyositis: its presentation, morbidity and mortality," *Brain*, vol. 98, no. 4, pp. 637–666, 1975.

[11] S. M. Sultan, Y. Ioannou, K. Moss, and D. A. Isenberg, "Outcome in patients with idiopathic inflammatory myositis: morbidity and mortality," *Rheumatology*, vol. 41, no. 1, pp. 22–26, 2002.

[12] M. C. Hochberg, D. Feldman, and M. B. Stevens, "Adult onset polymyositis/dermatomyositis: an analysis of clinical and laboratory features and survival in 76 patients with a review of the literature," *Seminars in Arthritis and Rheumatism*, vol. 15, no. 3, pp. 168–178, 1986.

[13] L. D. Kerr and H. Spiera, "Myocarditis as a complication in scleroderma patients with myositis," *Clinical Cardiology*, vol. 16, no. 12, pp. 895–899, 1993.

[14] S. Tabbutt, M. Leonard, R. I. Godinez et al., "Severe influenza B myocarditis and myositis," *Pediatric Critical Care Medicine*, vol. 5, no. 4, pp. 403–406, 2004.

[15] P. K. Paspalaki, E. P. Mihailidou, M. Bitsori, D. Tsagkaraki, and E. Mantzouranis, "Polyomyositis and myocarditis associated with acquired toxoplasmosis in an immunocompetent girl," *BMC Musculoskeletal Disorders*, vol. 2, no. 1, 2001.

[16] K. Greaves, J. S. Oxford, C. P. Price, G. H. Clarke, and T. Crake, "The prevalence of myocarditis and skeletal muscle injury during acute viral infection in adults," *Archives of Internal Medicine*, vol. 163, no. 2, pp. 165–168, 2003.

[17] M. P. Cheng, M. G. Kozoriz, A. A. Ahmadi, J. Kelsall, K. Paquette, and J. M. Onrot, "Post-vaccination myositis and myocarditis in a previously healthy male," *Allergy, Asthma & Clinical Immunology*, vol. 12, no. 1, p. 6, 2016.

[18] A. Malik, G. Hayat, J. S. Kalia, and M. A. Guzman, "Idiopathic inflammatory myopathies: clinical approach and management," *Frontiers in Neurology*, vol. 7, p. 64, 2016.

[19] P. A. Gordon, J. B. Winer, J. E. Hoogendijk, and E. H. S. Choy, "Immunosuppressant and immunomodulatory treatment for dermatomyositis and polymyositis," *Cochrane Database of Systematic Reviews*, no. 8, article CD003643, 2012.

Successful Rotational Atherectomy for an Angulated Calcified Lesion in an Anomalous Right Coronary Artery Using the "Mother-and-Child" Technique

Manabu Ogita,[1] Satoru Suwa,[1] Taketo Sonoda,[1] Shuta Tsuboi,[1] Katsumi Miyauchi,[2] and Hiroyuki Daida[2]

[1]*Department of Cardiology, Juntendo University Shizuoka Hospital, Izunokuni, Japan*
[2]*Department of Cardiovascular Medicine, Juntendo University Graduate School of Medicine, Tokyo, Japan*

Correspondence should be addressed to Manabu Ogita; m-ogita@sa2.so-net.ne.jp

Academic Editor: Hajime Kataoka

Percutaneous coronary intervention (PCI) involving the anomalous coronary artery is challenging with respect to difficulty in achieving stable catheterization. Rotational atherectomy (RA) can facilitate severely calcified lesions to improve stent delivery and stent expansion; however, its utility in tortuous and angulated coronary arteries is limited with difficulty in delivery of the RA burr. The mother-and-child technique is effective for complex PCIs with increased backup force for device delivery in such complicated cases. We report a case of successful rotational atherectomy using the "mother-and-child" technique with a Dio thrombus aspiration catheter for an angulated calcified lesion in an anomalous origin of the right coronary artery.

1. Introduction

Coronary artery anomalies are a diverse group of congenital disorders that are found in 5% of the population [1]. Anomalous origin of the right coronary artery (RCA) accounts for 10% of all anomalous coronary artery cases [2]. Percutaneous coronary intervention (PCI) involving the anomalous coronary artery is challenging with respect to selection of the guide catheter, insufficient backup force, and device delivery. The mother-and-child technique is useful for improving backup support and delivery of stents in such lesions [3]. Rotational atherectomy (RA) can facilitate lesion and stent expansion in severely calcified lesions especially in patients undergoing hemodialysis [4]; however, its utility is limited in tortuous and angulated coronary arteries, with an increased risk of vessel perforation and difficulty in delivery of the RA burr. We describe a case of successful rotational atherectomy for an angulated calcified lesion in the anomalous right coronary artery using the "mother-and-child" technique.

2. Case Presentation

A 46-year-old man with end-stage renal disease due to diabetic nephropathy was referred to our institution for percutaneous coronary intervention (PCI) for a severe calcified lesion in an anomalous right coronary artery. He had been undergoing hemodialysis three times a week for 3 years. Since patients with diabetic ESRD are at a high risk for coronary artery disease, coronary computed tomography angiography (CTA) had been performed at his previous hospital visit, which revealed multivessel disease. Coronary angiography (CAG) showed severe stenosis in the mid-portion of the left anterior descending (LAD) artery and a chronic total occlusion (CTO) in the proximal portion of the right coronary artery with an anomalous origin. Hence, PCI of the LAD lesion was first performed, and a bioresorbable polymer sirolimus-eluting stent (Ultimaster 3.0 × 38 mm and 3.0 × 33 mm, TERUMO, Tokyo, Japan) was successfully implanted at the previous hospital. Staged PCI for CTO of the RCA was performed with successful wire

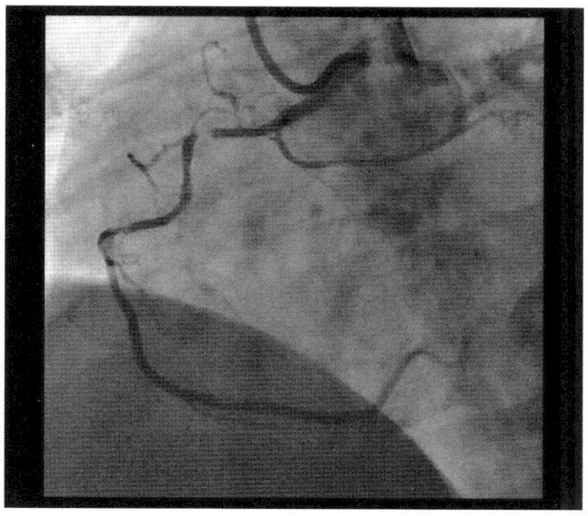

Figure 1: The left anterior oblique coronary angiography view showed severe calcified stenosis of the proximal segment of the right coronary artery (RCA) with anomalous origin.

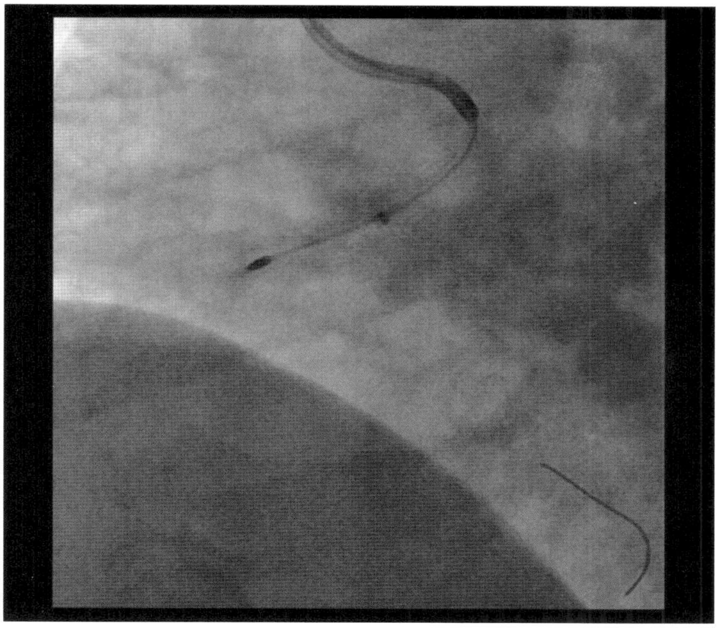

Figure 2: Advancement of a 1.5 mm burr through the Dio thrombus aspiration catheter.

crossing and recanalization. However, since subsequent standard balloon angioplasty was unsuccessful, he was referred to our hospital for PCI of the anomalous RCA.

CAG demonstrated residual severely calcified stenosis in the proximal RCA with patent antegrade coronary flow (Figure 1). We selected right femoral access with a long sheath using a 7 Fr Amplatz left 2 guiding catheter (Asahi Intecc, Tokyo, Japan) in consideration of size up to a 2.0 mm burr. A SION blue wire (Asahi Intecc) was advanced into the distal RCA using a microcatheter (Caravel, Asahi Intecc) and intravascular ultrasonography (IVUS; OptiCross, Boston Scientific Corp., MA, USA). Based on the IVUS findings, which indicated severe circumferential calcification with a minimal luminal diameter larger than 1.25 mm, we decided to perform rotational atherectomy with a 1.5 mm burr (Boston Scientific Corp., MA, USA). For this, the first wire was exchanged for an extrasupport RotaWire (Boston Scientific) using the microcatheter. To obtain greater backup force, a Dio thrombus aspiration catheter (Goodman Co. Ltd., Aichi, Japan) was inserted into the RCA. The burr was successfully delivered to the anomalous RCA with dynaglide because we had difficulty advancing the burr manually. Halfway ablation with a 1.5 mm burr at 200,000 rpm was attempted several times, taking care not to advance the burr beyond the angle [5], although subsequent CAG and IVUS did not show the effective lesion modification after ablation. Then, we switched to balloon angioplasty with a 2.5 mm high-pressure balloon (NC Emerge 2.5 × 12 mm, Boston Scientific) and a 2.5 mm cutting balloon (Flextome 2.5 × 10 mm, Boston Scientific), but it was not enough to dilate the lesion. Finally, we switched back to rotational atherectomy and were subsequently able to pass the burr beyond the angulated calcified lesion without complications (Figure 2) and confirmed a crack using IVUS. Following

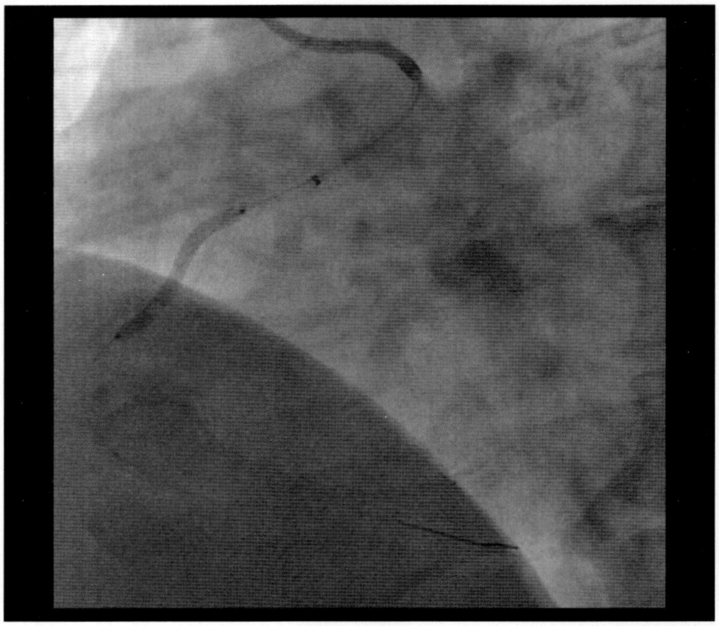

FIGURE 3: Successful stent deployment within the lesion.

effective dilation with a 3.0 mm high-pressure balloon (CELUSUS 3.0 × 8 mm, NIPRO, Osaka, Japan), we deployed a bioresorbable polymer everolimus-eluting stent (Synergy 2.5 × 24 mm, Boston Scientific) (Figure 3). The stent was additionally dilated with a noncompliance balloon (CELUSUS 3.0 × 8 mm, NIPRO, Osaka, Japan). A final coronary angiogram showed adequate and favorable dilatation of the culprit lesion (Figure 4).

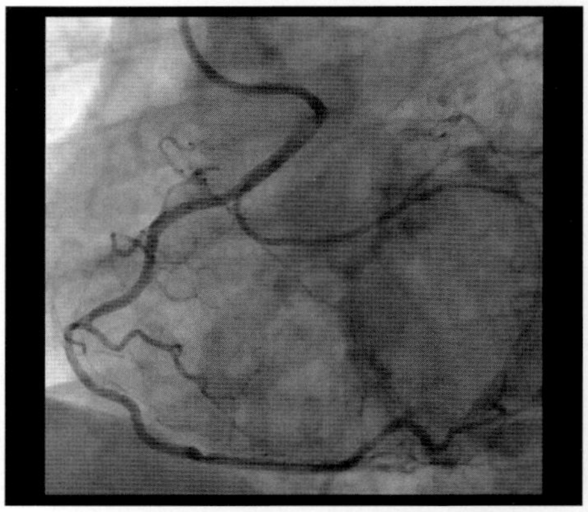

FIGURE 4: Final angiographic results after stent implantation and after dilatation.

3. Discussion

We report a case of successful rotational atherectomy for an angulated calcified lesion in an anomalous right coronary artery using the "mother-and-child" technique. PCI for the anomalous RCA can be associated with difficulty in achieving stable catheterization, leading to reduced backup support and device delivery failure. Rotational atherectomy (RA) can facilitate lesion and stent expansion in severely calcified lesions, although its utility is limited in tortuous and angulated coronary arteries, with an increased risk of complications. Appropriate guiding catheter selection is a key step to ensure successful PCI in such cases.

The mother-and-child technique is effective for complex PCIs, as it increases the backup force through deep catheterization of the target vessel and facilitates device delivery in tortuous or calcified lesions. Several mother-and-child catheters have been introduced in clinical practice (Table 1). The GuideLiner catheter is a guide extension catheter with the monorail system which permits rapid exchange and now is, hence, increasingly used [6]. Only a few cases have been previously reported of use of the mother-and-child technique to deliver rotational atherectomy burrs. Vo et al. first reported the use of the GuideLiner catheter to deliver rotational atherectomy burrs in tortuous vessels [7]. Costanzo et al. also reported GuideLiner-facilitated rotational atherectomy in calcified right coronary arteries [8]. However, the mother-and-child technique for rotablation has not been well established. To the best of our knowledge, this is the first report of RA using the mother-and-child technique in an RCA with anomalous origin.

In our case, we selected the conventional mother-child catheter, the 5 Fr Dio aspiration catheter for the following reasons. First, the 5 Fr Dio thrombus aspiration catheter has the RX-type inner catheter which facilitates smooth delivery and deep insertion of the outer catheter into the anomalous RCA. The relatively large inner lumen size of the outer catheter (1.51 mm) can provide the strong backup force for device delivery. Second, there is a concern that the rapid exchange transition zone of GuideLiner can lead to less backup support, difficulty in delivering the burr, and increase in the risk of burr entrapment. Thus, we thought that the Dio thrombus aspiration catheter can provide stronger backup support in our patient with rather complicated

Table 1: Design comparison of the guide extension catheter available in Japan and Dio thrombus aspiration catheter.

	Guidezilla II (Boston Scientific)	GuideLiner V3 (Lifeline)	Guideplus (NIPRO)	Dio (Goodman)
Sizes	6 Fr, 7 Fr, 8 Fr, and 6 Fr long	5.5 Fr, 6 Fr, 7 Fr	6 Fr	5 Fr
Inner lumen		1.30 mm (5.5 Fr)	1.30 mm (6 Fr)	1.51 mm (5 Fr)
	1.45 mm (6 Fr)	1.42 mm (6 Fr)		
	1.60 mm (7 Fr)	1.57 mm (7 Fr)		
	1.83 mm (8 Fr)	1.80 mm (8 Fr)		
Outer lumen		1.60 mm (5.5 Fr)	1.50 mm (6 Fr)	1.72 mm (5 Fr)
	1.45 mm (6 Fr)	1.70 mm (6 Fr)		
	1.60 mm (7 Fr)	1.90 mm (7 Fr)		
	2.11 mm (8 Fr)	2.16 mm (8 Fr)		
Guide segment length	25 cm/40 cm (6 Fr long)	25 cm	25 cm	
Working length	150 cm	150 cm	145 cm	124 cm
Coating	Z-glide (hydrophilic)	Silicon wipe (hydrophilic)	Hydrophilic	Hydrophilic

anatomy. Komatsu et al. reported successful PCI in an anomalous RCA using the Dio thrombus aspiration catheter [9]. This catheter allows not only stent delivery but also rotating burr delivery to severe calcified lesions in anomalous RCAs and can be a useful adjunctive device for rotational atherectomy. It is essential for operators to position the burr distal to the Dio thrombus aspiration catheter to prevent potential damage and shear of the child catheter. In summary, the "mother-and-child" technique is useful for rotational atherectomy in anomalous angulated RCAs. Rotablation with a Dio thrombus aspiration catheter is a potential therapeutic strategy in such complicated cases.

4. Conclusion

We report a case of successful rotational atherectomy using the "mother-and-child" technique with a Dio thrombus aspiration catheter for an angulated calcified lesion in an anomalous origin of the right coronary artery.

Acknowledgments

The authors thank all the nurses and technicians of the cath lab in Juntendo Shizuoka Hospital for their professional contributions and assistance.

References

[1] P. Angelini, "Coronary artery anomalies: an entity in search of an identity," *Circulation*, vol. 115, no. 10, pp. 1296–1305, 2007.

[2] O. Yamanaka and R. E. Hobbs, "Coronary artery anomalies in 126,595 patients undergoing coronary angiography," *Catheterization and Cardiovascular Diagnosis*, vol. 21, no. 1, pp. 28–40, 1990.

[3] S. Takahashi, S. Saito, S. Tanaka et al., "New method to increase a backup support of a 6 French guiding coronary catheter," *Catheterization and Cardiovascular Interventions*, vol. 63, no. 4, pp. 452–456, 2004.

[4] M. I. Tomey, A. S. Kini, and S. K. Sharma, "Current status of rotational atherectomy," *JACC: Cardiovascular Interventions*, vol. 7, no. 4, pp. 345–353, 2014.

[5] K. Sakakura, Y. Taniguchi, M. Matsumoto, H. Wada, S. I. Momomura, and H. Fujita, "How should we perform rotational atherectomy to an angulated calcified lesion?," *International Heart Journal*, vol. 57, no. 3, pp. 376–379, 2016.

[6] C. Cola, F. Miranda, B. Vaquerizo, A. Fantuzi, and J. Bruguera, "The GuideLiner™ catheter for stent delivery in difficult cases: tips and tricks," *Journal of Interventional Cardiology*, vol. 24, no. 5, pp. 450–461, 2011.

[7] M. Vo, K. Minhas, M. Kass, and A. Ravandi, "Novel use of the GuideLiner catheter to deliver rotational athetectomy burrs in tortuous vessels," *Case Reports in Cardiology*, vol. 2014, Article ID 594396, 5 pages, 2014.

[8] P. Costanzo, K. Aznaouridis, S. Hoye, and A. Alahmar, "GuideLiner-facilitated rotational atherectomy in calcified right coronary artery: the "child" makes the difference," *JACC: Cardiovascular Interventions*, vol. 9, no. 5, pp. e47–e48, 2016.

[9] T. Komatsu, I. Yaguchi, and T. Yufu, "Successful percutaneous coronary intervention of an anomalous right coronary artery with high anterior takeoff using a DIO thrombus aspiration catheter," *Journal of Invasive Cardiology*, vol. 24, no. 9, pp. E185–E187, 2012.

22

A Combination of Tachycardia-Mediated Heart Failure and Coronary Artery Vasospasm-Induced Silent Myocardial Infarction in a Patient with Severe Thyrotoxicosis

Serena Sert Kim Khoo,[1] **Chong Mow Chu**,[2] **and Yin Khet Fung**[1]

[1]*Endocrinology Unit, Queen Elizabeth Hospital II, Kota Kinabalu, Sabah, Malaysia*
[2]*Cardiology Department, Queen Elizabeth Hospital II, Kota Kinabalu, Sabah, Malaysia*

Correspondence should be addressed to Serena Sert Kim Khoo; sk_liv@rocketmail.com

Academic Editor: Manabu Shirotani

Severe thyrotoxicosis can present with a myriad of cardiovascular complications. It may be mild features such as palpitations, tachycardia, and exertional dyspnea or may progress to life-threatening consequences such as atrial fibrillation, tachyarrhythmias, heart failure, myocardial infarction, and shock. In rare cases, they may present with myocardial ischemia secondary to coronary artery vasospasm. We report a case of a 59-year-old Malay gentleman who presented with fast atrial fibrillation and tachycardia-mediated heart failure that evolved to a silent myocardial infarction secondary to severe coronary artery vasospasm with undiagnosed severe thyrotoxicosis. He had complete resolution of heart failure and no further recurrence of coronary artery vasospasm once treatment for thyrotoxicosis was initiated and euthyroidism achieved. This life-threatening consequence has an excellent prognosis if recognised early and treated promptly.

1. Introduction

The cardiovascular manifestations from hyperthyroidism are well described and may include palpitations, tachycardia, exercise intolerance, dyspnea on exertion, widened pulse pressure, and atrial fibrillation that can evolve to tachyarrhythmias, heart failure, cardiovascular collapse, and shock in the acute setting of thyroid storm [1]. In rare instances, patients with hyperthyroidism can experience angina suggestive of myocardial ischemia either due to known or suspected underlying ischemic heart disease or secondary to coronary artery vasospasm (CAS) [2].

We report the case of a patient with severe thyrotoxicosis who presented with a spectrum of cardiovascular complications of fast atrial fibrillation and congestive cardiac failure who developed silent acute myocardial infarction as a consequence of severe diffuse coronary artery vasospasm.

2. Case Report

A 59-year-old previously healthy Malay gentleman presented with progressive worsening dyspnea, orthopnea, and paroxysmal nocturnal dyspnea for 1 month. He had no angina, palpitations, or ankle oedema. He had a 20-pack-year smoking history but had no other cardiovascular risk factors. He also had epigastric discomfort and vomiting.

Physical examination revealed a thin, restless but oriented man. His vital signs were as follows: blood pressure of 130/87 mmHg, irregular pulse rate of 150 beats/min, respiratory rate of 32/min, and temperature of 37.3°C. Cardiovascular examination revealed a raised jugular venous pressure, displaced apex beat, bibasal crepitations, and minimal ankle oedema. His baseline laboratory findings on admission are listed in Table 1.

ECG on presentation showed fast atrial fibrillation with a ventricular rate of 156 beats per minute (Figure 1). Chest X-ray revealed signs of pulmonary congestion and cardiomegaly. Echocardiography showed mild to moderate left ventricular dysfunction with left ventricular ejection function of 40–50% with moderate mitral regurgitation, severe tricuspid regurgitation, and impaired right ventricular function. The mean estimated pulmonary artery pressure is 31 mmHg. No diastolic study was done in view of atrial fibrillation.

Table 1: Laboratory findings on admission.

	Result	Normal
FBC		
Hb	12.9 g/dl	13–17
Platelet	264	150–410
WBC	12.9	4–10
Renal		
Na^+	141 mmol/L	136–145
K^+	4.9 mmol/L	3.5–5.1
Urea	8.5 mmol/L	3–9.2
Creatinine	70 μmol/L	63.6–110.5
Liver function		
Total protein	73 g/L	64–83
Albumin	29 g/L	38–54
ALT	256 U/L	0–55
ALP	142 U/L	40–150
AST	269 U/L	5–34
Coagulation		
PT	18.9 s	12.2–14.3
PTT	43 s	34.1–45.8
Cardiac		
hs-Trop	74.4 pg/mL	<34.2
CK	26 U/L	30–200
LDH	230 U/L	125–220

He was admitted and stabilised in the CCU and commenced on intravenous frusemide infusion, spironolactone 12.5 mg daily, carvedilol 9.375 mg twice daily, perindopril 2 mg daily, and thiamine and anticoagulated with s/c Clexane. The next day, he was noted to have fluctuating ST segment elevation on the cardiac monitor but was asymptomatic. An immediate ECG revealed marked ST segment elevation in leads II, III, aVF, and V1–V4 with ST depression in I, aVL, and V5-V6 with atrial fibrillation and bradycardia (Figure 2). Minutes later, he developed cardiogenic shock with a blood pressure of 68/43 mmHg and bradycardia.

An immediate coronary angiography was performed which revealed diffuse coronary artery vasospasm. Diffuse small caliber vessels were demonstrated in the left coronary artery (Figure 3(a)) and the right coronary artery (Figure 3(b)). Following intracoronary injection of 200 mcg nitroglycerin, the caliber of the vessel improved significantly as visualized in Figure 3(c) for the left coronary artery and Figure 3(d) for the right coronary artery. There was improvement in myocardial brushing, and no coronary artery stenosis was seen. He was commenced on continuous nitroglycerin infusion, and ST elevation reduced remarkably after coronary angiogram.

He developed transient episodes of bradycardia after procedure and required IV atropine and IV adrenaline and brief cardiopulmonary resuscitation. The patient was treated with IV infusion of nitroglycerin and titrated according to the ECG and clinical symptoms.

Later, on further questioning, he had thyrotoxic symptoms of heat intolerance, sweating, weight loss, and muscle weakness for several months. He had not noticed any neck swelling, obstructive symptoms, or visual symptoms. On reexamination, he had fine tremors, lid retraction, lid lag, and bilateral mild proptosis to suggest Graves' ophthalmopathy. There was a grade II diffuse goiter with no thyroid bruit. His Burch-Wartofsky score was 65 (>45) (Table 2).

Thyroid function test results were as follows: free T_4 61.6 pmol/L (normal range: 9–25), free T_3 21.8 pmol/L (normal range: 3.5–6.5), and TSH 0.001 uIU/ml (normal range: 0.4–4.7). There was no TSH receptor antibody level.

He was commenced on IV hydrocortisone, carbimazole, oral Lugol's iodine, propranolol, Cardiprin, warfarin, and oral mononitrates. He improved remarkably with complete resolution of hyperthyroid and heart failure symptoms 3 weeks after. He reverted back to sinus rhythm, and his repeat echocardiogram showed marked improvement of his left ventricular and right ventricular function, LVEF 60–65%, and pulmonary pressure not raised demonstrated by no significant TR and PR. His thyroid function test 2 months after improved with FT_4 15.21 pmol/L (9–19) and TSH < 0.01 uIU/ml, and he was scheduled for a radioactive iodine therapy.

3. Discussion

This report highlights a spectrum of cardiac complications in a patient with delayed diagnosis of severe thyrotoxicosis presenting with fast atrial fibrillation and heart failure evolving into a painless acute myocardial infarction secondary to diffuse severe coronary vasospasm.

Thyrotoxicosis affects the cardiovascular system via T_3-mediated effects by increasing cardiac contractility, enhancing systolic and diastolic function, decreasing systemic vascular resistance and increasing circulating blood volume leading to increased preload, decreased afterload, and therefore increasing cardiac output by up to 300% from a euthyroid state [3].

This patient presented with classical tachycardia-mediated heart failure and fast atrial fibrillation. This mechanism led to an increased level of cytosolic calcium during diastole with reduced ventricular contractility and diastolic dysfunction. Increase in pulmonary artery pressure as in this case is contributory and a recognised cause of isolated right heart failure. In addition, 5% to 15% of thyrotoxic patients with atrial fibrillation are most likely to develop heart failure [3]. Beta-blockers can provide immediate relief of heart failure symptoms by slowing the heart rate and improving left ventricular function; however, cautious use in patients with true heart failure is advised. Marked symptoms resolution is seen upon attaining euthyroidism [4].

This case was further complicated with the development of painless acute myocardial infarction secondary to diffuse severe coronary vasospasm. The prevalence rate of coronary artery vasospasm with thyrotoxicosis is reported about 7.4% occurring more frequently in females, with age ranging between 44 and 75 years, and in Asians [5]. Smoking is a major risk factor for coronary artery vasospasm, and in this case it may be contributory [6].

Patients with coronary vasospasm with thyrotoxicosis typically present with either resting or exertional angina or syncope. However, it is important to note that the incidence of silent myocardial ischemia secondary to coronary vasospasm

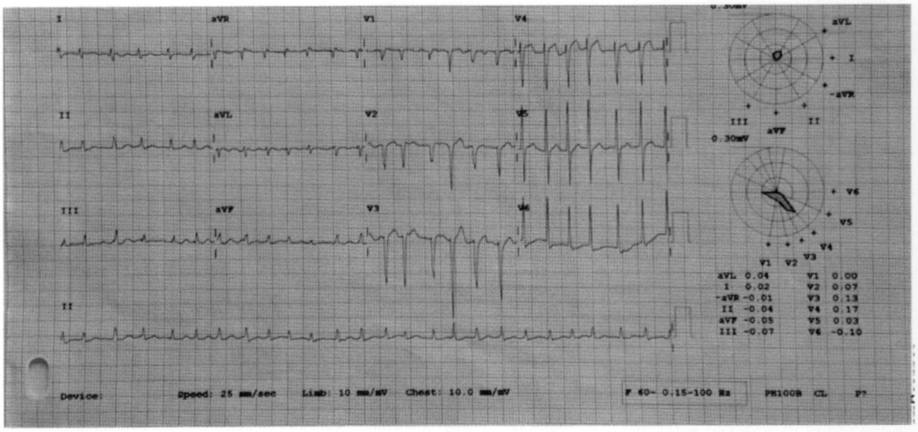

Figure 1: ECG on admission showing fast atrial fibrillation.

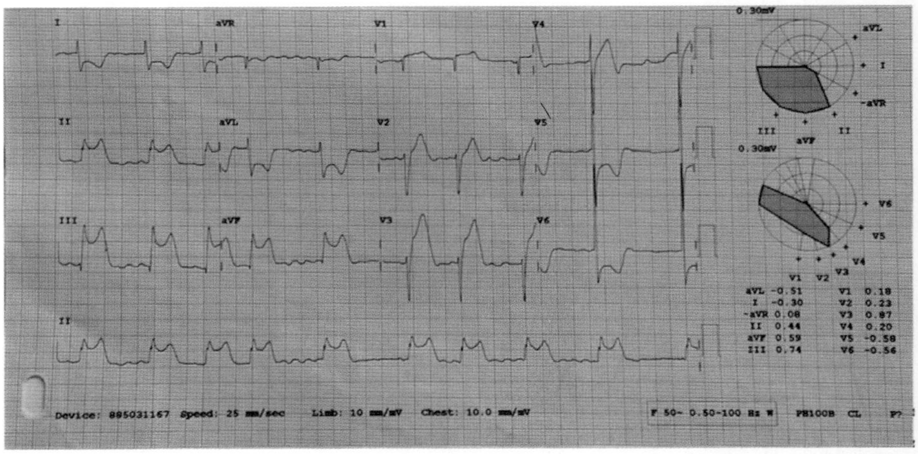

Figure 2: An immediate 12-lead ECG recorded atrial fibrillation with bradycardia and ST elevation in leads II, III, avF, and V1–V4 with ST depression in I, aVL, and V5-V6.

is more than twice than that of symptomatic ischemia [7] as in this case where the phenomenon was detected incidentally from ECG or cardiac monitoring.

Lee et al. described that coronary vasospasm with thyrotoxicosis presented with a higher incidence of acute myocardial infarction and angiographically had normal coronary arteries and were more spontaneous, diffuse, involving the left main vessel, and medically intractable compared to those without thyrotoxicosis [8]. This patient's presentation and angiographic findings were spontaneous, diffuse, and involving both coronary arteries and responded remarkably to intracoronary nitroglycerin.

The mechanism for the intensive spasm is still unclear. However, Napoli et al. demonstrated that vascular endothelium is a specific target of thyroid hormone evidenced by marked basal vasodilation contributed by excessive endothelial nitric oxide production coupled by exaggerated vascular reactivity because of enhanced sensitivity of the endothelial component and increased vasoconstrictory response to norepinephrine during the hyperthyroid state. This abnormal vasoconstrictory response reverses when euthyroidism is achieved [9]. This phenomenon not only involves the coronary arteries but also reported cerebrovascular occlusive disease (Moyamoya phenomenon) in uncontrolled Graves' disease that may share the same mechanism for acute vasospasm of the cerebral arteries [2].

Even though the clinical presentation of tachycardia-mediated heart failure along with CAS with thyrotoxicosis was severe, the clinical course became stable with excellent prognosis once the patient achieved euthyroidism [10, 11]. An important lesson to learn is the prompt clinical recognition and diagnosis of thyrotoxicosis as a cause of heart failure and coronary vasospasm. In this case, once the diagnosis of severe thyrotoxicosis was made and treatment initiated, the patient gradually improved with resolution of heart failure and hyperthyroid symptoms, reversion back to sinus rhythm, and improvement in echocardiogram findings and thyroid function levels.

4. Conclusion

Severe thyrotoxicosis can manifest with a myriad of cardiac complications. Tachycardia-mediated heart failure along with atrial fibrillation and coronary artery vasospasm is a life-threatening consequence of thyrotoxicosis, and the delay in diagnosis and treatment of hyperthyroidism in these patients may result in complications and unnecessary

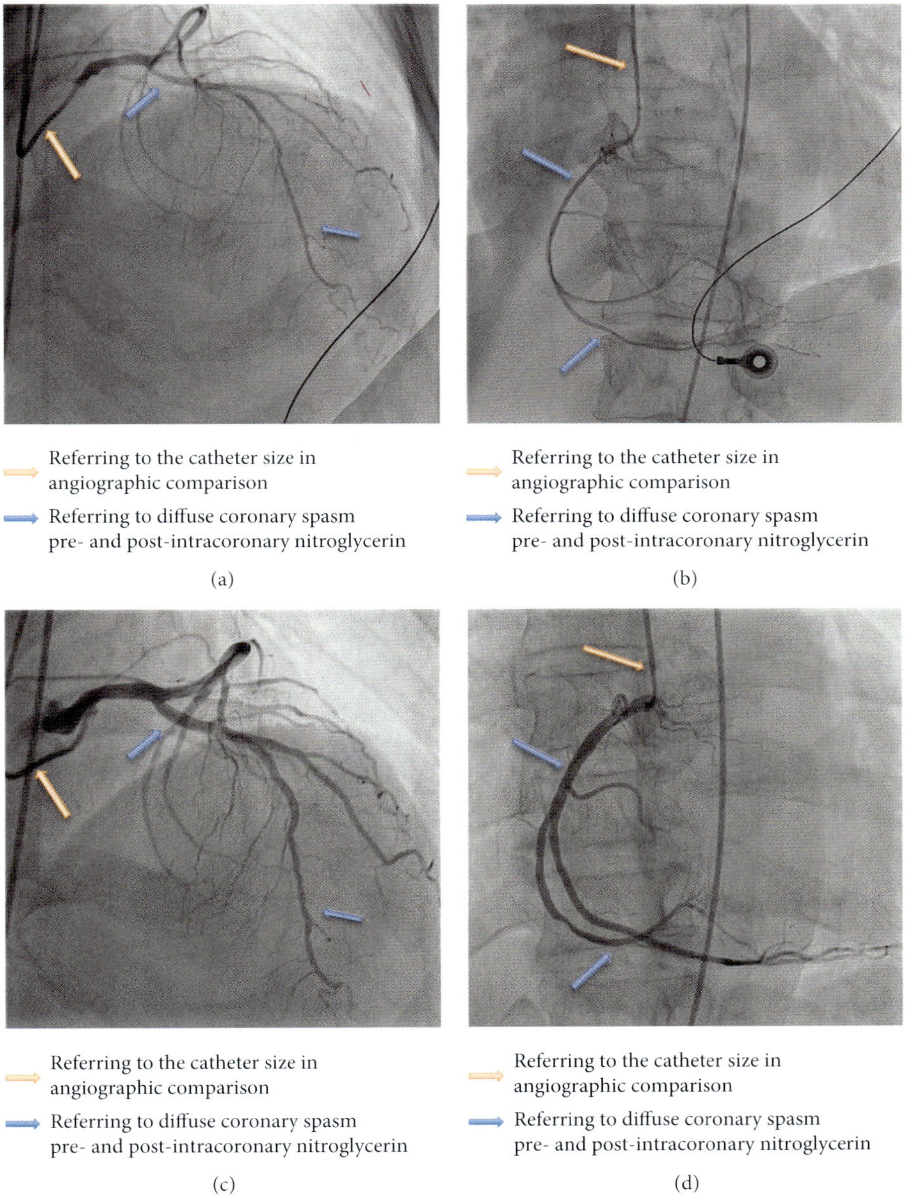

Figure 3: (a) Left coronary artery: diffuse coronary spasm involving proximal to distal of left anterior descending artery. (b) Right coronary artery: diffuse coronary spasm involving proximal to distal of right coronary artery, posterior descending artery, and posterior left ventricular branch. (c) Left coronary artery vasospasm resolved after intracoronary nitroglycerin. (d) Right coronary artery vasospasm resolved after intracoronary artery nitroglycerin.

Table 2: Burch-Wartofsky score.

Temperature	5
GI dysfunction	10
Central nervous system	0
Tachycardia	25
Congestive cardiac failure	10
Atrial fibrillation	10
History	0
Total	65

interventions. However, if recognised and treated early, it can lead to excellent prognosis.

References

[1] M. Chiha, S. Samarasinghe, and A. S. Kabaker, "Thyroid storm: an update review," *Journal of Intensive Care Medicine*, vol. 30, no. 3, pp. 131–140, 2015.

[2] R. Patel, G. Peterson, A. Rohatgi et al., "Hyperthyroidism-associated coronary vasospasm with myocardial infarction and subsequent euthyroid angina," *Thyroid*, vol. 18, no. 2, pp. 273–276, 2008.

[3] P. Dahl, S. Danzi, and I. Klein, "Thyrotoxic cardiac disease," *Current Heart Failure Reports*, vol. 5, no. 3, pp. 170–176, 2008.

[4] I. Klein and S. Danzi, "Thyroid disease and the heart," *Circulation*, vol. 116, no. 15, pp. 1725–1735, 2007.

[5] J. A. Jaber, H. Noor, S. Haque, B. Ibrahim, and J. A. Suwaidi, "Thyrotoxicosis and coronary artery spasm: case report and review of the literature," *Angiology*, vol. 61, no. 8, pp. 807–812, 2010.

[6] M. Sugiishi and F. Takatsu, "Cigarette smoking is a major risk factor for coronary spasm," *Circulation*, vol. 87, no. 1, pp. 76–79, 1993.

[7] H. Yasue, H. Nakagawa, T. Iyoh, E. Harada, and Y. Mizuno, "Coronary artery spasm–Clinical features, diagnosis, pathogenesis, and treatment," *Journal of Cardiology*, vol. 51, pp. 2–17, 2008.

[8] S. Y. Lee, C. W. Yu, Y. J. Choi et al., "A comparison of clinical features of coronary artery spasm with and without thyrotoxicosis," *Coronary Artery Disease*, vol. 25, no. 2, pp. 125–132, 2014.

[9] R. Napoli, B. Biondi, V. Guardasole et al., "Impact of hyperthyroidism and its correction on vascular reactivity in humans," *Circulation*, vol. 104, no. 25, pp. 3076–3080, 2001.

[10] J. Y. Wei, A. Genecin, H. L. Greene, and S. C. Achuff, "Coronary spasm with fibrillation during thyrotoxicosis: response to attaining euthyroid state," *American Journal of Cardiology*, vol. 43, no. 2, pp. 335–339, 1979.

[11] Y. H. Choi, J. H. Chung, S. W. Bae et al., "Severe coronary artery spasm can be associated with hyperthyroidism," *Coronary Artery Disease*, vol. 16, no. 3, pp. 135–139, 2005.

23

Time of Anderson-Fabry Disease Detection and Cardiovascular Presentation

K. Selthofer-Relatic[1,2]

[1]*Department for Cardiovascular Disease, Osijek University Hospital, J. Huttlera 4, 31000 Osijek, Croatia*
[2]*Department for Internal Medicine, Faculty of Medicine Osijek, Josip Juraj Strossmayer University of Osijek, Cara Hadrijana 10E, 31000 Osijek, Croatia*

Correspondence should be addressed to K. Selthofer-Relatic; selthofer.relatic@gmail.com

Academic Editor: Assad Movahed

Background. Anderson-Fabry disease is an X-linked inherited disease, which manifests in a different manner depending on gender and genotype. Making a working diagnosis of Anderson-Fabry disease is difficult because of several reasons: (a) that it is a multiorgan disease with wide variety of phenotypes, (b) different timelines of presentation, (c) gender differences, and (d) possible coexistence with other comorbidities. Late-onset/cardiac type of presentation with minimal involvement of other organs can additionally make diagnosis difficult. *Aim.* To describe different cardiac manifestations at different time points in the course of the disease: (1) 72-year-old female (echocardiography detection), heterozygote, significant left and mild right ventricular hypertrophy; (2) 62-year-old male (echocardiography detection), hemizygote, left ventricular hypertrophy, implanted cardiac pacemaker, a performed percutaneous coronary intervention after myocardial infarction, degenerative medium degree aortic valve stenosis; (3) 45-year-old female (asymptomatic/family screening), heterozygote, thickened mitral papillary muscle, mild left ventricular hypertrophy, first degree diastolic dysfunction; and (4) 75-year-old female (symptomatic/family screening), heterozygote, cardiomyopathy with reduced left ventricular ejection fraction after heart surgery (mitral valve annuloplasty and plastic repair of the tricuspid valve). *Conclusion.* All patients have Anderson-Fabry disease but with different clinical presentations depending on the gender, the type of mutation, and the time of detection. All these features can make the patients' profiles unique and delay the time of detection.

1. Introduction

Anderson-Fabry disease (AFD) is an X-linked disease of lysosomal metabolism resulting in attenuated activity or absence of the enzyme alpha-galactosidase A (a-Gal A). Impaired glycosphingolipid metabolism leads to systemic lysosomal globotriaosylceramide accumulation with multiorgan systemic involvement and complex clinical presentation: acroparesthesias, angiokeratoma, hypohidrosis, corneal and lenticular opacities, gastrointestinal and endocrine abnormalities, renal impairment, and neural and cardiovascular disease [1, 2].

AFD can affect both genders with 2 major phenotypes, the classic and the late-onset subtypes [3]. The classic phenotype has little or no a-Gal A activity and occurs with all typical AFD multiorganic presentations with renal failure development, hypertrophic cardiomyopathy, and cerebrovascular disease. Late-onset phenotype tends to have mutation-specific cardiac or kidney involvement, with slow progression and unknown underlying mechanisms [3]. Disease presentation of hemizygous males occurs more often as the classical type early in childhood or adolescence with typical symptoms, while heterozygous females can be affected as classical types, although the range of symptoms varies widely [2, 4]. So, it is more appropriate to describe AFD as a disease with a wide spectrum of heterogeneously progressive clinical phenotypes, from the classic severe phenotype in males to the asymptomatic disease course in females, with a variety of clinical presentations in-between. A high percentage of females develop vital organ involvement including the kidneys, heart, and/or brain about a decade later than the male patients [5, 6].

Table 1: Alpha-galactosidase levels and gene mutations of all cases.

	α-GAL level	Gene mutation
Case 1 (F)	**0.03** (normal range >0.185 nmol/spot/21 h)	c.[758T>C]
Case 2 (M)	**0.06** (normal range >0.185 nmol/spot/21 h)	c.[902G>T]
Case 3 (F)	0.2 (normal range >0.185 nmol/spot/21 h)	c.[902G>T]
Case 4 (F)	1.7 (normal range >1.2 μmol/L/h)	c.[902G>T]

The typical cardiac AFD manifestation is concentric left ventricular hypertrophy (LVH) in up to 50% of males and one-third of females, with or without right ventricular hypertrophy (RVH), as a result of the globotriaosylceramide accumulation in cardiomyocytes, endothelial cells, smooth muscle cells, conduction tissue, and valvular fibroblasts with consequent complex cellular cascades and a final result of hypertrophy and fibrosis [2, 7]. ECG abnormalities, echocardiographic findings, and arrhythmias are part of clinical presentations depending on the disease stage. A typical cardiac symptom is angina as a result of microvascular disease, while myocardial infarction is uncommon [2, 8–10].

Everyday clinical practice in AFD detection is challenging because of several reasons: various clinical manifestations depending on gender, age, time of detection, and type of disease [11]. Disease severity variations (symptoms, ECG changes, echocardiographic signs, and presence of arrhythmias), together with other organ involvement, can lead to disease presentations with unique profiles, especially if we take into account alpha-galactosidase activity levels, biomarker lyso-GL-3 levels, and results of genetic testing. This case series presents 4 patients with different cardiovascular presentations (Table 1).

2. Case Presentation

2.1. Case 1. A 72-year-old female presented with a personal history of hypohidrosis and acroparesthesia from childhood, started with antihypertensive medication, ramipril 1.25 mg, because of LVH and a mild level of hypertension 10 years ago. Also, laboratory analysis showed increased blood levels of creatinine (211 μmol/L) and endogenous creatinine clearance (22.8 mL/min/1.73 m^2) with proteinuria (174 mg/24 h). In 2013 and 2014, she had episodes of chest pain and dyspnea with increased levels of cardiac troponin and electrocardiogram changes (predominant left ventricular hypertrophy with negative T waves). On both occasions, she was admitted into the coronary unit with a working diagnosis of acute coronary syndrome. Coronary angiography was performed twice and showed no epicardial coronary artery stenosis, with developed smaller coronary arteries. During the past 2 years, she had several recidives of paroxysmal atrial fibrillation, started with oral anticoagulation. In last 10 years, echo examination was repeated several times, and every time significant LVH was described (LV mass calculated 305 g) while RVH was not. At the moment of detection, she had reduced ejection fraction of the left ventricle according to strain echo. Afterwards, testing for AFD was performed: alpha-galactosidase level was decreased (0.03 nmol/spot/21 h; normal range >0.185 nmol/spot/21 h) and a heterozygous mutation was detected (c.[758T>C]). Family screening test for sister and two sons were negative (Figures 1(a)–1(c)).

2.2. Case 2. A 62-year-old man presented with a personal history of hypohidrosis and acroparesthesia from childhood, hypertension over the last 20 years, started with cardiologic controls because of palpitations and dyspnea 20 years ago. At the moment of detection, he had persistent atrial fibrillation. He previously suffered an ischemic stroke, non-ST elevation myocardial infarction with percutaneous coronary intervention of the right coronary artery, had an implanted cardiac pacemaker because of sick sinus syndrome, increased blood levels of creatinine (116 μmol/L) and endogenous creatinine clearance (78.6 mL/min/1.73 m^2) with proteinuria (454 mg/24 h), without ophthalmological and dermatological manifestations of the disease. Repeated echo examination showed significant LVH without left ventricular outflow obstruction, decreased EF according to strain analysis, diastolic dysfunction of the first degree, and degenerative, moderate level of aortic valve stenosis. The patient was hospitalized for two more times because of chest pain with increased troponin levels. Afterwards, testing for Fabry disease was performed: alpha-galactosidase level was decreased (0.06 nmol/spot/21 h; normal range >0.12 nmol/spot/21 h), lyso-GL-3 was increased (36.1 ng/mL; normal range 0.0–3.5 ng/mL), and a hemizygous mutation was detected (c.[902G>T]) (Figures 2(a)–2(c)) [12].

2.3. Case 3. An asymptomatic 45-year-old female was detected to be heterozygous during family screening (AFD affected father). Echocardiographic examination showed thickened mitral papillary muscle, LV wall thickness 11/12 mm, and mild degree of diastolic dysfunction. Testing for AF disease was performed: alpha-galactosidase level was normal (0.2 nmol/spot/21 h; normal range >0.12 nmol/spot/21 h) and a heterozygous mutation was detected (c.[902G>T]). Thereafter, heart MRI was performed; there was no late gadolinium enhancement or signs of myocardial fibrosis, examination considered as completely normal. Furthermore, brain MRI was normal. Renal biopsy showed typical zebra bodies located in podocytes and partly in epithelial tubular cells. Laboratory analysis showed normal renal function: creatinine level 76 μmol/L, endogenous creatinine clearance 81 mL/min/1.73 m^2, albuminuria 5.1 mg/L, and proteinuria 78 mg/24 h (Figures 3(a) and 3(b)).

2.4. Case 4. A 75-year-old female, heterozygote for AFD, detected in family screening, had hypertension history for

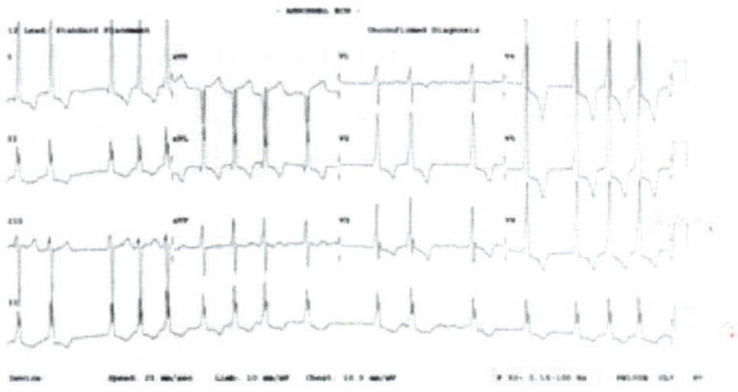

(a)

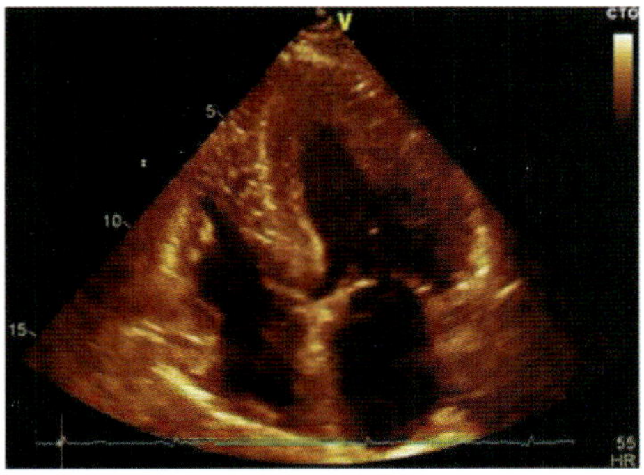

(b)

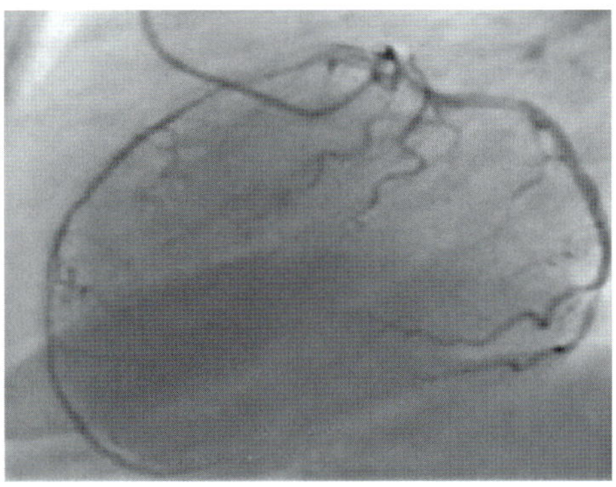

(c)

FIGURE 1: (a) Electrocardiogram: atrial fibrillation and left and right ventricular hypertrophy. (b) Two-dimensional transthoracic echocardiography (apical view): left and right ventricular hypertrophy. (c) Coronary angiography: normal findings of epicardial coronary artery.

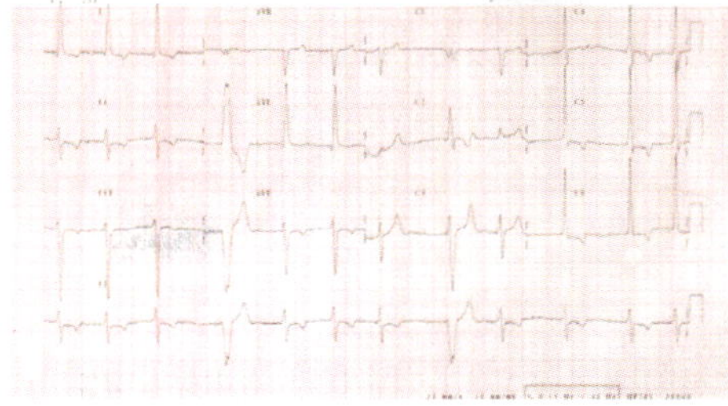

(a)

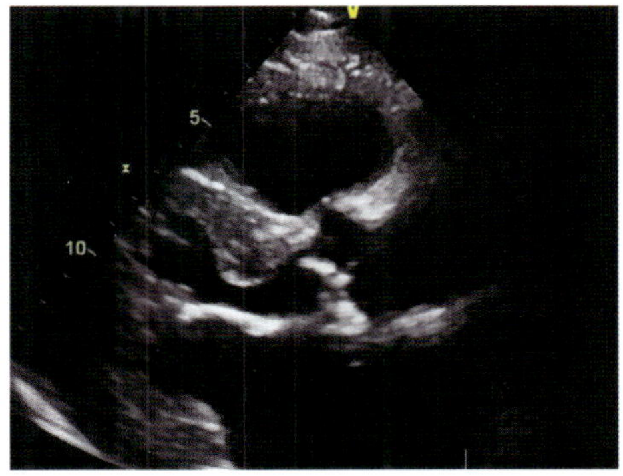

(b)

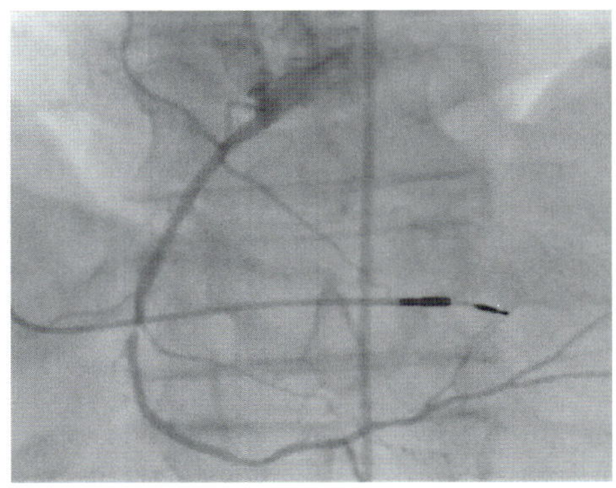

(c)

FIGURE 2: (a) Electrocardiogram: left ventricular hypertrophy and ventricular extrasystoles. (b) Two-dimensional transthoracic echocardiography (parasternal long-axis view): left ventricular hypertrophy and degenerative aortic valve changes. (c) Coronary angiography: significant right coronary artery stenosis and implanted cardiac electorstimulator.

over 20 years, atrial fibrillation, and dyspnea with signs of progressive heart failure of unknown cause during the past 10 years. Heart surgery was performed because of higher level of mitral and tricuspid regurgitation—mitral and tricuspid valve annuloplasty, before AFD detection. She had acroparestesia from childhood. According to earlier medical documentation, creatinine level was 125 μmol/L, and proteinuria was described a bit over the reference values. The patient was not interested in further examinations. Echocardiographic examination was performed before testing: there were no typical signs of AFD, and she had moderate LVH with hyperechogenic/hypokinetic LV walls and reduced ejection fraction of left ventricle 30% according to two-dimensional transthoracic. Testing for Fabry disease was performed: alpha-galactosidase level was normal (1.7 μmol/L/h; normal range >1.2 μmol/L/h), lyso-GL-3 was increased (7.5 ng/mL; normal range 0.0–3.5 ng/mL), and a heterozygous mutation was detected (c.[902G>T]) (Figures 4(a) and 4(b)).

3. Discussion

Patients with AFD are usually detected during different times of their life and in different stages of the disease when typical hypertrophic cardiomyopathy is not always present (early or late stages).

The typical cardiac type of AFD presents with concentric or sometimes asymmetric LVH, with or without RVH. ECG

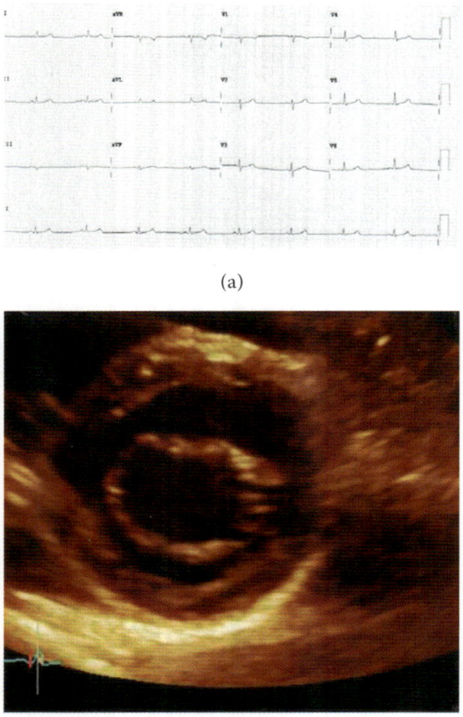

(a)

(b)

Figure 3: (a) Electrocardiogram: normal ECG. (b) Two-dimensional transthoracic echocardiography (short-axis view): normal mitral valve and partial thickened left ventricular walls.

changes include voltage signs of LVH/RVH, repolarization abnormalities, PR shortening, and different types of benign and malignant arrhythmias. Atherosclerotic coronary disease is not typical for AFD, but involvement of coronary microcirculation can lead to angina [2]. In the clinical routine, most patients are first evaluated with two-dimensional echocardiography. The echocardiographic determination is limited to morphology and function but without exact etiology determination. Cardiac magnetic resonance can evaluate the presence or absence of hyperenhancement and its location. Intramural or subepicardial areas of hyperenhancement, which are not related to any coronary perfusion territory, are typical for infiltrative disorders such as AFD. Additional valuable information can be gained by this examination, including information about the area of irreversible myocardial damage and prognosis, the amount of scarring, and the clinical risk for sudden death [13].

The hallmarks of AF cardiomyopathy (increasing wall thickness, regional functional abnormalities, and replacement fibrosis) during aging are not the same for both sexes. In male patients, the LV starts to hypertrophy during adolescence with concomitant reduction in longitudinal function. During aging, these two processes lead to replacement fibrosis. In females, the progression toward hypertrophy is prolonged, whereas the development of fibrosis and regional functional abnormalities progresses simultaneously [14]. Replacement

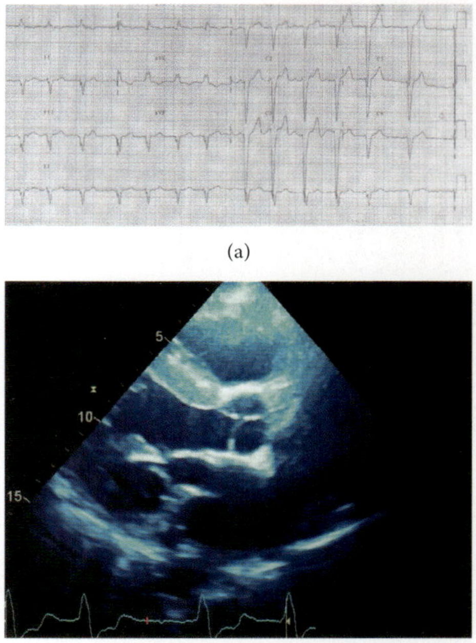

(a)

(b)

Figure 4: (a) Electrocardiogram: atrial fibrillation and left bundle branch block. (b) Two-dimensional echocardiography (parasternal long-axis view): hyperechogenic and hypertrophic interventricular septum; after mitral valve repair.

fibrosis may be a valid screening tool in females as opposed to males in the early stages of AFD [15].

Symptoms and results of cardiac imaging may be different than expected: echocardiogram after cardiac surgery, coronary angiogram after percutaneous coronary intervention, or electrocardiogram after pacemaker implantation, and this can delay clinical assumptions and the decision for genetic testing.

A cardiologist is usually the first person who can raise suspicion about an AFD etiology in HCM with the help of transthoracic echocardiography. Knowing and thinking about HCM differential diagnoses is crucial. According to ESC HCM guidelines, in over 60% of adults with HCM, the disease is an autosomal dominant trait caused by mutations in cardiac sarcomere protein genes; in 5–10%, it is caused by other genetic disorders including inherited metabolic and neuromuscular diseases, chromosome abnormalities, and genetic syndromes; and about 25–30% are still of unknown cause [16]. In routine practice, the most common conditions causing LVH are arterial hypertension, aortic stenosis, and obesity [2].

In differential diagnosis, it is obligatory to expand our thoughts on several more facts about Anderson-Fabry disease: (1) gender difference (inheritance); (2) age difference (time of clinical presentation); (3) disease burden (depending on the affected organs and degrees of changes); (4) individual manifestation (unique pathophysiologic personal profiles); (5) presence of comorbidities (coexistence of different cardiovascular diseases).

4. Conclusion

From a cardiac point of view, patients with unexplained ventricular hypertrophy should be tested for AFD, even without other organ affection because of different genotypes and phenotypes of the disease. Patients with atypical echocardiographic LVH findings, with other organ affection, should also be tested for AFD, especially after invasive/ operative cardiac therapeutic procedures.

References

[1] Y. A. Zarate and R. J. Hopkin, "Fabry's disease," *The Lancet*, vol. 372, pp. 1427–1435, 2008.

[2] Z. Yousef, P. M. Elliot, F. Cecchi et al., "Left ventricular hypertrophy in Fabry disease: a practical approach to diagnosis," *European Heart Journal*, vol. 34, no. 11, pp. 802–808, 2013.

[3] T. R. Hsu, S. C. Hung, F. P. Chang et al., "Later onset fabry disease, cardiac damage progress in silence: experience with a highly prevalent mutation," *Journal of the American College of Cardiology*, vol. 68, no. 23, pp. 2554–2563, 2016.

[4] C. Chimenti, M. Pieroni, E. Morgante et al., "Prevalence of Fabry disease in female patients with late-onset hypertrophic cardiomyopathy," *Circulation*, vol. 110, no. 9, pp. 1047–1053, 2004.

[5] W. R. Wilcox, J. P. Oliveira, R. J. Hopkin et al., "Females with Fabry disease frequently have major organ involvement: lessons from the Fabry Registry," *Molecular Genetics and Metabolism*, vol. 93, no. 2, pp. 112–128, 2008.

[6] D. P. Germain, "Fabry disease," *Orphanet Journal of Rare Diseases*, vol. 5, no. 1, p. 30, 2010.

[7] M. Namdar, "Electrocardiographic changes and arrhythmia in Fabry disease," *Frontiers in Cardiovascular Medicine*, vol. 3, p. 7, 2016.

[8] C. Kapmann, A. Linhart, F. Baehner et al., "Onset and progression of the Anderson-Fabry disease related cardiomyopathy," *International Journal of Cardiology*, vol. 130, no. 3, pp. 367–373, 2008.

[9] R. Schiffmann, D. Warnock, M. Banikazemi et al., "Fabry disease: progression of nephropathy, and prevalence of cardiac and cerebrovascular events before enzyme replacement therapy," *Nephrology Dialysis Transplantation*, vol. 24, no. 7, pp. 2102–2111, 2009.

[10] A. Linhart, C. Kampmann, J. L. Zamorano et al., "Cardiac manifestations of Anderson-Fabry disease: results from the international Fabry outcome survey," *European Heart Journal*, vol. 28, no. 10, pp. 1228–1235, 2007.

[11] M. Arends, M. Biegstraaten, D. A. Hughes et al., "Retrospective study of long-term outcomes of enzyme replacement therapy in Fabry disease: analysis of prognostic factors," *PLoS One*, vol. 12, no. 8, article e0182379, 2017.

[12] H. Roguljic and K. Selthofer-Relatic, "Different cardiovascular manifestations in a Fabry disease patient," Case Report. ESC Portal, 2017, http://learn.escardio.org/clinicalcase/casedetail/e8b6cb67-b909-4b1d-af2e-c1694c4e26af.

[13] H. Mahrholdt, A. Wagner, R. M. Judd, U. Sechtem, and R. J. Kim, "Delayed enhancement cardiovascular magnetic resonance assessment of non-ischaemic cardiomyopathies," *European Heart Journal*, vol. 26, no. 15, pp. 1461–1474, 2005.

[14] M. Niemann, S. Herrmann, K. Hu et al., "Differences in Fabry cardiomyopathy between female and male patients: consequences for diagnostic assessment," *JACC: Cardiovascular Imaging*, vol. 4, no. 6, pp. 592–601, 2011.

[15] S. Meyer, P. van der Meer, J. P. van Tintelen, and M. P. van den Berg, "Sex differences in cardiomyopathies," *European Journal of Heart Failure*, vol. 16, no. 3, pp. 238–247, 2014.

[16] P. M. Elliott, A. Anastasakis, M. A. Borger et al., "2014 ESC Guidelines on diagnosis and management of hypertrophic cardiomyopathy: the task force for the diagnosis and management of hypertrophic cardiomyopathy of the European Society of Cardiology (ESC)," *European Heart Journal*, vol. 35, no. 39, pp. 2733–2779, 2014.

24

Diagnosis of Anomalous Origin of the Left Coronary Artery from the Pulmonary Artery with Echocardiography and Digital Subtraction Angiography

Haiyan Yang,[1,2] Jinqing Li,[3] and Xiaojuan Ji[1,2]

[1]*Department of Cardiology, Children's Hospital of Chongqing Medical University, Chongqing 400014, China*
[2]*Ministry of Education Key Laboratory of Child Development and Disorders, Chongqing Key Laboratory of Child Infection and Immunity, China International Science and Technology Cooperation Base of Child Development and Critical Disorders, Chongqing 400014, China*
[3]*Department of Radiology, 324th Hospital of the PLA, Chongqing 400020, China*

Correspondence should be addressed to Xiaojuan Ji; jixiaojuan2003@163.com

Academic Editor: Assad Movahed

Anomalous origin of the left coronary artery from the pulmonary artery (ALCAPA) is a common coronary artery anomaly associated with high mortality and may lead to sudden death if left unrecognized and untreated. This report describes an 8-year-old female who had cardiac murmur but with no clinical symptoms. Electrocardiogram (ECG) was normal, but echocardiography made the diagnosis of ALCAPA. Digital subtraction angiography (DSA) with cardiac catheterization angiography (CAG) confirmed the diagnosis, and finally, the patient received surgery. This case demonstrates that echocardiography is a sensitive and convenient technique for establishing the initial diagnosis of ALCAPA in both symptomatic and asymptomatic patients.

1. Introduction

ALCAPA is a rare congenital cardiovascular malformation in which the left coronary artery originates from the pulmonary artery (PA) instead of the left coronary sinus [1]. The incidence is 1 in 300,000 live births and accounts for 0.25% to 0.5% of congenital heart disease cases. ALCAPA results in mortality as high as 90% in the first year of life if the patient is not treated in a timely fashion [2]. Here, we present a case of a female patient diagnosed with ALCAPA. The patient's medical records, such as clinical symptoms, electrocardiogram (ECG), echocardiography, and cardiac catheterization angiography (CAG) images, were analyzed retrospectively.

2. Case Report

An 8-year-old Chinese female with a cardiac murmur was initially diagnosed as having a ventricular septal defect (VSD) in the local hospital. She was asymptomatic, had no difficulty breathing, and displayed neither increased diaphoresis nor cyanosis, but she developed upper respiratory infections more often than her peers and had reduced exercise capacity compared to her peers. On physical examination, she had the following vital measurements: 24 kg weight, 121 cm height, blood pressure 115/51 mm·Hg, heart rate 92/min, respiratory rate of 22/min, and transcutaneous oxygen saturation (SpO_2) 96%. The results of physical examination were normal when compared with the same age of females within same race. On cardiac examination, her pulse and S1 and S2 were normal, but she had a grade 2/6 holosystolic murmur at the second left intercostal space.

ECG displayed normal sinus rhythm and no signs of myocardial ischemia. Chest X-ray revealed an enlarged cardiac silhouette. Echocardiography demonstrated ALCAPA, right coronary artery to right ventriclar fistula, right coronary artery aneurysm, collateral coronary circulation formation,

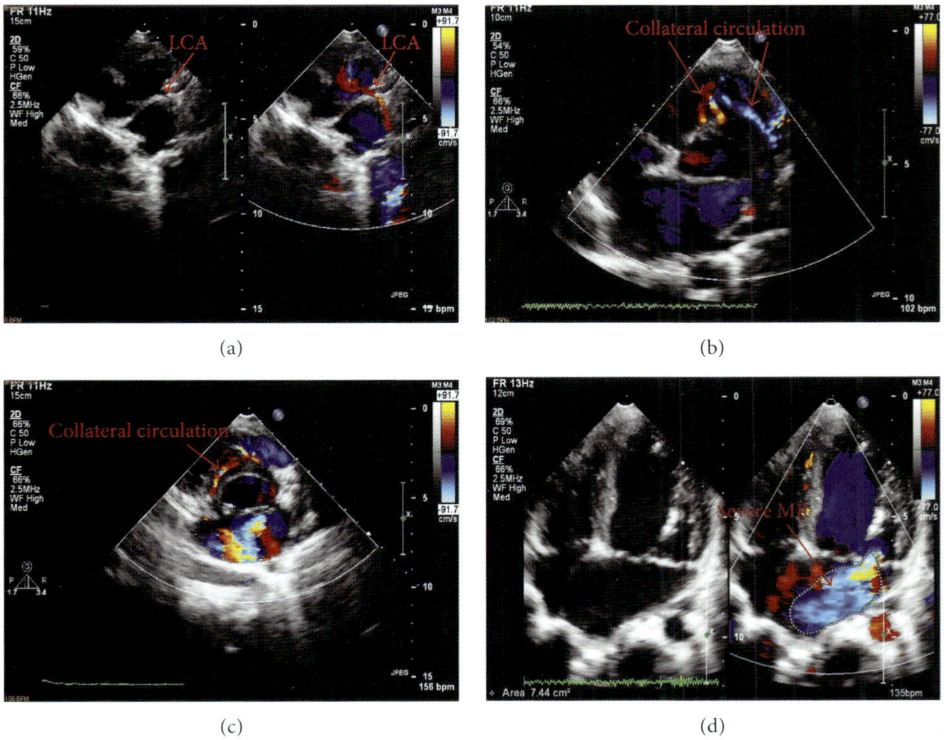

Figure 1: (a) The left coronary artery (LCA) originating from the pulmonary artery. (b) Reversal of blood flow in the left coronary artery (LCA) and abundant collateral circulation. (c) The abundant collateral circulation. (d) Severe mitral regurgitation (MR).

severe mitral regurgitation (MR), left ventricular ejection fraction (LVEF) of 61%, and left ventricular fractional shortening (LVFS) of 33% (Figure 1).

Subsequently, cardiac catheterization and left ventricular angiography demonstrated a dilated right coronary artery (RCA) and with delayed filling of a dilated left coronary artery (LCA). There was no shunt across the interventricular septum. Then, aortic root angiography showed the dilated RCA originating from the right coronary cusp (RCC), and delayed enhanced-imaging demonstrated the LCA filling via extensive intercoronary collateral circulation. Finally, PA angiography showed immediate filling of the LCA, which originated from the PA; then abundant collateral circulation and delayed RCA were imaged (Figure 2), confirming the diagnosis of ALCAPA.

The patient underwent direct reimplantation of the abnormal LCA into the aorta with general anesthesia under extracorporeal circulation through a median sternotomy. During the procedure, origin of the LCA from the PA trunk, a dilated and tortuous RCA from the RCC, extensive intercoronary collaterals, and anterior mitral valve prolapse were confirmed (Figure 3). Postoperative bedside echocardiography showed LCA connected to aorta sinus, bilateral coronary artery aneurysms (Figure 4), and moderate-to-severe MR with LVEF of 71%, LVFS of 39%. The chest was closed on postoperative day 2, and the patient was discharged on postoperative day 11 with an uneventful recovery. Postoperative chest X-ray showed inflammation and exudation in the lung and mild cardiomegaly. We followed the patient on the first month (bilateral coronary artery aneurysms and moderate MR with LVEF of 61%, LVFS of 32%), sixth month (right coronary artery aneurysms/dilated left coronary artery and mild-to-moderate MR with LVEF of 65%, LVFS of 35%), and first year (bilateral dilated coronary arteries and mild MR with LVEF of 67%, LVFS of 34%) after the surgery by echocardiography (Figure 5), and the patient showed good functional recovery.

3. Discussion

ALCAPA is also named Bland–White–Garland syndrome. Clinically, ALCAPA has been divided into adult and infant types according to intercoronary collateral circulation extent. Infant type usually survives only a few months for the reason of myocardial ischemia and heart failure, and only about 10% to 15% of patients survive to adolescence or adulthood [3]. On the other hand, extensive intercoronary collateral circulation usually exists in adult type, forming the "left to right shunt" and "coronary artery steal blood" phenomenon, which could induce to abnormal perfusion of myocardium and sudden death [4]. Our case was defined as the adult type, with relatively abundant collateral circulation and minimal symptoms and a heart murmur.

The incidence of adult type of ALCAPA is very low and often be asymptomatic, so it is usually being misdiagnosed,

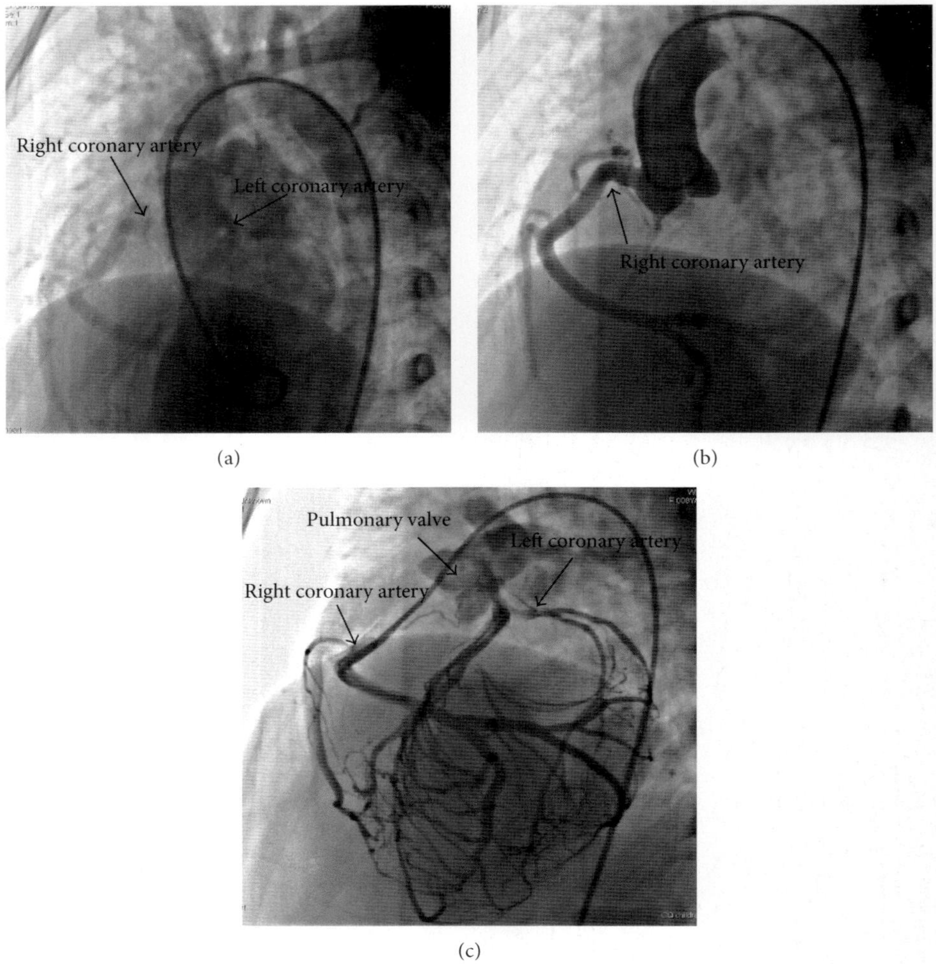

Figure 2: (a) Left ventricle angiography visualizing both right coronary artery (RCA) and delayed filling of the left coronary artery (LCA). (b) The aortic root angiography; only right coronary artery (RCA) originating from the right coronary cusp was imaged immediately. (c) Pulmonary arterial angiography; the left coronary artery (LCA) was imaged immediately, originating from the pulmonary artery; the RCA was then imaged via abundant collateral circulation.

especially when ECG shows no obvious ST-T change and V waves. Echocardiography is usually the initial diagnostic tool; when the echocardiographer found the imaging feature of the dilation and dysfunction of left ventricular with severe mitral regurgitation, abnormal flow-pattern in the ventricular septum and dilatation of the right coronary artery, and the wide enhancement and thickening of the endocardium, the echocardiographer should not only pay attention to idiopathic endocardial fibroelastosis (EFE) [5] and/or idiopathic dilated cardiomyopathy (DCM) [6] but also should check the origination of the coronary arteries to avoid being misdiagnosed. The typical and direct echocardiographic imaging feature is to show the LCA originating from the pulmonary artery when diagnosing ALCAPA and should also reveal the origin, size, and course of coronary arteries clearly. In addition, the reversal of blood flow in the left coronary artery and abundant collateral circulation are approval to the diagnosis of ALCAPA. Visibly, echocardiography is an indispensable diagnostic tool because of its noninvasive repeatability, low cost, and ability to clearly show the origin of the coronary artery. It can not only determine real-time hemodynamic change, but also can measure heart function in subclinical stage and postoperative follow-up, including the index of heart, resilience, myocardial wall motion, and strain rate [7]. The patient reported in this report was misdiagnosed as having a VSD in the local hospital mainly due to two reasons: first and most importantly, the fistula in the ventricular septum was diagnosed as a VSD; second, the echocardiographer may not have comprehensive knowledge of ALCAPA.

However, DSA with CAG is considered as the gold standard diagnosis of ALCAPA. The use of the contrast agent in severe infant patients remains controversial with regard to ionization radiation and potential allergic reaction [8]. Magnetic resonance angiography (MRA) and computed tomography angiography (CTA) have been increasingly employed for the diagnosis of ALCAPA. CTA is a noninvasive imaging technique with good density and spatial resolution, which has certain advantages to evaluate

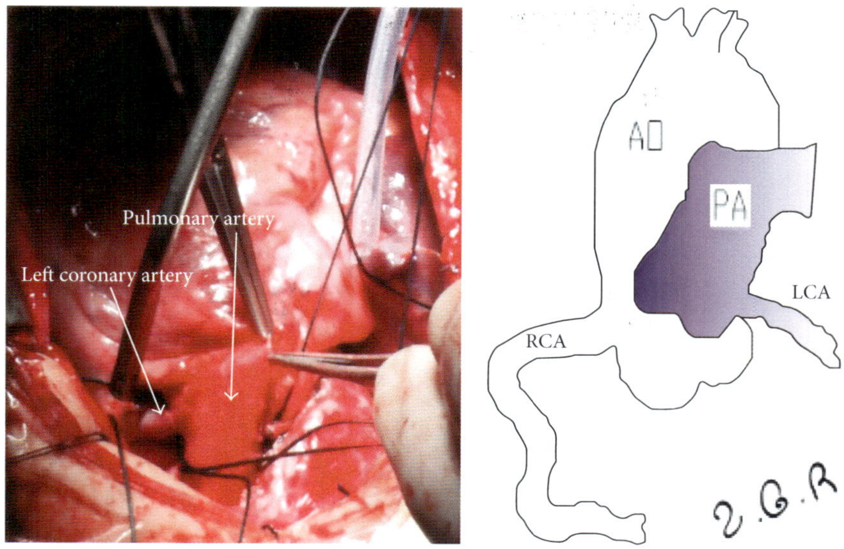

(a) (b)

FIGURE 3: The image in the surgery shows the left coronary artery originating from the pulmonary artery. The diagram displays the right coronary artery (RCA) originating from the aorta artery (AO) while the left coronary artery (LCA) from the pulmonary artery originating from the pulmonary artery (PA).

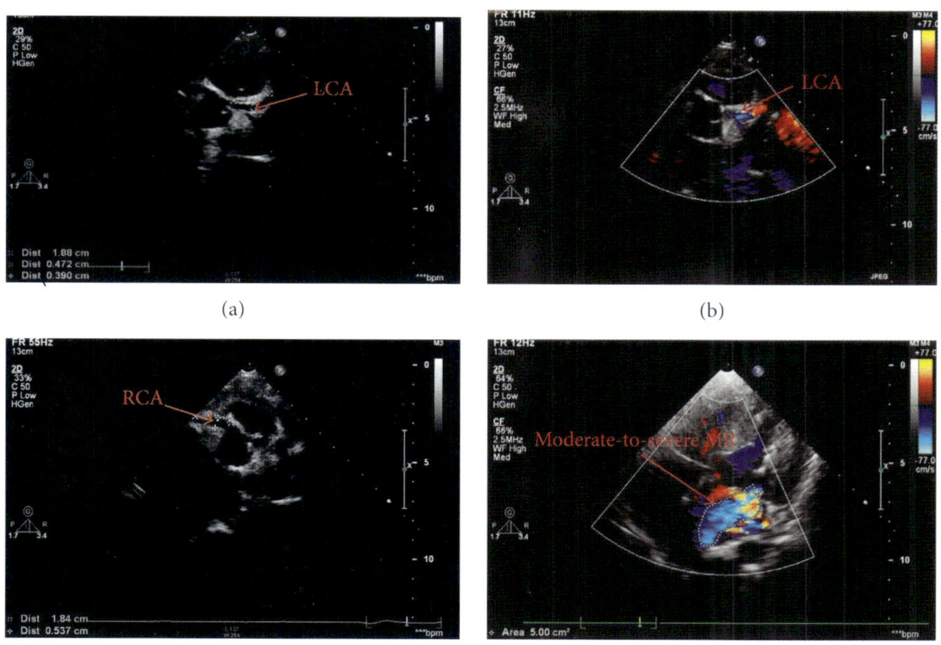

(a) (b) (c) (d)

FIGURE 4: (a, b) The dilated left coronary artery connected to the aorta in the two-dimensional and color doppler flow imaging(CDFI). (c) The dilated right coronary artery connected to the aorta. (d) Moderate-to-severe mitral regurgitation.

small blood vessels such as the coronary artery, but it cannot evaluate an intravascular blood flow condition. MRA can be used to diagnose postoperative left ventricular morphology and function in patients with suspected myocardial ischemia; its image quality can be easily influenced by heart rate.

4. Conclusion

ALCAPA is a rare congenital heart disease that carries a high mortality rate and may lead to sudden death if left untreated. Typical echocardiographic features and comprehension of ALCAPA are helpful for diagnosis and

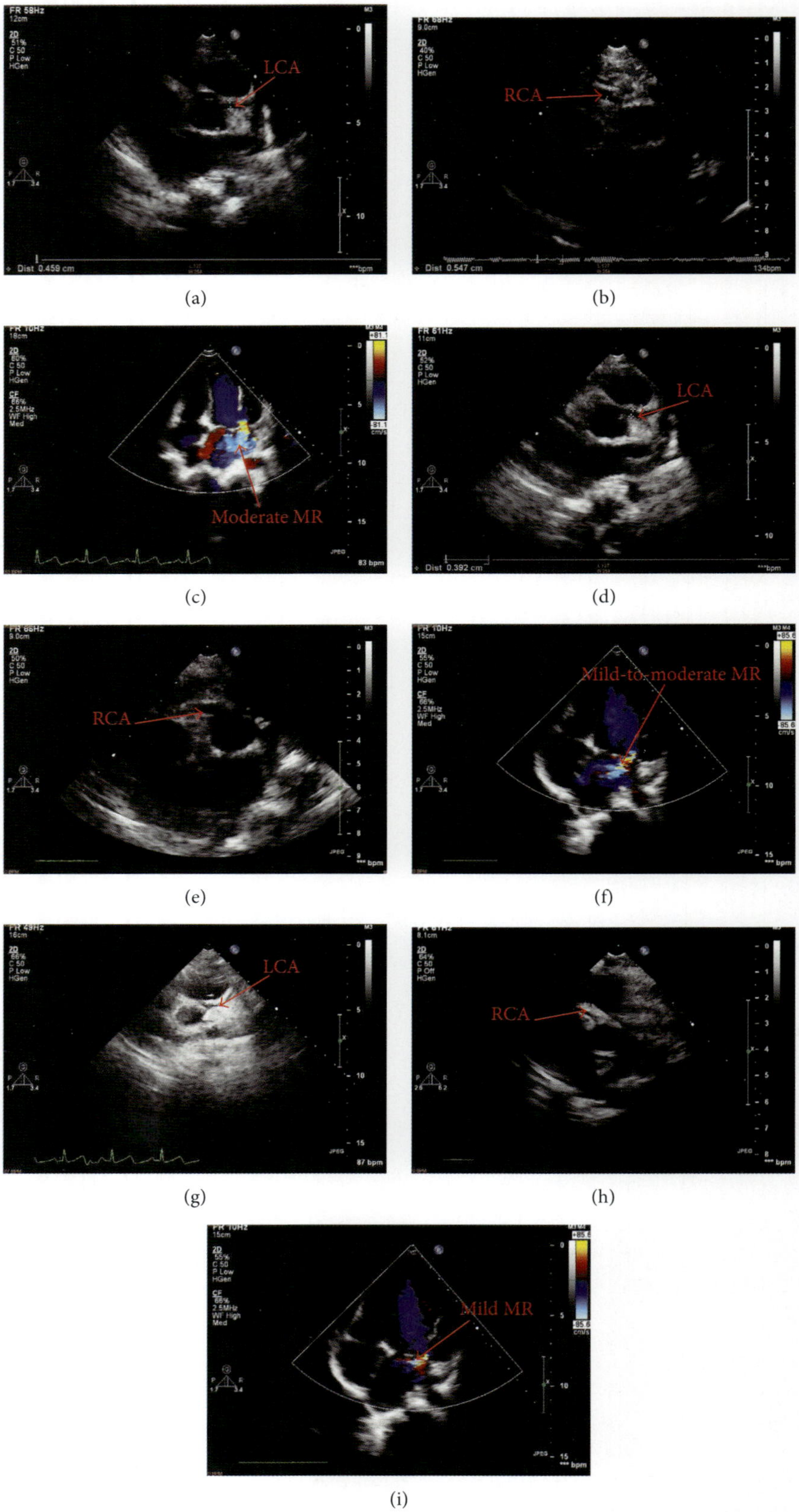

Figure 5: (a, b, c) Bilateral coronary artery aneurysms and moderate mitral regurgitation on the first month after the surgery. (d, e, f) The right coronary artery aneurysms/dilated left coronary artery and mild-to-moderate mitral regurgitation on the sixth month after the surgery. (g, h, i) Bilateral dilated coronary arteries and mild mitral regurgitation on the first year after the surgery.

differential diagnosis. The echocardiography can diagnose ALCAPA accurately and give sufficient information for heart function and operation.

Acknowledgments

The work was supported by National Natural Science Foundation of China (Grant no. 81301300); Natural Science Foundation of Chongqing, China (no. cstc 2014 jcyjA10011); and Chongqing Science and Technology Commission (cstc2016shmszx 130009).

References

[1] M. Kanoh, K. Inai, T. Shinohara, H. Tomimatsu, and T. Nakanishi, "Outcomes from anomalous origin of the left coronary artery from the pulmonary artery repair: long-term complications in relation to residual myocardial abnormalities," *Journal of Cardiology*, vol. 17, no. 5, pp. 498–503, 2017.

[2] M. Cauldwell, L. Swan, K. V. Klemperer, R. Patel, and P. Steer, "Management of ALCAPA in two pregnancies," *International Journal of Cardiology*, vol. 181, pp. 353-354, 2015.

[3] K. Takemoto, K. Hirata, T. Tanimoto et al., "Combined non-invasive doppler echocardiography and coronary computed tomography lead to diagnosis of anomalous left coronary artery from the pulmonary artery (ALCAPA) syndrome," *Circulation Journal*, vol. 79, no. 5, pp. 1136–1138, 2015.

[4] K. Nakanishi, S. Fukuda, K. Shimada et al., "Impaired coronary flow reserve as a marker of microvascular dysfunction to predict long-term cardiovascular outcomes, acute coronary syndrome and the development of heart failure," *Circulation Journal*, vol. 76, no. 8, pp. 1958–1964, 2012.

[5] S. G. Patel, M. A. Frommelt, P. C. Frommelt, S. Kutty, and J. W. Cramer, "Echocardiographic diagnosis, surgical treatment, and outcomes of anomalous left coronary artery from the pulmonary artery," *Journal of the American Society of Echocardiography*, vol. 17, no. 9, pp. 30383–30388, 2017.

[6] D. Giacomini, G. Romanucci, and S. Savastano, "CT diagnosis of a coronary-pulmonary baffle leak complicating Takeuchi repair procedure for ALCAPA syndrome," *Journal of Cardiovascular Computed Tomography*, vol. 10, no. 2, pp. 184-185, 2016.

[7] B. Castaldi, V. Vida, E. Reffo et al., "Speckle tracking in ALCAPA patients after surgical repair as predictor of residual coronary disease," *Pediatric Cardiology*, vol. 38, no. 4, pp. 749–800, 2017.

[8] N. DluzNiewska, M. Kostkiewicz, P. L. Tomkiewicz et al., "Noninvasive techniques for the diagnosis of anomalous origin of the left coronary artery from the pulmonary artery in adult patients," *Acta Cardiologica*, vol. 72, no. 1, pp. 41–46, 2017.

25

Multiple Culprit Coronary Artery Thrombosis in a Patient with Coronary Ectasia

Bruno da Silva Matte, Gustavo Neves de Araujo, Felipe Homem Valle, and Ana Maria Rocha Krepsky

Hospital de Clínicas de Porto Alegre, Federal University of Rio Grande do Sul, Porto Alegre, RS, Brazil

Correspondence should be addressed to Bruno da Silva Matte; bmatte@hcpa.edu.br

Academic Editor: Manabu Shirotani

We here report a case of ST-elevation myocardial infarction (STEMI) due to simultaneous acute coronary artery occlusions of two major coronary arteries in a patient with coronary ectasia. The patient had been previously submitted to percutaneous coronary angioplasty with bare metal stent implantation in both culprit vessels. Very late stent thrombosis could be the cause of the first occlusion, triggering the event in the other vessel. In addition, concomitant embolic sources were not identified. Although routine aspiration thrombectomy in STEMI was not proven to be beneficial in randomized clinical trials, it was of great value in this case. We also discuss the relation between coronary ectasia, chronic inflammatory status, and increased platelet activity which may have caused plaque disruption in another already vulnerable vessel.

1. Introduction

Multivessel acute thrombosis leading to ST-segment elevation myocardial infarction is rare, with a potentially devastating clinical presentation due to the vast myocardial area jeopardized [1]. Coronary artery ectasia (CAE) is characterized by abnormal dilatation of a localized or diffuse segment of epicardial coronary arteries, and its presence results in alterations in blood flow and stasis, predisposing to adverse coronary events [2]. On the one hand, current guidelines discourage routine thrombus aspiration techniques [3]. On the other hand, the performance of primary coronary angioplasty in the scenario of both high thrombotic burden and ectasic coronary artery may be facilitated by the adoption of aspirative thrombectomy approach. We present a case of ST-elevation myocardial infarction (STEMI) due to simultaneous thrombotic occlusions of two major coronary arteries in a patient with coronary ectasia, successfully treated with thromboaspiration followed by bare metal stent (BMS) implantation and chronic anticoagulation.

2. Case Presentation

A 56-year-old male patient with a history of current tobacco use and previous coronary artery disease was admitted to the emergency room with acute coronary syndrome. He had previous percutaneous coronary intervention (PCI) history in mid left anterior descendent (LAD) and proximal right coronary artery (RCA) with bare metal stents in a context of unstable angina two years before in another facility and was on aspirin 100 mg daily. Clopidogrel had been used for one year and then discontinued. He arrived at the hospital within five hours and thirty minutes from the onset of severe chest pain associated with nausea and diaphoresis. His blood pressure was 130/80 mmHg, heart rate was 80 bpm, cardiac auscultation was unremarkable, and his Killip class was II.

Admission ECG showed sinus rhythm with both anterior and inferior ST-segment elevation (Figure 1). Oral loading doses of antiplatelets (aspirin 300 mg and clopidogrel 600 mg) were administered, and coronary angiography was performed emergently. Surprisingly, thrombotic occlusions of both proximal RCA (Figure 2(a)) and mid LAD (Figure 2(b)) were disclosed. Unfractionated heparin

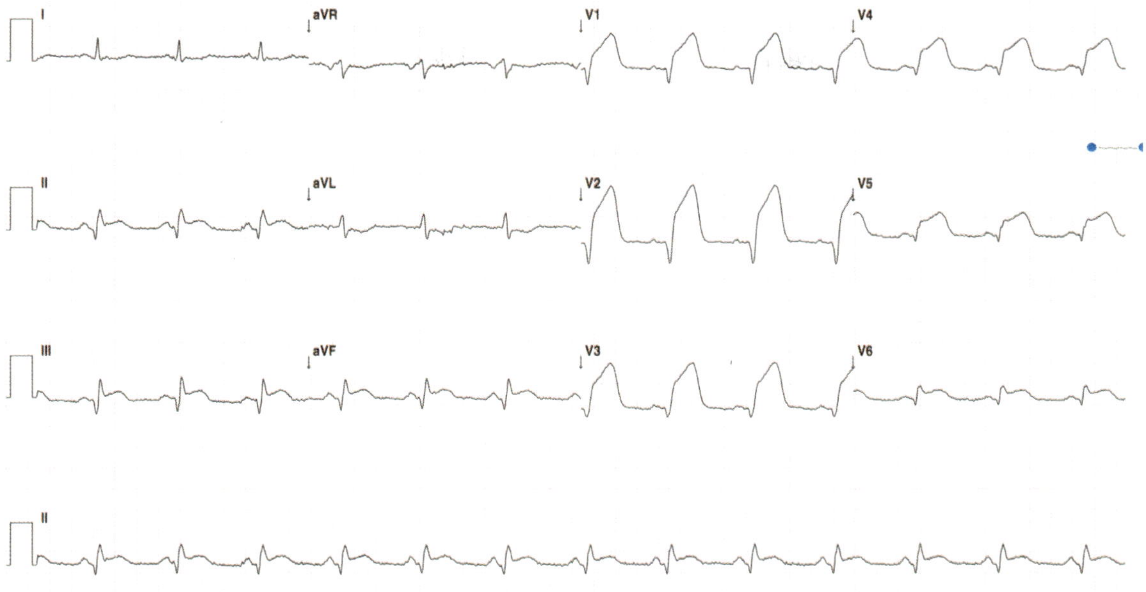

FIGURE 1: Admission electrocardiogram.

(100 UI/kg) and IIb/IIIa glycoprotein inhibitor (abciximab) were administered during the procedure, and the latter was continued up to 12 hours after the procedure. Both vessels were diffusely ectasic, and the occlusions occurred into pronounced ectasic spots. LAD thrombosis occurred just proximal to the previously implanted stent, and RCA thrombosis occurred in the proximal segment while the previously implanted stent was on the distal segment. There were only discrete collaterals from LAD to RCA after the first vessel was recanalized.

We decided to intervene first on LAD due to the larger myocardium area at risk. Guidewire easily surpassed the occluded segment, and LAD was predilated with 2.0×15 and 2.5×20 mm noncompliant balloons (NCB) without flow restoration despite several inflations. Manual thrombus aspiration with Export catheter was performed, and such approach allowed much better thrombus clearance and vessel delineation (Figure 2(d)). Kaname 3.0×28 mm BMS was then implanted and postdilated with a 3.5×15 mm NCB. RCA intervention was performed in the same procedure, and the vessel had a similar behavior, with easy guidewire navigation and no flow restoration with balloon angioplasty (2.5×20 mm and 3.0×20 mm). Manual aspiration also allowed better vessel delineation (Figure 2(c)). Multilink 4.0×33 mm and Prokinetic 4.0×20 mm BMS were implanted in distal and medial segments, respectively, with overlapping and was postdilated with a 5.0×20 mm NCB. Angiographic success (Figure 3) was achieved, and IIb/IIIa glycoprotein inhibitor was maintained for 12 hours in continuous infusion.

The patient was in sinus rhythm throughout hospitalization, and echocardiogram showed an ejection fraction of 34% with apical and septal akinesia. It did not show intracardiac thrombus or vegetation, making coronary embolization improbable as a cause of thrombosis. Outpatient hematologic evaluation was scheduled to investigate for possible thrombophilia. After a successful in-hospital evolution, the patient was discharged asymptomatic within six days. Discharge medications were aspirin 100 mg, metoprolol 50 mg BID, enalapril 10 mg BID, simvastatin 40 mg, clopidogrel 75 mg, and warfarin 5 mg. It was planned to use triple therapy for one month and then switch to dual therapy with clopidogrel and warfarin, indefinitely.

3. Discussion

Coronary artery ectasia (CAE) is characterized by abnormal dilatation of a localized or diffuse segment of the epicardial coronary arteries with a luminal diameter of at least 1.5-fold of normal adjacent segment or vessel diameter [4]. The incidence of CAE in patients investigated for coronary artery disease is between 1% and 2–5% [5]. It is caused by destruction of the vessel media and frequently coexists with coronary atherosclerosis. Even in the absence of obstructive disease, the presence of dilated coronary segments results in alterations in blood flow and stasis, predisposing to adverse coronary events like vasospasm, thrombosis, and dissection [4]. Recent study by Doi et al. showed higher incidence of major cardiac events, cardiovascular mortality, and nonfatal myocardial infarction in patients with CAE [6].

ST-segment elevation myocardial infarction caused by multiple culprit coronary arteries is rare, with the largest series of cases reporting 47 patients with this condition [7]. Clinical presentation can be devastating because of the vast myocardial area jeopardized, with a high rate of harmful outcomes such as ventricular arrhythmia, severe heart

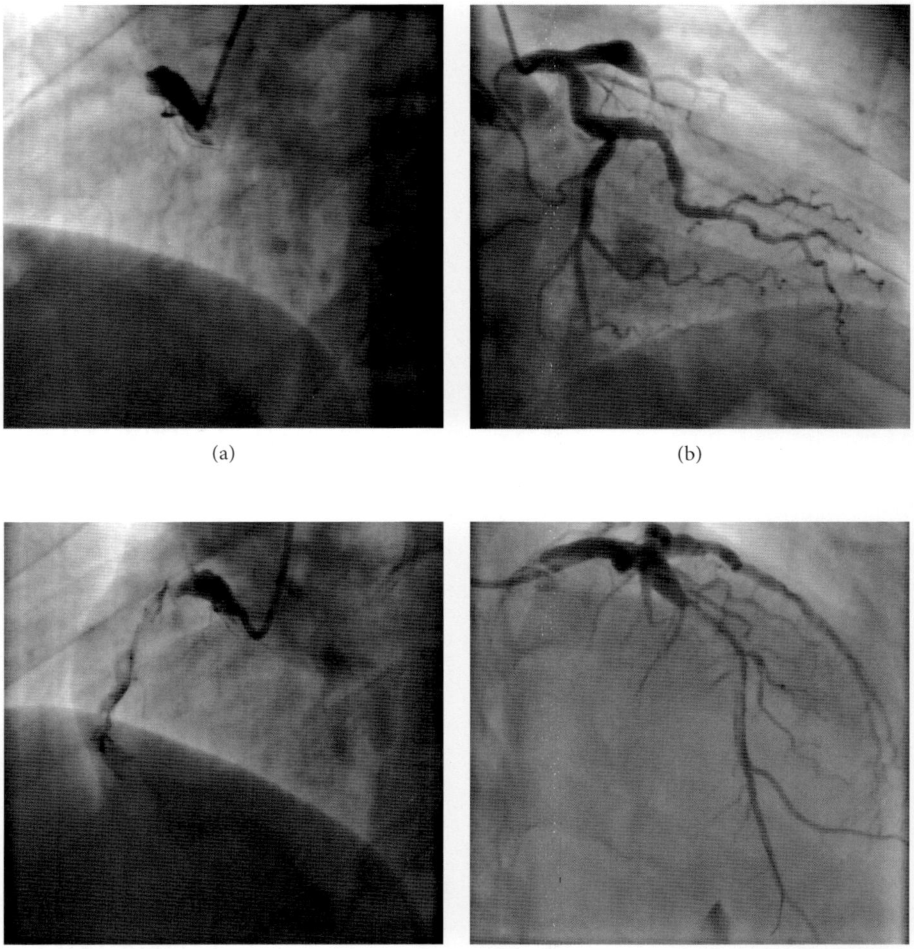

(a) (b)

(c) (d)

Figure 2: Coronary angiography. Marked ectasia and proximal occlusion of right coronary artery (a) and left anterior descending coronary artery (b). After initial ballon angioplasty, both vessels showed extensive thrombus burden and flow restriction (c and d).

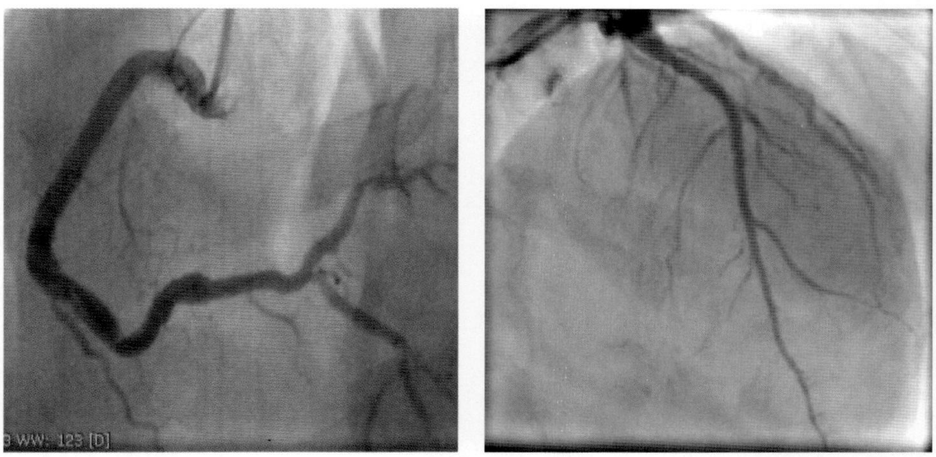

(a) (b)

Figure 3: Final angiographic result. Both right coronary artery (a) and left anterior descending coronary artery (b) showing good angiographic result, with TIMI 3 flow and no residual stenoses.

failure, and cardiogenic shock [5]. There are several etiologies of multivessel coronary thrombosis, all of them related to the Virchow's triad which include endothelial dysfunction, hemodynamic changes (i.e., stasis and turbulence), and hypercoagulability [7–9]. Factors probably involved with multiple coronary artery thrombosis in our patient include a proinflammatory state and blood turbulence caused by coronary ectasia, and heightened inflammatory response caused by the acute occlusion of the first vessel.

There are some considerations regarding the management of our patient that needs to be highlighted: First, the choice of the first vessel to be treated was made on the larger myocardium supplied by LAD, and hemodynamic collapse could have occurred if RCA had been treated first due to large delay that would have happened because of complexity of the RCA PCI. It is intriguing that cardiogenic shock did not occur in this case, possibly because of collateral recruitment from the previous coronary events. Second, the combination of coronary ectasia and high thrombus burden, such as in our patient, illustrates a potential scenario of clinical benefit of aspiration thrombectomy. Third, IIb/IIIa glycoprotein inhibitor therapy promptly initiated when anatomy was defined by angiography probably was of great value. Fourth, bare metal stenting was performed aiming chronic anticoagulation, allowing the use of triple antiplatelet therapy for a shorter period and reducing the risk of bleeding. Taken all together, the anatomical and technical issues in this case were very enlightening.

References

[1] T. Kanei, R. Janardhanan, J. T. Fox, and R. M. Gowda, "Multivessel coronary artery thrombosis," *Journal of Invasive Cardiology*, vol. 21, no. 2, pp. 66–68, 2009.

[2] P. S. Swaye, L. D. Fisher, P. Litwin et al., "Aneurysmal coronary artery disease," *Circulation*, vol. 67, no. 1, pp. 134–138, 1983.

[3] G. N. Levine, E. R. Bates, J. C. Blankenship et al., "2015 ACC/AHA/SCAI focused update on primary percutaneous coronary intervention or patients with ST-elevation myocardial infarction: an update of the 2011 ACCF/AHA/SCAI guideline for percutaneous coronary intervention and the 2013 ACCF/AHA guideline for the management of ST-elevation myocardial infarction: a report of the American College of Cardiology/American Heart Association task force on clinical practice guidelines and the Society for Cardiovascular Angiography and Interventions.," *Circulation*, vol. 133, no. 11, pp. 1135–1147, 2016.

[4] E. P. Bermudez, R. L. Oalop, I. L. Martinez-Luengas et al., "Coronary ectasia: prevalence, and clinical and angiographic characteristics," *Revista Española de Cardiología*, vol. 56, no. 5, pp. 473–479, 2003.

[5] G. G. Hartnell, P. M. Parnell, and R. B. Pridie, "Coronary artery ectasia, its prevalence and clinical significance in 4993 patients," *British Heart Journal*, vol. 54, no. 4, pp. 392–395, 1985.

[6] T. Doi, Y. Kataoka, T. Noguchi et al., "Coronary artery ectasia predicts future cardiac events in patients with acute myocardial infarction," *Arteriosclerosis, Thrombosis, and Vascular Biology*, vol. 37, no. 12, pp. 2350–2355, 2017.

[7] P. M. Pollak, S. V. Parikh, M. Kizilgul, and E. C. Keeley, "Multiple culprit arteries in patients with ST segment elevation myocardial infarction referred for primary percutaneous coronary intervention," *The American Journal of Cardiology*, vol. 104, no. 5, pp. 619–623, 2009.

[8] C. M. Tu, C. H. Hsueg, K. M. Chu, S. M. Cheng, and T. P. Tsao, "Simultaneous thombosis of double coronary arteries in a young male with antithrombin III deficiency," *The American Journal of Emergency Medicine*, vol. 27, no. 9, pp. 1169.e3–1169.e6, 2009.

[9] H. Meltser, D. Bhakta, and V. Kalaria, "Multivessel coronary thrombosis secondary to cocaine use successfully treated with multivessel primary angioplasty," *International Journal of Cardiovascular Interventions*, vol. 6, no. 1, pp. 39–42, 2004.

Successful Treatment of Occlusive Left Main Coronary Artery Dissection by Impella-Supported Stenting

James J. Glazier, Amir Kaki, and Theodore L. Schreiber

Detroit Medical Center Heart Hospital, Wayne State University, Detroit, MI, USA

Correspondence should be addressed to James J. Glazier; jamesjglazier@hotmail.com

Academic Editor: Assad Movahed

We report successful treatment of a patient, who, during diagnostic angiography, developed an ostial left main coronary artery dissection with stump occlusion of the vessel. First, mechanical circulatory support with an Impella CP device was established. Then, patency of the left coronary system was achieved by placement of stents in the left anterior descending, left circumflex, and left main coronary arteries. On completion of the procedure, left ventricular systolic function, as assessed by echocardiography, was normal. At 24-month clinical follow-up, the patient remains angina-free and well. This is the first reported case of the use of an Impella device to support treatment of iatrogenic left main coronary artery dissection.

1. Introduction

The Impella device is a percutaneously inserted miniaturized ventricular assist device that is being increasingly used in the treatment of patients with acute myocardial infarction complicated by cardiogenic shock (AMICS) [1–4]. It has also been found to have a potentially valuable role in increasing the safety and efficacy of high-risk coronary interventional procedures (PCI), such as stenting of unprotected left main stem coronary artery (ULMCA) [5]. Using a retrograde femoral (or, occasionally, axillary) artery access, it is generally placed using standard percutaneous techniques in the left ventricular chamber (LV) across the aortic valve. The device pumps blood from the left ventricle into the ascending aorta and systemic circulation at an upper rate between 2.5 and 5.0 L/min, depending on the particular model type. The device provides almost immediate and sustained unloading of the left ventricle while increasing overall systemic cardiac output with maintenance of mean arterial pressure [1, 2]. Recently, an increasing body of evidence has suggested that in AMICS, a strategy of first implanting the Impella device before performing PCI is associated with improved survival [3, 4]. In particular, a recent report by Meraj et al. [6] suggests that initiation of cardiac mechanical support by Impella prior to PCI on ULMCA culprit lesion in AMCIS is associated with significantly improved early survival compared to Impella support following PCI. We now report our application of these observations in the treatment of a patient with catheter-induced obliterative occlusion of the LMCA.

2. Case Report

A 58-year-old woman with a history of current cigarette smoking, hypertension, and hyperlipidemia presented to the emergency room at our center reporting recurrent episodes of severe central chest pain over the preceding 24 hours. While her ECG showed no significant ST segment shifts, troponin I levels were slightly increased (0.025 ng/mL). Accordingly, she was referred for coronary angiography in the setting of a non-ST segment elevation MI.

Catheterization was performed via the right radial artery using the 6 French (F) Amplatz R1 and 6F Judkins L 3.5 diagnostic catheters (Medtronic Inc., Minneapolis, MN, USA). The only angiographic abnormality noted was a moderate stenosis of the mid left anterior descending coronary artery (LAD) (Figure 1). To further assess the physiological significance of this stenosis, an iFFR PrimeWire (Volcano Corp, San Diego, CA, USA) was placed in the LAD, following exchange of the Judkins catheter for a 6F Extra Back-Up (EBU) 3.5 guiding catheter (Medtronic Inc., Minneapolis,

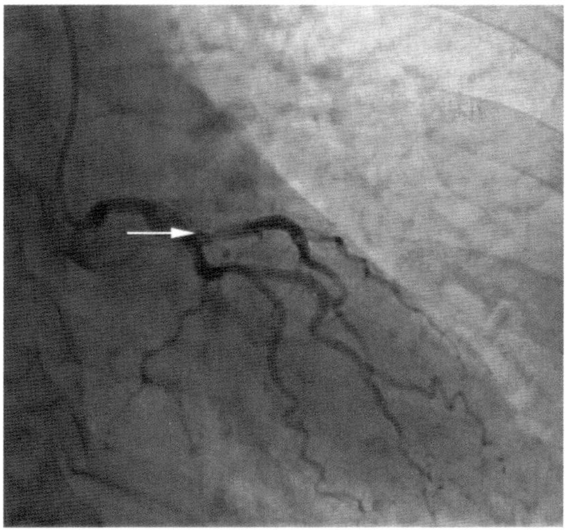

FIGURE 1: Left coronary angiogram showing a moderate stenosis (arrow) of the left anterior descending coronary artery.

MN, USA). Of note, initial angiography through the EBU guide catheter prior to advancing the wire showed good coronary flow. It was, however, not possible to advance the wire to the lesion. Accordingly, the PrimeWire was removed from the vessel and then an angiogram of the left coronary artery was taken. Angiography revealed only a stump of the left main coronary artery (LMCA) with occlusion of both the LAD and of the circumflex (LCx) coronary arteries (Figure 2). Marked (3 mm) anterior ST segment elevation then developed, and the patient became progressively hypotensive with systolic pressure falling to a nadir of 58 mmHg. Inotropic and pressor infusions were commenced.

We, at this point, decided to establish mechanical circulatory support with the Impella CP device (Abiomed, Danvers, MA, USA) prior to attempting to reestablish patency of the left coronary system with stents. We first placed a 6F sheath in the left femoral artery. Just as we gained access, the patient developed ventricular fibrillation. This was immediately treated with one 150-Joule biphasic nonsynchronized shock. Following this, the 6F sheath was changed out over a 0.35″ Wholey wire (Medtronic Inc., Minneapolis, MN, USA) for a long 8F arterial sheath. Then, a 6F multipurpose diagnostic catheter was advanced through the sheath to the LV. Next, the Impella 0.18″ deployment wire was advanced through the multipurpose catheter to the LV and the multipurpose catheter then withdrawn. The 8F sheath was then changed out for a 14F sheath, and the Impella CP device advanced over the wire to the LV. The wire was withdrawn, and satisfactory positioning of the device was confirmed by fluoroscopy with the inflow within the LV and the outflow above the aortic valve. The Impella device was then activated and placed on "auto mode" which allows the device to ramp to P9 level resulting in a cardiac output of 3.5 L/min. The mean arterial pressure increased to 80 mmHg, and there was no further occurrence of ventricular dysrhythmias.

Having initiated mechanical circulatory support, we then set out to reestablish patency of the left coronary system. A 0.014″ Runthrough guidewire (Terumo, Somerset, NJ,

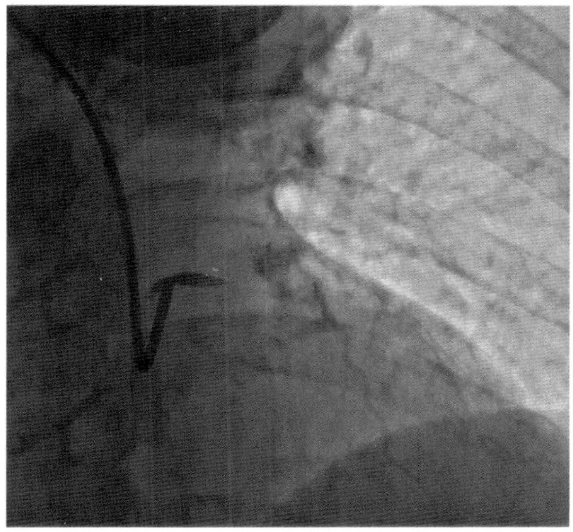

FIGURE 2: Occlusive dissection of the left main coronary artery.

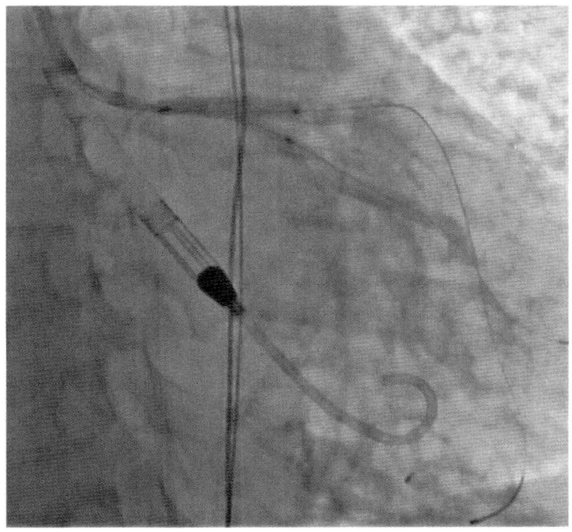

FIGURE 3: Final deployment of the left anterior descending and left circumflex coronary artery stents with a kiss.

USA) was advanced into the LCx artery, and a second 0.014″ Runthrough wire advanced into the LAD. The vessels were then dilated with 2.0 mm × 20 mm and 2.5 mm × 20 mm Trek (Abbott Vascular, Santa Clara, CA, USA) balloons with restoration of flow first in the LAD and then in the LCx.

We then placed a 3.0 mm × 18 mm Resolute stent (Medtronic Inc., Minneapolis, MN, USA) from the LM to the LAD. Next, we rewired the LCx through the LAD stent struts. We then stented the LCx with a 3.0 mm × 38 mm Resolute stent. After this, a 3.0 mm × 20 mm Trek balloon was placed within the LAD stent, and a 2.5 mm × 15 mm Trek balloon placed within the LCx stent. Final deployment of the stents was with simultaneous inflation of the 2 balloons (kissing balloon dilation) (Figure 3). Finally, a 4.0 mm × 9 mm Resolute stent was deployed from the shaft to the ostium of the LM. Angiography demonstrated reestablishment of patency of the LM, LAD, and LCx (Figure 4), and intravascular ultrasound of the LAD and LM showed good stent apposition in

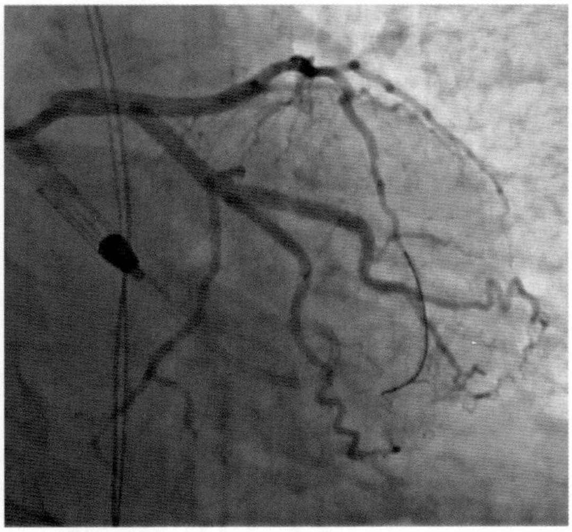

Figure 4: Final angiographic result demonstrating patency of the left coronary system.

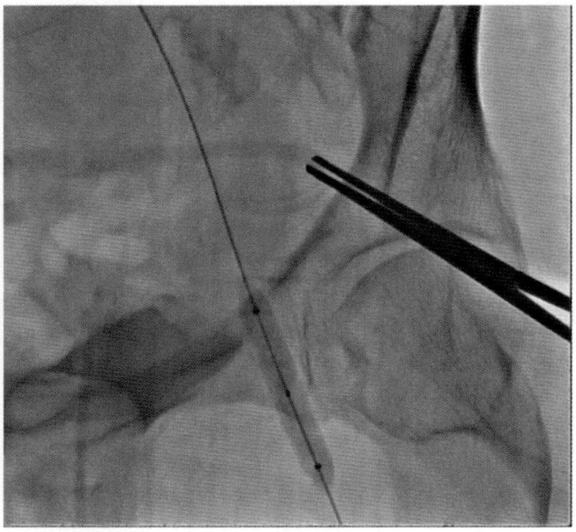

Figure 5: Crossover balloon tamponade of the left femoral artery following removal of the Impella device.

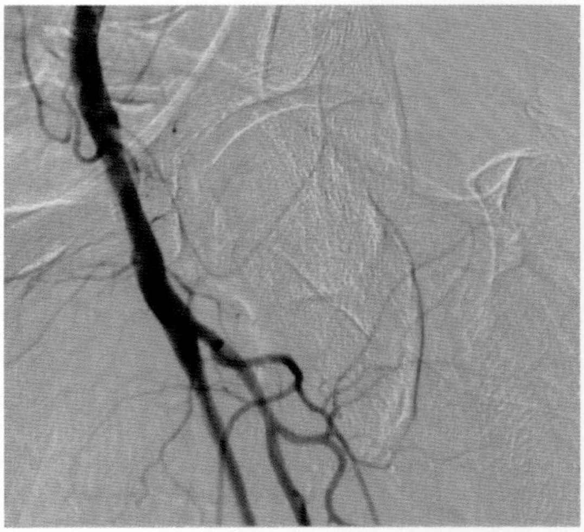

Figure 6: Final left femoral angiogram confirming hemostasis and absence of femoral artery abnormality or complication.

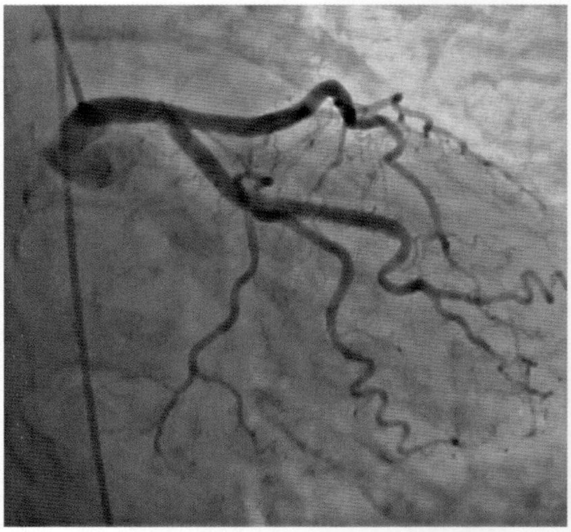

Figure 7: Left coronary angiogram at 6-month follow-up showing continued patency of the previously placed stents.

these vessels. Immediately on completion of the procedure, a 2D echocardiogram was performed in the lab. This showed normal LV systolic function (LVEF = 55%). By this time, all inotropic and pressor agents had been discontinued. The patient was then weaned from the Impella device, and the device was removed from the cardiac catheterization laboratory. At our center, the usual approach to device removal is with suture-mediated closure. Because of the emergent need for Impella support in our patient, a technique of crossover balloon tamponade was used (Figure 5) with completion angiography to confirm hemostasis and absence of femoral artery abnormality or complication (Figure 6). The general approach at our center to cases of primary PCI in the setting of cardiogenic shock is to retain the Impella hemodynamic support for a minimum of 24 hours to allow for myocardial recovery. However, in this case, because of the rapid identification of shock and the prompt recovery of mean arterial pressure and the ability to discontinue all pressor support, we elected to remove the device while in the cardiac catheterization laboratory. An additional parameter that supported the latter decision was demonstration of a mixed venous oxygen saturation ≥ 65% on P3 setting for 30 minutes.

Following her procedure, the patient did well with no recurrence of symptoms, hemodynamic abnormalities, or dysrhythmias, and she was discharged home 2 days later. Follow-up coronary angiography 6 months after the initial procedure (Figure 7) showed continuing patency of the left coronary system without any significant residual stenosis. At 24-month clinical follow-up, the patient remains angina-free and with continuing normal LV systolic function.

3. Discussion

Iatrogenic LMCA dissection, although rare, is a dreaded complication of diagnostic coronary angiography, often dubbed "the angiographer's nightmare." It has potentially devastating complications, including death on the cath lab table. It is usually treated with immediate stenting [7–10]. However, we judged that initial stenting might not be the optimal initial strategy in our patient. Most reports regarding iatrogenic LMCA dissection have described patients with a nonocclusive pattern with residual continued flow in the LAD and LCx. In contrast, our patient had an extreme form of dissection with amputation of the LMCA and no flow in the LAD or LCx. With such a dissection, successful advancement of guidewires first into the true lumen of the LMCA and then into the true lumina of the LAD and LCx can be technically challenging and time-consuming, with no guarantee of eventual success. Moreover, our patient was hemodynamically unstable and needed urgent institution of additional circulatory support to prevent development of refractory cardiogenic shock.

Of the available mechanical support devices, the Impella device seemed particularly suited to our patient. This device can be inserted quickly and provides almost immediate unloading of the LV and increased cardiac output and maintenance of mean arterial pressure. The particular Impella model used in our patient was the Impella CP. This pumps blood from the LV to the systemic circulation at a rate up to 4.0 L/min. This effect was demonstrated in our patient, who became hemodynamically stable within a few minutes of initiation of the Impella support. Thus, it allowed us to undertake, in a stable setting, the technically demanding and complex task of wiring and then performing bifurcation stenting using a two-stent technique of the occluded left coronary system. This stability was likely a key factor in achieving the excellent angiographic and durable clinical results out to 24 months seen in our patient. Without the Impella device, we would likely have had to attempt complex PCI on a background of recurrent malignant ventricular dysrhythmias and progressive hypotension despite escalating doses of inotropes and pressors. The Impella device also served as a potential valuable bridge to coronary bypass surgery in the event that we were unsuccessful in restoring left coronary patency by PCI.

Other authors [8, 10] have described the use of the intra-aortic balloon pump (IABP), as opposed to the Impella device, to provide hemodynamic support during coronary stent placement for left main dissection. However, in comparison to the Impella CP device, the ability of IABP to augment cardiac output is very modest: no more than 0.5 L/min [1]. The superior hemodynamic effect of the Impella device was a key factor in choosing this device over IABP in our patient. In addition, our large experience with the Impella (we implant >150 devices per year) allows us to implant this device in about the same time it takes to implant an IABP. However, we concede that there is a lack of evidence based on randomized controlled clinical trials to favor the use of the Impella over the IABP either in patients with cardiogenic shock [11] or in patients undergoing high-risk PCI [12].

Recently, an increasing body of evidence suggests that in patients with cardiogenic shock (as was the case for our patient), early initiation of Impella (i.e., initiation before PCI) (as was done in our patient) is associated with increased patient survival when compared with a strategy of initiating Impella after PCI [3, 4, 6]. In the reported data set, early initiation of Impella provides effective left ventricular unloading while maintaining adequate systemic and coronary perfusion and thus prevents the downward spiral of cardiogenic shock. These data provide further support for the interventional strategy used in the presently reported patient.

If the operator and cardiac catheterization laboratory have limited experience in Impella implantation, an excessive amount of time may be spent in attempting to implant the device. Accordingly, in such situations, it may be preferable that the operator proceeds directly to attempting to wire the occluded vessel.

The results of a recently reported study suggest that in non-CS patients undergoing LMCA PCI, prophylactic insertion of the Impella ventricular assist device may be associated with improved procedural success rates and reduced complication rates [5]. Accordingly, Impella insertion prior to LMCA stenting may also be considered in selected hemodynamically stable patients with iatrogenic LMCA dissection.

4. Conclusion

In the treatment of iatrogenic LMCA dissection, a strategy of initial insertion of the Impella device followed by LMCA stenting should be considered favorably in all those with hemodynamic instability as well as in selected hemodynamically stable patients.

References

[1] F. Burzotta, C. Trani, S. N. Doshi et al., "Impella ventricular support in clinical practice: collaborative viewpoint from a European expert user group," *International Journal of Cardiology*, vol. 201, pp. 684–691, 2015.

[2] N. A. Gilotra and G. R. Stevens, "Temporary mechanical circulatory support: a review of the options, indications, and outcomes," *Clinical Medicine Insights: Cardiology*, vol. 8-s1, article CMC.S15718, suppl 1, 2015.

[3] M. B. Basir, T. L. Schreiber, C. L. Grines et al., "Effect of early initiation of mechanical circulatory support on survival in cardiogenic shock," *The American Journal of Cardiology*, vol. 119, no. 6, pp. 845–851, 2017.

[4] M. P. Flaherty, A. R. Khan, and W. W. O'Neill, "Early initiation of Impella in acute myocardial infarction complicated by cardiogenic shock improves survival: a meta-analysis," *JACC: Cardiovascular Interventions*, vol. 10, no. 17, pp. 1805-1806, 2017.

[5] T. Schreiber, W. Wah Htun, N. Blank et al., "Real-world supported unprotected left main percutaneous coronary intervention with Impella device; data from the USpella registry," *Catheterization and Cardiovascular Interventions*, vol. 90, no. 4, pp. 576–581, 2017.

[6] P. M. Meraj, R. Doshi, T. Schreiber, B. Maini, and W. W. O'Neill, "Impella 2.5 initiated prior to unprotected left main PCI in acute myocardial infarction complicated by cardiogenic shock improves early survival," *Journal of Interventional Cardiology*, vol. 30, no. 3, pp. 256–263, 2017.

[7] P. Eshtehardi, P. Adorjan, M. Togni et al., "Iatrogenic left main coronary artery dissection: incidence, classification, manage-

ment, and long-term follow-up," *American Heart Journal*, vol. 159, no. 6, pp. 1147–1153, 2010.

[8] H. Kubota, T. Nomura, Y. Hori et al., "Successful bailout stenting strategy against lethal coronary dissection involving left main bifurcation," *Clinical Case Reports*, vol. 5, no. 6, pp. 894–898, 2017.

[9] F. Akgul, T. Batyraliev, F. Besnili, and Z. Karben, "Emergency stenting of unprotected left main coronary artery after acute catheter-induced occlusive dissection," *Texas Heart Institute Journal*, vol. 33, pp. 515–518, 2016.

[10] K. Onsea, P. Kayaert, W. Desmet, and C. L. Dubois, "Iatrogenic left main coronary artery dissection," *Netherlands Heart Journal*, vol. 19, no. 4, pp. 192–195, 2011.

[11] J. J. Glazier and A. Kaki, "Improving survival in cardiogenic shock: is Impella the answer?," *The American Journal of Medicine*, vol. 131, 2018.

[12] W. W. O'Neill, N. S. Kleiman, J. Moses et al., "A prospective, randomized clinical trial of hemodynamic support with Impella 2.5 versus intra-aortic balloon pump in patients undergoing high-risk percutaneous coronary intervention: the PROTECT II study," *Circulation*, vol. 126, no. 14, pp. 1717–1727, 2012.

Aortic Dissection Presenting as Acute Pancreatitis: Suspecting the Unexpected

Adam Hafeez, [1,2] Dillon Karmo, [1,2] Adrian Mercado-Alamo, [1,2] and Alexandra Halalau [2,3]

[1] *Internal Medicine Department, Beaumont Hospital, Royal Oak, MI, USA*
[2] *Oakland University William Beaumont School of Medicine, Rochester, MI, USA*
[3] *General Internal Medicine Division, Beaumont Hospital, Royal Oak, MI, USA*

Correspondence should be addressed to Adam Hafeez; adam.hafeez@beaumont.org

Academic Editor: Takatoshi Kasai

Aortic dissection is a life-threatening condition in which the inner layer of the aorta tears. Blood surges through the tear, causing the inner and middle layers of the aorta to separate (dissect). It is considered a medical emergency. We report a case of a healthy 56-year-old male who presented to the emergency room with sudden onset of epigastric pain radiating to his back. His blood pressure was 167/91 mmHg, equal in both arms. His lipase was elevated at 1258 U/L, and he was clinically diagnosed with acute pancreatitis (AP). He denied any alcohol consumption, had no evidence for gallstones, and had normal triglyceride level. Two days later, he endorsed new suprapubic tenderness radiating to his scrotum, along with worsening epigastric pain. A MRCP demonstrated evidence of an aortic dissection (AD). CT angiography demonstrated a Stanford type B AD extending into the proximal common iliac arteries. His aortic dissection was managed medically with rapid blood pressure control. The patient had excellent recovery and was discharged home without any surgical intervention.

1. Introduction

Aortic dissection remains the deadliest manifestation of acute aortic syndromes with mortality as high as 1% per hour for acute type A aortic dissections [1]. The classical clinical presentation of an aortic dissection is of a male in his 60s who presents to the emergency room with sudden onset tearing or ripping chest pain. Hypertension, noted on vitals and with physical exam maneuvers such as blood pressure discrepancies in the arms, can help make the diagnosis. However, more importantly, the presentation can vary, and the classical symptoms may be absent or inconsistent [2]. This can paint a diagnostic dilemma for the clinician.

Acute pancreatitis has been increasing in incidence, with estimates of an increase in 20% in admissions over the last 10 years in the United States [3]. Acute pancreatitis also presents with severe epigastric pain which often radiates to the back. Diagnosis can be made with two of the three following features: (1) abdominal pain, (2) elevated serum lipase or amylase at least three times the upper limit of normal, and (3) characteristic findings of acute pancreatitis on contrast-enhanced computed tomography (CT), magnetic resonance imaging (MRI), or even ultrasound [4]. Therefore, the diagnosis can be made clinically without imaging.

The presentation of acute pancreatitis in the setting of aortic dissection poses a diagnostic challenge, as some of the cardinal symptoms of aortic dissection, such as hypertension and pain, overlap with acute pancreatitis. Acute pancreatitis is a clinical diagnosis, but without an easily identifiable cause, such as gallstones, alcohol abuse, or hypertriglyceridemia, further imaging may be warranted if the patient does not clinically improve. Due to its lethal complications, physicians should be aware and should have a high index of suspicion for aortic dissection when evaluating a patient with presumed acute pancreatitis.

Acute pancreatitis presenting as acute aortic dissection is a rare entity with less than ten well-documented cases reported so far. It is hypothesized that the pancreas can be susceptible to hypoperfusion as seen in cardiopulmonary bypass surgery [3]. We present a case misdiagnosed as only

TABLE 1: Key laboratory investigations on admission.

Laboratory	Value	Normal	Laboratory	Value	Normal
Hemoglobin	14.4	13.6–17.6 g/dL	AST	59	10–37 U/L
Potassium	3.6	3.5–5.3 mmol/L	ALT	111	9–47 U/L
BNP	10	0–100 pg/mL	Cholesterol	220	70–199 mg/dL
BUN	16	8–23 mg/dL	Triglyceride	111	40–139 mg/dL
Creatinine	1.16	0.64–1.27 mg/dL	Troponin	0.03	0.00–0.05 ng/mL
Amylase	163	20–104 U/L	ANCA	<1 : 20	<1 : 20
Rheumatoid factor	Negative	Negative	ANA screen	Negative	Negative

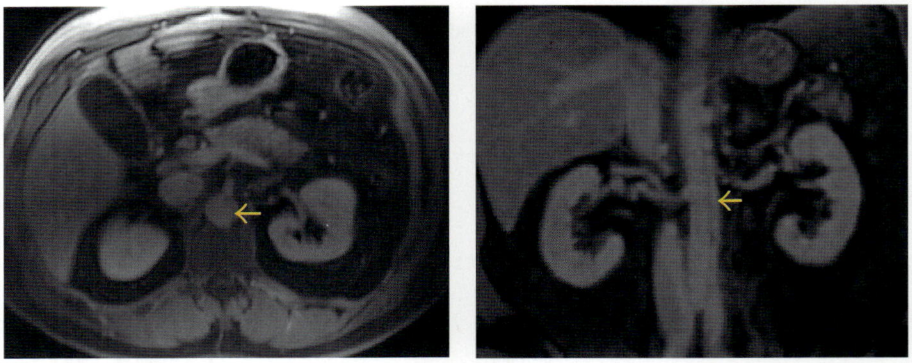

(a) (b)

FIGURE 1: Magnetic resonance cholangiopancreatography (MRCP). (a) Dissection can be seen extending to the origin of the iliac arteries. (b) MRCP demonstrating acute aortic dissection with narrowing of the true lumen (yellow arrow). Of note, there is no peripancreatic inflammatory changes or fluid collections noted.

acute pancreatitis based on clinical symptoms and later correctly diagnosed as an aortic dissection when symptoms did not improve.

2. Case Presentation

A 56-year-old male with no significant past medical history presented to the emergency room with the chief complaint of sudden onset of substernal chest pain radiating to his back. His family history was noncontributory. He denied tobacco, alcohol, or illicit drug use. The patient worked as a traveling musician. He denied any recent trauma. Initial vitals revealed hypertension (167/91 mmHg). Physical exam was significant for reproducible midepigastric pain, without guarding or rebound. Chest and abdominal radiographs were unremarkable. The patient had a mild leukocytosis (10.9 bil/L), elevated lipase (1258 U/L), elevated amylase (163 U/L), normal triglycerides, and negative autoimmune workup (Table 1). His EKG showed normal sinus rhythm with a rate of 80 beats/minute, normal axis, normal interval durations, and no signs of acute or chronic ischemia or left ventricular (LV) hypertrophy. Abdominal US was negative for cholelithiasis. He had no recent procedures performed and was on no medications prior to presentation. He was treated with IV fluids and bowel rest for presumed acute pancreatitis diagnosed clinically because of elevated lipase and epigastric pain. An abdominal CT scan to assess the severity of pancreatitis was not indicated to be performed as the patient's clinical symptoms were stable. Throughout his admission, his pain never fully resolved. On day 5, he developed a marked increase in blood pressure (194/112 mmHg). He was diaphoretic on exam with worsening of his epigastric pain. He also endorsed new suprapubic pain radiating to his scrotum along with dysuria and increased urinary frequency. Because of the acute worsening of the patient's condition, a MRCP was ordered to examine the pancreas and the hepatobiliary tree. Incidentally, the MRCP demonstrated evidence of a large aortic dissection (Figure 1). CT angiography demonstrated a Stanford type B AD (Figure 2) extending into the proximal common iliac arteries (Figure 3) that explained his new suprapubic and scrotum pain. There was no radiographic evidence of peripancreatic inflammatory changes or fluid collections.

The patient's pancreatitis was treated with bowel rest, IV fluids, and pain medication. The patient's aortic dissection was treated with IV labetalol and nitroprusside in the ICU with rapid lowering of his blood pressure. No surgical intervention was performed.

3. Discussion

Aortic dissection remains a devastating vascular catastrophe with a high mortality rate if not diagnosed and managed promptly. However, its signs and symptoms are unpredictable. As the dissection progresses, other organs can be affected and can obscure the inciting diagnosis.

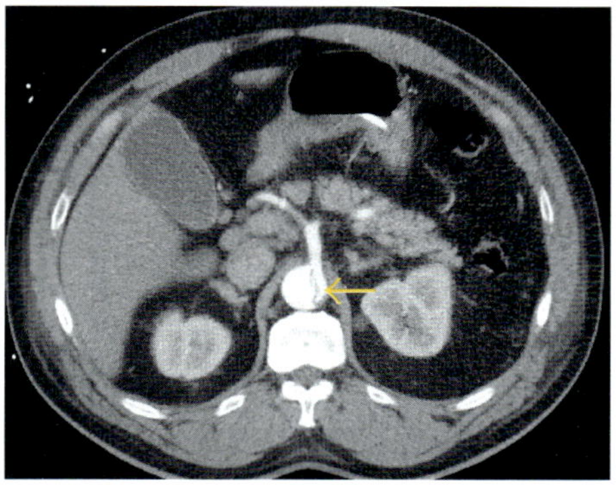

Figure 2: CT angiography showing acute type B aortic dissection with severe narrowing of the true lumen (yellow arrow).

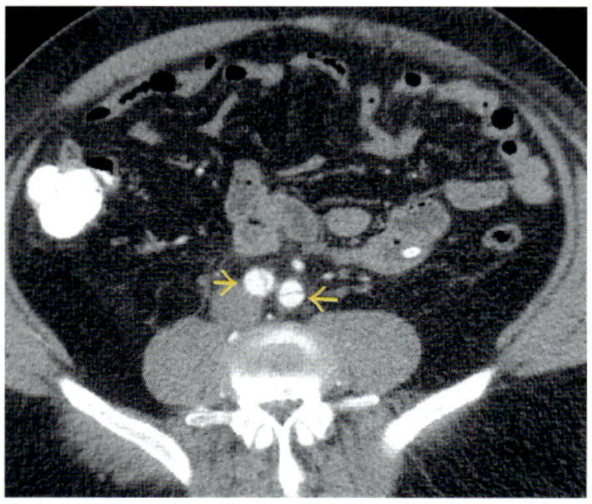

Figure 3: CT angiography showing acute type B aortic dissection extending into the proximal common iliac arteries (yellow arrows). This parallels with the patient's clinical complaints of scrotal pain and dysuria.

Pancreatitis remains a rare complication of aortic dissection, and the association between the two has yet to be elucidated. A retrospective study by Li et al. examining the forensic characteristics of patients who suffered sudden unexpected deaths due to an aortic dissection showed that 83.9% of the patients were misdiagnosed and the dissection was not recognized. Of these, only one case was diagnosed as acute pancreatitis, which highlights the rarity of this presentation [5]. To our knowledge, there are only ten well-documented cases reported worldwide. Recently, Pham and Nable described a case of a woman with an exacerbation of several months of abdominal pain that was clinically diagnosed with pancreatitis based on epigastric pain as well as elevated lipase (723 U/L). Unlike our case, the woman had a prior history of aortic aneurysmal repair. An abdominal CT was pursued to look for any complications of pancreatitis. She was found to have an incidental Stanford type B aortic dissection [6].

The International Registry of Acute Aortic Dissection (IRAD) database recognizes malperfusion in 21% of the patients with Stanford type B aortic dissection. However, acute pancreatitis is not described as an ischemic complication of acute aortic dissection in the IRAD [7]. Common risk factors for acute pancreatitis are gallbladder disease, chronic alcohol consumption, and recent procedures. Rarely, hypercalcemia, hyperlipidemia, autoimmune disorders, or medications can induce pancreatitis [3]. A limited number of case studies reported an association of acute aortic dissection with acute pancreatitis. Masaki reports a case of a middle-aged man diagnosed first with Stanford type B aortic dissection with the true lumen supplying the celiac trunk and splenic artery. Due to thrombosis of the false lumen, the true lumen became narrow. The patient developed upper abdominal pain as well as an elevation in pancreatic amylase. A CT showed peripancreatic fluid [8]. These findings were consistent with acute pancreatitis. As the acute pancreatitis developed hours after aortic dissection, it was thought that possible ischemia-reperfusion injury initiated the acute pancreatitis. A similar case was described by Zheng et al; however, the patient was found to have a type A aortic dissection when a CT scan was performed to confirm the diagnosis after management of acute pancreatitis had already begun [9].

Ischemic injury to the pancreas occurring in clinical situations such as shock or major cardiac surgery is rare. For example, ischemic injury to the pancreas following cardiopulmonary bypass surgery has been reported to occur with an incidence of less than 1% [10]. Similarly, resection or repair of an aortic aneurysm has been shown to induce pancreatitis [11]. Aortic dissection can, like cardiopulmonary bypass surgery or manipulation of the aorta, produce a hypoperfused state leading to ischemic injury to the pancreas. However, the injury seen in the pancreas may not be as severe as other organs, such as the kidney or liver. It is hypothesized that this can be due to rich collateral blood supply to the pancreas [12]. Notably, the pancreatic head receives blood supply from the superior mesenteric artery. The body and tail, on the other hand, can receive blood not only from branches of the splenic artery but also from branches originating from the celiac or superior mesenteric arteries as well as the splenic hilum itself [12]. This may explain why the acute pancreatitis caused by hypoperfusion may remain mild and not produce radiographic evidence of pancreatitis, as seen in our patient. Additionally, an acute aortic dissection is a dynamic process, and it is possible that transient malperfusion may take place as the dissection progresses. Therefore, the lipase may reflect ischemic injury that has resolved.

Due to the arterial collaterals supplying the pancreas, it is likely that hypoperfusion may not be the only factor at play. Another hypothesis comes from a case report of a patient that suffered severe necrotic pancreatitis caused by a type B aortic dissection [13]. It was hypothesized that cholesterol emboli from the dissecting aorta were the main cause of the pancreatic necrosis [13]. In our case, there was no such evidence for any embolic phenomena.

As noted, the kidney, heart, brain, and liver are commonly affected by shock. The pancreas is not regularly believed to be affected, although pathophysiologically can suffer ischemia like any other organ. Warshaw and O'Hara et al. retrospectively studied autopsies of patients who died due to shock after repair of abdominal aortic aneurysms or open heart surgery. He found a 9% incidence of pancreatic injury in this patient group. More interestingly, there was a strong positive correlation with presence of renal ischemic injury, with 50% concomitant pancreatic injury in the setting of acute tubular necrosis ($p < 0.001$) [14]. The author noted that it was ischemia, not operative trauma, which led to pancreatic injury. More so, all the patients with shock that were followed prospectively had elevated lipase levels but no signs or symptoms of pancreatitis. This is similar to our case report in the sense that the patient had elevated lipase and aortic dissection-related pain but no evidence of acute pancreatitis on imaging.

As the precise etiology of pancreatitis following aortic dissection continues to be elucidated, what remains is the diagnostic challenge of efficiently differentiating between the clinical manifestations of aortic dissection and other etiologies of acute abdominal pain such as acute cardiac ischemia, pancreatitis, or intestinal obstruction. Imaging remains at the heart of this differentiation, but this may not always be cost-effective, efficient, and noninvasive. Most patients with severe hypoperfusion will be having renal ischemia, and adding contrast agents for imaging may not be ideal. Wen et al. researched the role of matrix metalloproteinases (MMPs), proteases that have been indicated in aortic aneurysms to correlate with aortic-wall proteolysis, as a diagnostic tool for detection of aortic dissection. MMPs also have been shown to be elevated in patients with pancreatitis. They prospectively studied 20 patients each with aortic dissection and acute pancreatitis within 1 hour of symptom onset in the emergency room and found that MMPs were higher in patients with acute AD as compared to acute pancreatitis ($p < 0.05$) [15]. It is possible that, in the future, MMPs to be used as a marker to help differentiate between the two causes of severe epigastric pain. Although more research into optimal markers and imaging needs to be done, the burden rests on the clinician's shoulders to keep a wide differential diagnosis. If an etiology is not identified, further imaging must be pursued sooner rather than later to rule out rarer etiologies for pancreatitis and to also assess for other possible etiologies in the same anatomical region, that is, aortic dissection.

References

[1] M. A. Coady, J. A. Rizzo, L. J. Goldstein, and J. A. Elefteriades, "Natural history, pathogenesis, and etiology of thoracic aortic aneurysms and dissections," *Cardiology Clinics*, vol. 17, no. 4, pp. 615–635, 1999.

[2] F. J. Criado, "Aortic dissection: a 250-year perspective," *Texas Heart Institute Journal*, vol. 38, no. 6, pp. 694–700, 2011.

[3] C. E. Forsmark, S. Swaroop Vege, and C. M. Wilcox, "Acute pancreatitis," *New England Journal of Medicine*, vol. 375, no. 20, pp. 1972–1981, 2016.

[4] P. A. Banks, T. L. Bollen, C. Dervenis et al., "Classification of acute pancreatitis—2012: revision of the Atlanta classification and definitions by international consensus," *Gut*, vol. 62, no. 1, pp. 102–111, 2013.

[5] Y. Li, L. Li, H.-S. Mu, S.-L. Fan, F.-G. He, and Z.-Y. Wang, "Aortic dissection and sudden unexpected deaths: a retrospective study of 31 forensic autopsy cases," *Journal of Forensic Sciences*, vol. 60, no. 5, pp. 1206–1211, 2015.

[6] T. V. Pham and J. V. Nable, "Aortic dissection presenting with pancreatitis," *The American Journal of Emergency Medicine*, vol. 31, no. 7, pp. 1153. e1–1153. e2, 2013.

[7] T. Suzuki, R. H. Mehta, H. Ince et al., "Clinical profiles and outcomes of acute type B aortic dissection in the current era: lessons from the international registry of aortic dissection (IRAD)," *Circulation*, vol. 108, no. 1, pp. II312–II327, 2003.

[8] M. Hamamoto, "Acute ischemic pancreatitis associated with acute Type B aortic dissection: a case report," *Annals of Vascular Diseases*, vol. 5, no. 3, pp. 385–388, 2012.

[9] Z. Ziyu, J. Liu, Y. Huang et al., "Acute pancreatitis induced by acute Type A aortic dissection: a case report," *Journal of Cardiovascular Disease Research*, vol. 5, no. 4, pp. 64–66, 2014.

[10] A. T. Lefor, P. Vuocolo, F. B. Parker Jr., and L. F. Sillin, "Pancreatic complications following cardiopulmonary bypass. Factors influencing mortality," *Archives of Surgery*, vol. 127, no. 10, pp. 1225–1230, 1992.

[11] S. Sriussadaporn, "Acute pancreatitis following resection of juxtarenal abdominal aortic aneurysm," *Journal of the Medical Association of Thailand*, vol. 82, no. 12, pp. 1260–1264, 1999.

[12] M. Okahara, H. Mori, H. Kiyosue, Y. Yamada, Y. Sagara, and S. Matsumoto, "Arterial supply to the pancreas; variations and cross-sectional anatomy," *Abdominal Imaging*, vol. 35, no. 2, pp. 134–142, 2010.

[13] I. Umeda, T. Hayashi, H. Ishiwatari et al., "A case of severe acute pancreatitis and ischemic gastropathy caused by acute aortic dissection," *Nihon Shokakibyo Gakkai Zasshi*, vol. 108, no. 1, pp. 103–110, 2011, in Japanese.

[14] A. L. Warshaw and P. J. O'Hara, "Susceptibility of the pancreas to ischemic injury in shock," *Annals of Surgery*, vol. 188, no. 2, pp. 197–201, 1978.

[15] T. Wen, L. Liu, and G. Xiong, "Matrix metalloproteinase levels in acute aortic dissection, acute pancreatitis and other abdominal pain," *Emergency Medicine Journal*, vol. 26, no. 10, pp. 715–718, 2009.

Electromagnetic Interference from Left Ventricular Assist Device (LVAD) Inhibiting the Pacing Function of an Implantable Cardioverter-Defibrillator (ICD) Device

Sebhat Erqou,[1,2] Robert L. Kormos,[3] Norman C. Wang,[3] Dennis M. McNamara,[3] and Raveen Bazaz[3]

[1]*Department of Medicine, Alpert Medical School of Brown University, Providence, RI, USA*
[2]*Department of Medicine, Providence VA Medical Center, Providence, RI, USA*
[3]*Heart and Vascular Institute, University of Pittsburgh Medical Center, Pittsburgh, PA, USA*

Correspondence should be addressed to Sebhat Erqou; sebhaterqou@googlemail.com

Academic Editor: Nurten Sayar

There is an increasing prevalence of patients with concomitant implantable cardioverter-defibrillators (ICDs) and left ventricular devices (LVADs). The potential for negative interactions between these continually evolving technologies is a valid concern. Previously reported interactions include inappropriate ICD therapy and interference with ICD telemetry function. Understanding the nature of such interactions and developing a comprehensive strategy to approach such situations are important. In this report, we describe a case of electromagnetic interference from LVAD inhibiting the pacing function of an ICD that was corrected by reprograming the device. We would encourage investigators to review patients with ICD and LVAD in their institutions in order to help assess the frequency and nature of these and other interactions.

1. Background

Compared to medical therapy, the left ventricular assist device (LVAD) has been shown to prolong survival in patients with advanced heart failure who are awaiting or are not candidates for transplant [1]. Since most patients with advanced heart failure already have implantable cardioverter-defibrillators (ICDs) by the time they get LVAD implants, there is an increasing number of patients with a concomitant ICD and LVAD. With the increasing prevalence of coexistence between ICDs and LVADs, the potential for negative interactions between these devices would presumably increase. To date, a number of cases of adverse electromagnetic interference (EMI) between LVAD and ICD have been reported [2–6]. However, only two case series involving a total of 54 patients with implanted ICD and LVAD have assessed these interactions systematically [7, 8]. The reported interactions include inappropriate ICD therapy and interference with ICD telemetry function involving St. Jude Medical, Boston Scientific, and Sorin devices [2–8]. Understanding the nature of such interactions and developing a comprehensive strategy to approach them are important. In this case report, we describe a patient with an LVAD-ICD interaction that resulted in ventricular oversensing and subsequent inhibition of pacing.

2. Case Report

A 60-year-old female with history of ovarian cancer, doxorubicin-induced dilated cardiomyopathy, and advanced heart failure had a Medtronic cardiac resynchronization-defibrillator (CRT-D) device placed in May 2010. The patient had implantation of HeartWare LVAD for destination therapy in August 2011 due to progression of heart failure and functional decline. The postsurgical course was complicated by ventricular tachycardia and multiple episodes of pump thrombosis. Interrogation of the CRT-D device in December 2011 (as well as subsequent device checks) revealed that the patient had evidence of complete heart block with no escape rhythm at ventricular backup rate

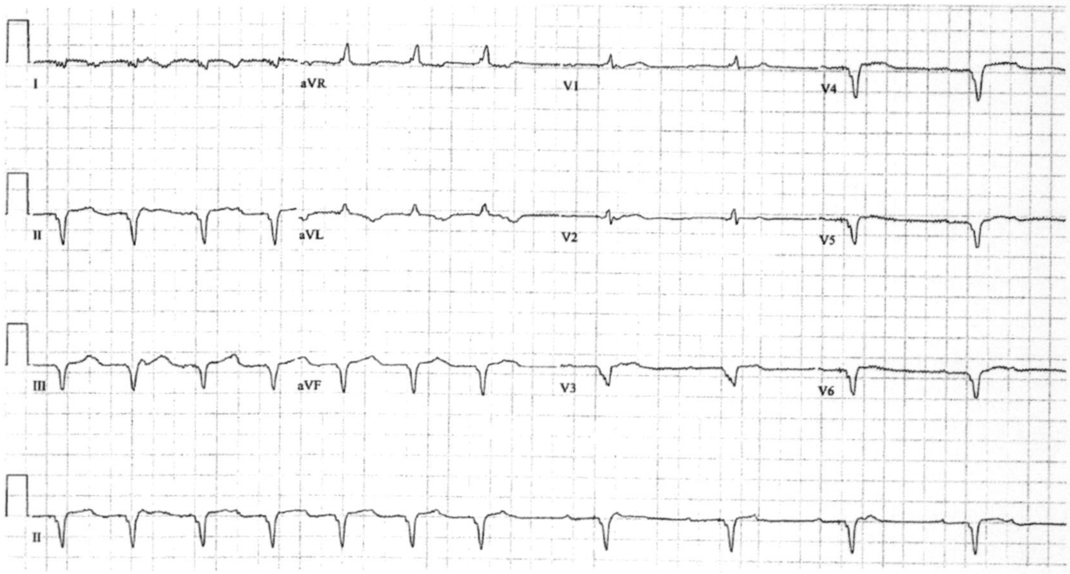

Figure 1: DDD pacing followed by VVI pacing showing an underlying rhythm of complete heart block.

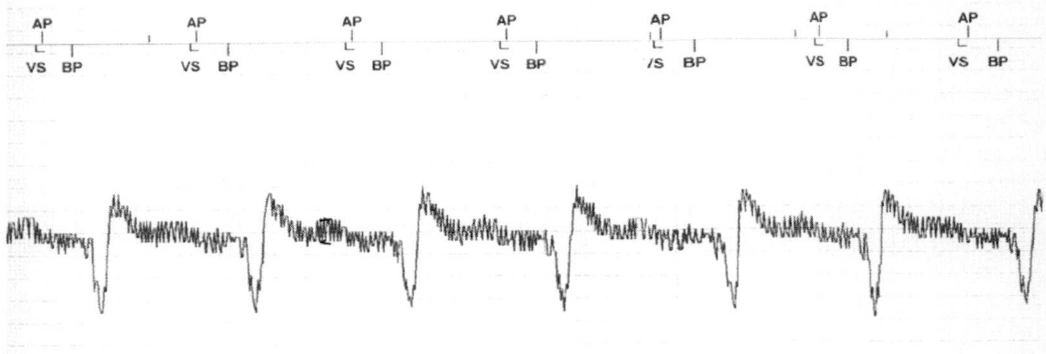

Figure 2: Pacing in asynchronous (DOO) mode with oversensing (marker annotations not affecting pacing mode) seen prior to the A paced marker.

of 40 (Figure 1 EKG). The CRT-D pulse generator was changed to a St. Jude Medical Assura model (3357-40C CRT-D) device in June 2014 once it reached its elective replacement indicator.

The patient was admitted to our hospital in November 2015 with concern for LVAD thrombosis. On this admission, the patient was treated with tissue-plasminogen activator (tPA) without improvement and was taken to the operating room for LVAD pump exchange on admission day 6. In the immediate postoperative period, it was noted that the patient's ICD was no longer consistently pacing. This prompted placement of epicardial pacing leads.

Device interrogation revealed stable right ventricle (RV), left ventricle (LV), and shock lead impedances. The RV lead pace threshold was increased to 1.75 V at 0.5 ms (previously <1 V at 0.5 ms), while the LV lead pace threshold was stable at 0.75 at 0.5 ms. There was a continuous external noise with a mean amplitude of 1 mV detected by the ventricular sense amplifier of the RV lead. The intracardiac electrograms (IEGMs) showed an increase in a baseline noise signal compared to prior device-based recordings—the amplitude of which correlated with the increase of the LVAD pump rotation speed. The device was reprogrammed to nonsensing mode (DOO) allowing consistent pacer function of the ICD (Figure 2 IEGM). These setting changes meant that the tachytherapy function of the ICD was mandatorily disabled, as the device was set to a nonsensing mode.

The EMI oversensing issue was resolved by turning off the "low-frequency attenuation" (LFA) filter, which had resulted in amplification of the high-frequency VAD signal. This allowed the device to function in a sensing/tracking mode (DDD) without inhibition by noise from the LVAD with RV sensitivity threshold of 0.3 mV and permitted functional tachytherapy.

The LFA filter is a proprietary option in St. Jude Medical devices that suppresses low-frequency signals with the intent to mitigate T-wave oversensing. As with any "band-pass filter," in addition to attenuating specific frequencies, they may also enhance or amplify other event frequencies, such as EMI, myopotential, R-waves, and far P-waves. The new VAD cannula position/orientation resulted in injection of the EMI signal more efficiently in the sensing antenna of the existing ICD lead. Additionally, the "sensibility" setting on the St. Jude device decays to baseline maximum sensitivity just prior to the A paced event—thus explaining why EMI was most consistently sensed in this window.

The patient underwent a successful defibrillation threshold (DFT) testing 10 days after her VAD exchange surgery. DFT testing showed that the ICD detected VF adequately with minimal dropout at a minimal sensitivity test setting of 1 mV. There was no further problem with the ICD, and the patient was discharged home one week later.

3. Discussion

To our knowledge, this is the first report where external noise from the LVAD device inhibited the pacer function of an ICD. This was caused by a combination of the new LVAD in-flow cannula position, as well as amplification of EMI by the LFA filter from the ICD. Previously reported interactions include inappropriate ICD therapy and interference with ICD telemetry function, as well as alteration RV sensing and pacing threshold [2–8]. Chhabra et al. [3] and Mozes et al. [6] have independently reported two cases of inappropriate tachytherapy delivery due to adverse EMI between HeartWare LVAD and ICD. Mozes et al. solved the problem by implanting a new pace-sense lead in the RV outflow tract "as far as possible" from the LVAD impeller and capping the pace-sense component of the old RV lead while continuing to use the existing atrial lead and defibrillation coils. A number of other case reports [2, 4, 5] as well as one case series of HeartMate II LVAD [8] have described loss of telemetry function of the ICD device after placement of LVAD, in some cases necessitating ICD replacement.

In the present case, we did observe an increase in RV lead pace threshold as was reported by Foo et al. [7]. The present case is unique, however, due to observation of significant adverse EMI causing external noise and leading to oversensing and resultant inhibition of pacing. This necessitated initial placement of epicardial wires in the operating room after the exchange of the LVAD pump. We were able to temporarily restore the pace function by reprogramming the device to nonsensed mode and decreasing the sensitivity of the RV lead to 1 mV, which unfortunately did not allow for the tachytherapy function to be turned on.

The HeartWare LVAD is a continuous flow system in which the impeller is suspended within the pump through magnetic and hydrodynamic forces. Electromagnetic forces power the rotational mechanism of the impeller. These electromagnetic forces could lead to adverse EMI with ICD as described above. While this inference may be nonconsequential in some cases, they may also lead to clinically significant problems such as inappropriate ICD shocks and loss of ICD-programmer telemetry, as well as inhibition of RV pacing as observed in our cases. Some of these cases have been corrected by using shielding techniques [4, 5], while others have necessitated ICD replacement. In the present case, we resolved the problem by changing device programming. Generally, it may be prudent to assess for these interactions intraoperatively to circumvent a subsequent ICD performance issue that may not be resolved by simple reprogramming.

There is paucity of systematic study into ICD-LVAD interactions. Data from the present and the previous case reports demonstrate that such interactions, albeit not very common, can be consequential. It is important to elucidate detailed mechanisms for ICD-LVAD interactions and describe the various types of interactions in sufficient detail. It will also be useful for investigators to review patients with ICD and LVAD in their institutions to assess the frequency and nature of such interactions.

4. Conclusion

There is accumulating evidence for potential adverse ICD-LVAD interactions. In this report, we described a case of EMI from LVAD inhibiting the pacing function of an ICD that was corrected by reprograming the device. We would encourage investigators to review patients with ICD and LVAD in their institutions to assess the frequency and nature of such interactions.

References

[1] E. A. Rose, A. C. Gelijns, A. J. Moskowitz et al., "Long-term use of a left ventricular-assist device for end-stage heart failure," *The New England Journal of Medicine*, vol. 345, no. 20, pp. 1435–1443, 2001.

[2] J. C. Matthews, D. Betley, F. Morady, and F. Pelosi, "Adverse interaction between a left ventricular assist device and an implantable cardioverter defibrillator," *Journal of Cardiovascular Electrophysiology*, vol. 18, no. 10, pp. 1107-1108, 2007.

[3] L. Chhabra, B. Hiendlmayr, and J. Kluger, "An adverse electrophysiological interaction between an implantable cardioverter-defibrillator and a ventricular assist device," *Connecticut Medicine*, vol. 79, no. 6, pp. 351–354, 2015.

[4] P. C. Netzler, N. Vasuki, J. L. Peura, and M. R. Gold, "Interactions between a left ventricular assist device and implantable cardioverter-defibrillator," *Pacing and Clinical Electrophysiology*, vol. 35, no. 9, pp. e272–e273, 2012.

[5] S. Jacob, P. K. Cherian, W. S. Ghumman, and M. K. Das, ""Pseudo" Faraday cage: a solution for telemetry link interaction between a left ventricular assist device and an implantable cardioverter defibrillator," *Journal of Interventional Cardiac Electrophysiology*, vol. 28, no. 3, pp. 221–225, 2010.

[6] A. Mozes, D. DeNofrio, D. T. Pham, and M. K. Homoud, "Inappropriate implantable cardioverter-defibrillator therapy due to electromagnetic interference in patient with a HeartWare HVAD left ventricular assist device," *Heart Rhythm*, vol. 8, no. 5, pp. 778–780, 2011.

29

Transcatheter Aortic Valve Implantation in a Nonagenarian with Aortic Aneurysm: Futility or Utility?

Evelyn Fennelly,[1] **Marcus Lee**,[1] **Mark Da Costa**,[2] **Sherif Sultan**,[3] **Faisal Sharif**,[1] **and Darren Mylotte**[1]

[1]*Department of Cardiology, University Hospital Galway, Galway, Ireland*
[2]*Department of Cardiothoracic Surgery, University Hospital Galway, Galway, Ireland*
[3]*Department of Vascular Surgery, University Hospital Galway, Galway, Ireland*

Correspondence should be addressed to Darren Mylotte; darrenmylotte@gmail.com

Academic Editor: Hajime Kataoka

Transcatheter aortic valve implantation (TAVI) has emerged as the standard of care for older patients with symptomatic severe aortic stenosis (AS) at high or excessive operative risk. There remain patients that are of such considerable risk that even TAVI can be futile. Such patients present ethical conundrums for institutional heart teams. Herein we present a case of a 90-year-old female patient with symptomatic severe AS and significant comorbidities including diffuse peripheral vascular disease and a large ascending aortic aneurysm. Would TAVI be utile or futile in this patient?

1. Introduction

While transcatheter aortic valve implantation (TAVI) is now the standard of care for elderly patients with symptomatic severe aortic stenosis (AS) at high or excessive operative risk, there remain, however, patients of such high risk that even TAVI may be futile. Such cases present the institutional Heart Team with many difficult considerations and ethical dilemmas. We illustrate these issues through the case presentation of a nonagenarian patient with severe symptomatic AS, multiple comorbid illnesses, and anatomical contraindications to TAVI.

2. Case Presentation

We present the case of a 90-year-old female with symptomatic severe AS. She described an episode of presyncope and progressive dyspnea on exertion (NYHA Class III). Medical history included hypertension, hypercholesterolemia, paroxysmal atrial fibrillation, stroke, peripheral vascular disease (PVD), and an ascending aortic aneurysm. She lived independently with Katz index of 6/6. Transthoracic echocardiogram (TTE) confirmed severe AS (mean gradient 40 mmHg; aortic valve area 0.8 cm^2), concomitant moderate aortic regurgitation, and preserved left ventricular function (ejection fraction 55%).

Given the patient's severe symptoms, advanced age, and associated comorbid illnesses, the patient was considered for TAVI. Multislice computed tomography (MSCT) showed a heavily calcified, tortuous iliofemoral vasculature (minimal lumen diameter (MLD) right: 5.7 mm; left: 5.8 mm), small subclavian arteries (MLD: 4.5 mm), and a bovine aortic arch (Figure 1). MSCT identified an infrarenal abdominal aortic aneurysm (AAA) (maximum diameter: 46 mm). The diameter of the ascending aortic aneurysm was 60 mm. The trileaflet aortic valve was heavily calcified (annular dimensions: mean diameter 26.4 mm; area 542 mm^2; perimeter 84.4 mm) (Figure 2).

The institutional Heart Team considered her to be at excessive risk for surgical aortic valve replacement (SAVR): EuroSCORE II 17.10%; Society of Thoracic Surgeons predicted risk of mortality 7.9%. A conservative management strategy was initially considered; however the patient and her family pressed for TAVI due to debilitating symptoms.

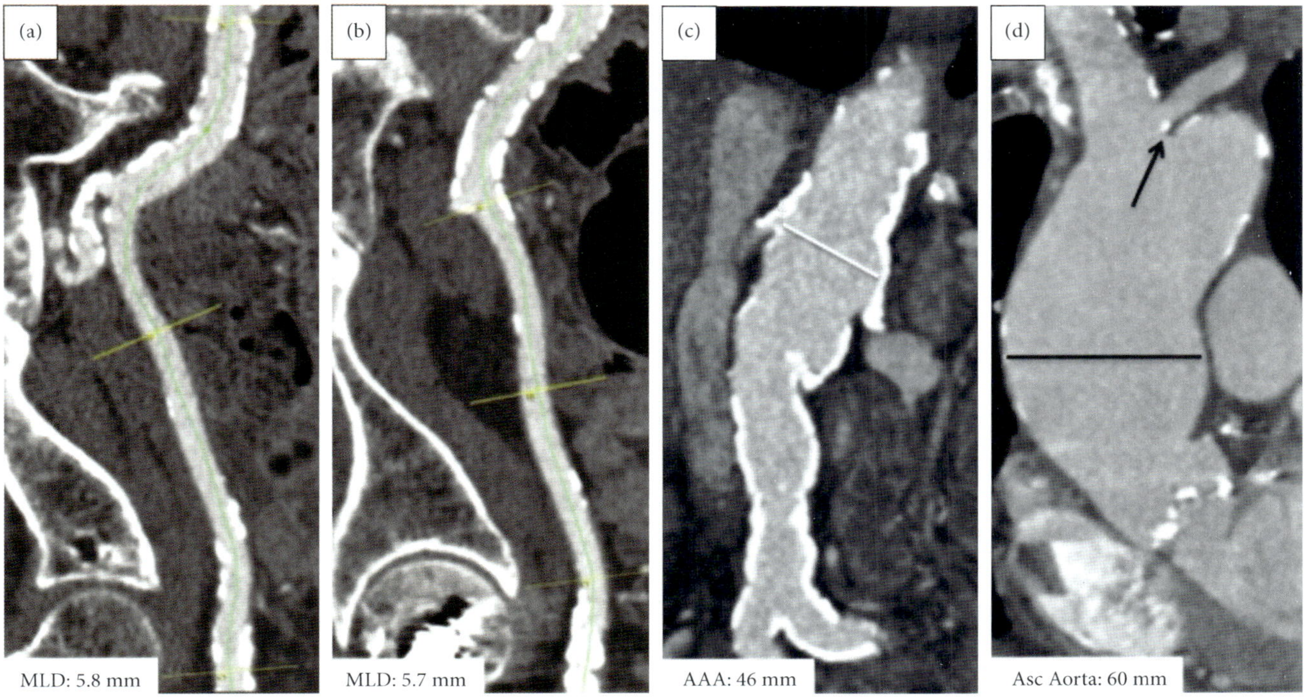

Figure 1: (a) MSCT of the right illiofemoral artery demonstrating an MLD of 5.8 mm. (b) MSCT of the left illiofemoral artery demonstrating heavy calcification just at the level of the femoral head and an MLD of 5.7 mm. (c) MSCT of the descending aorta. The white line denotes the maximum diameter of 46 mm. (d) MSCT of the ascending aorta. The black line denotes the maximum diameter of the ascending aorta aneurysm measuring 60 mm. The black arrow shows the left subclavian entering the right brachiocephalic trunk (the bovine arch).

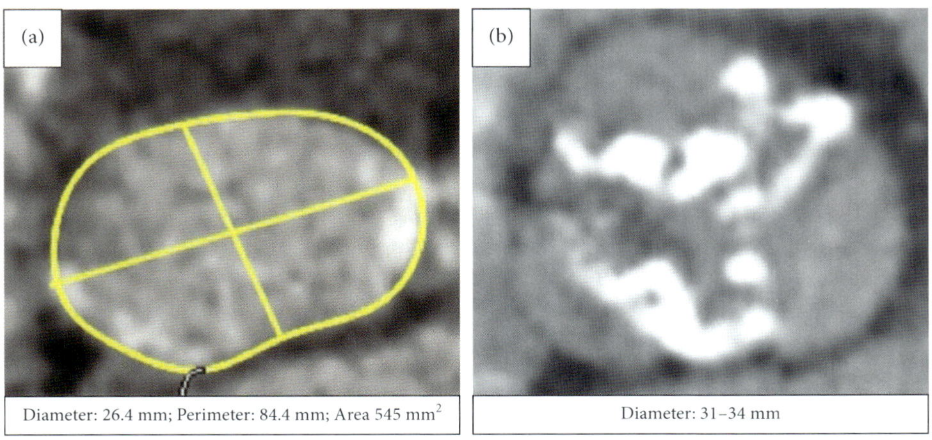

Figure 2: (a) MSCT of the aortic annulus with the diameter of 26.4 mm, perimeter of 84.4 mm, and aortic annular area of 542 mm^2. (b) MSCT of the aortic valve demonstrating a tricuspid aortic valve with heavy calcification of the aortic valve leaflets.

Given the ascending aorta and aortic branch anatomy, a transfemoral TAVI with a surgical femoral arterial cut-down was considered to be the most appropriate vascular access route for implantation of a self-expanding transcatheter heart valve (THV). The periprocedural plan did not include transition to cardiopulmonary bypass as the patient had been declined traditional cardiac surgery by the institutional Heart Team.

Under general anesthesia, the left common femoral artery was exposed, and an 18 Fr Cook (Cook Inc., Bloomington, IN, USA) vascular access sheath was inserted just cranial to a heavily calcified arterial segment. Sheath advancement to the descending aorta was challenging, though ultimately successful (Video 1). Heparin was administered to maintain an activated clotting time of >300 seconds. The stenotic aortic valve was crossed with some difficulty, and a stiff guide wire was placed in the left ventricle. Preimplant balloon aortic valvuloplasty was performed with an 18 mm NuMED balloon (NuMED Inc., Hopkinton, NY, USA) under rapid ventricular pacing. A 31 mm Medtronic CoreValve (Medtronic, Minneapolis, MN, USA) was deployed at an appropriate depth (3–6 mm), and transesophageal echocardiography and aortography suggested

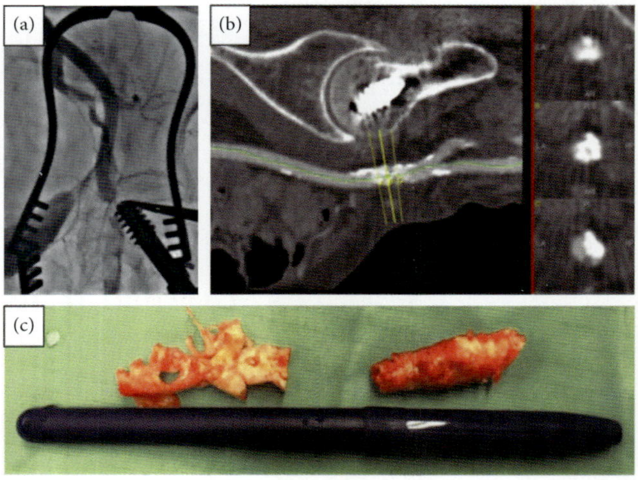

Figure 3: (a) Control angiography showing complete occlusion of the left femoral artery just distal to the puncture site. (b) MSCT of the left femoral artery showing heavy calcification at the level of the femoral head. Red arrow shows puncture site. (c) Calcific atheroma from the left common femoral artery during the femoral endarterectomy.

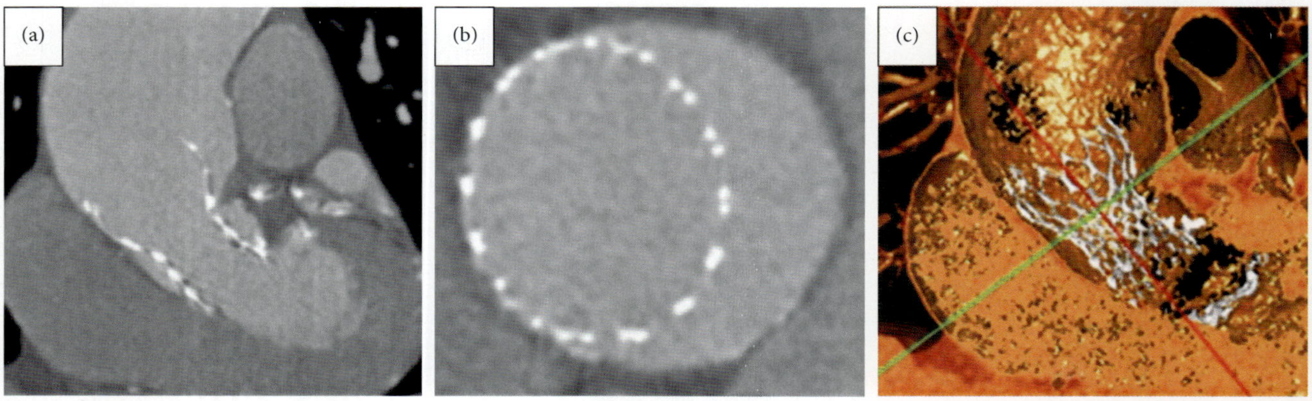

Figure 4: (a) MSCT of the 31 mm CoreValve in the aorta postimplant. (b) Aortic end of the CoreValve "floating" in the aorta. (c) 3D reconstruction of the CoreValve showing apposition to the greater curvature of the aorta.

excellent valve function with mild paravalvular aortic regurgitation (Videos 2 and 3).

Closure of the femoral arteriotomy was performed with a 6.0 Prolene. Control femoral angiography, however, showed occlusion of the common femoral artery just caudal to the puncture site (Figure 3(a); Video 4), and an area of extensive calcific plaque was observed on the screening MSCT (Figure 3(b)). In light of the extensive calcific disease, it was deemed that percutaneous recanalization of the artery would be impossible, and a common femoral endarterectomy was performed (Figure 3(c)). The patient subsequently required further surgical exploration for ongoing bleeding and needed transfusion with 10 units of packed red blood cells. She recovered quickly and was ambulating independently on discharge to respite care (postoperative day 8).

The patient underwent routine follow-up, including outpatient review and surveillance echocardiography. Follow-up TTE at 6 months showed normal valve function, mean gradient of 6 mmHg, and mild paravalvular leak. Repeat MSCT showed a well-positioned valve, with the outflow floating in the ascending aortic aneurysm, without evidence of in situ thrombus, and no expansion of the ascending or descending aortic aneurysms (Figure 4). The patient remains asymptomatic at 12-month follow-up and will continue to undergo surveillance echocardiography annually.

3. Discussion

We present a challenging case of a nonagenarian with severe symptomatic AS, multiple comorbid illnesses, and anatomical contraindications to TAVI. This case presented an ethical dilemma to the Heart Team, given the extreme patient risk. Initially, we preferred a conservative management strategy, but when faced with the patient's preference for definitive therapy, we elected to undertake transfemoral TAVI.

This case underscores the importance of a multidisciplinary approach to TAVI. The successful outcome for our patient was achieved with the collaboration of the cardiology, cardiothoracic, and vascular surgery teams, anesthesia, elderly medicine, and support services. The Heart Team model of care is recommended in both European and U.S. guidelines, which cite its role as essential in optimizing patient care [1, 2].

Vascular access was particularly challenging in this case; the extensive severe PVD left few options for insertion of an 18 Fr vascular access sheath. Percutaneous transfemoral, transaortic, and transcarotid approaches were ruled out due to the calcific nature and small caliber of the femoral arteries, the aneurysmal ascending aorta, and the bovine aortic arch, respectively [3]. Transapical TAVI could have been an option, though may be associated with inferior clinical outcomes [4]. Transcaval TAVI has also emerged as a possible access route for no-option patients, though experience is limited [5]. Ultimately, we elected to push the boundaries of the transfemoral approach using a surgical cut-down to try minimize patient risk. The left common femoral artery MLD of 5.7 mm yielded a sheath to femoral artery ratio (SFAR) of 0.95. In calcified vessels, a SFAR > 1.0 is recommended to avoid vascular complications [6]. When the complication was encountered, the vascular team was on hand to undertake emergent surgery.

Another major challenge in this case was the ascending aortic aneurysm. Aortic root dilation occurs in up to 3% of patients with severe AS [7]. Current American College of Cardiology recommendations suggest concomitant aneurysm repair during SAVR in those with an ascending aorta or aortic root > 45 mm in diameter [8]. Such recommendations do not apply to inoperable patients; the role of TAVI here remains unclear. Aortic root replacement aims to prevent future catastrophic dissection or rupture by restoring the normal dimension of the ascending aorta with a graft [9]. Untreated, such aneurysms remain exposed to the high velocity jet created by the stenotic valve, and this wall stress may induce dissection or rupture. The annual risk of death, rupture, or dissection for ascending aortic aneurysms of 60 to 69 mm in diameter is estimated to be 15.6% per year [10]. Critically, the risk of rupture increases 27-fold after 60 mm as there is an annual mean growth rate of 1 mm per year [10]. One could hypothesize that replacing the aortic valve alone (TAVI in this case) could reduce wall stress by removing the high-velocity jet caused by the stenotic valve [11, 12]. In contrast, the intervention itself could destabilize the aneurysm, and indeed the self-expanding prosthesis itself could exert forces on the aortic wall [9]. There are currently no published data on long-term changes in ascending aortic aneurysm sizes after TAVI.

Valve thrombosis has recently been identified as a complication of bioprosthetic valve replacement, occurring in up to 40% of recipients [13]. This entity may be prosthesis-dependent and may be associated with atrial fibrillation [14]. An ascending aortic aneurysm may increase the risk of valve thrombosis, according to the principles of Virchow's triad [15]. In this case, there was no evidence of valve thrombosis on MSCT after 6-month treatment with dual antiplatelet therapy.

The case presented here demonstrates the importance of the institutional Heart Team in optimizing patient outcome with TAVI. We suggest cautiously that CoreValve implantation for inoperable older patients with ascending aortic root aneurysms is feasible and safe and in our patient was associated with symptomatic improvement.

Authors' Contributions

All authors contributed significantly to the concept, preparation, and editing of the manuscript.

References

[1] A. Vahanian, H. Baumgartner, J. Bax et al., "Guidelines on the management of valvular heart disease," *Revista española de cardiología*, vol. 60, no. 6, pp. 1e–50e, 2007.

[2] R. A. Nishimura, C. M. Otto, R. O. Bonow et al., "2014 AHA/ACC guideline for the management of patients with valvular heart disease: executive summary: a report of the American College of Cardiology/American Heart Association Task Force on Practice Guidelines," *Circulation*, vol. 129, no. 23, pp. 2440–2492, 2014.

[3] M. Pozzi, D. Grinberg, J.-F. Obadia et al., "Transcatheter aortic valve implantation using the left transcarotid approach in patients with previous ipsilateral carotid endarterectomy," *Catheterization and Cardiovascular Interventions*, vol. 85, no. 7, pp. E203–E209, 2015.

[4] F. Biancari, S. Rosato, P. D'Errigo et al., "Immediate and intermediate outcome after transapical versus transfemoral transcatheter aortic valve replacement," *American Journal of Cardiology*, vol. 117, no. 2, pp. 245–251, 2016.

[5] I. Ott, A. B. Greenbaum, H. Schunkert, A. Kastrati, and M. Kasel, "First use of an expandable sheath and transcaval access for transcatheter Edwards SAPIEN 3 aortic valve implantation," *EuroIntervention*, vol. 11, no. 7, pp. 782–784, 2015.

[6] K. Hayashida, T. Lefèvre, B. Chevalier et al., "Transfemoral aortic valve implantation: new criteria to predict vascular complications," *JACC: Cardiovascular Interventions*, vol. 4, no. 8, pp. 851–858, 2011.

[7] M. H. Crawford and C. A. Roldan, "Prevalence of aortic root dilatation and small aortic roots in valvular aortic stenosis," *American Journal of Cardiology*, vol. 87, no. 11, pp. 1311–1313, 2001.

[8] L. F. Hiratzka, G. L. Bakris, J. A. Beckman et al., "2010 ACCF/AHA/AATS/ACR/ASA/SCA/SCAI/SIR/STS/SVM guidelines for the diagnosis and management of patients with thoracic aortic disease: executive summary: a report of the American College of Cardiology Foundation/American Heart Association Task Force on Practice Guidelines, American Association for Thoracic Surgery, American College of Radiology, American Stroke Association," *Circulation*, vol. 121, no. 13, pp. 1544–1579, 2010.

[9] R. Erbel, V. Aboyans, C. Boileau et al., "2014 ESC guidelines on the diagnosis and treatment of aortic diseases," *European Heart Journal*, vol. 35, no. 41, pp. 2873–2926, 2014.

[10] R. R. Davies, L. J. Goldstein, M. A. Coady et al., "Yearly rupture or dissection rates for thoracic aortic aneurysms: simple prediction based on size," *Annals of Thoracic Surgery*, vol. 73, no. 1, pp. 17–28, 2002.

[11] A. Garnham and S. Khogali, "Critical aortic stenosis in a patient with a large saccular abdominal aortic aneurysm: simultaneous transcatheter aortic valve implantation and drive-by endovascular aortic aneurysm repair," *Catheterization and Cardiovascular Interventions*, vol. 80, no. 6, pp. 1014–1018, 2012.

[12] M. Chen, Y. Feng, D. Mazzitelli et al., "Transcatheter aortic valve implantation in a patient with severe bicuspid aortic valve stenosis and ascending aortic aneurysm," *JACC: Cardiovascular Interventions*, vol. 7, no. 7, pp. e83–e84, 2014.
[13] R. R. Makkar, G. Fontana, H. Jilaihawi et al., "Possible subclinical leaflet thrombosis in bioprosthetic aortic valves," *New England Journal of Medicine*, vol. 373, no. 21, pp. 2015–2024,
[14] A. C. Egbe, S. V. Pislaru, P. A. Pellikka et al., "Bioprosthetic valve thrombosis versus structural failure: clinical and echocardiographic predictors," *Journal of the American College of Cardiology*, vol. 66, no. 21, pp. 2285–2294, 2015.
[15] L. S. Costanzo, *Physiology, Board review series,* vol. 13, p. 314, Wolters Kluwer Health/Lippincott Williams & Wilkins, Philadelphia, PA, USA, 5th edition, 2011.

30

Complex Recanalization of Chronic Total Occluison Supported by Minimal Extracorporeal Circulation in a Patient with an Aortic Valve Bioprothesis in Extraanatomic Position

Ruben Jansen,[1,2] Brigitte Bathgate,[1,2] Alexander Bufe,[1,2,3] and Jan-Erik Guelker[1,2]

[1]Department of Cardiology, Heartcentre Niederrhein, Helios Clinic Krefeld, Krefeld, Germany
[2]Institute for Heart and Circulation Research, University of Cologne, Cologne, Germany
[3]University of Witten/Herdecke, Witten, Germany

Correspondence should be addressed to Jan-Erik Guelker; jan-erik.guelker@helios-kliniken.de

Academic Editor:

Percutaneous coronary intervention (PCI) of chronic total occlusion (CTO) still remains a major challenge in interventional cardiology. This case describes a complex PCI of the left main coronary artery and of a CTO of the right coronary artery using a minimal extracorporeal circulation system (MECC) in a patient with an aortic valve bioprothesis in extraanatomic position. It illustrates that complex recanalization strategies can be solved combining it with mechanical circulatory support technologies.

1. Introduction

Recanalization of chronic total occlusion (CTO) remains a complex procedure in interventional cardiology. CTO of a coronary artery can be identified in up to 20% among patients with a clinical indication for coronary angiography. With the advent of novel recanalization techniques and emerging devices, percutaneous coronary interventions (PCIs) have become a promising treatment option for these patients [1–5].

The minimal extracorporeal circulation (MECC) system (Maquet, Hirrlingen, Germany) is a preconnected closed system with a centrifugal pump and a membrane oxygenator. It is a tip-to-tip heparin coated system which needs less than 500 ml priming volume. Venous blood returns through active drainage with a centrifugal pump instead of a roller pump to a membrane diffusion oxygenator. Venous reservoir and cardiotomy suction of shed blood is not necessary [6]. We report a case of complex coronary recanalizations using the MECC support in a patient with a calcified coronary artery disease.

2. Case Report

We present a case of a 66-year-old woman with advanced coronary artery disease (CAD). In 2013, she underwent coronary artery bypass graft (CABG) surgery with an IMA bypass to the left anterior descending (LAD) and implantation of an aortic valve bioprothesis in extraanatomic position with a conduit from the apex of the left ventricle to the descending aorta for treatment of a symptomatic aortic valve stenosis. This procedure was chosen as a "porcelain" aorta did not allow an implantation in a regular position.

Due to recurrent angina pectoris (CCS III) and dyspnoe (NYHA III), a coronary angiography was performed exhibiting an occlusion of the IMA bypass graft, a high-grade stenosis of the left main coronary artery (LCA) and a chronic total occlusion (CTO) of the right coronary artery (RCA).

Transoesophageal and transthoracal echocardiography revealed a reduced left ventricular function with an ejection fraction of 45% with mild hypokinesia of the inferior wall. The function of the bioprothesis was regular. This was also confirmed by magnet resonance imaging (MRI) of the heart. The prothesis was positioned 8 cm distal in the conduit (Figures 1 and 2).

The local heart team decided to perform a percutaneous coronary intervention (PCI) of the left main coronary artery and a PCI of the RCA-CTO assisted by a MECC system.

Before starting the procedure, anesthesia and mechanical ventilation were installed. To prevent thrombembolic

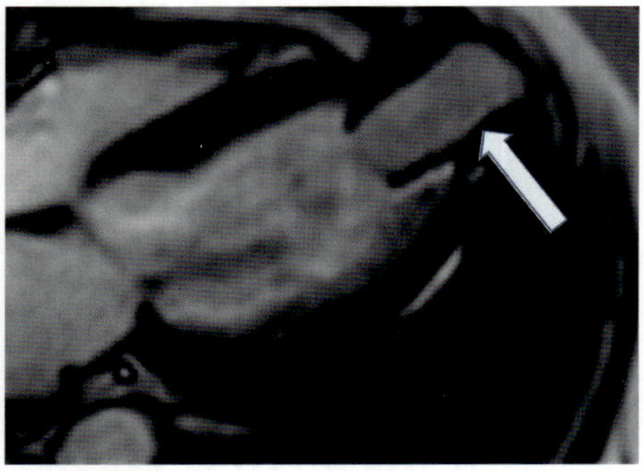

Figure 1: MRI shows a conduit from the apex of the left ventricle (arrow).

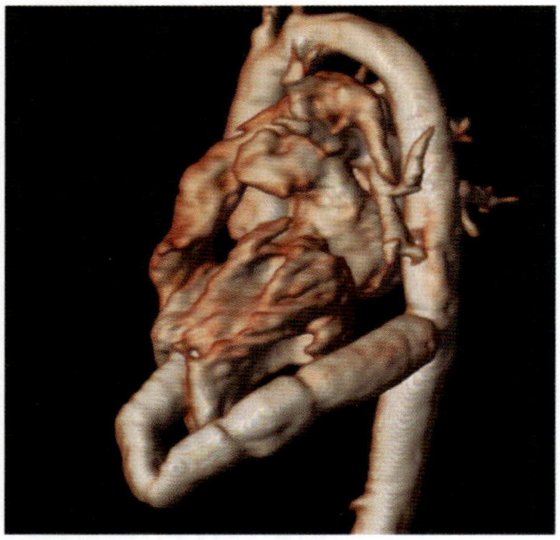

Figure 2: MRI shows a conduit from the apex of the left ventricle to the descending aorta.

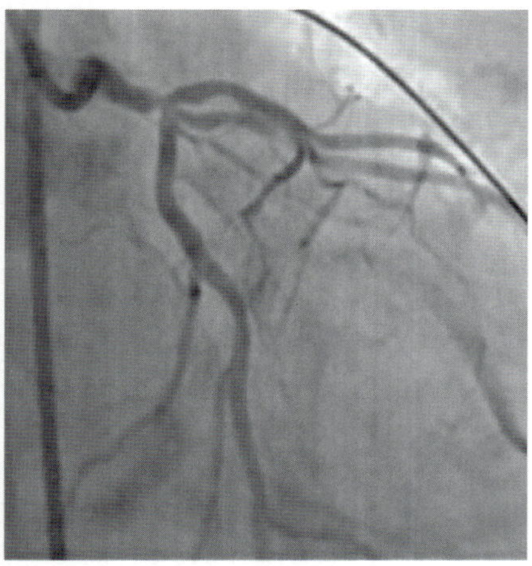

(a)

Figure 3: Continued.

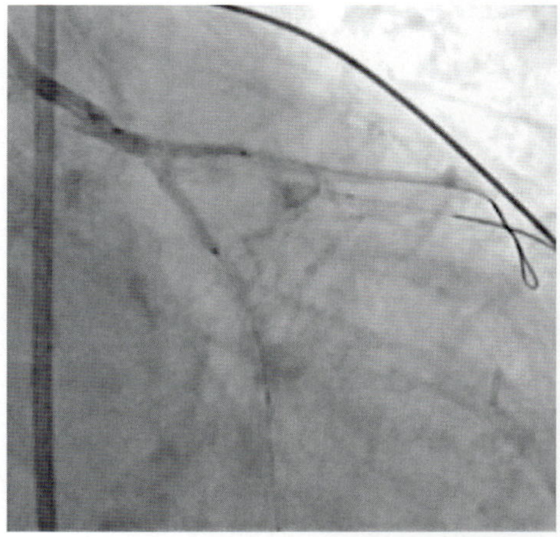

(b)

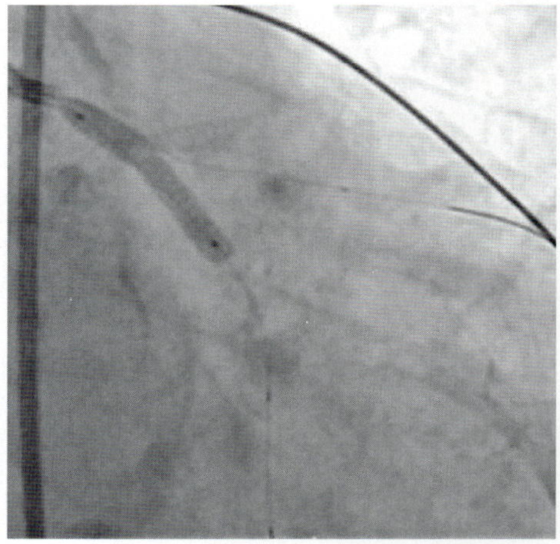

(c)

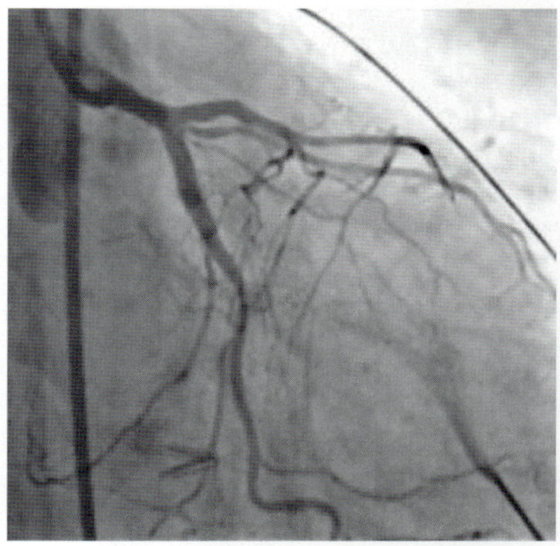

(d)

Figure 3: Complex recanalization of the left main coronary artery (a–d).

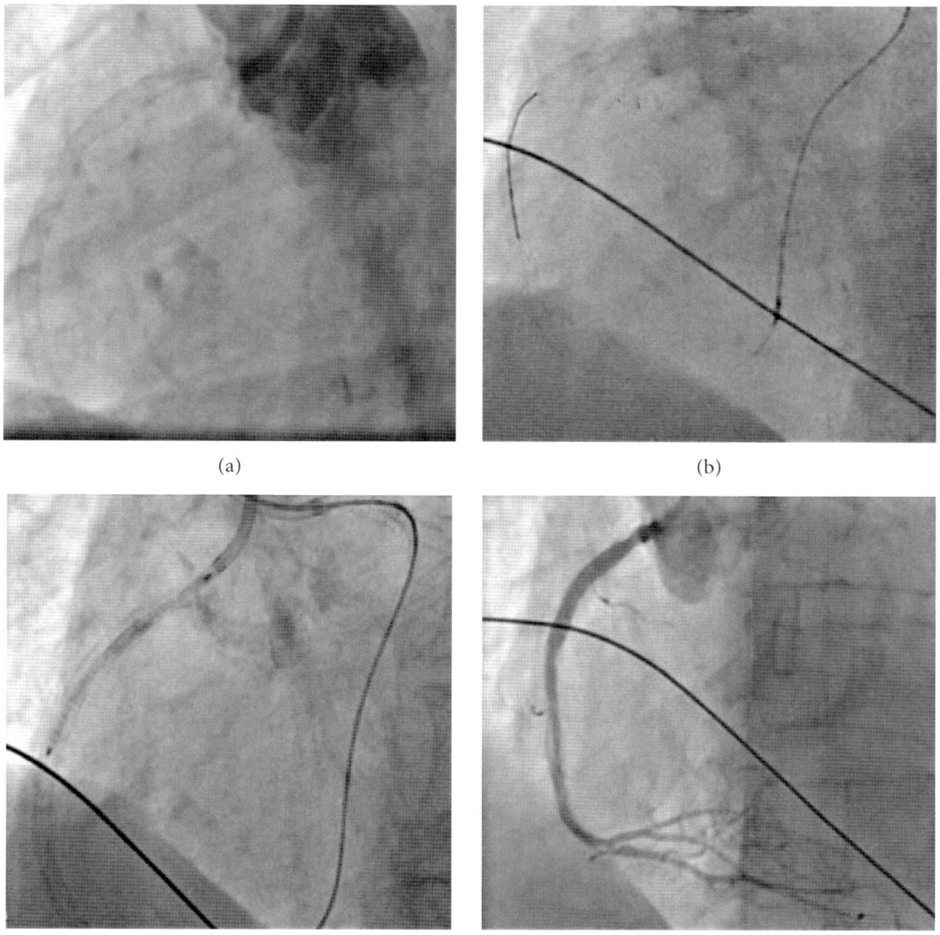

(a) (b) (c) (d)

FIGURE 4: Retrograde recanalization of the RCA (a–d).

complications, heparin was given during the interventions guided by the activated clotting time (>300 sec). To introduce the minimal extracorporeal circulation system, an arterial 14 French and a venous 21 French access were established. Following a loading dose of 600 mg clopidogrel, a 7F JL4 guiding catheter was advanced to the left main coronary artery, and 0.014" floppy guide wires were introduced into the LAD, left circumflex artery (LCX), and ramus intermedius.

The left main coronary artery was stented in the direction of the LAD and LCX using the mini-crush technique; a 2.75 × 15 mm and a 3.5 × 23 mm drug-eluting stent (DES) were deployed at 18 and 20 atmospheres, respectively (Figure 3).

After two failed antegrade attempts in the past, the retrograde CTO technique was applied to recanalize the RCA. For recanalization, a Sion wire (Asahi Intecc, Japan) and a Corsair microcatheter (Asahi Intecc, Japan) were used. Wire and microcatheter passed the occluded segment, and after multiple balloon dilatations, a 3.5 × 38 mm DES was implanted (Figure 4). After the procedure, we checked the result with intravascular ultrasound (IVUS). A dual antiplatelet therapy consisting of 100 mg of aspirin once daily and 75 mg of clopidogrel daily for at least 6 months was continued. Artificial ventilation was stopped on the same day, and the patient could leave the hospital five days later.

3. Discussion

The MECC system has been introduced in clinical practice in 1999. Initially, it was applied in aortic valve surgery as well as in other cardiac surgical procedures [7, 8].

Complex interventional procedures like PCI of the left main or of the CTO often require a hemodynamic support. The advantages of the MECC system in comparison to other mechanical circulatory support technologies like the intra-aortic balloon pump (IABP) or the left ventricular assist device (LVAD) are an immediate hemodynamic stabilization and additional support by unloading the right ventricle [9]. As a potential alternative, the Impella CP microaxial pump (Abiomed, USA) has been introduced. Several trials have shown before that cardiac survival was higher in patients with complete revascularization when compared to patients with incomplete revascularization [10, 11].

Our case demonstrates that by combining advanced recanalization techniques and the MECC system complex, coronary conditions which are so far considered as intractable by interventional means can be treated successfully. The combination of both, high-standard CTO-PCI and an extracorporeal circulation support system, allows us to pursue the interventional procedure. A profound knowledge and a confident command of CTO techniques are required for this kind of intervention. Nevertheless, a strong cooperation between interventional cardiologists and cardiac surgeons is still necessary as part of the heart team [12].

References

[1] P. Fefer, M. L. Knudtson, A. N. Cheema et al., "Current perspectives on coronary chronic total occlusions. The Canadian multicenter chronic total occlusions registry," *Journal of the American College of Cardiology*, vol. 59, no. 11, pp. 991–997, 2012.

[2] S. D. Tomasello, M. Boukhris, S. Giubilato et al., "Management strategies in patients affected by chronic total occlusions: results from the Italian registry of chronic total occlusions," *European Heart Journal*, vol. 36, no. 45, pp. 3189–3198, 2015.

[3] A. Bufe, G. Haltern, W. Dinh et al., "Recanalisation of coronary chronic total occlusions with new techniques including the retrograde approach via collaterals," *Netherlands Heart Journal*, vol. 19, no. 4, pp. 162–167, 2011.

[4] A. R. Galassi, S. D. Tomasello, N. Reifart et al., "In-hospital outcomes of percutaneous coronary intervention in patients with chronic total occlusion: insights from the ERCTO (European registry of chronic total occlusion) registry," *EuroIntervention*, vol. 7, no. 4, pp. 472–479, 2011.

[5] B. E. Stähli, C. Gebhard, M. Gick et al., "Impact of body mass index on long-term mortality in women and men undergoing percutaneous coronary intervention for chronic total occlusion," *International Journal of Cardiology*, vol. 224, pp. 305–309, 2016.

[6] K. Anastasiadis, P. Antonitsis, A. B. Haidich, H. Argiriadou, A. Deliopoulos, and C. Papakonstantinou, "Use of minimal extracorporeal circulation improves outcome after heart surgery; a systematic review and meta-analysis of randomized controlled trials," *International Journal of Cardiology*, vol. 164, no. 2, pp. 158–169, 2013.

[7] A. Castiglioni, A. Verzini, F. Pappalardo et al., "Minimally invasive closed circuit versus standard extracorporeal circulation for aortic valve replacement," *Annals of Thoracic Surgery*, vol. 83, no. 2, pp. 586–591, 2007.

[8] K. Anastasiadis, O. Chalvatzoulis, P. Antonitsis et al., "Use of minimized extracorporeal circulation system in non-coronary and valve cardiac surgical procedures-a case series," *Artificial Organs*, vol. 35, no. 10, pp. 960–963, 2011.

[9] K. Anastasiadis, S. Hadjimiltiades, and P. Antinitsis, "Successful high-risk percutaneous coronary intervention with the use of minimal extracorporeal circulation system," *Catheterization and Cardiovascular Interventions*, vol. 80, no. 5, pp. 845–849, 2012.

[10] R. Valenti, A. Migliorini, U. Signorini et al., "Impact of complete revascularization with percutaneous coronary intervention on survival in patients with at least one chronic total occlusion," *European Heart Journal*, vol. 29, no. 19, pp. 2336–2342, 2008.

[11] Z. Gao, B. Xu, Y. J. Yang et al., "Long-term outcomes of complete versus incomplete revascularization after drug-eluting stent implantation in patients with multivessel coronary disease," *Catheterization and Cardiovascular Interventions*, vol. 82, no. 3, pp. 343–349, 2013.

[12] P. Kolb, W. Wijns, N. Danchin et al., "Guidelines on myocardial revascularization," *European Journal of Cardio-Thoracic Surgery*, vol. 38, pp. S1–S52, 2010.

Early Response after Catheter Ablation of the Epicardial Substrate in a Patient with Brugada Syndrome Can Be Predicted by High Precordial Leads

Yae Min Park,[1] Mi Sook Cha,[1] Hanul Choi,[1] Woong Chol Kang,[1] Seung Hwan Han,[1] In Suck Choi,[1] Eak Kyun Shin,[1] and Young-Hoon Kim[2]

[1]*Cardiology Division, Department of Internal Medicine, Gachon University Gil Medical Center, Incheon, Republic of Korea*
[2]*Cardiology Division, Department of Internal Medicine, Korea University Anam Hospital, Seoul, Republic of Korea*

Correspondence should be addressed to Young-Hoon Kim; yhkmd@unitel.co.kr

Academic Editor: Hajime Kataoka

A 52-year-old male with Brugada syndrome presented with repeated and appropriate shock from an implantable cardioverter defibrillator (ICD). Catheter ablation for substrate elimination targeting low-voltage, complex, and fractionated electrocardiograms and late potentials in the epicardial right ventricular outflow tract was successfully performed. Brugada phenotype in the right precordial leads from the third intercostal space disappeared in the early stage after catheter ablation and that from the standard fourth intercostal space disappeared later. He remained free from ventricular fibrillation over the next fourteen months. We suggest that this novel ablation strategy is effective in Brugada syndrome patients with ICD, and early response after catheter ablation can be predicted by high precordial leads.

1. Introduction

Brugada syndrome is characterized by a typical electrocardiogram (ECG) abnormality in the right precordial leads and a high risk of ventricular fibrillation- (VF-) related sudden cardiac death. The cornerstone to prevent sudden cardiac death is implantation of an implantable cardioverter defibrillator (ICD) in the high-risk patients [1]. Recently, a novel approach of substrate modification in the anterior epicardial region of the right ventricular outflow tract (RVOT) reduces VF episodes and even eliminates the Brugada phenotype in ECG [2]. The ST segment elevation in a Brugada syndrome patient is the most prominent in the leads overlying the RVOT and closely follows its anatomic position. Here, we present the case of successful substrate elimination in the epicardial RVOT in a patient with Brugada syndrome whose Brugada phenotype of high precordial leads in ECG disappeared in the early stage after catheter ablation.

2. Case Report

A 52-year-old male presented with aborted sudden cardiac arrest and was referred to our electrophysiology department for further workup. The initial ECG at the emergency room revealed VF. Biphasic 200-Joule defibrillation restored sinus rhythm, and cardiopulmonary function recovered without neurologic sequelae. He suffered from several episodes of the agonal breathing pattern and generalized tonic-clonic movement prior to admission. The family history and past history including structural heart disease, syncope, or sudden cardiac death were unremarkable. His ECG after stabilization showed sinus rhythm with type I Brugada pattern (Figure 1). Echocardiography demonstrated no structural heart disease with normal left ventricular ejection fraction, and cardiac magnetic resonance imaging scan demonstrated normal biventricular function with no late gadolinium enhancement. Laboratory findings did not show any electrolyte abnormalities. He received ICD implantation

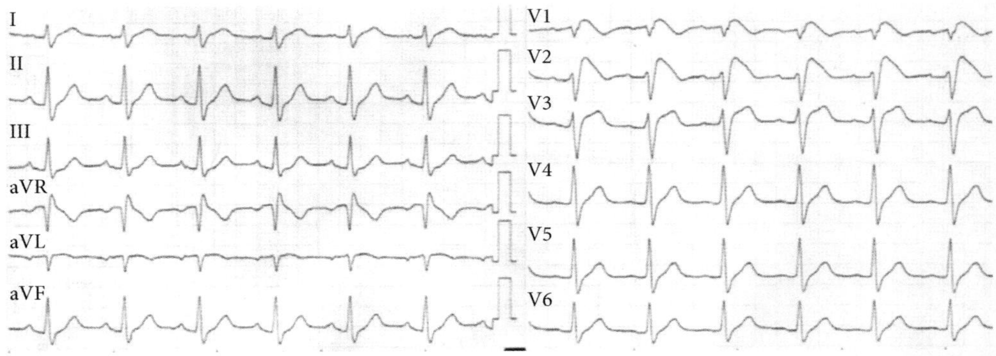

FIGURE 1: ECG after stabilization showed sinus rhythm with type I Brugada pattern, resulting in the diagnosis of Brugada syndrome. ECG = electrocardiogram.

for the secondary prevention of sudden cardiac death. Genetic studies were recommended, although declined by his family due to high cost.

Later, regular ECG exams showed consistently unprovoked type I Brugada pattern. Six months after the ICD implantation, he experienced appropriate shock due to VF. Medication with quinidine was started, and the dose was titrated up to 200 mg tid. However, he suffered from repeated appropriate shocks 10 months after starting quinidine. Premature ventricular complexes (PVCs) were rare during continuous ECG monitoring, and VF-triggering PVCs were absent. Therefore, he was offered radiofrequency catheter ablation for substrate elimination.

In conscious sedation with intravenous propofol and midazolam, a VF induction test was attempted with programmed ventricular stimulation with three basal cycle lengths (600–500–400 ms) with up to three extra stimuli decremented to ventricular refractoriness or 200 ms from the RV apex prior to the ablation procedure, and VF was reproducibly inducible. Endocardial substrate mapping of the RV and RVOT was performed (NavX System; St. Jude Medical Inc., St. Paul, MN, USA), which showed no significant low-voltage area or fragmented potential. Epicardial access was obtained using fluoroscopy-guided subxiphoid puncture, and a long sheath (SL1; St. Jude Medical Inc., St. Paul, MN, USA) was introduced. Epicardial mapping (173 points) including RV and left ventricular areas was performed, revealing an extensive area of low voltage defined as bipolar signal amplitude <0.5 mV with wide duration (>80 ms) and fragmentation (≥3 distinct components) and late potential in the anterior RVOT. These areas were measured at 34.4 mm^2, with the longest total duration of abnormal fractionated potential up to 468 ms and up to 326 ms after the end of the surface QRS. Unipolar mapping showed J-point elevation identical to the typical Brugada pattern (Figure 2(a)). Epicardial ablation was performed by an open irrigated tip catheter (Coolflex; St. Jude Medical, Minnetonka, MN, USA) targeting these areas (35 W; total ablation time: 19.8 minutes) (Figure 2(b)). This resulted in elimination of the fractionated potentials and drastic reduction of the local amplitude.

Remapped epicardial voltage mapping revealed that these areas were replaced with scar tissue (<0.1 mV; Figure 2(c)). Slight changes in morphologies of V1–V3 were detected, although the Brugada pattern remained in surface ECG right after the ablation procedure. An evaluation for the remnant substrate was performed after flecainide infusion (2 mg/kg for 10 minutes), revealing no significant changes in local amplitude in epicardial RVOT, although coved-type ST elevation in surface ECG was accentuated. The programmed ventricular stimulation was repeated, resulting in noninducibility of VF. The patient was discharged on the third day after the procedure with resumed quinidine therapy.

Right precordial leads from the third intercostal space showed disappearance of coved-type ST elevation on the third day after ablation, while those from the fourth intercostal space still showed the Brugada pattern. One month later, the Brugada pattern of precordial leads from either the third or fourth intercostal space disappeared (Figures 3(a)–3(c)). The flecainide provocative test (2 mg/kg for 10 minutes) was performed after three months of catheter ablation which revealed unmasking of type I Brugada pattern (Figure 3(d)). He remained free from palpitations, fainting, or syncopal episodes over the next fourteen months without quinidine treatment. There was no ventricular arrhythmia detected by the ICD.

3. Discussion

We report the case of Brugada syndrome patient with successful substrate elimination in the epicardial RVOT, who had been suffering from repeated appropriate ICD shocks. The Brugada phenotype in the high right precordial leads disappeared in the early stage after catheter ablation and that in the standard precordial leads disappeared later. Epicardial ablation in the anterior RVOT suppressed further VF episodes and completely eliminated the Brugada phenotype in this patient.

Catheter ablation for the management of Brugada syndrome has not been extensively reported. The epicardial ablation technique targeting the potential substrate in the RVOT for the Brugada syndrome was first introduced by Nademanee et al. in 2011 [3]. Delayed depolarization over the anterior aspect of the RVOT epicardium was suggested as the underlying electrophysiological mechanism in Brugada syndrome, and catheter ablation over this abnormal area

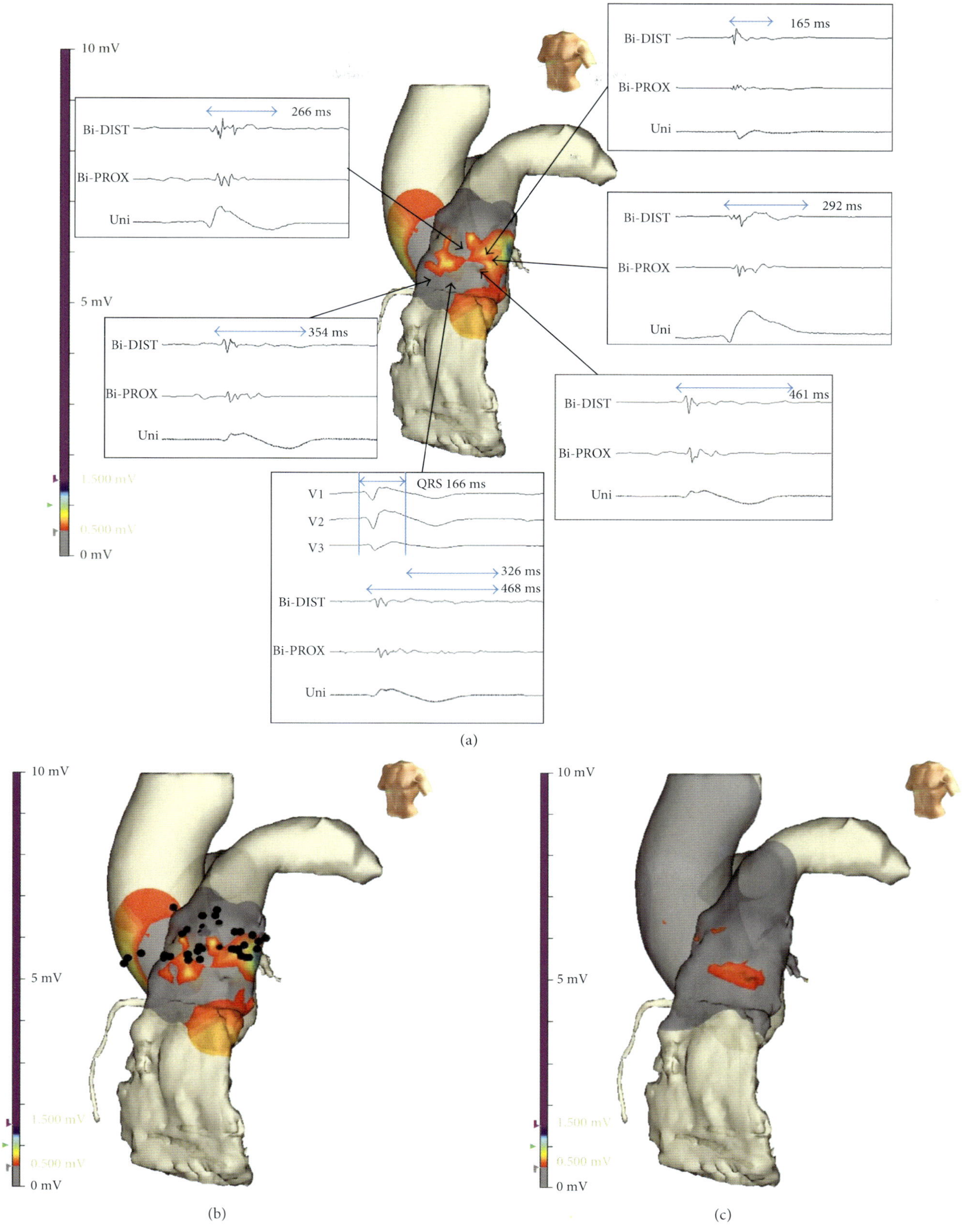

Figure 2: (a) Epicardial mapping revealed an extensive area of low voltage with fragmented and late potential in the anterior RVOT. Gray color of 3D mapping indicates scar tissue, and these areas were measured at 34.4 mm^2, with the longest total duration of abnormal fractionated potential up to 468 ms and up to 326 ms after the end of the surface QRS. (b) Epicardial ablation was performed targeting the area of low voltage with fragmented and late potential in the anterior epicardial RVOT. (c) Remapped epicardial voltage mapping revealed that these areas were substituted with a scar. RVOT = right ventricular outflow tract.

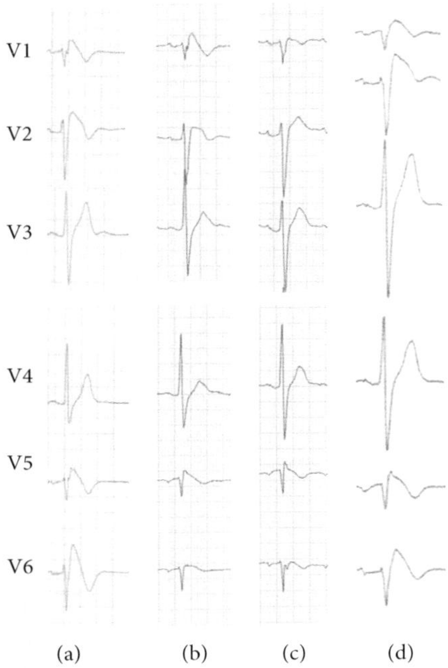

FIGURE 3: ECGs of the Brugada syndrome patient showing recordings of the anterior precordial leads: V1-2 leads from the 4th intercostal space and high precordial leads (V5 and V6 positioned cranially from V1 and V2) from the 3rd intercostal space. (a) Baseline before catheter ablation; (b) three days after ablation; (c) one month after ablation. Note the disappearance of the Brugada pattern at high precordial leads (V5-6) in the early stage and then at standard precordial V1-2 leads after catheter ablation. (d) The flecainide provocative test after three months of ablation revealed unmasking of type I Brugada pattern. ECG = electrocardiogram.

resulted in normalization of the Brugada ECG pattern and prevented VF episodes [3]. A combined epicardial and endocardial ablation strategy for Brugada syndrome targeting low-voltage, fractionated late potentials in the RVOT was reported recently [4]. We performed endocardial substrate mapping before attempting the epicardial approach; however, there were no abnormal electrocardiograms to target.

The ST segment elevation in a Brugada syndrome patient is the most prominent in the leads overlying the RVOT and closely follows its anatomic position [5, 6]. Recording ECGs by placing the right precordial leads at higher intercostal spaces increases the sensitivity for detecting Brugada syndrome. Regional epicardial fibrosis and electrocardiogram abnormalities affecting the RVOT correspond to the high precordial leads where the Brugada phenotype is best seen and also an ablation effect is best seen in our patient.

We confirmed noninducibility of VF by programmed electric stimulation at the end of the procedure. However, noninducibility might not be the proper endpoint because of several shortcomings of the induction test. Recently, Pappone et al. published the catheter ablation of Brugada syndrome with endpoints of elimination of all abnormal electric ventricular potentials before and after ajmaline, leading to ECG normalization and noninducibility of VT/VF [7]. However, acute normalization of the Brugada ECG pattern during the ablation procedure needs further evaluation as an endpoint [8]. Despite normalization of spontaneous type I Brugada patterns after successful ablation, VF recurrence persisted in 27% of patients [9], and a substantial number of patients showed normalization of the Brugada pattern within three months of ablation [3]. Previous studies demonstrated that elimination of the arrhythmogenic substrate associated with disappearance of the Brugada ECG pattern as confirmed by flecainide testing indicates successful outcome [2, 7]. However, our patient showed unmasking of type I Brugada pattern by flecainide testing after three months of catheter ablation even though we ablated all abnormal substrates confirmed by the sodium channel blocker at the time of the ablation procedure. Currently, the best endpoint is to eliminate all substrate areas that harbor abnormal low-voltage fractionated signals detected after the sodium channel blocker challenge [8]. And we suggest that early disappearance of the Brugada pattern at high precordial leads is helpful to assess the success of ablation before disappearance of the Brugada pattern at standard precordial leads.

Epicardial ablation was effective in eliminating the substrate and the Brugada phenotype in our patient, and early successful response after catheter ablation can be predicted by high precordial leads.

References

[1] K. Nademanee, G. Veerakul, M. Mower et al., "Defibrillator versus beta-blockers for unexplained death in Thailand (DEBUT): a randomized clinical trial," *Circulation*, vol. 107, no. 17, pp. 2221–2226, 2003.

[2] J. Brugada, C. Pappone, A. Berruezo et al., "Brugada syndrome phenotype elimination by epicardial substrate ablation," *Circulation: Arrhythmia and Electrophysiology*, vol. 8, no. 6, pp. 1373–1381, 2015.

[3] K. Nademanee, G. Veerakul, P. Chandanamattha et al., "Prevention of ventricular fibrillation episodes in Brugada syndrome by catheter ablation over the anterior right ventricular outflow tract epicardium," *Circulation*, vol. 123, no. 12, pp. 1270–1279, 2011.

[4] S. A. Saha, K. Krishnan, C. Madias, and R. G. Trohman, "Combined right ventricular outflow tract epicardial and endocardial late potential ablation for treatment of Brugada storm: a case report and review of the literature," *Cardiology and Therapy*, vol. 5, no. 2, pp. 229–243, 2016.

[5] C. Veltmann, T. Papavassiliu, T. Konrad et al., "Insights into the location of type I ECG in patients with Brugada syndrome: correlation of ECG and cardiovascular magnetic resonance imaging," *Heart Rhythm*, vol. 9, no. 3, pp. 414–421, 2012.

[6] S. Savastano, R. Rordorf, A. Vicentini et al., "A comprehensive electrocardiographic, molecular, and echocardiographic study of Brugada syndrome: validation of the 2013 diagnostic criteria," *Heart Rhythm*, vol. 11, no. 7, pp. 1176–1183, 2014.

[7] C. Pappone, J. Brugada, G. Vicedomini et al., "Electrical substrate elimination in 135 consecutive patients with Brugada syndrome," *Circulation: Arrhythmia and electrophysiology*, vol. 10, no. 5, p. e005053, 2017.

32

A Long-Term Survivor with Tetralogy of Fallot Treated Only with the Classical Blalock-Taussig Shunt

Yu Yamada,[1] Tomoko Ishizu,[1] Hidekazu Tsuneoka,[1] Yutaka Eki,[2] and Hitoshi Horigome[3]

[1]*Department of Cardiology, Faculty of Medicine, University of Tsukuba, Ibaraki, Japan*
[2]*Department of Cardiology, Hitachi General Hospital, Ibaraki, Japan*
[3]*Department of Pediatrics, University of Tsukuba, Ibaraki, Japan*

Correspondence should be addressed to Tomoko Ishizu; tomoco@md.tsukuba.ac.jp

Academic Editor: Tayfun Sahin

The prognosis of tetralogy of Fallot (TOF) treated only with Blalock-Taussig shunt (BTS) operation is unclear. A woman with TOF underwent classic BTS operation at 10 years of age. Despite no medication, she delivered two children and worked without apparent heart failure. At 72 years of age, she complained of dyspnea on exertion and leg edema. The cardiac angiogram revealed a well-patent BTS and severely stenotic right ventricular outflow tract. Right heart catheterization showed adequately maintained pulmonary blood flow with slight pulmonary arterial hypertension. Her unexpected yet favorable outcome reaffirms the importance of structural and functional self-adaptation even with cyanosis. If she had undergone a valve-sparing corrective surgery in adolescence, much better quality of life and outcome could have been expected.

1. Introduction

Tetralogy of Fallot (TOF) is the most common cause of cyanotic congenital heart disease, and Blalock-Taussig shunt (BTS) operation is considered the first-step management for maintaining pulmonary blood flow in TOF patients. Complete transventricular repair of TOF is the standard surgical treatment that should be performed in infancy or early childhood [1]. Long-term survival has improved because it is associated with lower operative mortality [2, 3]. However, the prognosis of patients with TOF treated by only palliative operation remains unclear. We describe a patient with TOF treated by classic BTS operation who lived a productive life without obvious symptoms in the long term.

2. Case Presentation

A woman with TOF underwent left classic BTS operation by the late cardiac surgeon Professor Shigeru Sakakibara at the Tokyo Women's Medical College, Tokyo, Japan, in the 1950s when she was 10 years old. She stopped visiting the hospital a few years postoperatively because she did not have difficulty performing daily activities. Subsequently, she got married at 25 years of age and gave birth to two children at 29 years of age without special gynecological care at a local hospital. She kept working on a production line while raising her children without experiencing symptoms of heart failure.

At 70 years of age, she was found to have a low oxygen saturation during a health examination program, but she did not seek hospital care. She developed dyspnea and leg edema when she was 72 years old, and then diuretic was started for a diagnosis of heart failure at a local clinic. When she was referred to our hospital for further evaluation, her symptoms of heart failure were comparable with the New York Heart Association (NYHA) functional class III. Her oxygen saturation was 88% on room air at rest. Her heart examination revealed a continuous murmur (Levine III/VI) and systolic ejection murmur (IV/VI) in the second right sternal border. Laboratory data showed the following values (reference ranges): hemoglobin level 15.7 g/dl, hematocrit 44.5%, platelet count $19.7 \times 10^4/\mu l$, prothrombin time 11.4 seconds, 98.5%, D-dimer level $1.2\,\mu g/dl$ ($<1.0\,\mu g/dl$),

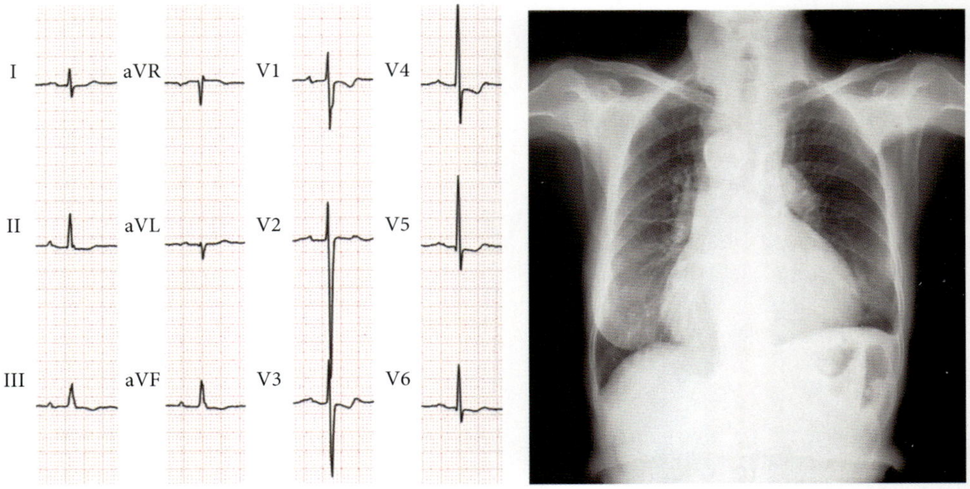

(a) (b)

Figure 1: Electrocardiography and the chest X-ray. (a) Electrocardiogram shows normal sinus rhythm at 75 beats/min with a prolonged PR interval; negative T in leads II, III, and aVF; and ST depression in V1 and V4–6. (b) Chest radiograph reveals a cardiothoracic ratio of 66%, right-sided aortic arch, and dilated pulmonary arteries.

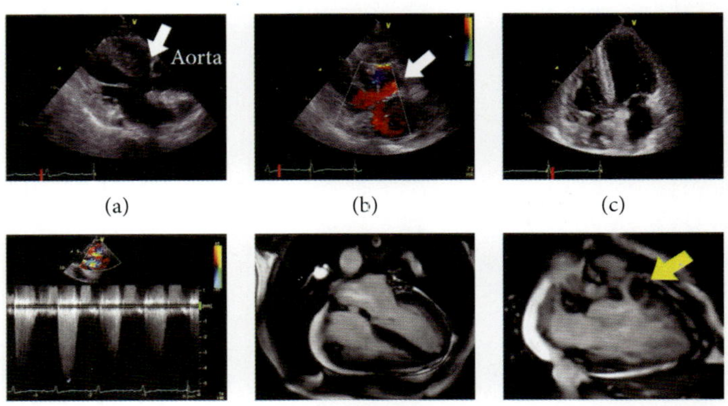

(a) (b) (c)

(d) (e) (f)

Figure 2: Transthoracic echocardiogram and cardiac magnetic resonance imaging (CMRI). (a) Parasternal long-axis view shows the ventricular septal defect (VSD) (white arrow) and overriding of the aorta. (b) Color Doppler image in the long-axis view shows two shunts through the VSD (white arrow). (c) Apical four-chamber view shows the hypertrophic right ventricle. (d) There is an RV outflow obstruction with a peak velocity of 4.9 m/s. (e) Analysis of CMRI reveals a normal RV end-diastolic volume (76 ml), reduced RV ejection fraction of 28%, and preserved left ventricular ejection fraction of 60%. (f) CMRI scan shows subvalvular pulmonary stenosis (yellow arrow).

creatinine level 1.35 mg/dl (0.4–0.8 mg/dl), and serum brain-type natriuretic peptide level 210 pg/ml (<18.4 pg/ml). A chest radiograph revealed a cardiothoracic ratio of 66%, right-sided aortic arch, and prominently dilated PA without pulmonary congestion (Figure 1(a)). The electrocardiogram showed sinus rhythm with a prolonged PR interval and ST-T segment abnormalities (Figure 1(b)). The echocardiogram showed a large ventricular septal defect with a bidirectional, mainly left-to-right shunt, overriding the aorta, right ventricular (RV) hypertrophy, and a stenotic RV outflow tract with a peak velocity of 4.9 m/s (Figure 2). Left ventricular (LV) diastolic indices of echocardiogram were as follows: peak E velocity 80 cm/s, E/A 0.72, septal E′ velocity 4.1 cm/s, lateral E′ velocity 3.5 cm/s, and average E/E′ 21. Abnormal relaxation pattern of transmitral flow, low E′ velocity, and high E/E′ suggested the existence of LV diastolic dysfunction. The cardiac magnetic resonance imaging scan showed reduced RV ejection fraction (EF) of 28% and preserved LVEF of 60% with a LV end-diastolic volume index of 103 ml/m^2 (Figures 2(e) and 2(f)). There was no abnormality in the pulmonary valve (PV), and the diameter of the PV annulus was 24 mm. The catheter angiogram revealed a patent BTS and severe stenosis at the ostium of the left PA (Figure 3). Right heart catheterization showed a normal PA wedge pressure (systolic/diastolic/mean pressure: 15/9/8 mmHg), mildly elevated PA pressure (systolic/diastolic/mean pressure: 35/20/30 mmHg), elevated RV systolic and end-diastolic pressure (135/20 mmHg), mean right atrial pressure (11 mmHg), and systolic and end-diastolic LV pressure (149/23 mmHg). The pressure gradient between the PA and right ventricle was 117 mmHg. Cardiac output calculated by the Fick principle

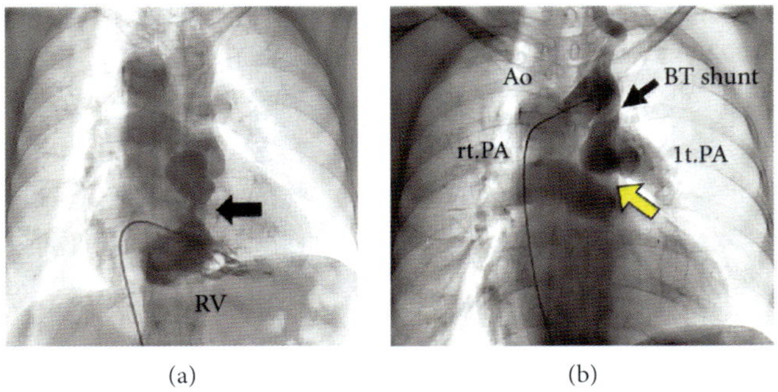

FIGURE 3: Catheter angiography. (a) Right ventriculogram shows subvalvular pulmonary stenosis (black arrow). (b) Aortogram shows a right-sided aortic arch and patent Blalock-Taussig shunt. There is stenosis at the ostium of the left pulmonary artery (yellow arrow) and both pulmonary artery aneurysms. Ao: Aorta; BT shunt; Blalock-Taussig shunt; lt.PA: left pulmonary artery; rt.PA: right pulmonary artery; RV: right ventricle.

TABLE 1: Previous reports in PubMed of unoperated TOF surviving over 70 years old.

Number	Author (year)	Age	Gender	Symptom or reason of admission	Other cardiac complications
1	Thomas et al. (1987) [5]	77	Male	Dyspnea	Ductus arteriosus, mitral regurgitation
2	Fernicola et al. (1993) [6]	74	Male	Dyspnea	Mitral prolapse
3	Ishida et al. (2001) [7]	71	Male	Dyspnea	None
4	Bielik et al. (2005) [8]	74	Male	Syncope	None
5	Tanaka et al. (2005) [9]	72	Female	Dyspnea	None
6	Yang et al. (2005) [10]	73	Male	Dyspnea	None
7	Alonso et al. (2007) [11]	86	Male	Chest pain	Coronary artery disease
8	Nieves et al. (2007) [12]	70	Female	Dyspnea	None
9	Stanescu et al. (2008) [13]	75	Male	Dyspnea	Quadricuspid aortic valve
10	Subhawoang et al. (2009) [14]	87	Female	Cerebral infraction	None
11	Sousa et al. (2013) [15]	72	Female	Dyspnea	Endocarditis

was 2.9 l/min, and pulmonary vascular resistance index was 5.95 Wood units·m^2. The brain's magnetic resonance imaging scan showed no significant abnormalities. She started to take diuretics and home oxygen inspiration therapies; her heart failure symptom improved to NYHA II. Based on the clinical and hemodynamic assessments and her age, we decided not to perform radical operation.

3. Discussion

The patient was fortunate to have a patent right ventricular outflow tract (RVOT) that allowed her to live for ten years without surgery. The combination of the classic BTS at age 10 and the patent RVOT provided enough pulmonary blood flow to allow her to survive into her seventies. The use of the left classic BTS in the setting of a right aortic arch created a source of pulmonary blood flow that could grow along with her. Also, the RVOT must have grown along with her somatic growth [4].

Previous reports in PubMed of unoperated TOF surviving over 70 years old are shown in Table 1 [5–15]. There are rarely reported studies on long-term outcome about patients with TOF treated by only palliative operation.

Prolonged survival of patients with uncorrected TOF is often associated with a well-developed left ventricle, initially mild pulmonary stenosis, or well-maintained pulmonary blood flow by such as systemic to pulmonary collaterals or persistent patent ductus arteriosus. Furthermore, in our case, there was no history of significant organ dysfunction due to hypoxia, and no major complication of adult patients with uncorrected TOF such as brain abscess or infective endocarditis. Compared to previous reports (Table 1), it is an important thing that she gave birth to two children without significant symptoms of heart failure. In the case reported by Sousa et al. [15], the patient gave birth to one child without complications; however, her subpulmonary stenosis was very mild (maximum gradient of 31 mmHg) and her pulmonary blood flow was well maintained (Qp/Qs = 0.9). In our case, appropriately adjusted pulmonary blood flow by BTS might enable her to give birth to two children safely.

This patient had favorable anatomy that allowed her to live for a long time, but there was evidence of biventricular dysfunction accompanied with elevated right and left ventricular end-diastolic pressure. It might be caused by long-term pressure overload and cyanotic state. Although the diameter of the PV annulus was measured in her seventies, the size of 24 mm must have been acceptable for valve-sparing corrective surgery [16–18]. If she had undergone a valve-sparing corrective surgery in adolescence, much better quality of life and outcome could have been expected.

4. Conclusion

This case shows that classical BTS has a potential of long-term patency with good functional capacity. Appropriately adjusted pulmonary blood flow by BTS may cause long-term survival and a productive life in patients with TOF.

References

[1] G. S. Van Arsdell, G. S. Maharaj, J. Tom et al., "What is the optimal age for repair of tetralogy of Fallot?," *Circulation*, vol. 102, Supplement 3, pp. III-123–III-129, 2000.

[2] G. Nollert, T. Fischlein, S. Bouterwek, C. Böhmer, W. Klinner, and B. Reichart, "Long-term survival in patients with repair of tetralogy of Fallot: 36-year follow-up of 490 survivors of the first year after surgical repair," *Journal of the American College of Cardiology*, vol. 30, no. 5, pp. 1374–1383, 1997.

[3] E. J. Hickey, G. Veldtman, T. J. Bradley et al., "Late risk of outcomes for adults with repaired tetralogy of Fallot from an inception cohort spanning four decades," *European Journal of Cardio-Thoracic Surgery*, vol. 35, no. 1, pp. 156–164, 2009.

[4] E. T. Ross, J. M. Costello, C. L. Backer, L. M. Brown, and J. D. Robinson, "Right ventricular outflow tract growth in infants with palliated tetralogy of Fallot," *The Annals of Thoracic Surgery*, vol. 99, no. 4, pp. 1367–1372, 2015.

[5] S. H. Thomas, P. Bass, H. Pambakian, and J. H. Marigold, "Cyanotic tetralogy of Fallot in a 77 year old man," *Postgraduate Medical Journal*, vol. 63, no. 739, pp. 361-362, 1987.

[6] D. J. Fernicola, V. R. Boodhoo, and W. C. Roberts, "Prolonged survival (74 years) in unoperated tetralogy of Fallot with associated mitral valve prolapse," *The American Journal of Cardiology*, vol. 71, no. 5, pp. 479–483, 1993.

[7] Y. Ishida, M. Kawasuji, N. Sakakibara et al., "A case report of total repair in a 71-year-old patient with tetralogy of Fallot," *Kyobu Geka*, vol. 54, no. 3, pp. 225–227, 2001.

[8] H. Bielik, M. A. Ohlow, B. Hügl, K. Reinig, R. Gröger, and B. Lauer, "First diagnosis of Fallot tetralogy in a 74-year-old man," *Zeitschrift für Kardiologie*, vol. 94, no. 3, pp. 205–210, 2005.

[9] S. Tanaka, N. Kikuchi, N. Hirakawa et al., "Prolonged survival in a female with untreated tetralogy of Fallot," *Journal of UOEH*, vol. 27, no. 2, pp. 189–195, 2005.

[10] X. Yang, L. J. Freeman, and C. Ross, "Unoperated tetralogy of Fallot: case report of a natural survivor who died in his 73rd year; is it ever too late to operate?," *Postgraduate Medical Journal*, vol. 81, no. 952, pp. 133-134, 2005.

[11] A. Alonso, B. C. Downey, and J. T. Kuvin, "Uncorrected tetralogy of Fallot in an 86-year-old patient," *The American Journal of Geriatric Cardiology*, vol. 16, no. 1, pp. 38–41, 2007.

[12] O. N. Nieves and J. E. López, "Uncorrected tetralogy of Fallot with agenesis of the left pulmonary artery in a 70-year-old elderly female," *Boletin de la Asociacion Medica de Puerto Rico*, vol. 99, no. 3, pp. 226–229, 2007.

[13] C. Stanescu and K. Branidou, "A case of 75-year-old survivor of unrepaired tetralogy of Fallot and quadricuspid aortic valve," *European Journal of Echocardiography*, vol. 9, no. 1, pp. 167–170, 2008.

[14] T. K. Subhawong and O. Teytelboym, "Survival to the age of 87 years in a woman with unoperated tetralogy of Fallot," *Journal of Radiology Case Reports*, vol. 3, no. 8, pp. 14–17, 2009.

[15] P. Sousa, W. Santos, N. Marques et al., "A 72-year-old woman with an uncorrected tetralogy of Fallot presenting with possible pulmonary endocarditis: a case report," *Journal of Medical Case Reports*, vol. 7, no. 1, p. 150, 2013.

[16] R. D. Stewart, C. L. Backer, L. Young, and C. Mavroudis, "Tetralogy of Fallot: results of a pulmonary valve-sparing strategy," *The Annals of Thoracic Surgery*, vol. 80, no. 4, pp. 1431–1439, 2005.

[17] M. Nathan, A. C. Marshall, J. Kerstein et al., "Technical performance score as predictor for post-discharge reintervention in valve-sparing tetralogy of Fallot repair," *Seminars in Thoracic and Cardiovascular Surgery*, vol. 26, no. 4, pp. 297–303, 2014.

[18] T. Hoashi, K. Kagisaki, Y. Meng et al., "Long-term outcomes after definitive repair for tetralogy of Fallot with preservation of the pulmonary valve annulus," *The Journal of Thoracic and Cardiovascular Surgery*, vol. 148, no. 3, pp. 802–809, 2014.

33

Transcutaneous Puncture of an Undeflatable Coronary Angioplasty Balloon Catheter

Gregor Leibundgut,[1] **Christian Degen**,[2] **and Florian Riede**[1]

[1]*Department of Cardiology, Medizinische Universitätsklinik, Kantonsspital Baselland, Rheinstrasse 26, 4410 Liestal, Switzerland*
[2]*Departement of Internal Medicine, Medizinische Universitätsklinik, Kantonsspital Baselland, Rheinstrasse 26, 4410 Liestal, Switzerland*

Correspondence should be addressed to Gregor Leibundgut; kardiologie@mac.com

Academic Editor: Man-Hong Jim

This case report describes a quick and safe method to successfully retrieve an undeflatable angioplasty balloon via the transradial access site. The article also presents potential mechanisms of contrast media entrapment and bench tests of guidewire-assisted balloon puncture. After successful stent implantation in the proximal right coronary artery in a 74-year-old female patient referred for acute coronary syndrome, the balloon catheter became undeflatable for an unknown reason. Several attempts to burst the balloon in the guide catheter and the aorta failed. After a pullback into the radial artery, the still inflated balloon became stuck again and was unable to be retrieved through the sheath. Finally, transcutaneous puncture and aspiration of contrast media with a 23 gauge syringe needle through the skin in the right forearm allowed deflation and successful removal the balloon.

1. Introduction

Transradial access for percutaneous coronary interventions (PCI) has become more frequent in recent years [1]. In particular, patients presenting with ST-segment elevation myocardial infarction (STEMI), non-STEMI (NSTEMI), and cardiogenic shock benefit from the radial approach [2–8]. Based on these studies, the latest ESC guidelines recommend the transradial access for the management of acute coronary syndromes (ACS) (class I, level A) [9]. Radial access is also associated with reduced incidence of acute kidney injury after PCI [10].

Optimized guide support, the latest guidewire and balloon technologies, and additional accessories such as extension catheters provide enough backup to successfully cross severely calcified lesions via the radial route. However, more complex procedures inevitably result in more complications. Smaller-sized guide catheters with the radial approach may limit the ability to remove damaged gear through the access site. Undeployed or lost stents, broken guidewires, twisted guiding catheters, trapped balloon catheters, and other interventional tools have been successfully removed by the femoral access or cardiac surgery [11]. Only a few reports describing true transradial bailout methods have been published [12]. The use of large balloon diameters and lengths concurrently with smaller guiding catheters may further increase complication rates.

This case report describes an easy method for successful transradial retrieval of an undeflatable 3.5/48 balloon catheter using transcutaneous puncture and contrast aspiration in the forearm.

2. Case Report

A 74-year-old female patient with an acute non-ST-segment elevation myocardial infarction (NSTEMI) was referred for coronary angiography. Transradial access was established with a 10 cm 6F Introducer sheath (Glidesheath, Terumo Medical Corporation). Coronary angiography with a 6F Judkins right 4 diagnostic catheter revealed a long and heavily calcified lesion of the proximal segment and ostium of the right coronary artery (RCA). During the retrieval of

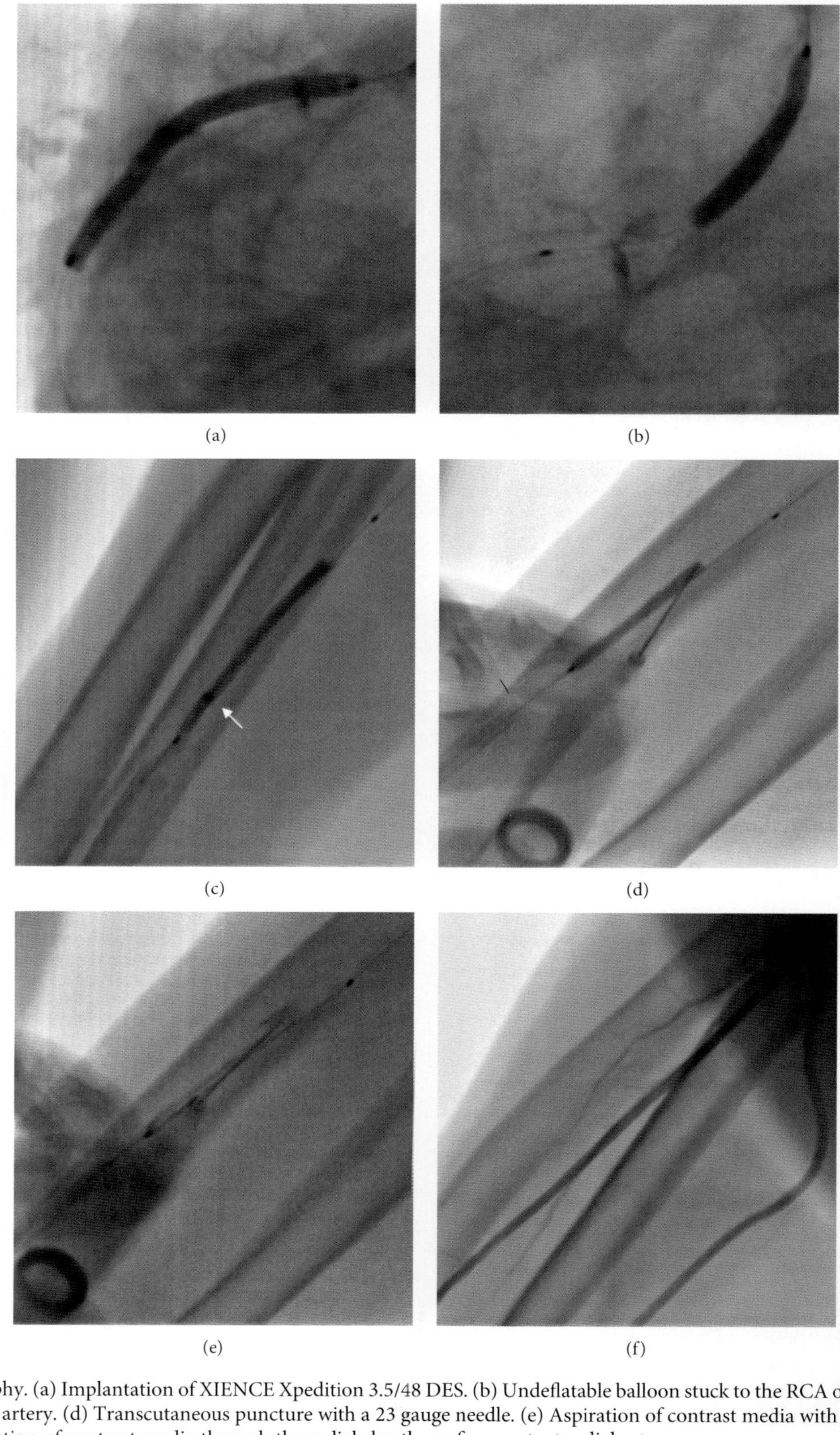

Figure 1: Angiography. (a) Implantation of XIENCE Xpedition 3.5/48 DES. (b) Undeflatable balloon stuck to the RCA ostium. (c) Undeflated balloon in the radial artery. (d) Transcutaneous puncture with a 23 gauge needle. (e) Aspiration of contrast media with complete deflation of the balloon. (f) Injection of contrast media through the radial sheath confirms patent radial artery.

the diagnostic catheter, the patient complained of severe pain in her right arm due to spasm of the radial artery. After repetitive intravenous administration of midazolam up to 8 mg and nitroglycerine through the radial sheath, retrieval of the catheter was finally possible. PCI of the lesion in the proximal RCA was then performed over a 5F Amplatz left 1 guiding

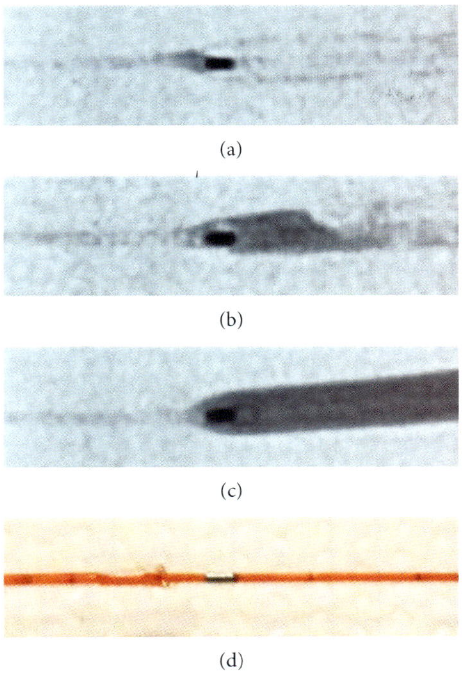

FIGURE 2: Exit/Entrance port of contrast media. (a), (b), and (c) show entrance of contrast media filling the angioplasty balloon by X-ray. (d) Photograph of a balloon catheter with the balloon cut from the rest of the catheter.

catheter (Launcher, Medtronic) using an extra support guidewire (Galeo ES, Biotronik) and a 3.0/15 semi compliant balloon (Across HP, Acrostak) for predilatation. A 3.5/48 drug-eluting stent (DES) (XIENCE Xpedition, Abbot Vascular) was then placed in the predilated coronary segment and inflated to 18 atm (Figure 1(a)). A mixture of contrast media and saline at a ratio of 1 : 1 was used for all balloon inflations. After a second more proximal inflation, the balloon catheter did not deflate completely and the operator was unable to pull it back into the 5F guiding catheter (Figure 1(b)). Excessive inflation and deflation with the indeflator and forced aspiration with a 50 ml syringe were unable to deflate the balloon that was stuck at the RCA ostium. The operator then decided to pull back the entire equipment including the guiding catheter, guidewire, and stent balloon at once. Finally, the balloon catheter became released from the stent remaining in place in the coronary artery. An attempt to burst the balloon in the ascending aorta by inflation well over rated burst pressure (RBP), as well as puncturing the balloon within the guide catheter with multiple stiff guidewires, also failed.

During a further pullback of the system, the still inflated balloon became stuck again in the small and vasospastic radial artery. The operator was unable to pull or push the balloon in any direction and was unable to wedge the balloon into the 6F radial sheath. Moreover, a forced pullback of the partially inflated balloon catheter resulted in invagination of the distal part of the balloon (Figure 1(c), white arrow). After injecting local anesthesia on the middle forearm, transcutaneous puncture of the balloon through the skin and the radial artery wall was performed with a 23 gauge syringe needle using fluoroscopy for guidance (Figure 1(d)), and contrast media were aspirated with the syringe (Figure 1(e)). Retrieval of the deflated balloon was then possible through the radial sheath. Reintubation of the RCA with a fresh guiding catheter revealed a good angiographic result in the proximal segment and relevant acute recoil at the ostium of the calcified RCA. Implantation of a second short 4.0/9 mm DES (BMX-Alpha, Biosensors) was necessary to mechanically stabilize the lesion. Injection of contrast media through the sheath confirmed the integrity of the radial artery at the puncture site (Figure 1(f)). Radial compression was used to close the 6F access site. The clinical follow-up remained uneventful.

3. Discussion

The presented case describes a quick and safe method to successfully retrieve an undeflatable angioplasty balloon via the transradial access site. Transcutaneous puncture can easily be performed by palpation of the balloon or using fluoroscopy for guidance. Puncture of the balloon catheter alone may be sufficient for retrieval through the sheath; however, aspiration of contrast media with the syringe facilitates balloon deflation and may be beneficial.

Contrast media exit the balloon at the proximal end (Figure 2) and flows through the flexible distal part of the catheter shaft and then through the metallic hypotube. Viscosity plays an important role with deflation time depending on the mixing ratio between contrast media and saline solution [13]. Potential mechanisms of contrast media entrapment in angioplasty balloons are illustrated in Figure 3 and include (A) acute recoil of a severely calcified lesion after balloon inflation with compression of the deflating balloon around the entry port; (B) strangulation of the proximal end of the balloon by the guiding catheter after the early pullback of the balloon catheter before complete deflation; and (C) damage to the hypotube. The final common scenario is that the balloon can only be partially deflated due to the entrapment of contrast media, which further complicates retrieval of the balloon catheter. In the first two situations, contrast media collect in the distal part of the balloon and this can complicate balloon retrieval. Only the third mechanism explains all features observed in the current case including distal deflation of the balloon and inability to inflate the balloon again. In the present case, however, a collection of contrast media in the proximal part could also have been a result from incomplete deaeration prior to initial inflation. The heavily calcified ostium and the acute recoil after stent implantation were very likely the reason for the balloon entrapment. Longitudinal stent compression (LSC) is frequently found in ostial lesions and may further complicate acute recoil and removal of the distally placed gear [14]. However, no angiographic characteristics of LSC were found in the present case.

A classic bailout method for undeflatable angioplasty balloons includes prolonged/forced balloon inflation well above rated burst pressures (RBP) to intentionally burst the balloon. This maneuver should be performed in a large vessel such as the ascending aorta or subclavian artery to avoid

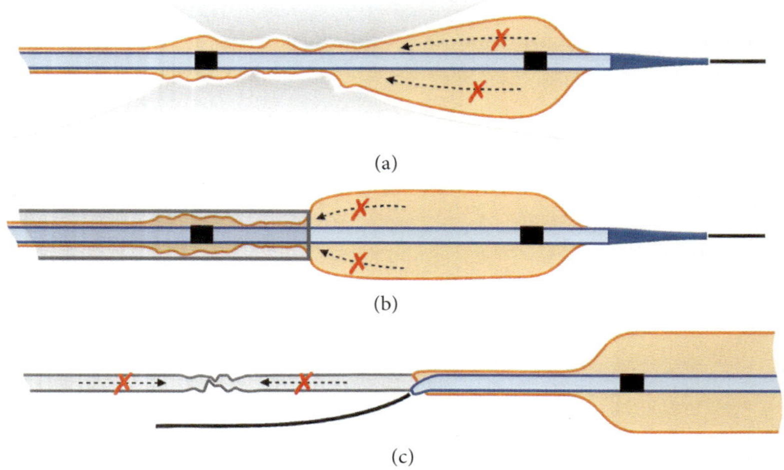

FIGURE 3: Mechanisms of contrast media entrapment. Several potential mechanisms can result in the contrast media being trapped inside the balloon. (a) Acute recoil of calcified lesion or stent and (b) strangulation of the balloon in the guide catheter. (c) Damage to the hypotube (kink or break). Dotted arrows and red X indicate compromised contrast media flow from the balloon into the hypotube.

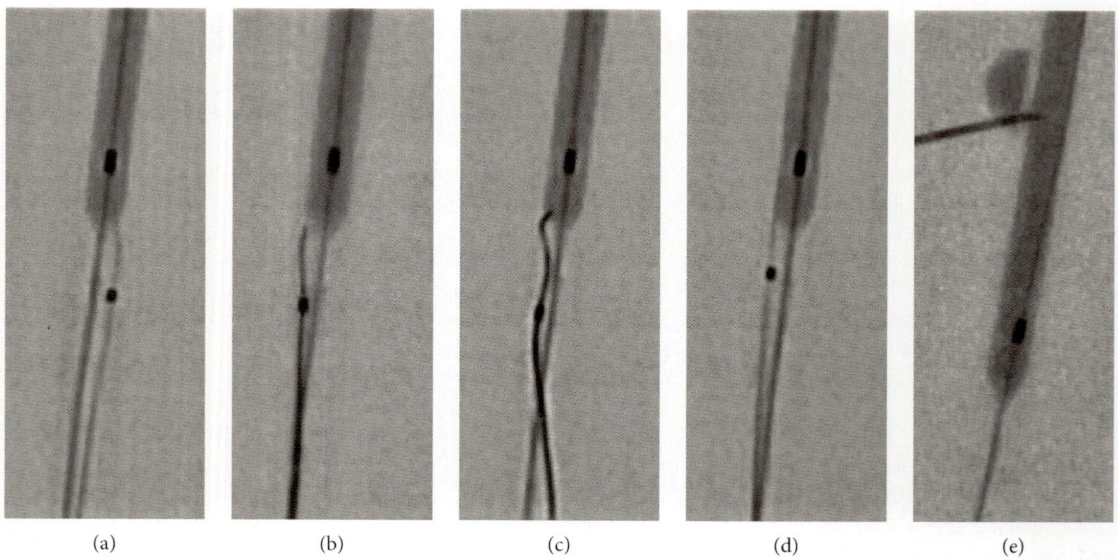

FIGURE 4: Transluminal balloon puncture. Inflated balloon from a XIENCE Xpedition 3.5/48 DES in a 6F guide catheter. Microcatheter placed proximal to the balloon for optimal guidewire support. Serial failed attempts to puncture the balloon with (a) Conquest Pro 12, (b) Stingray guidewire, (c) Gaia 3, and (d) opposite side of a work horse guidewire. (e) Successful balloon puncture with a 23G syringe needle through the guide catheter wall.

rupture of the coronary artery. This can be difficult with noncompliant (NC) and other high and very high-pressure balloons such as the OPN NC (SIS Medical, Switzerland) that can withstand up to 50 atm. The fact that inflation was also impossible suggests that the hypotube was obstructed or damaged and no contrast was able to flow in or out of the balloon. However, a close examination of the balloon catheter did not reveal a definite mechanism of failure in this case.

Other potential methods such as transluminal puncture of the balloon at its proximal end within the guide catheter with hard wires like the Gaia 3rd, Confianza Pro 12, Stingray guidewire (stiff wire with 0.0035-inch distal taper), or even the back end of a guidewire failed in bench tests (Figure 4). Even increasing the penetration force with the use of an additional microcatheter failed and is therefore not recommended in such cases. Similar to the present case, Watt and associates also were unable to puncture the balloon using a stiff guidewire and instead had to cut the kinked hypotube to passively let the balloon deflate [15]. Finally, successful balloon puncture is only feasible with a pointed and cut 23 gauge syringe needle and does not leave any damage to the radial artery wall.

Balloon catheters becoming undeflatable are extremely rare complications of PCI. A forced pullback of the balloon catheter of an undeflated balloon may cause the outer body of the distal shaft to shrink, forming a seal with the underlying tube of the distal shaft. At this stage, inflation may help to overcome this seal but may remain permanent once the distal shaft has ruptured. Ruptured balloon shafts leave the balloon behind in the coronary artery, and these cases cannot be resolved with this method.

An easy pullback into large sheaths commonly used in femoral access may account for the rare complication reports. In one published case, the operators were able to retrieve the balloon from the coronary artery and pull it into a 6F femoral sheath [16]. The present case, however, describes a true transradial bailout method without additional access. Using a 5F guide catheter may likely have contributed to the damage of the hypotube in this case. The use of sheathless catheters with a larger lumen may facilitate PCI and further reduce these complications with the radial approach.

4. Conclusion

Transcutaneous puncture of an undeflatable balloon catheter in the forearm is feasible and safe and may be considered a true/primary transradial retrieval method.

References

[1] K. Ratib, M. A. Mamas, S. G. Anderson et al., "Access site practice and procedural outcomes in relation to clinical presentation in 439,947 patients undergoing percutaneous coronary intervention in the United Kingdom," *JACC: Cardiovascular Interventions*, vol. 8, no. 1, Part A, pp. 20–29, 2015.

[2] S. S. Jolly, S. Yusuf, J. Cairns et al., "Radial versus femoral access for coronary angiography and intervention in patients with acute coronary syndromes (RIVAL): a randomised, parallel group, multicentre trial," *The Lancet*, vol. 377, no. 9775, pp. 1409–1420, 2011.

[3] P. Généreux, R. Mehran, T. Palmerini et al., "Radial access in patients with ST-segment elevation myocardial infarction undergoing primary angioplasty in acute myocardial infarction: the HORIZONS-AMI trial," *EuroIntervention*, vol. 7, no. 8, pp. 905–916, 2011.

[4] E. Romagnoli, G. Biondi-Zoccai, A. Sciahbasi et al., "Radial versus femoral randomized investigation in ST-segment elevation acute coronary syndrome," *Journal of the American College of Cardiology*, vol. 60, no. 24, pp. 2481–2489, 2012.

[5] S. R. Mehta, S. S. Jolly, J. Cairns et al., "Effects of radial versus femoral artery access in patients with acute coronary syndromes with or without ST-segment elevation," *Journal of the American College of Cardiology*, vol. 60, no. 24, pp. 2490–2499, 2012.

[6] W. Karrowni, A. Vyas, B. Giacomino et al., "Radial versus femoral access for primary percutaneous interventions in ST-segment elevation myocardial infarction patients: a meta-analysis of randomized controlled trials," *JACC: Cardiovascular Interventions*, vol. 6, no. 8, pp. 814–823, 2013.

[7] M. Valgimigli, A. Gagnor, P. Calabró et al., "Radial versus femoral access in patients with acute coronary syndromes undergoing invasive management: a randomised multicentre trial," *The Lancet*, vol. 385, no. 9986, pp. 2465–2476, 2015.

[8] S. B. Pancholy, G. Palamaner Subash Shantha, E. Romagnoli et al., "Impact of access site choice on outcomes of patients with cardiogenic shock undergoing percutaneous coronary intervention: a systematic review and meta-analysis," *American Heart Journal*, vol. 170, no. 2, pp. 353–361.e6, 2015.

[9] M. Roffi, C. Patrono, J. P. Collet et al., "2015 ESC Guidelines for the management of acute coronary syndromes in patients presenting without persistent ST-segment elevation: task force for the management of acute coronary syndromes in patients presenting without persistent ST-segment elevation of the European Society of Cardiology (ESC)," *European Heart Journal*, vol. 37, no. 3, pp. 267–315, 2016.

[10] G. Andò, B. Cortese, F. Russo et al., "Acute kidney injury after radial or femoral access for invasive acute coronary syndrome management: AKI-MATRIX," *Journal of the American College of Cardiology*, vol. 69, no. 21, pp. 2592–2603, 2017.

[11] K. Alexiou, U. Kappert, M. Knaut, K. Matschke, and S. M. Tugtekin, "Entrapped coronary catheter remnants and stents: must they be surgically removed?," *Texas Heart Institute Journal*, vol. 33, no. 2, pp. 139–142, 2006.

[12] G. Leibundgut, N. Löffelhardt, and F.-J. Neumann, "Percutaneous retrieval of a twisted guide catheter using a longer second radial sheath," *Catheterization and Cardiovascular Interventions*, vol. 83, no. 4, pp. 560–563, 2014.

[13] O. Mogabgab, V. G. Patel, T. T. Michael et al., "Impact of contrast agent viscosity on coronary balloon deflation times: bench testing results," *Journal of Interventional Cardiology*, vol. 27, no. 2, pp. 177–181, 2014.

[14] G. Leibundgut, M. Gick, A. Toma et al., "Longitudinal compression of the platinum-chromium everolimus-eluting stent during coronary implantation: predisposing mechanical properties, incidence, and predictors in a large patient cohort," *Catheterization and Cardiovascular Interventions*, vol. 81, no. 5, pp. E206–E214, 2013.

[15] J. Watt, A. Khurana, J. M. Ahmed, and I. F. Purcell, "Simple solution for an undeflatable stent balloon in the left main stem," *JACC: Cardiovascular Interventions*, vol. 8, no. 14, pp. e245–e246, 2015.

[16] M. Bostan, O. Satiroğlu, T. Erdoğan, M. E. Durakoğlugil, and Y. Uğurlu, "A rare complication: undeflatable balloon of the stent," *Interventional Medicine and Applied Science*, vol. 5, no. 1, pp. 43–45, 2013.

STEMI in a Young Male after Use of Synephrine-Containing Dietary Supplement

Dileep Unnikrishnan, Radhika Annam, Aasems Jacob, Braghadheeswar Thyagarajan, and Peter Farrugia

Department of Internal Medicine, Monmouth Medical Center, Long Branch, NJ, USA

Correspondence should be addressed to Dileep Unnikrishnan; drdileepunni@gmail.com

Academic Editor: Assad Movahed

A twenty-two-year-old male with no significant past medical history who presented with chest pain was found to have ST-segment elevation in leads II, III, aVF, and V4–V6. On subsequent EKGs, patient had new ST-segment elevations in anterolateral leads with dynamic changes. Cardiac catheterization showed acute dissection with thrombosis of the distal left main coronary artery leading into the ostial left anterior descending artery. The patient had no cardiac risk factors including hypertension, hyperlipidemia, diabetes, or family history of early cardiac disease. On further inquiry, the patient was found to be on two separate performance-enhancing supplements which contained synephrine, a sympathomimetic chemical which was later attributed as the cause of his acute coronary syndrome. Synephrine acts on alpha-1 adrenergic receptors causing peripheral and coronary vasoconstriction, hypertension, and hyperglycemia. Increased hemodynamic stress on the coronary arteries can lead to fatal dissections. Ours is an atypical case of synephrine-induced nonatherosclerotic spontaneous coronary artery dissection which helps caution the physicians about the importance of dietary supplement use in the history and possible side effects of such performance-enhancing additives.

1. Introduction

Several weight-loss and performance-enhancing dietary supplements are available over the counter in the US markets. Adding sympathomimetic chemicals like ephedra-containing compounds are highly effective in performance enhancement with the potential of causing fatal cardiac and respiratory side effects. Ephedra-containing compounds were banned by the FDA. However, this has led to the use of alternative sympathomimetic compounds like synephrine in these dietary supplements [1]. These selective alpha blockers can potentially be dangerous due to their effects like elevated systemic blood pressure, coronary vasospasm, and arterial dissections. Nonatherosclerotic spontaneous coronary artery dissection (NA-SCAD) is a rare cause of nontraumatic coronary dissection in young adults due to weakening of the arterial wall from hemodynamic stress. Most commonly associated factors include fibromuscular dysplasia, postpartum status, connective tissue disorders, and hormonal therapy [2]. Here, we report a case of a massive STEMI in a young African American male secondary to the use of synephrine-containing dietary supplement. On review of literature, we were able to find only one other similar case of young STEMI attributed to sympathomimetic dietary supplement administration [3].

2. Case Presentation

A 22-year-old African American male presented to the ER with acute onset of "pressure-like" substernal, nonradiating chest pain. His symptoms started while playing basketball. The pain was associated with shortness of breath and nausea. He had no significant past medical history or family history of coronary artery disease or sudden deaths. He denied excessive caffeine use, smoking, or alcohol intake. There was no reported use of any illicit drugs such as cocaine or amphetamines and was physically very active. Vital signs on admission included blood pressure of 138/89 mmHg, heart

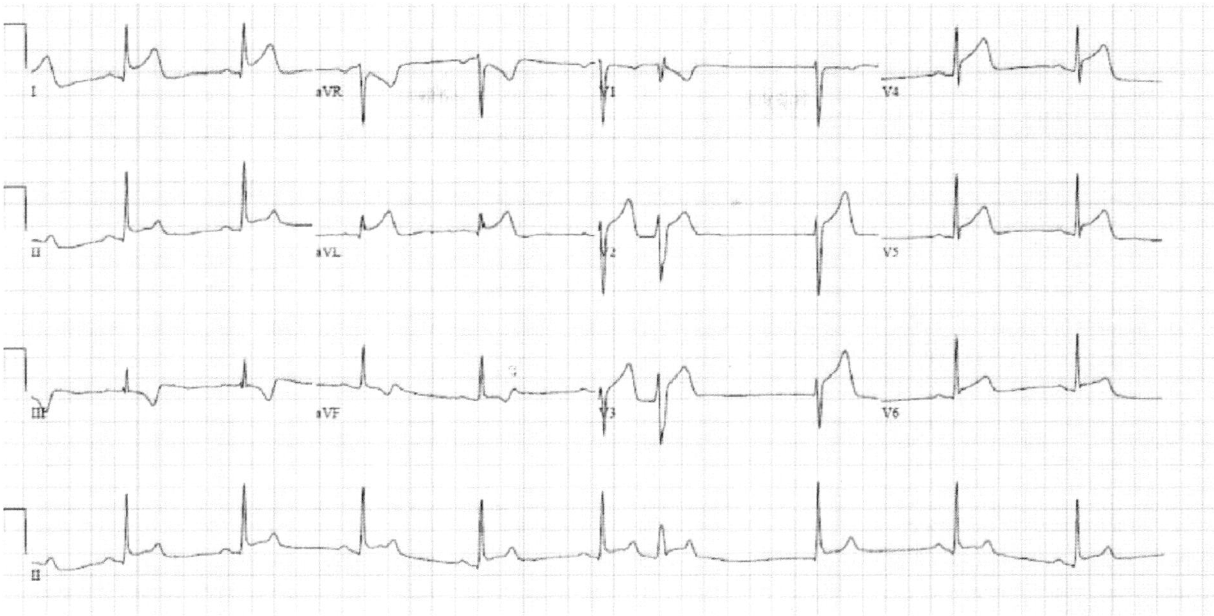

FIGURE 1: EKG of the patient showing ST elevation in leads I, avL, II, III, and V2–V6.

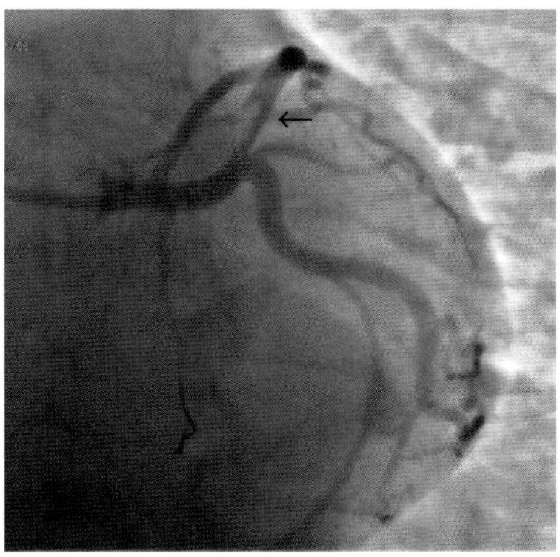

FIGURE 2: Coronary angiogram: left anterior oblique view of LAD prior to percutaneous coronary intervention showing dissection and clot in the proximal LAD (black arrow).

rate of 94/min, and respiratory rate of 22 breaths/min. His BMI was 28. Physical examination was unremarkable with no chest tenderness on palpation and no jugular venous distention. Heart sounds were normal with no murmurs or additional sounds. The electrocardiogram showed ST-segment elevation myocardial infarction (STEMI) in leads II, III, aVF, and V4–V6 (Figure 1). On subsequent EKGs, the patient had new ST-segment elevations in anterolateral leads with dynamic changes. Laboratory studies were pertinent for a troponin-I level of 0.83 ng/ml. The patient was given aspirin and ticagrelor loading doses, metoprolol succinate 25 mg, intravenous morphine, intravenous heparin drip, and sublingual nitroglycerin which did not relieve his chest pain.

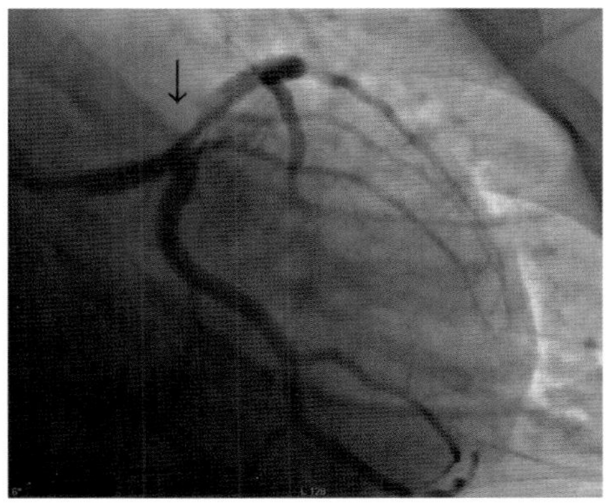

FIGURE 3: Coronary angiogram: right anterior oblique view of LAD prior to percutaneous coronary intervention showing dissection with clot in proximal LAD with TIMI 2 flow distally (black arrow).

The patient was taken for emergent cardiac angiography within 60 minutes of presentation and revealed acute dissection with thrombosis of the distal left main coronary artery (LCA) leading into the proximal left anterior descending artery (LAD) (Figures 2 and 3). An EBU 3.5 guide catheter was advanced over the wire with repeat injection of the left main performed revealing persistence of acute occlusion. Repeat angiography after balloon inflation revealed significant improvement in flow from TIMI 2 to TIMI 4. An extending thrombus was noted in the distal LAD which was suctioned out. Following this, a bare metal stent was inserted in the distal LCA ostial and the proximal LAD (Figures 4 and 5).

After catheterization, the patient was pain-free and hemodynamically stable. He was on epitifibatide infusion for a total of 18 hours. Other medications including carvedilol,

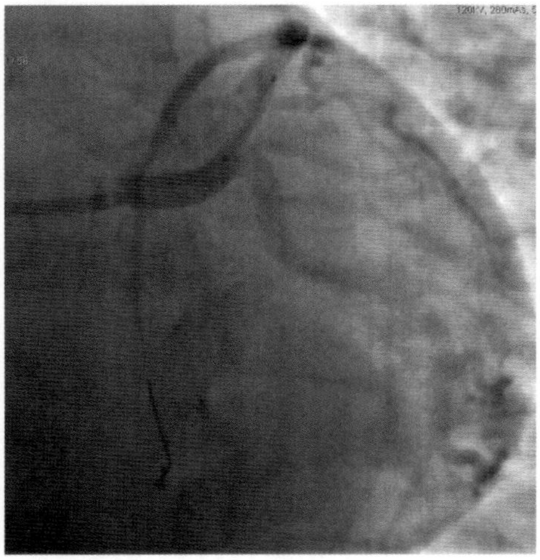

Figure 4: Coronary angiogram: left anterior oblique view of LAD during intervention with bare metal stent in the proximal LAD.

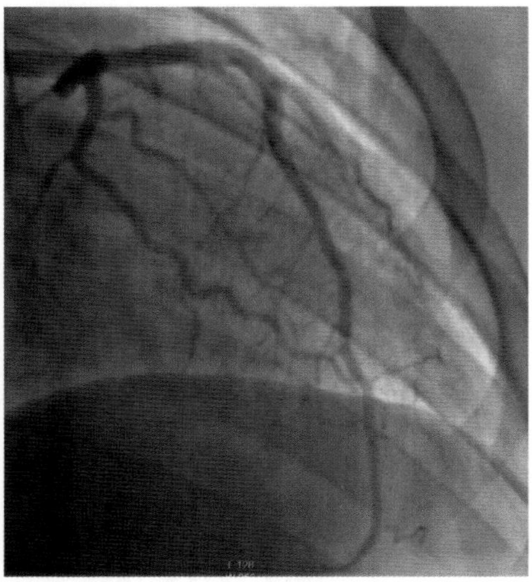

Figure 5: Coronary angiogram: right anterior oblique view of LAD after intervention showing bare metal stent in the proximal LAD with TIMI 4 flow distally.

lisinopril, aspirin, ticagrelor, and atorvastatin were initiated. The patient's peak troponin went up to 48.56 ng/ml in less than 24 hrs of initial laboratory studies and subsequently was trending down. Additional laboratory studies including hemoglobin A1c and lipid profile were normal. He was also worked up for thrombotic conditions which might lead to arterial thrombi such as homocystinemia and anti-phospholipid antibody syndrome both of which were negative. Transthoracic echocardiography performed revealed preserved left ventricular systolic function normal with ejection fraction estimated to be 0.50 to 0.54%. There was no patent foramen ovale that might have led to paradoxical embolus. A urine and serum toxicology screen was also done on the patient who came back as negative for cocaine or methamphetamine.

After the procedure, the patient was further questioned to elicit any history that might shine light to the etiology of his STEMI. He admitted to the use of two different weight-loss products (Performix™ stim-free; Performix SST) for the past 1 year, taking one capsule up to three times a day as indicated on the product label. However, he took Performix SST for the first time on the afternoon of presentation, drinking 3 scoops mixed with water, approximately 2 hours before started playing basketball. On reviewing, the contents of the supplement, it was noted to contain synephrine, an epinephrine analogue. Other contents of the mixture consisted of anhydrous caffeine, sensoril ashwagandha extract, bitter orange extract, n-methyltyramine, hordenine, tyramine, octopamine, huperzine A, yohimbine HCL, mucuna pruriens, and Bioperine. The patient was advised to avoid the use of the supplements. He was discharged home from the hospital with outpatient cardiology follow-up and advice to be maintained on dual antiplatelet therapy for at least one year.

3. Discussion

This is an interesting case of a young active male with no apparent past medical or familial risk factors who presented with STEMI secondary to dissection with thrombosis of distal left main coronary artery extending to proximal LAD. The patient's condition could be attributed to his use of synephrine-containing weight-loss and performance-enhancing supplements. Administration of beta-blockers preprocedure might also have led to the unimpeded alpha action of the adrenergics in this case. Synephrine is a naturally occurring alkaloid which has been used in combination with caffeine in several weight-loss and dietary supplements. Pharmacologically synephrine has its action on alpha-1 adrenergic receptors causing effects such as peripheral vasoconstriction, hypertension, and hyperglycemia [4]. Unsupervised use of such supplements could be risky and even fatal. In addition, mixing several stimulants and natural compounds such as caffeine and bitter orange extract with synephrine can lead to increase in the adverse effects profile of each [5]. A definitive causal relation between the dietary supplement intake and coronary dissection cannot be drawn in this case; however, given the paucity of any other likely risk factors, the event is presumably secondary to the hypertension and sympathetic overactivity from synephrine. Dietary supplement and weight reduction drug industries are highly lucrative, and the unscrupulous and potentially dangerous practice of adding sympathomimetic compounds for quick results is rampant [6]. More FDA regulations have to be implemented in this regard for the safety of the users. For any such patients presenting with acute coronary syndrome, the use of beta-blockers should be avoided [7]. Furthermore, it is important for physicians to be cognizant of sympathomimetics in the dietary supplements and elicit such history in atypical cases such as the one presented here in order to avoid diagnostic confusion and inadvertent harm to the patient.

References

[1] Anon, 2017, http://www.fda.gov/Food/DietarySupplements/GuidanceComplianceRegulatoryInformation/RegulationsLaws/ucm079733.htm.

[2] J. W. Saw, E. Aymong, C. Buller et al., "Non-atherosclerotic spontaneous coronary artery dissection association with predisposing and precipitating conditions and cardiovascular outcomes," *Journal of the American College of Cardiology*, vol. 12, no. 63, p. A4, 2014.
[3] J. E. Thomas, J. A. Munir, P. Z. McIntyre, and M. A. Ferguson, "STEMI in a 24-year-old man after use of a synephrine-containing dietary supplement, of a synephrine-containing dietary supplement: a case report and review of the literature," *Texas Heart Institute Journal*, vol. 36, no. 6, pp. 586–590, 2009.
[4] A. B. Stockton, P. T. Pace, and M. L. Tainter, "Some clinical actions and therapeutic uses of racemic synephrine," *Journal of Pharmacology and Experimental Therapeutics*, vol. 41, no. 1, pp. 11–20, 1931.
[5] G. C. Schmitt, M. D. Arbo, A. L. Lorensi et al., "Toxicological effects of a mixture used in weight loss products: p-synephrine associated with ephedrine, salicin, and caffeine," *International Journal of Toxicology*, vol. 31, no. 2, pp. 184–191, 2012.
[6] C. A. Haller and N. L. Benowitz, "Adverse cardiovascular and central nervous system events associated with dietary supplements containing ephedra alkaloids," *New England Journal of Medicine*, vol. 343, no. 25, pp. 1833–1838, 2000.
[7] B. G. Schwartz, S. Rezkalla, and R. A. Kloner, "Cardiovascular effects of cocaine," *Circulation*, vol. 122, no. 24, pp. 2558–2569, 2010.

Mediastinal Hematoma and Tracheal Compression following Transradial Percutaneous Coronary Intervention

Nathaniel R. Smilowitz, Muhamed Saric, Michael J. Attubato, and James N. Slater

Division of Cardiology, Department of Medicine, NYU School of Medicine, NYU Langone Health, New York, NY, USA

Correspondence should be addressed to Nathaniel R. Smilowitz; nathaniel.smilowitz@nyumc.org

Academic Editor: Ramazan Akdemir

Vascular complications from transradial percutaneous coronary intervention (PCI) are rare. We report an unusual case of stridor after PCI due to brachiocephalic artery perforation, pseudoaneurysm formation, and development of a large mediastinal hematoma with tracheal compression. Endovascular repair of the brachiocephalic artery was achieved with covered stent placement at the neck of the pseudoaneurysm. This case highlights the importance of careful guide catheter placement from the right radial approach. Ultimately, rapid diagnosis of vascular perforation, appropriate airway management, and prompt endovascular repair of the injured vessel is critical to the successful management of this life-threatening condition.

1. Introduction

Percutaneous coronary intervention (PCI) via the radial artery is an effective approach to treat patients with coronary artery disease. In large randomized trials of transradial versus transfemoral arterial access, patients who underwent transradial catheterization had fewer major adverse cardiovascular events, fewer access site bleeding events, and lower mortality than those who underwent transfemoral coronary intervention [1–3]. Thus, transradial access has been hailed as the preferred approach to minimize vascular complications associated with cardiac catheterization. Major vascular complications of transradial arterial access, although rare, occur in approximately 0.2% of coronary procedures [4, 5]. Vascular perforation, one of the most severe complications of radial PCI, can occur following aggressive manipulation of guidewires or catheters as they are advanced through the radial, brachial, subclavian, and brachiocephalic arteries. Complications typically occur when wires or catheters shear the arterial wall in looped, tortuous, or small caliber arterial segments. In this report, we present an unusual case of stridor after PCI due to brachiocephalic artery perforation, pseudoaneurysm formation, and development of a large mediastinal hematoma with tracheal compression.

2. Case Report

A 69-year-old man with a history of hypertension, dyslipidemia, and type 2 diabetes mellitus presented with lifestyle-limiting angina. He underwent diagnostic coronary angiography that revealed stenoses of the left anterior descending (LAD) coronary artery, ramus intermedius coronary artery, and the distal right coronary artery (RCA). Coronary artery bypass grafting was recommended, but the patient refused surgery and elected for percutaneous coronary intervention (PCI) instead. Initially, transradial PCI of the LAD and ramus coronary arteries was performed with placement of drug-eluting stents in each vessel. The patient was discharged on aspirin and ticagrelor with a plan for staged coronary intervention of the distal RCA at a later date.

Three months after the initial coronary intervention, the patient returned for planned PCI of the distal RCA stenosis. Access was again obtained in the right radial artery with a short 6 French slender sheath. After routine diagnostic coronary angiography confirmed a severe stenosis in the distal RCA (Figure 1(a)), bivalirudin was administered. A 6 French AL 0.75 guide catheter (Medtronic, Minneapolis, MN, USA) was advanced over an exchange length 0.035″ J-wire, but could not be delivered to the ascending aorta due to resistance in the brachiocephalic artery. The guide was

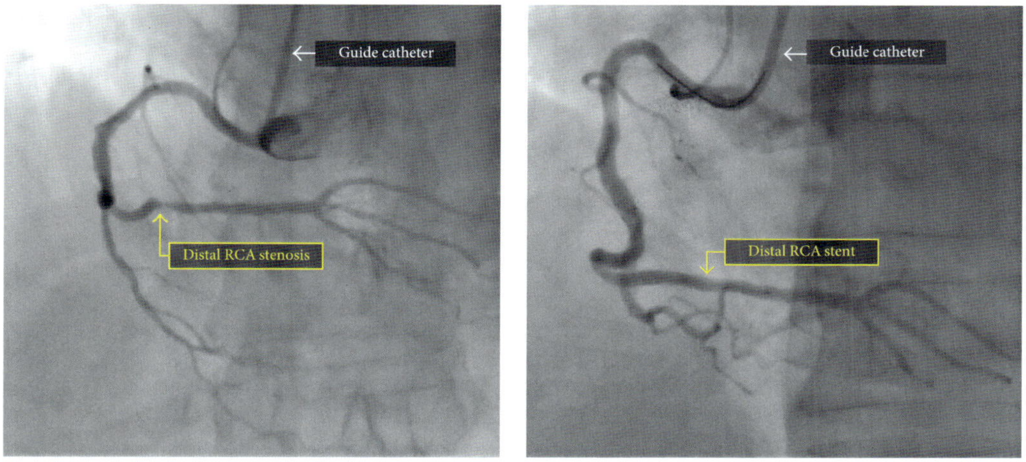

(a) (b)

FIGURE 1: Coronary angiography of the right coronary artery in the left anterior oblique view before (a) and after (b) percutaneous coronary intervention and drug-eluting stent placement.

removed and exchanged for a 6 French JR 4 guide catheter (Medtronic, Minneapolis, MN, USA), which was easily advanced into the ascending aorta and used to engage the ostium of the RCA without complication. Next, a standard 0.014″ RunThrough coronary guidewire (Terumo, Tokyo, Japan) was placed in the distal RCA, and percutaneous coronary intervention was performed. The lesion was pre-dilated with a 2.0 mm Maverick compliant balloon (Boston Scientific, Marlborough, MA, USA) inflated to 10 ATM, and a Xience Alpine 2.75 × 12 mm cobalt chromium everolimus drug-eluting stent (Abbot Vascular, Abbott Park, IL, USA) was delivered to the lesion and deployed at 16 ATM. There was a good angiographic result of the distal RCA with no residual stenosis (Figure 1(b)). Immediately following completion of the procedure, the patient reported an episode of chest discomfort, a new cough, bilateral expiratory wheezes, and respiratory stridor. A transient episode of hypotension was noted but resolved without intervention. The patient was rapidly administered IV methylprednisolone, famotidine, diphenhydramine, and inhaled racemic epinephrine for presumed allergic reaction to iodinated contrast. Although his symptoms largely improved, stridor persisted. Urgent otolaryngology consultation was obtained for the evaluation of possible laryngeal edema, but flexible fiber-optic laryngoscopy was unremarkable. Next, chest radiography was promptly obtained, which revealed a markedly widened superior mediastinum (Figure 2).

Based on the findings on chest radiography, transesophageal echocardiography (TEE) was urgently performed. Echocardiography revealed no evidence of aortic dissection, but vague echodensities were noted anterior to the right heart suggestive of a hematoma. Thus, computed tomography (CT) of the chest without intravenous contrast was performed to obtain cross-sectional imaging of the mediastinum. The chest CT revealed a large hyperdense region surrounding the trachea suggestive of an anterior mediastinal hematoma, resulting in severe airway compression (Figure 3(a)). Due to the severity of tracheal compression, the decision was made to perform

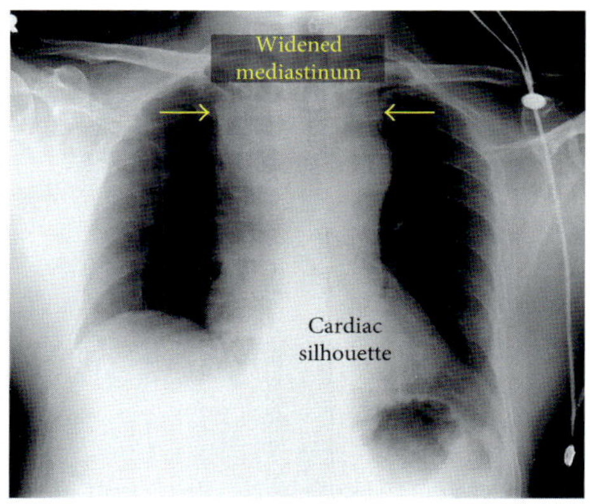

FIGURE 2: Chest radiography (AP orientation) demonstrating a widened superior mediastinum.

endotracheal intubation and mechanical ventilation and transfer to the intensive care unit. After intubation, a repeat CT of the chest with administration of intravenous contrast was notable for a small pseudoaneurysm arising from the inferior aspect of the brachiocephalic artery, as well as significant narrowing of the distal trachea below the endotracheal tube (Figure 3(b)).

After consultation with cardiothoracic and vascular surgery, the decision was made to pursue endovascular repair of the brachiocephalic artery pseudoaneurysm and presumed site of vascular perforation. Access was obtained in the left common femoral artery, and angiography of the brachiocephalic artery was performed, which confirmed the presence of a brachiocephalic artery pseudoaneurysm (Figure 4(a)). Next, a SupraCore wire (Abbot Vascular, Abbott Park, IL, USA) was placed in the right subclavian artery and a 10 × 40 mm iCAST covered stent (Atrium Medical, Hudson, NH, USA) was deployed across the neck of the pseudoaneurysm. The covered stent was postdilated with a 12 × 20 mm Armada balloon (Abbot Vascular, Abbott Park,

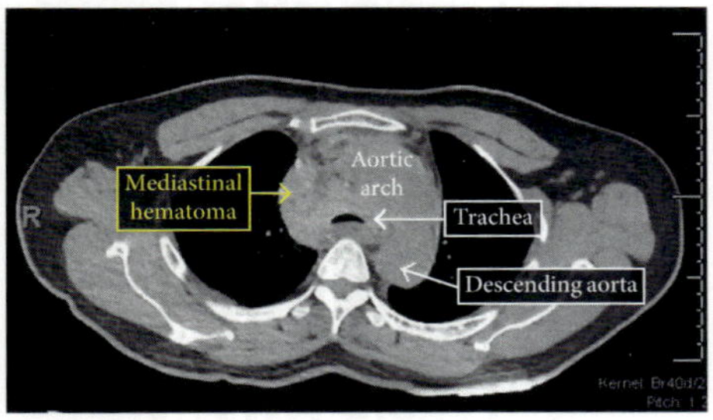

(a)

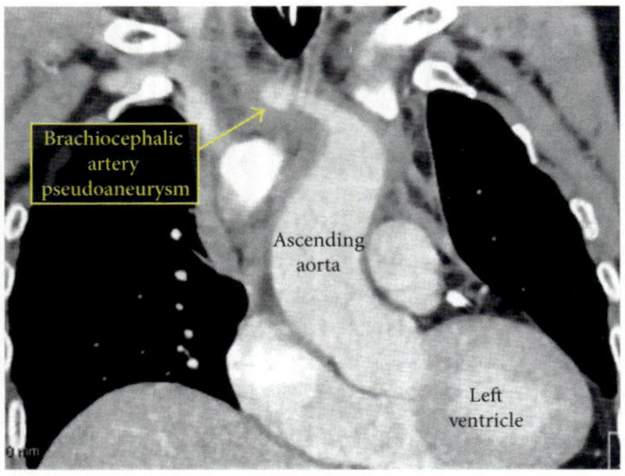

(b)

FIGURE 3: Computed tomography (CT) of the chest without intravenous contrast demonstrating a hyperdense region surrounding the trachea suggestive of an anterior mediastinal hematoma (a). Computed tomography (CT) of the chest with intravenous contrast demonstrating a small pseudoaneurysm arising from the inferior aspect of the brachiocephalic artery (b).

IL, USA). Following the intervention, there was an excellent angiographic result with preserved subclavian and carotid runoff (Figure 4(b)). Aspirin was continued; P2Y12 inhibitors were temporarily withheld.

Due to persistent tracheal compression after endovascular repair of the brachiocephalic artery, a Tracheobronxane Dumon silicone tracheal stent (Novatech, La Ciotat, France) was inserted by interventional pulmonology to maintain airway patency while the mediastinal hematoma resorbed. Over the ensuring days, serial imaging demonstrated no further enlargement of the mediastinal hematoma, and dual antiplatelet agents were resumed. The tracheal stent was retrieved and removed after 12 days. The patient was ultimately discharged to inpatient rehabilitation on hospital day 19.

3. Discussion

Vascular perforation associated with delivery of a 6 French guide catheter in the subclavian and brachiocephalic arteries is rare, with few cases reported in the literature [6–8]. In this case, brachiocephalic artery perforation resulted in pseudoaneurysm formation and a large mediastinal hematoma with tracheal compression and stridor. This highlights the importance of careful guide catheter placement from the right radial approach. When guide catheters are advanced through tortuous subclavian and brachiocephalic arteries, the application of forward pressure against resistance can lead to vascular complications, even when a guidewire is appropriately positioned in the ascending aorta. If resistance is encountered, fluoroscopy should be used to confirm the relative positions of the distal guidewire and guide catheter, and care should be taken to ensure appropriate guidewire position before advancing the guide further. Abduction of the arm and deep inspiration may also facilitate advancement of guide catheters to the ascending aorta. When the guide catheter cannot be easily advanced, balloon-assisted tracking (or similar techniques employing a low-profile 0.035″ compatible support catheter protruding through the lumen of a standard 6 Fr guiding catheter) can smooth the transition at the distal tip of the guide catheter. This can prevent vessel shearing from the "razor effect" at the distal tip of the guide catheter and minimize vascular trauma. Hydrophilic guiding catheters may also be used to pass tortuous subclavian or brachiocephalic anatomy. Rigid guide catheters, larger French sizes, and those with a more tortuous or curved shape at the distal tip may be most likely to cause trauma during catheter delivery. In the present case, the Amplatz shape of the initial guiding catheter may have played a role in the resulting perforation.

This report also illustrates the importance of maintaining a broad differential diagnosis when respiratory distress occurs after PCI. In this case, an allergic reaction to iodinated contrast was initially suspected when stridor and wheezing developed after completion of the procedure. Reactions to contrast media affect approximately 1 in every 500 patients undergoing coronary angiography in the cardiac catheterization laboratory, and the clinical presentation can range from urticaria to laryngeal edema and bronchospasm to cardiovascular shock and respiratory arrest [9]. The likelihood of an anaphylactoid reaction to contrast media is not necessarily related to contrast media dose, nor is it always an immediate response to contrast media exposure. When angioedema is suspected, patients require prompt airway evaluation and may require tracheal intubation to maintain airway patency. In this case, flexible fiber-optic laryngoscopy was urgently performed to exclude this dangerous diagnosis. Once it was evident that laryngeal edema was absent and anaphylactoid reaction to contrast media was unlikely, alternate diagnoses were considered. Ultimately, this rare vascular complication of PCI was only identified after a series of diagnostic imaging studies, including chest radiography, transesophageal echocardiography, computed tomography, and finally, invasive angiography. Therefore, all providers in the cardiac catheterization laboratory should be aware of procedural risks specific to the transradial approach.

In conclusion, vascular perforations due to guide catheter advancement from the right radial artery are rare. In this case, a 6 French AL 0.75 guide catheter led to brachiocephalic artery perforation, pseudoaneurysm formation, and a large mediastinal hematoma with tracheal compression. Prompt recognition, appropriate airway management, and endovascular repair of the injured vessel is critical to the successful management of this potentially life-threatening condition.

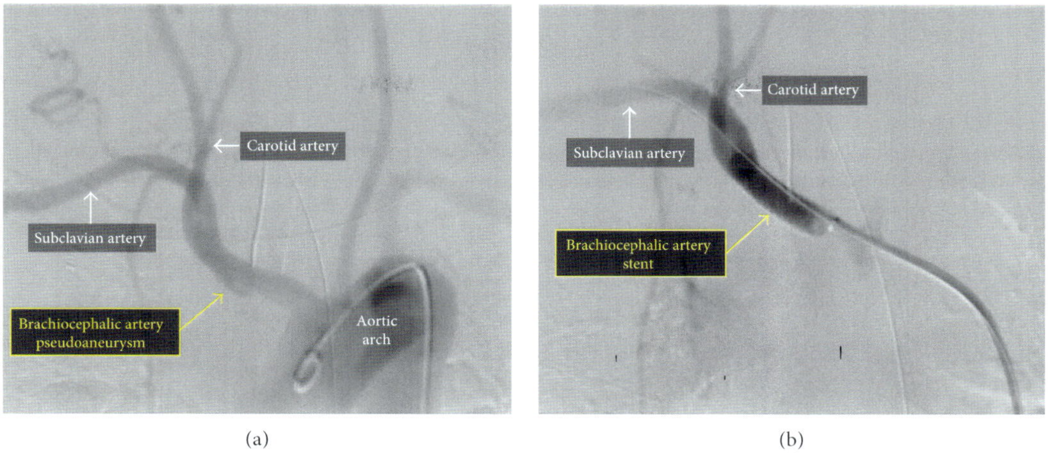

Figure 4: Angiography of the brachiocephalic artery demonstrating a small pseudoaneurysm (a). There was an excellent angiographic result after deployment of a covered stent (b).

References

[1] M. Valgimigli, A. Gagnor, P. Calabro et al., "Radial versus femoral access in patients with acute coronary syndromes undergoing invasive management: a randomised multicentre trial," *The Lancet*, vol. 385, no. 9986, pp. 2465–2476, 2015.

[2] G. Ferrante, S. V. Rao, P. Juni et al., "Radial versus femoral access for coronary interventions across the entire spectrum of patients with coronary artery disease: a meta-analysis of randomized trials," *JACC: Cardiovascular Interventions*, vol. 9, no. 14, pp. 1419–1434, 2016.

[3] G. Ando and D. Capodanno, "Radial access reduces mortality in patients with acute coronary syndromes: results from an updated trial sequential analysis of randomized trials," *JACC: Cardiovascular Interventions*, vol. 9, no. 7, pp. 660–670, 2016.

[4] E. Tatli, A. Buturak, A. Cakar et al., "Unusual vascular complications associated with transradial coronary procedures among 10,324 patients: case based experience and treatment options," *Journal of Interventional Cardiology*, vol. 28, no. 3, pp. 305–312, 2015.

[5] T. Patel, S. Shah, K. Sanghavi, and S. Pancholy, "Management of radial and brachial artery perforations during transradial procedures–a practical approach," *Journal of Invasive Cardiology*, vol. 21, no. 10, pp. 544–547, 2009.

[6] N. Habib, A. Jerzewski, E. M. Koomen et al., "Subclavian artery perforation complicating coronary angiography," *Netherlands Heart Journal*, vol. 20, no. 6, pp. 288–290, 2012.

[7] F. Farooqi, J. Alexander, and A. Sarma, "Rare vascular perforation complicating radial approach to percutaneous coronary angioplasty," *BMJ Case Reports*, vol. 2013, p. bcr2012007732, 2013.

[8] M. A. Abdool, S. Morrison, and H. Sullivan, "Iatrogenic perforation of subclavian artery as a complication of coronary angiography from the radial route, endovascularly repaired with a covered stent-graft," *BMJ Case Reports*, vol. 2013, p. bcr2012007602, 2013.

[9] J. E. Goss, C. E. Chambers, and F. A. Heupler Jr., "Systemic anaphylactoid reactions to iodinated contrast media during cardiac catheterization procedures: guidelines for prevention, diagnosis, and treatment. Laboratory Performance Standards Committee of the Society for Cardiac Angiography and Interventions," *Catheterization and Cardiovascular Diagnosis*, vol. 34, no. 2, pp. 99–104, 1995.

Should de Winter T-Wave Electrocardiography Pattern Be Treated as ST-Segment Elevation Myocardial Infarction Equivalent with Consequent Reperfusion? A Dilemmatic Experience in Rural Area of Indonesia

Raymond Pranata,[1,2] **Ian Huang**,[1] **and Vito Damay**[1,3]

[1]*Faculty of Medicine, Universitas Pelita Harapan, Tangerang, Banten, Indonesia*
[2]*Tabanan General Hospital, Tabanan, Bali, Indonesia*
[3]*Siloam Hospitals Lippo Village, Tangerang, Banten, Indonesia*

Correspondence should be addressed to Vito Damay; vito.damay@uph.edu

Academic Editor: Hajime Kataoka

Background. Although de Winter T-wave electrocardiography pattern is rare, it signifies proximal left anterior descending artery occlusion and is often unrecognized by physicians. The aim of this case report was to highlight the dilemma in the management of a patient with de Winter T-wave pattern in the hospital without interventional cardiology facility. *Case Presentation.* A 65-year-old male presented with typical chest pain since 2 hours before admission, and ECG showed sinus rhythm of 57 bpm and >1 mm upsloping ST depression with symmetric tall T in lead $V_{2\text{-}3}$ characteristic of de Winter T-wave ECG pattern. He was given dual antiplatelet therapy, nitrate, statin, and anticoagulant. He refused referral to interventional cardiology available hospital. 3 hours after admission, the electrocardiography transformed into Q-waves consistent with final stages of acute STEMI and ST-segment elevation that barely meets the threshold in the guideline, and thrombolytic was administered and successful. There is a suggestion that de Winter T-wave electrocardiography should be treated as ST-segment myocardial infarction equivalent and should undergo coronary angiography; however, not every hospital has the luxury of interventional cardiology facility. The other modality for reperfusion is thrombolysis; however, without a clear guideline and scarcity of study, we prefer to resort to conservative treatment. "Fortunately," transformation into ST-segment elevation helps us to determine the course of action which is reperfusion using thrombolytic. *Conclusions.* de Winter T-wave ECG pattern is not mentioned in any guidelines regarding acute coronary syndromes, and there are no clear recommendations. Physicians in rural area without interventional cardiology facility face a dilemma with the lack of evidence-based guideline. Fibrinolytic may be appropriate in those without contraindications with strong chest pain consistent with acute coronary occlusion, less than 3 hours of symptoms, and convincing de Winter T-wave ECG pattern for a rural non-PCI hospital far away from PCI capable hospital.

1. Background

In 2008, de Winter et al. reported an electrocardiography (ECG) pattern that is found in about 2% of patients with proximal left anterior descending artery occlusion (acute anterior myocardial infarction) and is often unrecognized by physicians [1, 2]. Although de Winter T-wave ECG pattern was suggested to be managed as STEMI equivalent [3], it was not mentioned in recent guidelines by the European Heart Society (ESC) and the American Heart Association (AHA) [4, 5]. Hence, a question arises regarding whether or not this pattern be treated with fibrinolytic in an area where cardiac catheter laboratory (cath lab) is not readily available. The aim of this case report was to highlight the dilemma in the management of a patient with de Winter T-wave pattern in hospital without interventional cardiology facility (non-PCI hospital).

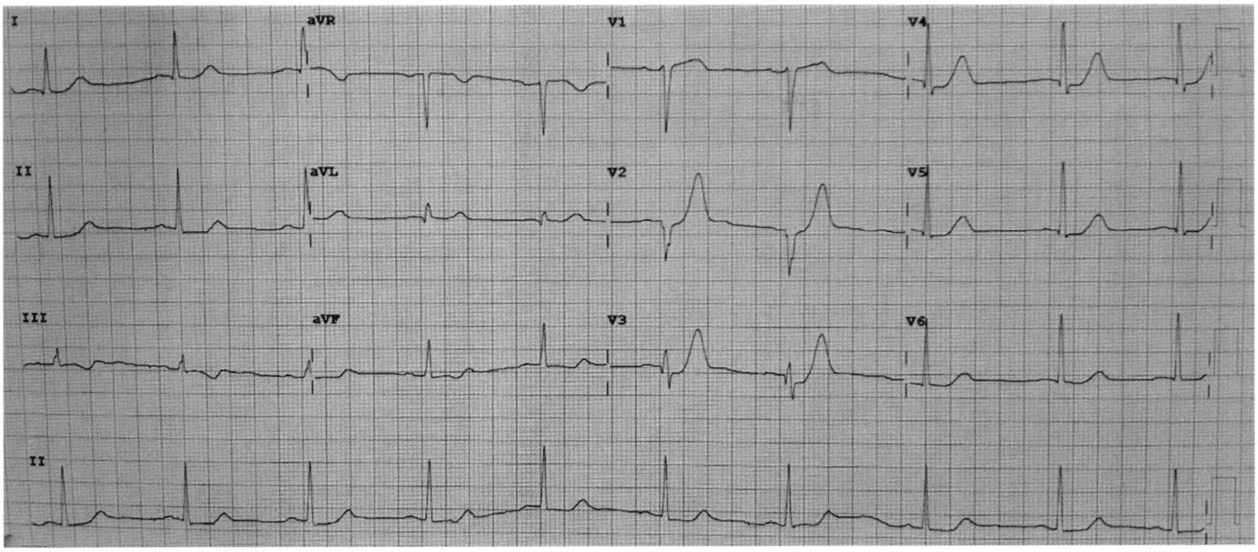

FIGURE 1: Initial ECG showing >1 mm upsloping ST depression with symmetric tall T in lead V_{2-6} characteristic of de Winter ECG pattern.

2. Case Presentation

A 65-year-old male presented to the emergency department with typical chest pain at rest since 2 hours before admission after eating. The patient denied shortness of breath and previous episode of chest pain before admission. He had a past medical history of poorly controlled hypertension and was taking captopril. History of diabetes, smoking, and previous stroke or myocardial infarction was denied. On physical examination, blood pressure was 150/90 mmHg, heart rate was 57x/minute, and respiratory rate was 20x/minute, and the cardiopulmonary examination was within normal limits. ECG showed sinus rhythm of 57 bpm and >1 mm upsloping ST depression with symmetric tall T in lead V_{2-3} characteristic of de Winter T-wave ECG pattern (Figure 1). Routine blood examination, AST/ALT, BUN, and serum creatinine were within normal limits. Sodium was 137 mmol/L, and potassium was 3.4 mmol/L denoting that tall T was not due to hyperkalemia. Troponin at the 2nd hour after onset was negative. The patient was diagnosed with acute coronary syndrome with suspected de Winter T-wave ECG pattern. Aspirin 160 mg, clopidogrel 300 mg, sublingual isosorbide dinitrate, simvastatin 20 mg (atorvastatin was not available), and enoxaparin 0.4 mg subcutaneous were administered. The patient refused referral to the interventional cardiology capable hospital due to distance and socioeconomic causes. Repeat ECG was done 3 hours later showing Q-waves developing in V_{2-4}, consistent with the final stages of acute STEMI accompanied with ST-segment elevation in lead V_{2-4} which barely meets the 2 mm threshold for those precordial leads as per the guidelines (Figure 2). Elevated troponin at the 5th hour confirmed the presence of myocardial infarction. The patient still experienced sustained and severe chest pain although not as intense as initial presentation. Streptokinase (1.5 million units) was administered, and chest pain subsided with a resolution of ST-segment elevation (Figure 3). The patient was discharged on the 5th day after admission.

3. Discussion

The de Winter T-wave ECG pattern may signify proximal left anterior descending artery occlusion and was suggested as ST-segment elevation myocardial infarction (STEMI) equivalent [1–3]. The de Winter T-wave ECG pattern was also shown to have positive predictive values of 95.2% (95% confidence interval: 76.2–99.9%), 100% (69.2–100.0%), and 100% (51.7–100%) for acute coronary occlusions in the three diagnostic studies [6]. Verouden et al. also reported that approximately 50% of those with de Winter T-wave ECG pattern had a wraparound LAD which is associated with larger area of ischemia [2]. However, despite these findings, de Winter T-wave ECG pattern is yet to be included in ESC guidelines for management of acute coronary syndromes in both persistent (2017) or without persistent ST-elevation (2015) and ACC/AHA guidelines regarding STEMI (2013) and NSTEMI (2014) [4, 5].

Ideally, the presence of de Winter T-wave ECG should be treated as urgent as STEMI with catheter lab activation for coronary angiography and possible stenting. This was not possible in our case due to a limited facility in the region [3]. Thrombolysis was initially avoided because de Winter T-wave ECG is currently not an indication for fibrinolysis even in latest guidelines, and there was no clear-cut evidence of acute coronary occlusion. The lack of the evidence-based guidelines for the aforementioned condition compelled us to choose dual antiplatelet therapy and anticoagulant for the initial mainstay of therapy. Evolution from suspected de Winter T-wave pattern to the final stage of acute STEMI was observed three hours after admission. This helped us in ushering the direction of management, as the guideline for STEMI is straightforward in terms of reperfusion. Thrombolysis was initiated, and repeat ECG showed resolution of chest pain and elevated ST-Segment which proves the acute coronary occlusion (anterior myocardial infarction).

Whether de Winter T-wave ECG pattern can evolve into STEMI is debatable, and there are arguments that de Winter

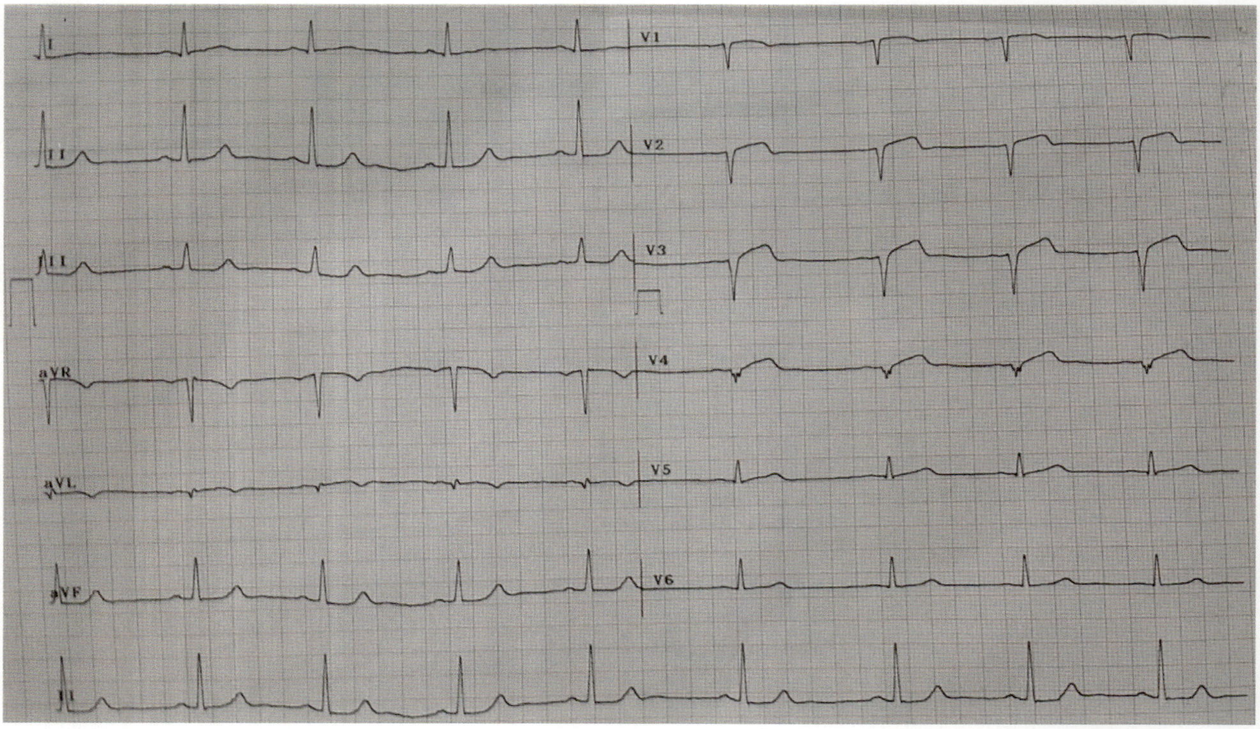

FIGURE 2: ECG showing progression into ST-segment elevation myocardial infarction.

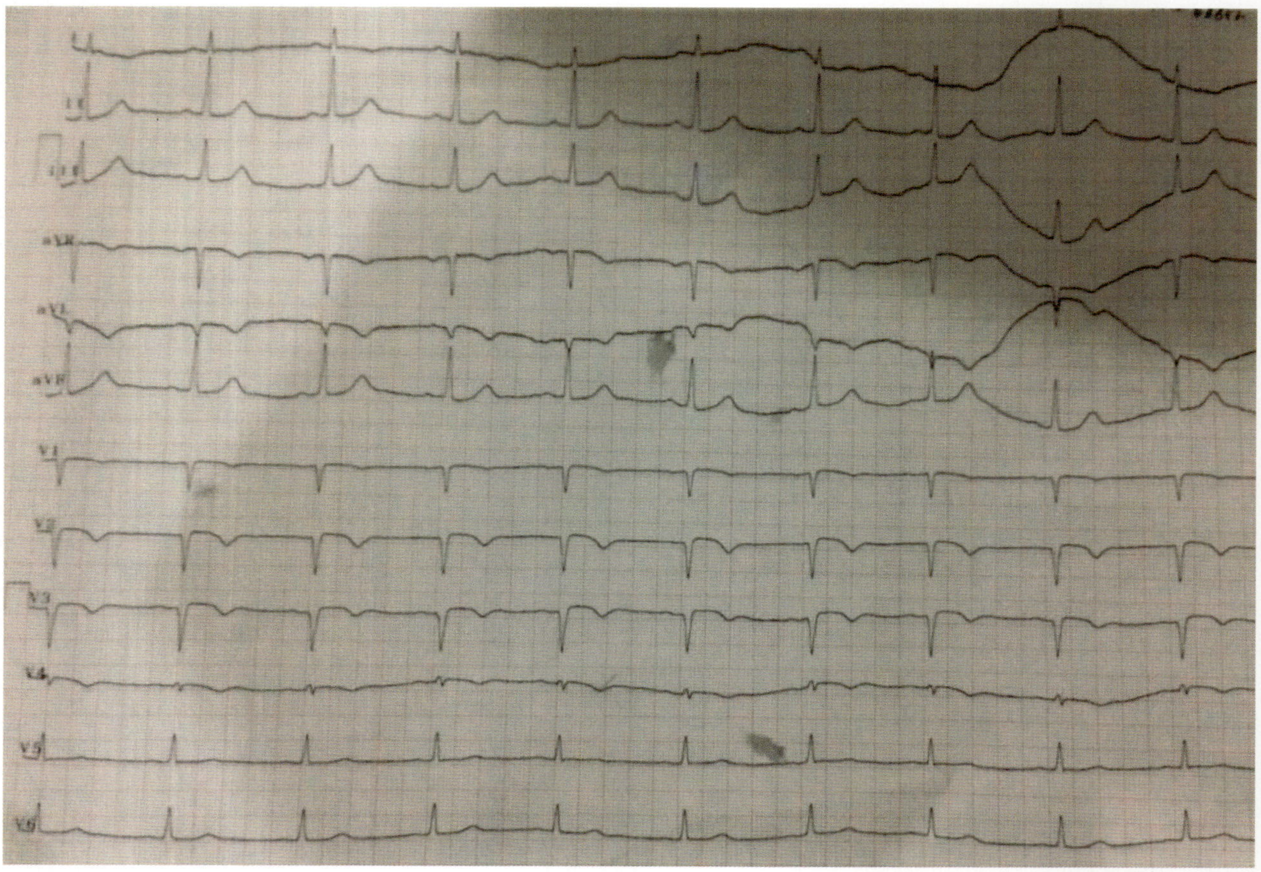

FIGURE 3: ECG after fibrinolysis showing resolution of ST-segment elevation.

T-wave pattern is a part of STEMI evolution which was impeded with aggressive antithrombotic/antiplatelet therapy [7]. Another opinion states that ECG evolution into STEMI was actually indicative of hyperacute T-wave instead of de Winter T-wave ECG pattern, in which the latter usually progresses directly to sign of transmural infarction on ECG [3, 8]. A more diplomatic view was the categorization of de Winter T-wave ECG pattern into those 2 debated groups, respectively [9]. The presence of Q-waves in our patient with ST-segment elevation which barely meets 2 mm suggests transformation into final stages of acute STEMI; hence, our patient showed both evolution into STEMI and signs of transmural infarction (Q-wave).

Regardless of the debate, the most important issue is to recognize this ECG pattern and prevent the delay in management. Delay leads to a higher total ischemic time which is related to higher mortality in STEMI; however, whether the same applies to de Winter T-wave ECG is unclear [10].

4. Conclusions

The de Winter T-wave ECG pattern is not mentioned in any guidelines regarding acute coronary syndromes, and there are no clear recommendations. Physicians in rural area without interventional cardiology facility face a dilemma with the lack of evidence-based guideline and prefer to resort to a conservative strategy rather than potentially doing harm. Such approach may or may not lead to the best possible outcome but is the only choice in the middle of scarcity. Fibrinolysis may be considered in a young patient (without usual contraindications) who arrives with strong chest pain consistent with acute coronary occlusion, less than 3 hours of symptoms, and with convincing de Winter T-wave ECG pattern (especially if a prior baseline ECG is available for comparison) for a rural non-PCI hospital far away from PCI capable hospital. Discussion with the interventional cardiologist at the PCI hospital whenever possible should also be done in these challenging cases to optimize real-time decision-making.

Abbreviations

AST:	Aspartate aminotransferase
ALT:	Alanine aminotransferase
BUN:	Blood urea nitrogen
ECG:	Electrocardiogram
STEMI:	ST-segment elevation myocardial infarction
NSTEMI:	Non-ST-segment elevation myocardial infarction.

Authors' Contributions

Raymond Pranata admitted, evaluated, and treated the patient. He also planned and drafted the manuscript. Ian Huang performed extensive research on the topic and helped in giving another point of view based on theory and experience. Vito Damay supervised and gave expert advice regarding the manuscript. All authors read and approved the final manuscript.

References

[1] R. J. de Winter, N. J. Verouden, H. J. Wellens, and A. A. Wilde, "A new ECG sign of proximal LAD occlusion," *New England Journal of Medicine*, vol. 359, no. 19, pp. 2071–2073, 2008.

[2] N. J. Verouden, K. T. Koch, R. J. Peters et al., "Persistent precordial "hyperacute" T-waves signify proximal left anterior descending artery occlusion," *Heart*, vol. 95, no. 20, pp. 1701–1706, 2009.

[3] I. C. Rokos, W. J. French, A. Mattu et al., "Appropriate cardiac cath lab activation: optimizing electrocardiogram interpretation and clinical decision-making for acute ST-elevation myocardial infarction," *American Heart Journal*, vol. 160, no. 6, pp. 995–1003, 2010.

[4] B. Ibanez, S. James, S. Agewall et al., "2017 ESC guidelines for the management of acute myocardial infarction in patients presenting with ST-segment elevation," *European Heart Journal*, vol. 39, pp. 119–177, 2017.

[5] P. T. O'Gara, F. G. Kushner, D. D. Ascheim et al., "ACCF/AHA guideline for the management of ST-elevation myocardial infarction: a report of the American College of Cardiology Foundation/American Heart Association task force on practice guidelines," *Circulation*, vol. 127, no. 4, pp. e362–e425, 2013.

[6] N. P. Morris and R. Body, "The de winter ECG pattern: morphology and accuracy for diagnosing acute coronary occlusion: systematic review," *European Journal of Emergency Medicine*, vol. 24, no. 4, pp. 236–242, 2017.

[7] M. F. Sala, A. B. de Luna, A. C. López, and J. Garcia-Niebla, "The "De Winter Pattern" can progress to ST-segment elevation acute coronary syndrome," *Revista Española de Cardiología*, vol. 68, no. 11, pp. 1042-1043, 2015.

[8] I. Stankovic, I. Ilic, M. Panic, A. Vlahovic-Stipac, B. Putnikovic, and A. N. Neskovic, "The absence of the ST-segment elevation in acute coronary artery thrombosis: what does not fit, the patient or the explanation?," *Journal of Electrocardiology*, vol. 44, no. 1, pp. 7–10, 2011.

[9] Y. T. Zhao, L. Wang, and Z. Yi, "Evolvement to the de Winter electrocardiographic pattern," *American Journal of Emergency Medicine*, vol. 34, no. 2, pp. 307–337, 2016.

[10] A. E. Denktas, H. V. Anderson, J. McCarthy, and R. W. Smalling, "Total ischemic time: the correct focus of attention for optimal ST-segment elevation myocardial infarction care," *JACC: Cardiovascular Interventions*, vol. 4, no. 6, pp. 599–604, 2011.

37

Cardiac Aspergilloma: A Rare Case of a Cardiac Mass Involving the Native Tricuspid Valve, Right Atrium, and Right Ventricle in an Immunocompromised Patient

Christina S. Chen-Milhone,[1] Kalyan Chakravarthy Potu,[2] and Sudhir Mungee[2]

[1]*Department of Internal Medicine and Pediatrics, University of Illinois College of Medicine at Peoria, Peoria, IL, USA*
[2]*Department of Cardiology, University of Illinois College of Medicine at Peoria, Peoria, IL, USA*

Correspondence should be addressed to Christina S. Chen-Milhone; cschen@uicomp.uic.edu

Academic Editor: Tayfun Sahin

Aspergillus can cause devastating opportunistic infections in immunocompromised patients. Rarely does this fungus invade the heart, and when it does, survival is especially poor despite optimal medical and surgical treatment. We report a case of cardiac aspergilloma with involvement of the tricuspid valve and both the right atrium and ventricle found on a transthoracic echocardiogram in an immunocompromised patient after developing atrial fibrillation with rapid ventricular rate. The findings from this case suggest that early clinical suspicion is critical in early diagnosis and thus early treatment.

1. Introduction

Aspergillus is a common fungus in the environment that can cause fatal diseases in humans. The *Aspergillus* spores are easily inhaled, and immunocompromised individuals are known to be more susceptible to its disease. Acute invasive aspergillus of the heart is particularly uncommon. *Aspergillus* endocarditis accounts for 20–25% of all cases of fungal endocarditis, and fungal endocarditis only comprises <2% of all cases of endocarditis [1, 2]. Invasive aspergillus involving heart valves and chambers is even rarer with only a handful of cases reported in the literature. In this report, we present a case of cardiac aspergilloma involving the native tricuspid valve and both the right atrium and ventricle that initially presented as a cardiac mass in an immunocompromised patient.

2. Case Report

A 62-year-old male presented to an outlying hospital with a one-month history of productive cough, shortness of breath, and intermittent fevers, and a syncopal episode one week before. His past medical history was significant for hypertension, prostatic adenocarcinoma with bone metastasis, atrial fibrillation, and bilateral pulmonary embolism. The prostatic adenocarcinoma was diagnosed 11 months before, and he developed the bilateral pulmonary embolism approximately 8 months before. He completed 40 cycles of radiation, and medications included Zytiga in conjunction with prednisone, Lupron, and Eliquis. He was a former smoker and smoked a maximum of 5 cigarettes daily for 35 years. His social history was otherwise negative for high-risk sexual behavior, intravenous (IV) drug use, recent travel, and occupational exposure. He was subsequently admitted with a diagnosis of anemia with hemoglobin of 7.1 g/dL and sepsis secondary to presumed pneumonia.

On admission, the patient received 4 units of packed red blood cells for anemia. The patient was also noted to have thrombocytopenia with platelet count of 48,000/mcL; thus, Eliquis was held. Chest X-ray revealed a 7.4 cm opacity in the right lung base as well as multiple right pulmonary nodules (Figure 1). A CT chest showed similar findings with the addition of extensive bone metastasis. The patient was started on vancomycin and Zosyn for sepsis while awaiting blood culture results. Infectious workup was positive for *Aspergillus fumigatus* IgG, *Aspergillus galactomannan* antigen

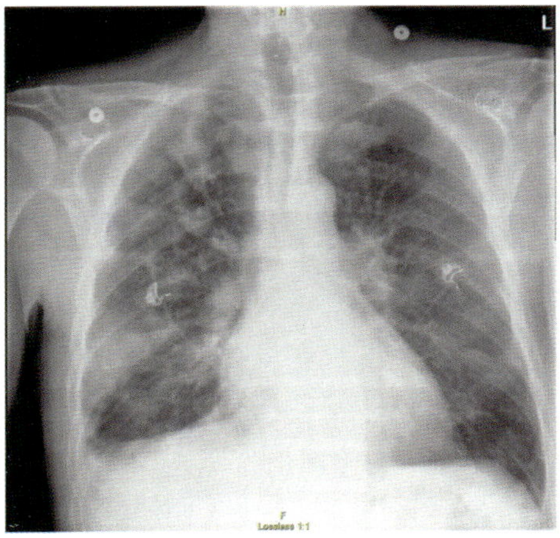

Figure 1: CXR showing multiple right pulmonary nodules.

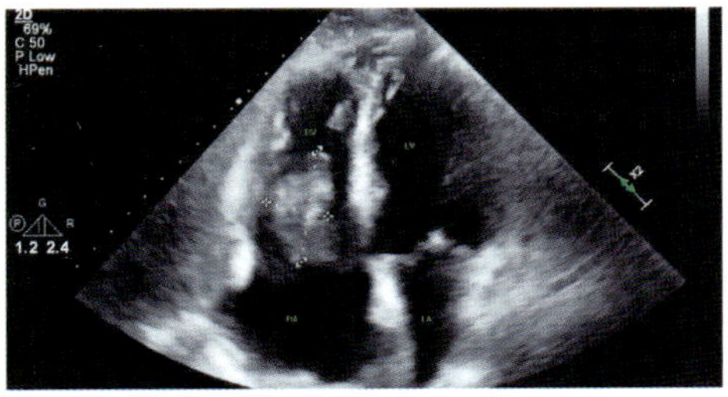

Figure 2: Transthoracic echocardiogram showing a mass involving the tricuspid valve and both the right atrium and ventricle.

(Ag), *Histoplasma* Ag, Fungitell, and *Blastomyces* antibody (Ab). Human immunodeficiency virus (HIV), herpes simplex virus (HSV), and influenza A and B serologies were negative. Blood cultures were negative for viruses, bacteria, and fungi. Infectious diseases were consulted. The patient subsequently underwent a bronchoscopy, with lavage specimens returning positive for *Aspergillus* Ag but negative for pneumocystis pneumonia, HSV, bacteria, fungus including *Histoplasma*, and malignant cells. The patient was then diagnosed with presumed subacute invasive pulmonary aspergillus. Antibiotics were then discontinued, and the patient was discharged with voriconazole for a 6-week duration.

Two days after discharge, he was admitted for atrial fibrillation with rapid ventricular rate. A transthoracic echocardiogram (TTE) was performed and showed a highly mobile 5 cm mass involving the tricuspid valve with variable involvement of the right atrium and right ventricle (Figure 2). The ejection fraction was preserved. Infectious diseases and oncology were then consulted. The patient remained on voriconazole, and Zytiga was discontinued as his prostate cancer was castration sensitive, per oncology. CT surgery was consulted and performed sternotomy with resection of the mass, portions of the right atrium and ventricle, and tricuspid valve on day 2 of admission. The excised mass was pale yellow and pink, irregularly shaped, fragmented, bulky, and approximately $3 \times 2 \times 1.3$ cm (Figure 3). Pathology from the mass and tricuspid valve showed necrotic debris with acute inflammation and abundant fungal hyphae (Figure 4).

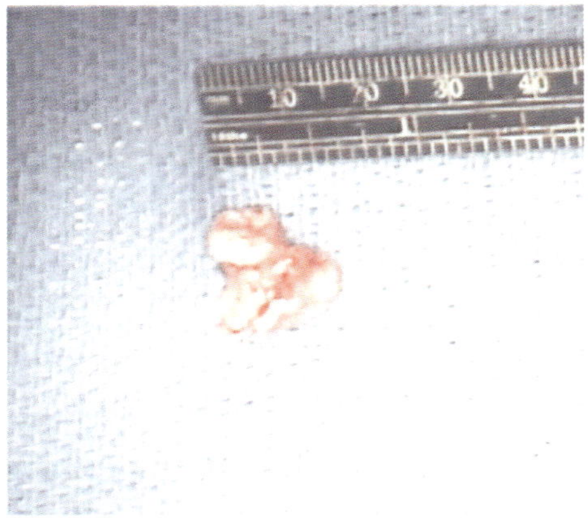

Figure 3: Right atrial and tricuspid ventricular mass.

Cultures obtained from tissue in the operating room were positive for *Aspergillus fumigatus* and negative for bacteria and viruses.

The patient did well postoperatively. He was extubated to nasal cannula within 12 hours; however, he remained on pressor support. Voriconazole was continued. On day 4 of admission, he developed septic shock, renal failure with oliguria and acidosis, and shock liver requiring increased pressor support. He continued to deteriorate the next day requiring endotracheal intubation and ventilator support. On day 5 of admission, the patient developed ventricular tachycardia followed by pulseless electrical activity. Shortly thereafter, he was pronounced dead. The cause of death was invasive aspergillosis-induced septic shock with multiorgan failure.

3. Discussion

Aspergilloma of the heart is a rare disease that carries a very poor prognosis. On review of the current literature, only a small number of cases have been reported. These cases include an invasive aspergillus of the interventricular septum in an allogenic stem cell transplant patient [3], aspergilloma involving all four chambers of the heart [4], aspergillosis presenting as a pedunculated mass with multiple nodules on the left ventricular wall in an acute lymphoblastic leukemia patient [5], a large right ventricular aspergilloma in a young man on chemotherapy for acute myelogenous leukemia [6], an incidental finding of a tricuspid valve aspergilloma after abdominal surgery [7], and the three cases described in the correspondence by Wiwanitkit and Wiwanitkit [8]. Of note, all except for one of the aforementioned cases resulted in death within days to weeks after diagnosis.

Fungal endocarditis alone, without involvement of the surrounding cardiac structure, is associated with a mortality rate of at least 50% with an average survival period of 11 days [9]. Fungal endocarditis has also recently been shown to have increasing prevalence with medical and surgical advancements [1, 2]. Historically, the main risk factors for developing fungal endocarditis included previous valve surgery, history of prosthetic valve endocarditis, prolonged use of antibiotics, rheumatic heart disease, and IV drug use [1].

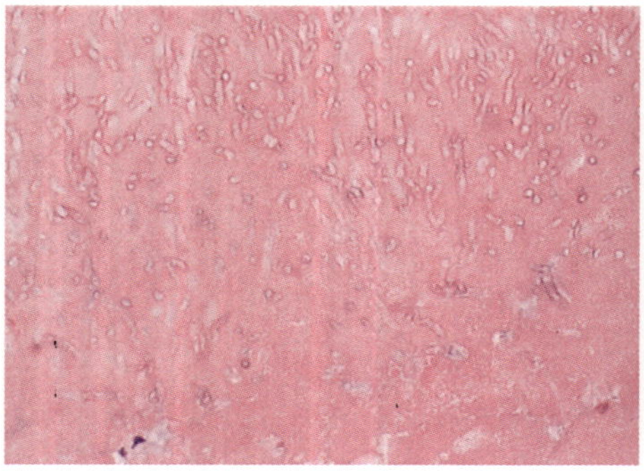

(a)

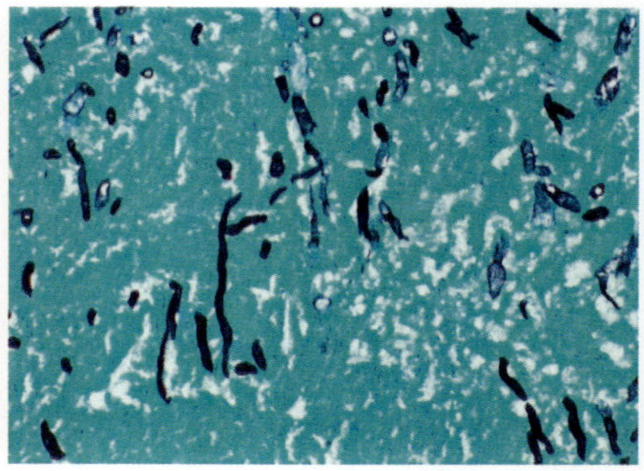

(b)

FIGURE 4: Specimen of the mass with H&E stain (a) and GMS stain highlighting fungal elements (b).

Most recent studies suggest that these characteristics have changed and that fungal endocarditis now more commonly affects immunocompromised patients, patients with prosthetic valves and central venous catheters, and those on broad-spectrum antibiotics [1, 2]. Of note, *Aspergillus* endocarditis is mostly found on aortic or mitral prosthetic valves [10] and has a mortality rate of approximately 80% [2].

Prolonged fever, as seen in the described case, is the most common presenting feature; however, some patients may present with new or changing heart murmur, chest pain, cough, dyspnea, hemoptysis, weakness, or generalized pain. Hemorrhagic black skin lesions have been reported in *Aspergillus* endocarditis [11]. Such symptoms in combination with leukocytosis, anemia, and thrombocytopenia may also be suggestive of fungal septicemia. As discussed earlier, an immunocompromised state, neutropenia, recent history of long-term central venous catheter, prosthetic heart valve, steroid use, prolonged antibiotic therapy, recent prolonged hospitalization, parenteral nutrition, immunocompromised status, and IV drug use predispose patients to an invasive fungal infection.

With the diverse symptoms and risk factors, the diagnosis of fungal endocarditis is rather challenging and can be easily delayed without a high clinical suspicion, especially given that fungal pathogens are slow growing. Diagnosis is further complicated as the majority of fungi are not detected in blood cultures. *Aspergillus*, in particular, is positive in 4–30% of blood cultures in cases of *Aspergillus* endocarditis [2, 12]. Some reviews have also suggested testing for galactomannan antigen, which is released when *Aspergillus* proliferates [1, 12]. TTE is a valuable diagnostic tool in diagnosing endocarditis and has been shown to identify 89% and 76.5% of the vegetations in native and prosthetic valves, respectively [2]. Although vegetations seen on TTE may not distinguish between bacterial versus fungal etiology, fungal vegetations are typically characterized as a large, bulky, highly mobile mass, as seen in the described case, and cause an increased risk of embolic events, more commonly affecting the brain. Still, many cases of fungal endocarditis are diagnosed during surgery or autopsy.

Upon diagnosing fungal invasion of the heart, a multidisciplinary team involving cardiology, infectious diseases, and cardiovascular surgery is necessary. Most recent reviews as well as Infectious Diseases Society of America (IDSA) guidelines favor a combined medical and early surgical intervention for treatment of *Aspergillus* endocarditis, pericarditis, and myocarditis. Surgical valve replacement in addition to systemic antifungal therapy was noted to be pertinent to survival due to poor prognosis and risk of relapse in patients receiving only pharmacological therapy, decreased effect of antifungal medication on fungal vegetations, large vegetations possibly compromising cardiac function, and the risk of embolic events [1, 12]. Per IDSA, the recommended initial antifungal agents are voriconazole or liposomal amphotericin B 3–5 mg/kg/day, followed by lifelong antifungal treatment postsurgical valve replacement [13]. Amphotericin B is preferred for patients with hepatic insufficiency [12]. Some have proposed using caspofungin in addition to voriconazole and amphotericin [14]; however, the use of combining antifungal therapies has not been shown to be superior to monotherapy [13]. In the described case, the patient was already on voriconazole and underwent surgical resection.

The differential diagnosis for the cardiac mass beyond a fungal etiology includes thrombus, primary cardiac tumor, myxoma, metastatic lesion, and lymphoma. Though the patient had new-onset atrial fibrillation, a thrombus was unlikely as he had been on apixaban for approximately 6-7 months. Prostate cancer does not typically metastasize to the heart; thus, metastasis was also unlikely. Given the patient's immunocompromised state, being on steroids, and recent diagnosis of invasive pulmonary aspergillosis, the clinical suspicion for a fungal mass was high. Hematogenous spread of invasive pulmonary aspergillus was considered in the development of cardiac aspergilloma. The spread of invasive pulmonary aspergillus to the heart is very rare and is associated with a high mortality estimated to be as high as 80–90% [15], which is approximately the same mortality rate of having *Aspergillus* endocarditis alone, despite aggressive pharmacological and surgical interventions [2]. However, the hematogenous spread of invasive pulmonary aspergillus would be expected to invade the left cardium rather than the right, as seen in our patient.

In considering the described case, prior to discovering the cardiac aspergilloma, the patient was already on antifungal therapy. Furthermore, once a fungal mass was suspected, the patient underwent surgery and continued antifungal treatment as per recommendations. The overall outcome, nonetheless, was grim.

Cardiac aspergilloma remains a rare yet deadly disease that carries a high mortality rate despite aggressive pharmacological and surgical interventions. Decreasing the mortality rate remains a challenging task, given the nature of the disease and diagnostic barriers to detecting the disease early on. While innovative molecular methods can detect the diagnosis sooner than was previously possible, clinical suspicion remains the key to diagnosing the disease. Early clinical suspicion will lead to early treatment, and earlier treatment will presumably result in decreased mortality.

Acknowledgments

The authors thank Dr. Janeen N. Buonaccorsi for assistance with providing the pathology slides for the case report and Dr. Matthew Mischler, Assistant Professor at University of Illinois College of Medicine at Peoria, for comments that greatly helped with the manuscript.

References

[1] P. Tattevin, M. Revest, A. Lefort, C. Michelet, and O. Lortholary, "Fungal endocarditis: current challenges," *International Journal of Antimicrobial Agents*, vol. 44, no. 4, pp. 290–294, 2014.

[2] L. C. Pierrotti and L. M. Baddour, "Fungal endocarditis, 1995–2002," *Chest*, vol. 122, no. 1, pp. 302–310, 2002.

[3] M. Paul, A. Schuster, S. T. Hussain, E. Nagel, and A. Chiribiri, "Invasive aspergillosis, extensive cardiac involvement demonstrated by cardiac magnetic resonance," *Circulation*, vol. 126, no. 14, pp. 1780–1783, 2012.

[4] S. O. Soman, G. Vijayaraghavan, N. P. Padmaja, A. R. Warrier, and M. Unni, "Aspergilloma of the heart," *Indian Heart Journal*, vol. 66, no. 2, pp. 238–240, 2014.

[5] J. Alvarez Rubiolvarez, J. Sierra Quiroga, C. Rubio Taboada, A. Fernandez Gonzalez, F. Martinon Torres, and J. Garcia-Bengochea, "Cardiac aspergillosis with pedunculated mass in the left ventricle," *Texas Heart Institute Journal*, vol. 31, no. 4, pp. 439–441, 2004.

[6] H. W. Chou, M. K. Chuang, and Y. S. Chen, "Rapid recurrence of right ventricular aspergilloma," *European Journal of Cardio-Thoracic Surgery*, vol. 44, no. 5, p. 965, 2013.

[7] M. K. Singla, A. Shrivastava, K. C. Mukherjee, and K. Sodhi, "Potentially fatal tricuspid valve aspergilloma detected after laparoscopic abdominal surgery," *Southern African Journal of Anaesthesia and Analgesia*, vol. 17, no. 3, pp. 266–268, 2011.

[8] S. Wiwanitkit and V. Wiwanitkit, "Cardiac aspergilloma," *Indian Heart Journal*, vol. 67, no. 3, p. 288, 2015.

[9] M. E. Ellis, H. Al-Abdely, A. Sandridge, W. Greer, and W. Ventura, "Fungal endocarditis: evidence in the world literature 1965–1995," *Clinical Infectious Diseases*, vol. 32, no. 1, pp. 50–62, 2001.

[10] A. C. Pasqualotto and D. W. Denning, "Post-operative aspergillosis," *Clinical Microbiology and Infection*, vol. 12, no. 11, pp. 1060–1076, 2006.

[11] G. M. Varghese and J. D. Sobel, "Fungal endocarditis," *Current Infectious Disease Reports*, vol. 10, no. 4, pp. 275–279, 2008.

[12] A. K. Pasha, J. Z. Lee, S. W. Low, H. Desai, K. S. Lee, and M. Al Mohajer, "Fungal endocarditis: update on diagnosis and management," *The American Journal of Medicine*, vol. 129, no. 10, pp. 1037–1043, 2016.

[13] T. F. Patterson, G. R. Thompson III, D. W. Denning et al., "Practice guidelines for the diagnosis and management of aspergillosis: 2016 Update by the Infectious Diseases Society of America," *Clinical Infectious Diseases*, vol. 63, no. 4, pp. e1–e60, 2016.

[14] S. M. Yuan, "Fungal endocarditis," *Brazilian Journal of Cardiovascular Surgery*, vol. 31, no. 3, pp. 252–255, 2016.

[15] B. Sulik-Tyszka, P. Kacprzyk, K. Madry, B. Ziarkiewicz-Wroblewska, W. Jedrzejczak, and M. Wroblewska, "Aspergillosis of the heart and lung and review of published reports on fungal endocarditis," *Mycopathologia*, vol. 181, no. 7-8, pp. 583–588, 2016.

Safety and Efficacy of Triple Therapeutic Targets with Rivaroxaban after Acute Myocardial Infarction Complicated by Left Ventricular Thrombi in a Case of Nonvalvular Atrial Fibrillation

Francesco Summaria, Gregory A. Sgueglia, Fabrizio D'Errico, Antonella De Santis, Fabiana Piccioni, Gaetano Gioffrè, and Achille Gaspardone

Department of Cardiology, San Eugenio Hospital, Rome, Italy

Correspondence should be addressed to Francesco Summaria; f.summaria@gmail.com

Academic Editor: Nurten Sayar

We present the complex case of a high-risk patient with nonvalvular atrial fibrillation, who experienced a non-ST elevation myocardial infarction complicated by left ventricular (LV) thrombi and underwent percutaneous coronary intervention with drug-eluting stent implantation. The patient was initially treated with short-term triple therapy including aspirin, clopidogrel, and rivaroxaban 15 mg/die. Following aspirin dropping one month after discharge, the patient continued on dual therapy with clopidogrel and rivaroxaban, and a clinical and imaging follow-up at 6 and 12 months confirmed the LV thrombi resolution, with no thromboembolic episodes and a good safety profile.

1. Introduction

Among acute coronary syndrome (ACS) patients undergoing percutaneous coronary intervention (PCI), approximately 5% to 22% have concomitant atrial fibrillation (AF) [1]. Among ACSs, AF is 2-fold more frequent during non-ST elevation myocardial infarction (NSTEMI) than during STEMI [2]. Despite the overlap in the occurrence of these syndromes, the pharmacotherapies used to manage AF and ACSs differ.

Left ventricular (LV) thrombi often represent an unexpected echocardiographic finding [3], accurately detected by cardiovascular magnetic resonance (CMR) [4]. Although the occurrence of this complication has declined significantly since the advent of primary PCI, its incidence is not negligible, ranging between 5% and 17% [5, 6].

According to current guidelines, despite an increased rate of bleeding complications, warfarin is considered the anticoagulant of choice to prevent thromboembolic sequelae. As an advantageous alternative, the novel oral anticoagulants (NOACs) have been implemented in the setting of nonvalvular AF (NVAF) [7–9]. Yet, the evidence about their role in combination with antiplatelet agents in the management of LV thrombi for ACS patients undergoing PCI is poor, and mostly limited to case reports. Hence, their efficacy can be only extrapolated [10–13]. At present, two randomized trials (PIONEER AF-PCI and RE-Dual PCI) [14, 15] have demonstrated that the use of NOACs plus a P2Y12 inhibitor was associated with a lower rate of clinically significant bleeding, compared to VKAs plus dual antiplatelet therapy, thus ensuring a dual target of ischemic and thromboembolic protection against coronary and cerebrovascular events.

2. Case Report

We report the case of a 66-year-old woman, hypertensive, and smoker, referred to our Emergency Department for prolonged chest pain. Due to permanent NVAF, she was on warfarin and rate-control therapeutic strategy. At admission, electrocardiogram showed AF and a ST segment depression of 2 mm in V5-V6. The creatine kinase-MB was of 10 and

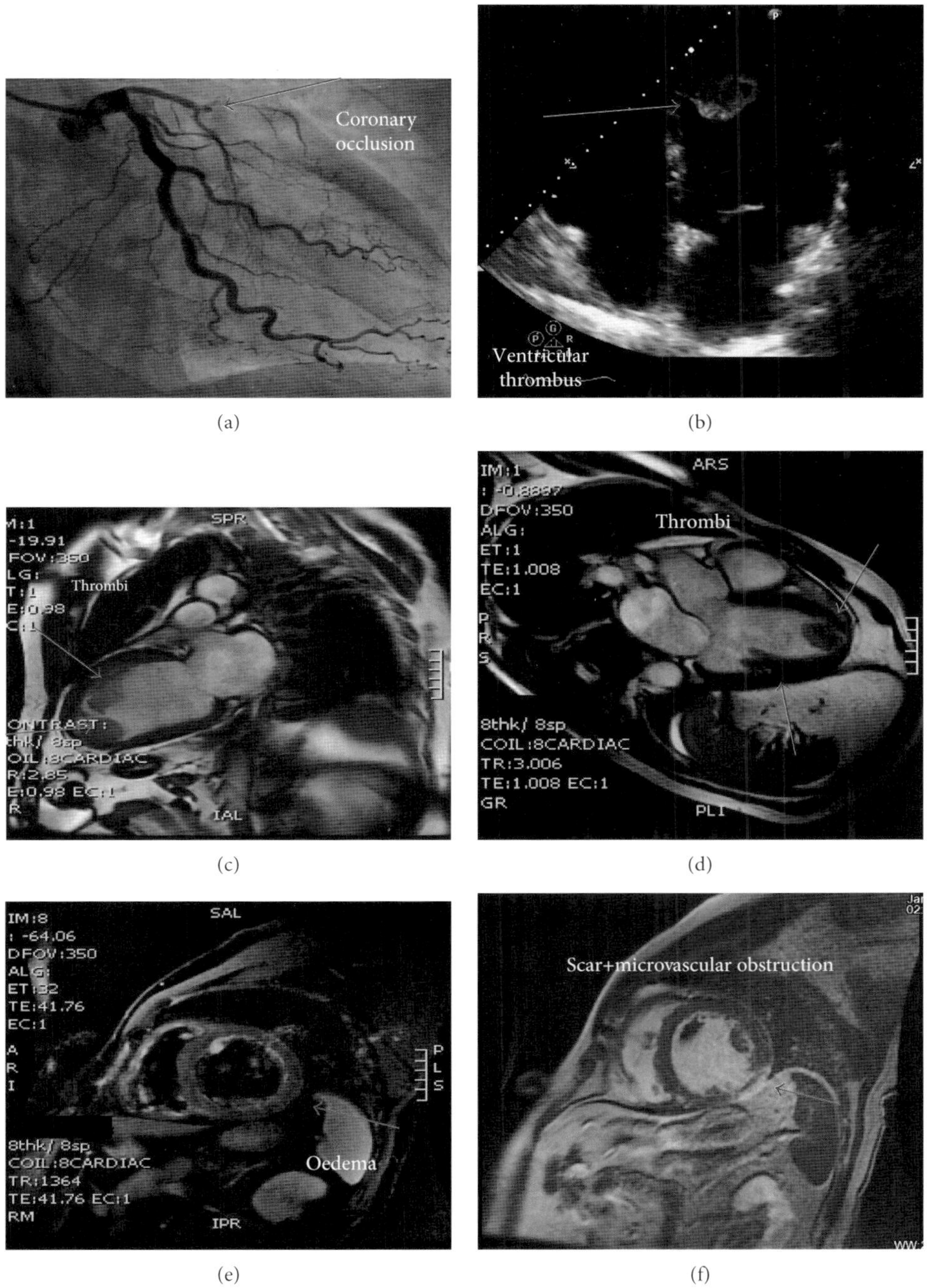

(a) (b) (c) (d) (e) (f)

Figure 1: Continued.

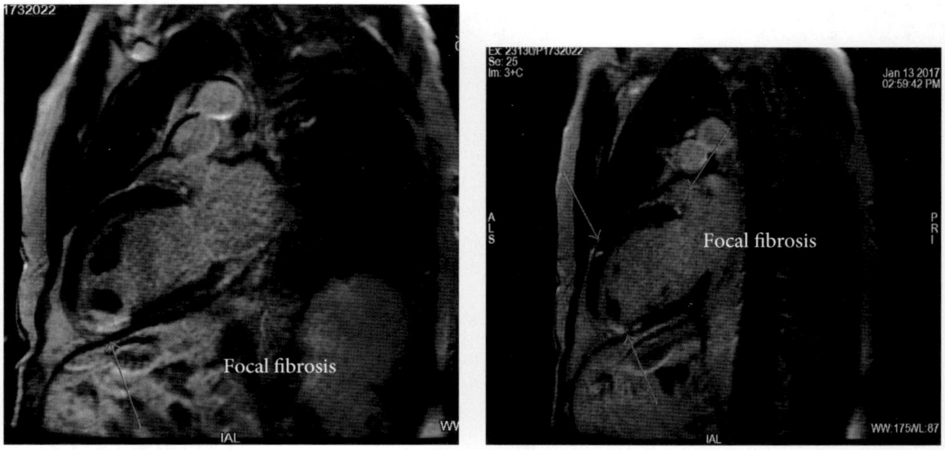

(g) (h)

Figure 1: (a) Coronary angiography showing the occlusion of the left descending artery in the proximal segment (arrow); (b) transthoracic 2-D echocardiography showing an apical ventricular thrombus; (c, d) cardiac magnetic resonance (CMR) unveiling the presence of two large left ventricular thrombi in the apex and along the anterior wall; (e) CMR TIR-T2 sequences showing myocardial edema involving the anterior wall of the left ventricle; (f, g) delay enhancement revealing scar, microvascular obstruction, and fibrosis (arrows); (h) CMR imaging: three hyperenhancement focal areas of fibrosis.

high-sensitivity troponin I was of 6.0 ng/mL, with normal hemoglobin level and INR of 1.9. At baseline, a combined thromboembolic and bleeding scoring system evaluation was performed, resulting in a CHA_2DS_2-VASc of 4 and HAS-BLED of 3 [16–18]. A NSTEMI diagnosis was made, and an antiplatelet therapy with aspirin 300 mg, clopidogrel 600 mg loading dose, and intravenous unfractionated heparin 5000 IU was administered, while an early invasive strategy with a transradial approach was planned. The coronary angiography showed a normal right coronary artery and the occlusion of the left descending artery in the proximal segment (Figure 1(a)). An IVUS-guided PCI was performed, with the implantation of two overlapped last-generation DES (Xience Alpine, Abbott), 2.75×28 mm and 3.0×28 mm, respectively, both expanded up to 16 atmospheres. In order to optimize expansion and avoid malapposition, the stents were overexpanded, with noncompliant balloons of 3.5×15 mm (NC Quantum, Boston), up to 20 atmospheres, according to IVUS-guided vessel sizing.

Considering the clinical setting (NSTEMI + AF) and the procedure (PCI with DES implantation), the antiplatelet therapy with aspirin 100 mg/day plus clopidogrel 75 mg/day was continued and anticoagulation with rivaroxaban 15 mg/day was started immediately after PCI. The transthoracic 2-D echocardiography revealed a hypokinesia of the apex and anterior wall with moderate reduction of the ejection fraction. Two mobile masses were found in the apex and in the anterior wall of the left ventricle, respectively (Figure 1(b)). A CMR was performed at day three, confirming apex and anterior wall hypokinesia and 40% ejection fraction. CMR unveiled the presence of two LV thrombi in the apex and along the anterior wall, respectively (Figures 1(c) and 1(d)). TIR-T2 sequences showed myocardial oedema (Figure 1(e)) involving the LV anterior wall; delay enhancement (Figures 1(f) and 1(g)) revealed a thickness fibrosis in the same segment, with a hypoenhanced internal area suggesting microvascular obstruction. Three hyperenhancement focal areas were detected (Figure 1(h)): a transmural area at inferior apical septum, just beneath one thrombus, and two subepicardial areas, at anterior basal septum and at midanterior wall, respectively.

The patient was discharged 7 days after admission. A clinical and cardiovascular imaging follow-up was planned at 1 month, 6 months, and 1 year. According to current guidelines and expert consensus knowledge [19, 20], the antithrombotic/anticoagulant therapy was managed as follows: at 1 month, the thromboembolic and bleeding risk scores (CHA_2DS_2-VASc of 4 and HAS-BLED of 3) were rechecked, the antiplatelet therapy with clopidogrel together with the anticoagulant therapy with rivaroxaban 15 mg/day was confirmed, and aspirin was stopped considering the high bleeding risk. At 6 months, no ischemic thromboembolic or bleeding events were reported. The echo and CMR imaging confirmed the resolution of the LV thrombi. Despite the fact that MRI are not necessary to confirm the thrombi resolution documented by echocardiogram, in our institution CMR facility together with an internal protocol in the case of a newer therapeutic strategy led us to perform this modality of cardiac imaging for speculative purpose. The dual therapy with clopidogrel plus rivaroxaban was confirmed [14].

At 1 year, a clinical follow-up confirmed the good clinical results: the patient was asymptomatic, and neither ischemic coronary events nor thromboembolic or bleeding events were reported. After 1 year, considering the CHA_2DS_2-VASc score, the high rate of recurrence of events after NSTEMI, the use of DES, the absence of bleeding events during previously dual antiplatelet therapy, a treatment with rivaroxaban plus aspirin was confirmed.

3. Discussion

The optimal antithrombotic strategy for patients with NVAF and ACS undergoing PCI is still controversial, and the role of NOACs in this setting is poorly documented [10–14].

The guidelines of ACS and AF report how to manage the antiplatelet and anticoagulant therapies in overlapped situations, but, frequently, the indication and level of evidence are strong only when the conditions are considered alone [19, 20]. Many different combinations have been proposed based on the use of different agents and for varying duration, but as the final target must balance the risk of bleeding and ischemic events in each patient, it is difficult to make a definitive decision especially when other potential thromboembolic complications (e.g., LV thrombi) occur. NOACs are at least as effective as warfarin in terms of thromboembolic complications, but safer in terms of bleeding complications [8, 9]. As for the dose, in the dual or triple therapy, guidelines recommend the lower available dose of NOACs [19, 20]. Based on the recent results of the PIONEER AF-PCI trial [14], the more effective and safer ratio is clopidogrel 75 mg plus rivaroxaban 15 mg, or either clopidogrel or ticagrelor plus dabigatran at 110 mg or 150 mg (RE-DUAL PCI) [21]. In contrast with the currently available data in which the evidence of the efficacy and safety of NOACs in patients with ACS and AF undergoing PCI is limited to a low HAS-BLED score, our patient had a high bleeding risk; therefore, despite this acute setting, a triple therapy was used for 4 weeks only, followed by dual therapy with clopidogrel plus rivaroxaban 15 mg/die for 12 months [14].

The use of aspirin has been reconsidered in the subgroup of patients at high risk of bleeding: for 6 months only in case of low bleeding risk, while for one month in case of high bleeding risk [19, 20]. However, given the results of PIONEER and RE-Dual PCI, it is likely that aspirin will be definitively abandoned.

Periprocedural and technical cautions are crucial to minimize either the risk of access site bleeding or the risk of stent thrombosis and recurrence of coronary events. The transradial approach is mandatory also because it shortens the time to restart oral anticoagulation. In our case, the use of the latest-generation fluoro-passivated everolimus-eluting stent, as recently documented [22], lowers the rate of stent thrombosis and thrombotic complications. Intracoronary imaging with an IVUS-guided stent implantation reduces vessel wall malapposition and, consequently, stent thrombosis, thus improving a tailored pharmacological management.

Our combined interventional and pharmacological strategy aimed at balancing the ischemic and bleeding risk was also based on the use of the lower dose of NOAC tested for stroke prevention, and clopidogrel instead of the more potent ticagrelor and prasugrel, as suggested by guidelines and expert consensus [19, 20].

Although coronary DES significantly reduced the recurrences during the follow-up, the likelihood of a new event is not negligible. In this context, the use of NOACS seems to be a safe and effective option when the patient complexity and frailty due to higher combined thromboembolic and bleeding risk require to achieve multiple therapeutic targets.

Disclosure

Bayer HealthCare was not involved in the collection, analysis, and interpretation of data. In case of acceptance for publication, Bayer HealthCare will pay the article processing fee.

Acknowledgments

The authors would like to thank Clara Ricci, PhD (Primula Multimedia SRL, Pisa, Italy), who provided skillful editorial assistance. Financial support for editorial services was provided by Bayer HealthCare, Italy.

References

[1] A. Rubboli, M. Colletta, J. Valencia et al., "Periprocedural management and in-hospital outcome of patients with indication for oral anticoagulation undergoing coronary artery stenting," *Journal of Interventional Cardiology*, vol. 22, no. 4, pp. 390–397, 2009.

[2] L. De Luca, S. Leonardi, C. Cavallini et al., "Contemporary antithrombotic strategies in patients with acute coronary syndrome admitted to cardiac care units in Italy: the EYESHOT study," *European Heart Journal: Acute Cardiovascular Care*, vol. 4, no. 5, pp. 441–452, 2015.

[3] F. Chiarella, E. Santoro, S. Domenicucci, A. Maggioni, and C. Vecchio, "Predischarge two-dimensional echocardiographic evaluation of left ventricular thrombosis after acute myocardial infarction in the GISSI-3 study," *American Journal of Cardiology*, vol. 81, no. 7, pp. 822–827, 1998.

[4] C. Lanzillo, M. Di Roma, A. Sciahbasi et al., "Cardiac magnetic resonance detection of left ventricular thrombus in acute myocardial infarction," *Acute Cardiac Care*, vol. 15, no. 1, pp. 11–16, 2013.

[5] G. Pizzetti, G. Belotti, A. Margonato et al., "Thrombolytic therapy reduces the incidence of left ventricular thrombus after anterior myocardial infarction. Relationship to vessel patency and infarct size," *European Heart Journal*, vol. 17, no. 3, pp. 421–428, 1996.

[6] D. Nayak, W. S. Aronow, R. Sukhija, J. A. McClung, C. E. Monsen, and R. N. Belkin, "Comparison of frequency of left ventricular thrombi in patients with anterior wall versus non-anterior wall acute myocardial infarction treated with antithrombotic and antiplatelet therapy with or without coronary revascularization," *American Journal of Cardiology*, vol. 93, no. 12, pp. 1529-1530, 2004.

[7] H. Heidbuchel, P. Verhamme, M. Alings et al., "European Heart Rhythm Association, European Heart Rhythm Association Practical Guide on the use of new oral anticoagulants in patients with non-valvular atrial fibrillation," *Europace Journal*, vol. 15, no. 5, pp. 625–651, 2013.

[8] M. R. Patel, K. W. Mahaffey, J. Garg et al., "Rivaroxaban versus warfarin in nonvalvular atrial fibrillation," *New England Journal of Medicine*, vol. 365, no. 10, pp. 883–891, 2011.

[9] C. T. Ruff, R. P. Giugliano, E. Braunwald et al., "Comparison of the efficacy and safety of new oral anticoagulants with warfarin in patients with atrial fibrillation: a meta-analysis of randomised trials," *The Lancet*, vol. 383, no. 9921, pp. 955–962, 2014.

[10] C. A. Makrides, "Resolution of left ventricular postinfarction thrombi in patients undergoing percutaneous coronary intervention using rivaroxaban in addition to dual antiplatelet therapy," *BMJ Case Reports*, vol. 2016, p. bcr2016217843, 2016.

[11] Y. Mano, K. Koide, H. Sukegawa, M. Kodaira, and T. Ohki, "Successful resolution of a left ventricular thrombus with apixaban treatment following acute myocardial infarction," *Heart and Vessels*, vol. 31, no. 1, pp. 118–123, 2016.

[12] R. Seecheran, V. Seecheran, S. Persad, and N. A. Seecheran, "Rivaroxaban as an antithrombotic agent in a patient with ST-segment elevation myocardial infarction and left ventricular thrombus: a case report," *Journal of Investigative Medicine High Impact Case Reports*, vol. 5, no. 1, p. 2324709617697991, 2017.

[13] C. Hammerstingl, B. Pötzsch, and G. Nickenig, "Resolution of giant left atrial appendage thrombus with rivaroxaban," *Thrombosis and Haemostasis*, vol. 109, no. 4, pp. 583-584, 2013.

[14] C. M. Gibson, R. Mehran, C. Bode et al., "Prevention of bleeding in patients with atrial fibrillation undergoing PCI," *New England Journal of Medicine*, vol. 375, no. 25, pp. 2423–2434, 2016.

[15] C. P. Cannon, D. L. Bhatt, J. Oldgren et al., "Antithrombotic therapy with dabigatran after PCI in atrial fibrillation," *New England Journal of Medicine*, vol. 377, no. 16, pp. 1513–1524, 2017.

[16] G. Y. H. Lip, R. Nieuwlaat, R. Pisters, D. A. Lane, and H. J. G. M. Crijns, "Refining clinical risk stratification for predicting stroke and thromboembolism in atrial fibrillation using a novel risk factor-based approach: the euro heart survey on atrial fibrillation," *Chest*, vol. 137, no. 2, pp. 263–272, 2010.

[17] G. Y. H. Lip, L. Frison, J. L. Halperin, and D. A. Lane, "Comparative validation of a novel risk score for predicting bleeding risk in anticoagulated patients with atrial fibrillation: the HAS-BLED (hypertension, abnormal renal/liver function, stroke, bleeding history or predisposition, labile inr, elderly, drugs/alcohol concomitantly) score," *Journal of the American College of Cardiology*, vol. 57, no. 2, pp. 173–180, 2011.

[18] S. Apostolakis, D. A. Lane, H. Buller, and G. Y. H. Lip, "Comparison of the CHADS2, CHA2DS2-VASc and HAS-BLED scores for the prediction of clinically relevant bleeding in anticoagulated patients with atrial fibrillation: the AMADEUS trial," *Thrombosis and Haemostasis*, vol. 110, no. 5, pp. 1074–1079, 2013.

[19] G. Y. H. Lip, S. Windecker, K. Huber et al., "Management of antithrombotic therapy in atrial fibrillation patients presenting with acute coronary syndrome and/or undergoing percutaneous coronary or valve interventions: a joint consensus document of the European Society of Cardiology Working Group on Thrombosis, European Heart Rhythm Association (EHRA), European Association of Percutaneous Cardiovascular Interventions (EAPCI) and European Association of Acute Cardiac Care (ACCA) endorsed by the Heart Rhythm Society (HRS) and Asia-Pacific Heart Rhythm Society (APHRS)," *European Heart Journal*, vol. 35, no. 45, pp. 3155–3179, 2014.

[20] M. Roffi, C. Patrono, J.-P. Collet et al., "2015 ESC guidelines for the management of acute coronary syndromes in patients presenting without persistent ST-segment elevation," *European Heart Journal*, vol. 37, no. 3, pp. 267–315, 2016.

[21] C. P. Cannon, S. Gropper, D. L. Bhatt et al., "Design and rationale of the RE-DUAL PCI trial: a prospective, randomized, phase 3b study comparing the safety and efficacy of dual antithrombotic therapy with dabigatran etexilate versus warfarin triple therapy in patients with nonvalvular atrial fibrillation who have undergone percutaneous coronary intervention with stenting," *Clinical Cardiology*, vol. 39, no. 10, pp. 555–564, 2016.

[22] T. Palmerini, U. Benedetto, G. Biondi-Zoccai et al., "Long-term safety of drug-eluting and bare-metal stents: evidence from a comprehensive network meta-analysis," *Journal of the American College of Cardiology*, vol. 65, no. 23, pp. 2496–2507, 2015.

A 66-Year-Old Female with Apical Hypertrophic Cardiomyopathy Presenting with Hypertensive Crises and Type 2 Myocardial Infarction and a Normal Coronary Angiogram

Vineet Meghrajani ,[1] Karan Wats,[2] Abhinav Saxena,[2] and Bilal Malik[2]

[1]*Department of Internal Medicine, Maimonides Medical Center, 4802 10th Avenue, Brooklyn, New York 11219, USA*
[2]*Department of Cardiology, Maimonides Medical Center, 4802 10th Avenue, Brooklyn, New York 11219, USA*

Correspondence should be addressed to Vineet Meghrajani; vineetmeghrajani@gmail.com

Academic Editor: Konstantinos P. Letsas

A 66-year-old female presented to the emergency room with an episode of chest pain that lasted for a few minutes before resolving spontaneously. Electrocardiogram showed a left bundle branch block, left ventricular hypertrophy, and T wave inversions in the lateral leads. Initial cardiac troponin level was 0.15 ng/ml, with levels of 4 ng/ml and 9 ng/ml obtained 6 and 12 hours later, respectively. The peak blood pressure recorded was 195/43 mmHg. Echocardiogram with DEFINITY showed a small left ventricular cavity with apical hypertrophy, and coronary angiogram showed no stenotic or occluding lesions in the coronary arteries. The patient was admitted for a type 2 myocardial infarction with hypertensive crises. She was diagnosed with having apical hypertrophic cardiomyopathy, which is a variant of hypertrophic cardiomyopathy (HCM) in which the hypertrophy predominantly involves the apex of the left ventricle resulting in midventricular obstruction, as opposed to the left ventricular outflow tract obstruction seen in HCM. Patients with apical HCM may present with angina, heart failure, myocardial infarction, syncope, or arrhythmias and are typically managed with medications like verapamil and beta-blockers for those who have symptoms and antiarrhythmic agents like amiodarone and procainamide for treatment of atrial fibrillation and ventricular arrhythmias. An implantable cardioverter defibrillator (ICD) is recommended for high-risk HCM patients with a history of previous cardiac arrest or sustained episodes of ventricular tachycardia, syncope, and a family history of sudden death.

1. Introduction

There are several causes of troponin elevation other than acute coronary syndromes. Some of the common noncoronary ischemia-related causes include chronic renal failure, advanced heart failure, acute pulmonary embolism, acute inflammatory myocarditis, and coronary artery vasospasm. Apical hypertrophic cardiomyopathy (HCM) is one of the rare cardiomyopathies which can also present like an acute myocardial infarction (MI). We present a case of 66-year-old female who presented with chest pain to our emergency room and was found to have apical hypertrophic cardiomyopathy.

2. Case Presentation

A 66-year-old independently functioning woman presented to the emergency room with an episode of midepigastric and left sternal chest pain. Her medical history included hypertension, hyperlipidemia, glaucoma, and multiple previous episodes of chest pain similar to her current episode that necessitated three separate coronary angiograms which showed no stenotic or occluding lesions in the coronary arteries. The patient described her chest pain as a sensation of burning that started suddenly at 11 pm in the night while she was resting comfortably at home after having dinner. The pain was mild in intensity, nonradiating,

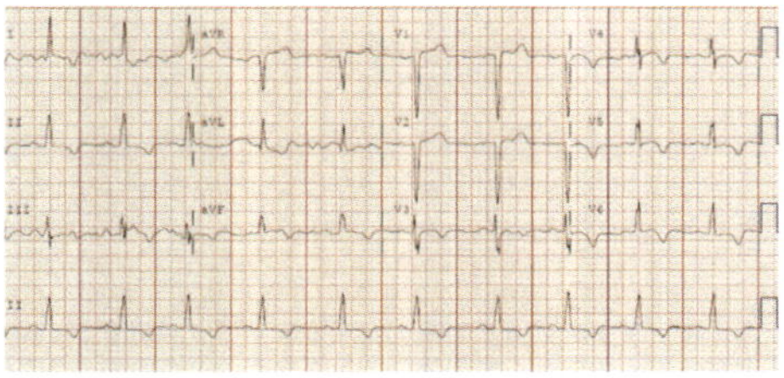

Figure 1: Initial EKG showing normal sinus cardiac rhythm with a left bundle branch block, possible left ventricular hypertrophy, and T wave inversions in the lateral leads. No ST segment changes were noted.

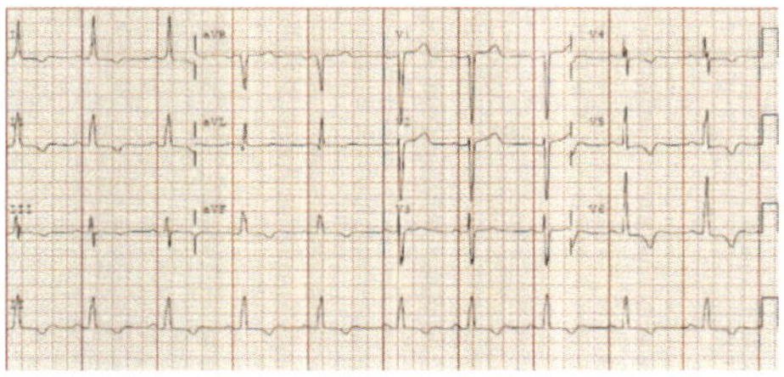

Figure 2: Follow-up EKG showing no changes compared to the first EKG.

and lasted for a few minutes before resolving spontaneously. She denied having any dyspnea, palpitations, dizziness, or loss of consciousness during this episode. She had no history of smoking or illicit drug use. Her home medications included felodipine extended release 5 mg once daily, isosorbide mononitrate extended release 30 mg once daily, atorvastatin 80 mg once daily, losartan 100 mg once daily, hydrochlorothiazide 25 mg once daily, and metoprolol succinate extended release 100 mg once daily. The patient activated emergency medical services immediately after onset of her symptoms, who brought the patient to the emergency room. On arrival in the emergency room, the patient was asymptomatic. Her vital signs were as follows: blood pressure of 168/46 mmHg (right arm, supine position), heart rate of 66/min, respiratory rate of 19/min, and an oral temperature of 97.9 F. An electrocardiogram was obtained which showed a normal sinus cardiac rhythm with a left bundle branch block, possible left ventricular hypertrophy, and T wave inversions in the lateral leads. No ST segment changes were noted (Figure 1). There were no prior electrocardiograms available for comparison. Her laboratory data included a cardiac troponin level of 0.15 ng/ml. Follow-up cardiac troponin levels obtained 6 and 12 hours later were 4 ng/ml and 9 ng/ml, respectively. The patient continued to be asymptomatic during this time, and a follow-up EKG showed no changes compared to the first EKG (Figure 2). Her blood pressure, however, continued to remain high during her time in the emergency room with a peak blood pressure recording of 195/43 mmHg. Based on the elevated troponin level up to 9 ng/ml with the absence of ST segment changes on the EKG and the significantly elevated blood pressure, it was decided to admit the patient to the cardiac intensive care unit for treatment of a hypertensive crisis with elevated troponin levels possibly due to a

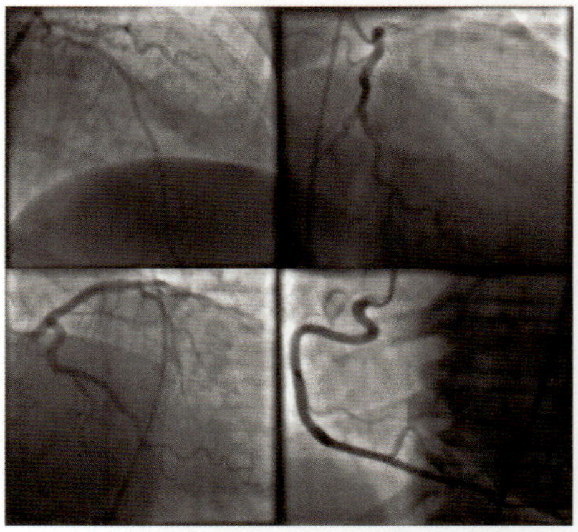

Figure 3: Coronary angiogram showing normal left main, left anterior descending, left circumflex, and right coronary arteries with no stenotic or occluding lesions.

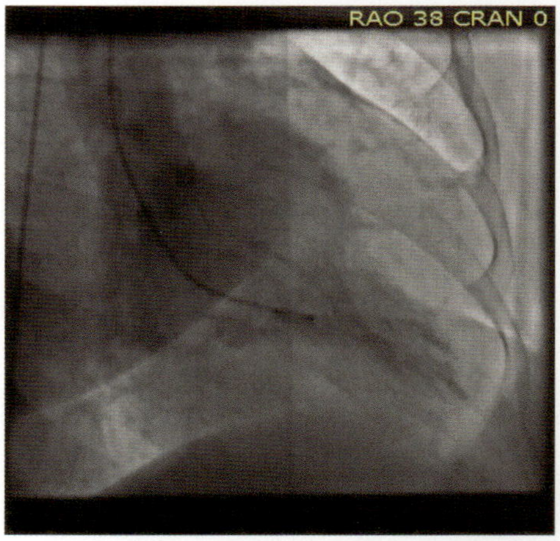

Figure 4: Cardiac left ventriculogram done by cardiac chamber catheterization confirming the echocardiographic finding of apical hypertrophy.

type 2 myocardial infarction. She was given a loading dose of aspirin 325 mg and clopidogrel 300 mg orally and was started on an intravenous heparin drip at 12 units/kg/hour. A onetime dose of hydralazine 5 mg was administered intravenously which was followed by an improvement in the blood pressure to 150/46 mmHg. An echocardiogram was ordered with DEFINITY which showed a small left ventricular cavity with apical hypertrophy, an impaired relaxation pattern during left ventricular diastolic filling, and a left ventricular ejection fraction of 76–80%. The patient subsequently underwent a coronary angiogram the next day through right femoral artery access which showed normal left main, left anterior descending, left circumflex, and right coronary arteries with no stenotic or occluding lesions (Figure 3). A cardiac left ventriculogram was done by cardiac chamber catheterization during the procedure, which confirmed the echocardiographic finding of apical hypertrophy (Figure 4). Based on the finding of apical hypertrophic cardiomyopathy, it was decided to start the patient on metoprolol succinate extended release 100 mg daily and verapamil sustained release 180 mg daily. The remainder of the patient's hospitalization was uneventful, with an optimally controlled blood pressure and a downtrend in her cardiac troponin levels, and she was subsequently discharged on the 3rd hospital day.

3. Case Discussion

Apical hypertrophic cardiomyopathy is a variant of hypertrophic cardiomyopathy in which the hypertrophy of the myocardium predominantly involves the apex of the left ventricle resulting in midventricular obstruction, as opposed to the left ventricular outflow tract obstruction seen in HCM [1–3]. It occurs due to autosomal dominant mutations in one of nine genes encoding sarcomeric proteins, most commonly the sarcomere gene ACTC 1 (actin, alpha, cardiac muscle 1)—Glu101Lys missense mutation [4, 5]. Apical HCM is also known as Yamaguchi syndrome after the person who first described its imaging features in Japan and is more common in East Asian populations—representing 41 percent of Chinese patients with HCM and 15 percent of Japanese patients, but only 1–3 percent of non-Asian populations with HCM [1, 6–8]. The mean age at presentation has been variable in different studies, it was 41.4 ± 14.5 years in one study [3] and 58 ± 17 years in another [9]. Most patients with apical HCM are asymptomatic, and those who do develop symptoms usually present with angina, heart failure, myocardial infarction, presyncope, syncope, atrial fibrillation, or ventricular fibrillation. These occur usually due to diastolic dysfunction with low cardiac output [3]. The typical clinical and diagnostic features of apical HCM include audible fourth heart sound, "giant" negative T waves on EKG, particularly in left precordial leads, apical wall motion abnormalities including hypokinesis and aneurysm formation, and "spade-like" configuration of left ventricular cavity at end-diastole on imaging [3, 10, 11]. Among these findings, the "giant" negative T wave has been identified as a predictor of favorable outcome [8]. The diagnosis of apical HCM can be made with echocardiography, left ventriculography, computed tomography, or most accurately with cardiac MRI [1, 12, 13]. Lladó et al. showed that MRI allowed better overall assessment of the degree and extent of LVH in HCM patients than did echocardiogram [12]. The apical segment was adequately visualized in all patients by MRI but only in 60% of the patients by echo, and MRI allows the early diagnosis of apical HCM by identifying even a small quantity of hypertrophied myocardium in different apical locations in a "non-spade" variety of apical HCM [12, 14]. While apical HCM has a better mortality prognosis than other forms of HCM, with one retrospective study of 105 patients having a total cardiovascular mortality rate of 1.9% over 13.6 ± 8.3 years [3] and overall estimated survival of 95 percent at 15 years, it is still associated with a relatively high rate of important cardiac events—30 percent of patients experienced a serious cardiac complication, most commonly atrial fibrillation (12 percent) or a myocardial infarction (10 percent) [3]. In the same study, apical myocardial infarction in the presence of normal coronary arteries, a presentation similar to the patient in our case, was found in about 10% of patients. The possible mechanisms responsible for ischemia in apical HCM include limitation in coronary flow reserve, decreased capillary myocardial ratio, small vessel disease, and other mechanisms [15–17]. Severe clinical manifestations, including sudden cardiac death, severe arrhythmias, and apical infarction with apical aneurysm, are uncommon with apical HCM, although they have been described [3]. Among the subtypes of HCM, the "true apical" phenotype (hypertrophy of only the apical segments) has been shown to have improved survival over a "distal-dominant" phenotype (cases in which hypertrophy extended into the middle LV segments) [18]. In another study of 193 patients in Minnesota, the observed versus expected 20-year survival was 47% versus 60% [9]. Sudden cardiac death, resuscitated cardiac arrest, and/or defibrillator discharge was observed in 6% of patients during follow-up.

While apical HCM is low on the list of suspected differentials for patients presenting with chest pain and elevated cardiac troponin levels on laboratory testing, the more common causes of such a presentation being STEMI or NSTEMI, this case still demonstrates the importance of following the proper testing protocol for patients who present with these findings to the emergency room—namely, an EKG, followed by testing for cardiac troponin levels, a bedside echocardiogram, and an urgent coronary angiogram if EKG changes are seen along with elevated cardiac troponin levels. For patients with no EKG changes and elevation in cardiac troponin levels, they should still be treated as an NSTEMI with anticoagulation and an early coronary angiogram preferably within 24 hours of presentation, especially if they have clinical findings that are strongly suggestive of an NSTEMI, i.e., symptoms of ischemic chest pain on presentation and prior risk factors of coronary artery disease.

The approach to the management of apical HCM is the same as for most patients with HCM; symptomatic patients are initially treated with medical therapy, which includes medications like verapamil and beta-blockers [3, 19, 20]. Antiarrhythmic agents such as amiodarone and procainamide are used in the treatment of atrial fibrillation and ventricular arrhythmias [21]. Since apical HCM does not involve LVOT obstruction, septal reduction therapy is almost never used to treat apical HCM. Similarly, the risk of ventricular tachyarrhythmias and sudden cardiac death is low in apical HCM, and an implantable cardioverter defibrillator (ICD) is only recommended for high risk HCM patients with a history of previous cardiac arrest or sustained episodes of ventricular tachycardia, syncope, a family history of sudden death, or episodes of nonsustained ventricular tachycardia on serial Holter monitoring [22].

4. Conclusion

Apical HCM is a variant of HCM in which the hypertrophy of the myocardium predominantly involves the apex of the left ventricle resulting in midventricular obstruction, as opposed to the left ventricular outflow tract obstruction seen in HCM. While apical HCM has a better mortality prognosis than other forms of HCM, it is still associated with a relatively high rate of important cardiac events like atrial fibrillation or myocardial infarction. Apical HCM is low on the list of suspected differentials for patients presenting with chest pain and elevated cardiac troponin levels on laboratory testing, the more common causes of such a presentation being STEMI or NSTEMI. This case demonstrates the importance of following the proper testing protocol for patients who present with these findings to the emergency room—namely, an EKG, followed by testing for cardiac troponin levels, a bedside echocardiogram, and an urgent coronary angiogram if EKG changes are seen along with elevated cardiac troponin levels. The approach to the management of apical HCM is similar to most patients with HCM—medical therapy for symptomatic patients, which includes medications like verapamil and beta-blockers and antiarrhythmic agents such as amiodarone and procainamide for treatment of atrial fibrillation and ventricular arrhythmias. Since apical HCM does not involve LVOT obstruction, septal reduction therapy is almost never used to treat apical HCM. The risk of ventricular tachyarrhythmias and sudden cardiac death is low in apical HCM, and an implantable cardioverter defibrillator (ICD) is only recommended for high-risk HCM patients with a history of previous cardiac arrest or sustained episodes of ventricular tachycardia, syncope, a family history of sudden death, or episodes of nonsustained ventricular tachycardia on serial Holter monitoring.

References

[1] M. S. Maron, J. J. Finley, J. M. Bos et al., "Prevalence, clinical significance, and natural history of left ventricular apical aneurysms in hypertrophic cardiomyopathy," *Circulation*, vol. 118, no. 15, pp. 1541–1549, 2008.

[2] T. Sakamoto, "Apical hypertrophic cardiomyopathy (apical hypertrophy): an overview," *Journal of Cardiology*, vol. 37, Supplement 1, pp. 161–178, 2001.

[3] M. J. Eriksson, B. Sonnenberg, A. Woo et al., "Long-term outcome in patients with apical hypertrophic cardiomyopathy," *Journal of the American College of Cardiology*, vol. 39, no. 4, pp. 638–645, 2002.

[4] G. Bonne, L. Carrier, P. Richard, B. Hainque, and K. Schwartz, "Familial hypertrophic cardiomyopathy: from mutations to functional defects," *Circulation Research*, vol. 83, no. 6, pp. 580–593, 1998.

[5] C. Seidman, "Hypertrophic cardiomyopathy: from man to mouse," *The Journal of Clinical Investigation*, vol. 106, pp. S9–13, 2000.

[6] H.-H. Ho, K. L. F. Lee, C.-P. Lau, and H.-F. Tse, "Clinical characteristics of and long-term outcome in Chinese patients with hypertrophic cardiomyopathy," *The American Journal of Medicine*, vol. 116, no. 1, pp. 19–23, 2004.

[7] H. Kitaoka, Y. Doi, S. A. Casey, N. Hitomi, T. Furuno, and B. J. Maron, "Comparison of prevalence of apical hypertrophic cardiomyopathy in Japan and the United States," *The American Journal of Cardiology*, vol. 92, no. 10, pp. 1183–1186, 2003.

[8] H. G. Klues, A. Schiffers, and B. J. Maron, "Phenotypic spectrum and patterns of left ventricular hypertrophy in hypertrophic cardiomyopathy: morphologic observations and significance as assessed by two-dimensional echocardiography in 600 patients," *Journal of the American College of Cardiology*, vol. 26, no. 7, pp. 1699–1708, 1995.

[9] K. W. Klarich, C. H. Attenhofer Jost, J. Binder et al., "Risk of death in long-term follow-up of patients with apical hypertrophic cardiomyopathy," *The American Journal of Cardiology*, vol. 111, no. 12, pp. 1784–1791, 2013.

[10] T. Sakamoto, C. Tei, M. Murayama et al., "Giant T wave inversion as a manifestation of asymmetrical apical hypertrophy (AAH) of the left ventricle: echocardiographic and ultrasono-cardiotomographic study," *Japanese Heart Journal*, vol. 17, no. 5, pp. 611–629, 1976.

[11] H. Yamaguchi, T. Ishimura, S. Nishiyama et al., "Hypertrophic nonobstructive cardiomyopathy with giant negative T waves (apical hypertrophy): ventriculographic and echocardiographic features in 30 patients," *The American Journal of Cardiology*, vol. 44, no. 3, pp. 401–412, 1979.

[12] G. Pons-Lladó, F. Carreras, X. Borrás, J. Palmer, J. Llauger, and A. Bayés de Luna, "Comparison of morphologic assessment of hypertrophic cardiomyopathy by magnetic resonance versus echocardiographic imaging," *The American Journal of Cardiology*, vol. 79, no. 12, pp. 1651–1656, 1997.

[13] J. C. Moon, N. G. Fisher, W. J. McKenna, and D. J. Pennell, "Detection of apical hypertrophic cardiomyopathy by cardiovascular magnetic resonance in patients with non-diagnostic echocardiography," *Heart*, vol. 90, no. 6, pp. 645–649, 2004.

[14] J.-I. Suzuki, R. Shimamoto, J.-I. Nishikawa et al., "Morphological onset and early diagnosis in apical hypertrophic cardiomyopathy: a long term analysis with nuclear magnetic resonance imaging," *Journal of the American College of Cardiology*, vol. 33, no. 1, pp. 146–151, 1999.

[15] M. E. Bertrand, P. Y. Tilmant, J. M. Lablanche, and F. A. Thieuleux, "Apical hypertrophic cardiomyopathy: clinical and metabolic studies," *European Heart Journal*, vol. 4, Supplement F, pp. 127–133, 1983.

[16] E. D. Wigle, Z. Sasson, M. A. Henderson et al., "Hypertrophic cardiomyopathy. The importance of the site and the extent of hypertrophy. A review," *Progress in Cardiovascular Diseases*, vol. 28, no. 1, pp. 1–83, 1985.

[17] S. Ishiwata, S. Nishiyama, S. Nakanishi, and A. Seki, "Two types of left ventricular wall motion abnormalities with distinct clinical features in patients with hypertrophic cardiomyopathy," *European Heart Journal*, vol. 14, no. 12, pp. 1629–1639, 1993.

[18] T. Kubo, H. Kitaoka, M. Okawa et al., "Clinical profiles of hypertrophic cardiomyopathy with apical phenotype–comparison of pure-apical form and distal-dominant form," *Circulation Journal*, vol. 73, no. 12, pp. 2330–2336, 2009.

[19] S. C. Chen, K. T. Wang, C. J. Y. Hou, Y. S. Chou, and C. H. Tsai, "Apical hypertrophic cardiomyopathy with severe myocardial bridging in a syncopal patient," *Acta Cardiologica Sinica*, vol. 19, pp. 179–184, 2003.

[20] D. Ridjab, M. Koch, M. Zabel, H. P. Schultheiss, and A. J. Morguet, "Cardiac arrest and ventricular tachycardia in Japanese-type apical hypertrophic cardiomyopathy," *Cardiology*, vol. 107, no. 2, pp. 81–86, 2007.

[21] K. Okishige, T. Sasano, K. Yano, K. Azegami, K. Suzuki, and K. Itoh, "Serious arrhythmias in patients with apical hypertrophic cardiomyopathy," *Internal Medicine*, vol. 40, no. 5, pp. 396–402, 2001.

Emergency Valve-in-Valve Transcatheter Aortic Valve Implantation for the Treatment of Acute Stentless Bioprosthetic Aortic Insufficiency and Cardiogenic Shock

Ivan D. Hanson[1], **Pratik K. Dalal**[1], **Brian M. Renard**[1], **George S. Hanzel**[1] **and Alessandro Vivacqua**[2]

[1]*Department of Cardiovascular Medicine, Beaumont Health System, Royal Oak, MI, USA*
[2]*Department of Cardiovascular Surgery, Beaumont Health System, Royal Oak, MI, USA*

Correspondence should be addressed to Ivan D. Hanson; ivan.hanson@beaumont.org

Academic Editor: Markus Ferrari

Bioprosthetic aortic valve degeneration may present as acute, severe aortic regurgitation and cardiogenic shock. Such patients may be unsuitable for emergency valve replacement surgery due to excessive risk of operative mortality but could be treatable with transfemoral valve-in-valve transcatheter aortic valve implantation (TAVI). There is a paucity of data regarding the feasibility of valve-in-valve TAVI in patients presenting with cardiogenic shock due to acute aortic insufficiency from stentless bioprosthetic valve degeneration. We present one such case, highlighting the unique aspects of valve-in-valve TAVI for this challenging patient subset.

1. Introduction

Acute severe aortic regurgitation is an emergency necessitating immediate intervention due to the inability of the left ventricle to adapt to the sudden increase in preload and left ventricular diastolic pressure, which ultimately results in pulmonary edema and cardiogenic shock. Pharmacologic preload and postload reduction can temporize clinical deterioration, but only valve replacement can abort the inevitable hemodynamic collapse. We present a case of successful valve-in-valve transcatheter aortic valve implantation (TAVI) for a structurally deteriorated Medtronic Freestyle stentless bioprosthesis in a patient presenting with severe aortic regurgitation and cardiogenic shock. Due to clinical presentation in extremis and presence of stentless bioprosthetic degeneration, the case presented unique challenges that highlight important aspects of preprocedural care, heart team collaboration, imaging guidance, and implantation technique.

2. Case Report

The patient is a 72-year-old female with a history of diabetes mellitus, hypertension, and bicuspid aortic valve status post aortic valve and root replacement using a 23 mm Freestyle (Medtronic, Minneapolis, MN) aortic valve and root bioprosthesis implanted by root inclusion method 12 years prior to admission. She was transferred from an outside hospital with acute-onset chest pain and shortness of breath. She denied fever and chills. Physical examination was notable for blood pressure 100/30 mmHg and hypoxia. Grade 3/6 systolic and diastolic murmurs were heard at the right 2nd intercostal space. Subsequently, she developed pulmonary edema and shock necessitating mechanical ventilation and vasopressor support. A transthoracic echocardiogram suggested flail aortic valve leaflet (Video 1), and transaortic Doppler signal was suggestive of wide-open aortic regurgitation (Figure 1).

Due to rapid deterioration of the patient, the heart team was immediately organized. Two cardiac surgeons deemed her unsuitable for redo surgical aortic valve replacement (Society of Thoracic Surgeons predicted operative mortality >50%). Therefore, valve-in-valve TAVI was considered. After review of the operative report and manufacturer product information, the inner diameter of the Freestyle valve was confirmed to be 20 mm. A 23 mm S3 valve (Edwards Lifesciences,

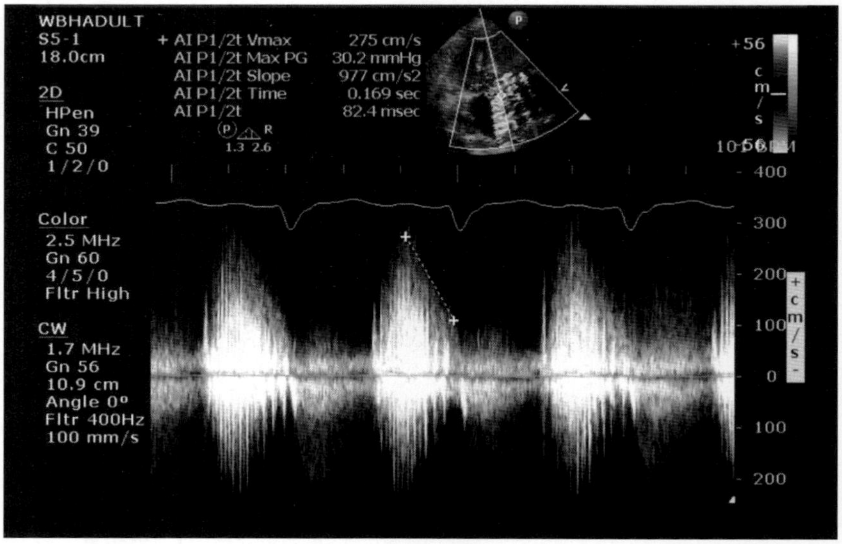

Figure 1: Transaortic Doppler demonstrating dense aortic regurgitation signal with markedly reduced pressure half time, suggestive of severe aortic insufficiency.

Irvine, CA) was selected. Images from a remote contrast-enhanced CT scan suggested absence of peripheral arterial calcification and adequate caliber of iliofemoral arteries for large-bore sheath insertion.

Transesophageal echocardiography (TEE) was used to guide the procedure. The etiology of valve deterioration was confirmed to be leaflet flail; no vegetations were identified. Arterial and venous access was obtained followed by placement of a transvenous pacemaker. Aortography was performed (Video 2), followed by insertion of a 14 F × 36 cm E sheath (Edwards Lifesciences, Irvine, CA). The 23 mm S3 valve was implanted during rapid pacing, using nominal inflation volume (Video 3). Of note, wide pulse pressure was observed even during pacing at 200 beats per minute. Pre-TAVI central aortic pressure was 114/30 mmHg, and left ventricular pressure was 120/30 mmHg (Figure 2(a)). Post-TAVI central aortic pressure was 90/40 mmHg with a left ventricular pressure of 90/13 mmHg (Figure 2(b)). The final TEE images and aortogram showed trivial aortic regurgitation (Figures 2(c)–2(f)). Blood cultures, which had been obtained at presentation, were negative. The patient was discharged home in stable condition after 7 days. At a 30-day postprocedure follow-up visit, she was asymptomatic and had returned to working as a teacher. An echocardiogram at that time revealed normal left ventricular size and function, no aortic insufficiency, mean transaortic gradient 12 mmHg, and calculated aortic valve area 1.0 cm^2 (Video 4, Figure 3).

3. Discussion

Several large, multicenter registries have demonstrated that valve-in-valve TAVI is safe and effective in stable patients with degenerated aortic bioprostheses [1–4]. In an analysis from the Global Valve-in-Valve Registry, Dvir and colleagues demonstrated excellent 1-year survival in such patients (83.2%; 95% CI, 80.8%–84.7%) [2]. One-year survival for patients with pure insufficiency as the mode of bioprosthetic failure was even more favorable (91.2%; 95% CI, 85.7%–96.7%). Of patients with pure insufficiency, 36.7% had New York Heart Association (NYHA) 4 symptoms (number of patients in shock was not reported), and 29.6% had stentless valve degeneration.

In contrast to more stable patients with failed *stented* bioprostheses, valve-in-valve TAVI for acute, severe aortic insufficiency and cardiogenic shock due to *stentless* bioprosthetic degeneration represents a particularly challenging TAVI subset, and published data are limited to a few case reports. Bagur and colleagues [5] treated a patient with 15-year old degenerated 23 mm Medtronic Freestyle (Minneapolis, Minnesota) who presented with hemodynamically unstable pulmonary edema. They used a 23 mm Edwards SAPIEN XT (Edwards Lifesciences Inc., Irvine, California). Since there was relative lack of calcification in the body of the prosthesis, valve positioning was facilitated by a pigtail catheter left in the right sinus of Valsalva until the SAPIEN XT was half deployed, and the operators used a very slow deployment technique. Chevalier and colleagues [6] treated a patient presenting with shock and acute aortic insufficiency due to a deteriorated 19 mm Freestyle valve with a 23 mm SAPIEN XT valve with 5 cc less than nominal inflation volume; a transcatheter valve with a smaller diameter was not used due to patient-prosthesis mismatch at baseline. The hemodynamic result was acceptable (shock resolved, residual 25 mmHg mean transaortic gradient with no aortic insufficiency), and the patient was free of heart failure at 6-month follow-up. Finally, Duncan et al. [7] reported a series of valve-in-valve TAVI in 22 patients with failing stentless bioprostheses, one of which had a failed 25 mm homograft and presented with acute aortic insufficiency and cardiogenic shock. Extracorporeal circulatory support was used before and after TAVI, which utilized a 29 mm Medtronic Corevalve (Minneapolis, Minnesota). The Corevalve was 4.4% oversized based on the perimeter of the homograft annulus. All patients in the series, including this one, were alive at 30 days.

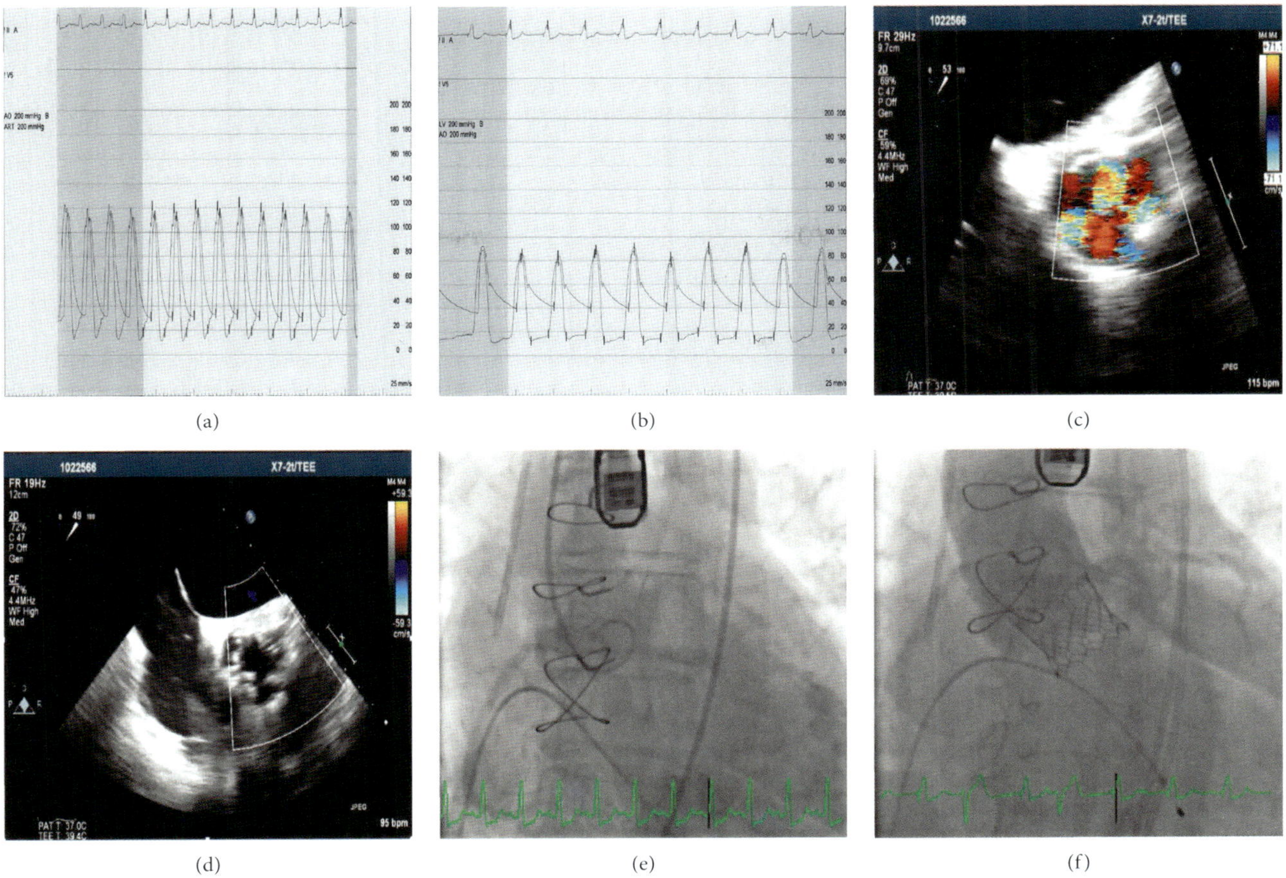

FIGURE 2: (a) Pre-TAVI simultaneous aortic and left ventricular pressures demonstrating equalization of Ao diastolic LV end-diastolic pressures. (b) Post-TAVI hemodynamics revealing normal diastolic LV-Ao gradient and no systolic LV-Ao gradient. (c) Pre-TEE image of the bioprosthetic aortic valve during diastole shows three large regurgitant jets. (d) Post-TEE short axis of the TAVI valve during diastole shows absence of regurgitant flow. (e) Pre-TAVI aortogram shows 4+ aortic insufficiency. (f) Post-TAVI aortogram shows no aortic insufficiency and acceptable implantation depth. TAVI = transcatheter aortic valve replacement; Ao = aortic; LV = left ventricular; TEE = transesophageal echocardiogram.

Emergency valve-in-valve TAVI in a patient with *acute, severe aortic insufficiency* and *cardiogenic shock* presents unique technical challenges. Preprocedural stabilization in the crucial moments prior to TAVI must include airway intubation and hemodynamic support. Pharmacologic vasopressor support may be necessary in the short term to increase central aortic pressure and perfuse vital organs. Intra-aortic balloon pump and transaortic axial flow pumps (such as Impella (Danvers, Massachusetts)) are generally contraindicated. Extracorporeal membrane oxygenation may be effective as a temporizing measure, as was reported by Duncan et al. [7], but an arterio-venous circuit in a beating heart would be expected to ultimately lead to worsening aortic regurgitation and pump failure [8]. Therefore, timely aortic valve replacement is the key to survival. With the airway secured, TEE can confirm the etiology of leaflet degeneration (i.e., whether due to a purely mechanical problem or endocarditis), visualize the sewing ring of the stentless valve (invisible by fluoroscopy), and may be helpful in coordinating the appropriate TAVI implant height. Preprocedural CT angiography, while ideal for planning stentless (or stented) valve-in-valve TAVI in more stable patients, is not feasible for patients in shock. Transfemoral access is the least invasive and likely to be the best tolerated large-bore vascular access for hemodynamically unstable patients. Although low mean systemic blood pressure was achieved with pacing at 200 bpm, pulse pressure remained relatively wide. This was likely the result of hyperdynamic ventricular contractility and stroke volume due to inotropic agents and severe aortic insufficiency, respectively. Despite this, the balloon-expandable transcatheter valve remained in a stable position throughout deployment.

In contrast to *stented* aortic prostheses, *stentless* prostheses do not have radiopaque markings to fluroscopically guide transcatheter valve implantation depth. The exception may be if there is heavy calcification in the body of the prosthesis. Importantly, the sewing ring may be more ventricular than the calcium landmarks in the body of the prosthesis, so a combination of TEE and aortography, with one or two pigtail catheters to locate the sewing ring relative to the root, may be useful [9]. For stable patients with stentless valve degeneration, self-expanding, recapturable transcatheter valves have been successfully used for valve-in-valve TAVI

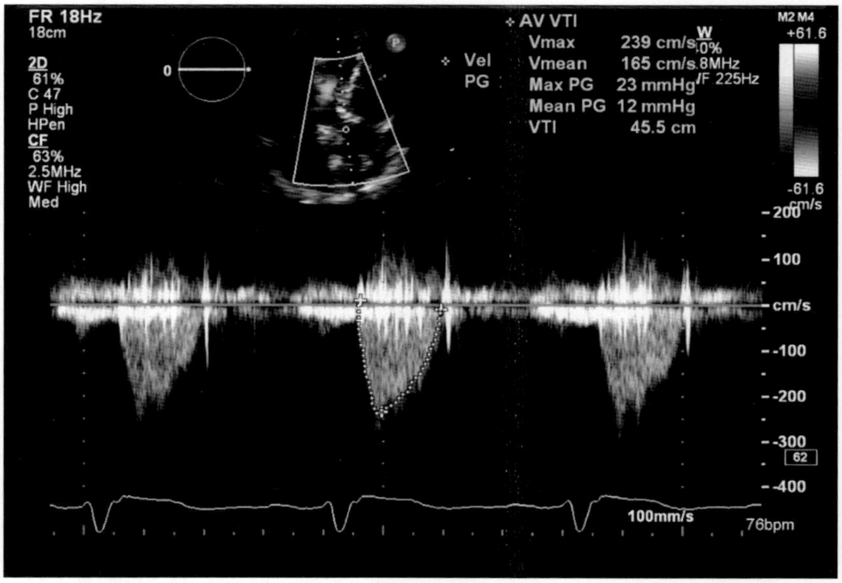

Figure 3: Transaortic Doppler at 30 days after TAVI reveals mean systolic gradient of 12 mmHg and no aortic insufficiency. TAVI = transcatheter aortic valve replacement.

[10–12]. However, balloon-expandable valves have also been used with good results [5]. In the present case, oversizing of the S3 valve relative to the Freestyle inner diameter (23 mm versus 20 mm, resp.) provided some reassurance that device migration or embolization would be unlikely. Furthermore, baseline echocardiography and aortography (in lieu of CT angiography) suggested that the sinuses of Valsalva appeared to be sufficiently spacious and the height of the coronary ostia from the annulus appeared grossly adequate to accommodate the 23 mm S3 valve without causing coronary artery obstruction from the degenerated prosthetic valve leaflets. Fortunately, the aortogram (double the normal contrast volume was used for the injection) nicely opacified the sewing ring of the Freestlye prosthesis which was approximately 2 mm below the bottom of the pigtail catheter in the aortic root. Alignment of the middle marker of the S3 balloon catheter with this plane resulted in perfect implantation depth.

4. Conclusion

We present a challenging case of emergency valve-in-valve TAVI in a stentless bioprosthesis for a patient presenting with severe aortic regurgitation and cardiogenic shock using a balloon-expandable transcatheter valve. This case adds to the experience of the few reported cases of valve-in-valve TAVI for this uniquely challenging patient subset. Prompt diagnosis, preprocedural airway and hemodynamic stabilization, immediate heart team collaboration, and skillful use of invasive and noninvasive imaging were all instrumental in achieving a successful outcome.

Acknowledgments

The authors would like to acknowledge Drs. Nathan Kerner, Marc Sakwa, and Francis Shannon for their contributions to the care of the patient.

References

[1] J. G. Webb, M. J. Mack, J. M. White et al., "Transcatheter aortic valve implantation within degenerated aortic surgical bioprostheses: partner 2 valve-in-valve registry," *Journal of the American College of Cardiology*, vol. 69, no. 18, pp. 2253–2262, 2017.

[2] D. Dvir, J. G. Webb, S. Bleiziffer et al., "Transcatheter aortic valve implantation in failed bioprosthetic surgical valves," *JAMA*, vol. 312, no. 2, pp. 162–170, 2014.

[3] G. M. Deeb, S. J. Chetcuti, M. J. Reardon et al., "1-year results in patients undergoing transcatheter aortic valve replacement with failed surgical bioprostheses," *JACC: Cardiovascular Interventions*, vol. 10, no. 10, pp. 1034–1044, 2017.

[4] D. Dvir, J. Webb, S. Brecker et al., "Transcatheter aortic valve replacement for degenerative bioprosthetic surgical valves: results from the global valve-in-valve registry," *Circulation*, vol. 126, no. 19, pp. 2335–2344, 2012.

[5] R. Bagur, J. Rodes-Cabau, R. De Larochelliere, D. Doyle, M. Rheault, and E. Dumont, "Transfemoral aortic valve-in-valve implantation with a balloon-expandable valve for the treatment of stentless xenograft severe aortic regurgitation," *JACC: Cardiovascular Interventions*, vol. 4, no. 11, pp. 1248-1249, 2011.

[6] F. Chevalier, J. Leipsic, and P. Genereux, "Valve-in-valve implantation with a 23-mm balloon-expandable transcatheter heart valve for the treatment of a 19-mm stentless bioprosthesis severe aortic regurgitation using a strategy of

"extreme" underfilling," *Catheterization and Cardiovascular Interventions*, vol. 84, no. 3, pp. 503–508, 2014.

[7] A. Duncan, S. Davies, C. Di Mario, and N. Moat, "Valve-in-valve transcatheter aortic valve implantation for failing surgical aortic stentless bioprosthetic valves: a single-center experience," *Journal of Thoracic and Cardiovascular Surgery*, vol. 150, no. 1, pp. 91–98, 2015.

[8] F. Pappalardo, D. Regazzoli, A. Mangieri et al., "Hemodynamic and echocardiographic effects of aortic regurgitation on femoro-femoral veno-arterial ECMO," *International Journal of Cardiology*, vol. 202, pp. 760–762, 2016.

[9] A. Halapas, M. Chrissoheris, and K. Spargias, "Challenging transfemoral valve-in-valve implantation in a degenerated stentless bioprosthetic aortic valve," *Journal of Invasive Cardiology*, vol. 26, no. 8, pp. E106–E108, 2014.

[10] J. Cockburn, M. Dooley, J. Parker et al., "Transcatheter aortic valve-in-valve treatment of degenerative stentless supra-annular Freedom Solo valves: a single centre experience," *Catheterization and Cardiovascular Interventions*, vol. 89, no. 3, pp. 438–444, 2017.

[11] G. P. Ussia, M. Barbanti, and C. Tamburino, "Treatment of severe regurgitation of stentless aortic valve prosthesis with a self-expandable biological valve," *Journal of Invasive Cardiology*, vol. 21, no. 3, pp. E51–E54, 2009.

[12] D. Attias, D. Himbert, U. Hvass, and A. Vahanian, ""Valve-in-valve" implantation in a patient with stentless bioprosthesis and severe intraprosthetic aortic regurgitation," *Journal of Thoracic and Cardiovascular Surgery*, vol. 138, no. 4, pp. 1020–1022, 2009.

41

The Wire Rendezvous and Chasing Wire Technique in the Bidirectional Approach for the Percutaneous Coronary Intervention for Chronic Total Occlusion with a Single Guiding Catheter

Keisuke Nakabayashi, Daisuke Sunaga, Nobuhito Kaneko, Akihiro Matsui, Kazuhiko Tanaka, Hiroshi Ando, and Minoru Shimizu

Kasukabe Chuo General Hospital, Heart Center, Saitama, Japan

Correspondence should be addressed to Keisuke Nakabayashi; keisuke2018@gmail.com

Academic Editor: Man-Hong Jim

A bidirectional approach for percutaneous coronary intervention for chronic total occlusion (CTO-PCI) using ipsilateral collaterals with a single guiding catheter limits procedural choices. The CTO of the left circumflex artery with ipsilateral collateral artery was treated by the bidirectional approach using a single guiding catheter. While the retrograde wire directly crossed the CTO lesion, the microcatheter could not pass the CTO lesion despite the conventional strategies. Therefore, we performed the wire rendezvous and chasing wire techniques. The wire rendezvous technique enables deeper retrograde guidewire progression, and the antegrade microcatheter can reach the CTO entry. The chasing wire technique enables the antegrade guidewire to pass the route made by the retrograde guidewire. These techniques might offer a possible solution for bidirectional CTO-PCI using a single guiding catheter. However, this technique should be considered as a last resort because of the risk of rapid reocclusion.

1. Introduction

Percutaneous coronary intervention (PCI) for chronic total occlusion (CTO) has improved not only patients' symptoms [1] and left ventricular function [2] but also long-term mortality [3, 4]. The advancement of techniques [5] and devices [6, 7] for CTO-PCI has contributed to this development. In addition, the procedural steps in current CTO-PCI have also been established [8]. Although the antegrade approaches, including the manipulation of stiff wires, knuckle wire technique, parallel wire technique, subintimal tracking and reentry (STAR) technique [9], contrast-guided STAR technique [10], or reentry devices [11, 12], are important, the retrograde approach is a particularly promising strategy in this era. The most commonly used collateral artery for the retrograde approach is the contralateral collateral artery, e.g., the right coronary artery (RCA) for the left coronary artery. However, some CTO lesions involve the ipsilateral collateral artery, such as the left anterior descending artery (LAD) to the left circumflex artery (LCX) or bridge collateral arteries. CTO-PCI with ipsilateral collateral channels is challenging [13]. A double guiding-catheter strategy, the so called "ping-pong" technique, could be one possible option, which leads to the smooth manipulation of the retrograde approach without interference from the antegrade system. This technique was reported for treating complications [14, 15] and CTO-PCI [16]. On the other hand, the single guiding-catheter strategy could be a less invasive option but limits the procedure choices because of the interferences in both systems. Herein, we present a novel strategy named the wire rendezvous and chasing wire technique. "Wire rendezvous" indicates full insertion of the retrograde wire into the antegrade microcatheter to advance the antegrade microcatheter tracking on the retrograde wire. "Chasing wire" indicates pushing the antegrade guidewire and pulling the retrograde guidewire simultaneously to let

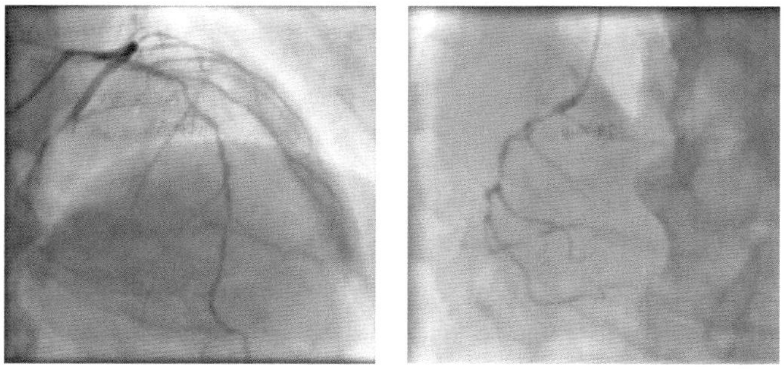

(a) (b)

FIGURE 1: Angiography after the compensation of heart failure reveals severe stenosis with heavy calcification of the left anterior descending artery, chronic total occlusion of the left circumflex artery (a), and hypoplasty of the right coronary artery (b).

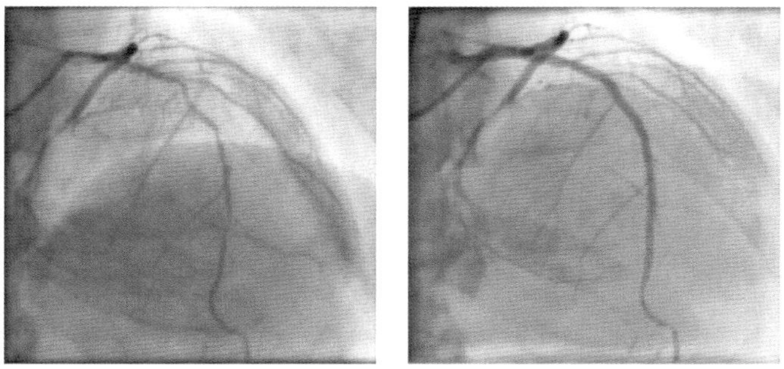

(a) (b)

FIGURE 2: Angiographies before and after the percutaneous coronary intervention to the left anterior descending artery.

the antegrade guidewire track the route made by the retrograde guidewire before reocclusion. These techniques result in antegrade CTO crossing. These techniques could be options in the bidirectional approach for CTO-PCI using the single guiding catheter.

2. Case Presentation

A 78-year-old man with heart failure and low ejection fraction was referred to our institution. Electrocardiogram showed sinus rhythm, heart rate of 82 beats, and complete left branch bundle block. Laboratory data indicated 1.04 mg/dL of creatinine, 7.0% of HbA1c, and 268 pg/mL of brain natriuretic protein. Echocardiography showed an ejection fraction of 30%, left ventricle diastolic diameter of 60 mm, diffuse hypokinesis, and apical akinesis. Angiography after compensated heart failure revealed hypoplasty of the right coronary artery, severe stenosis with heavy calcification of the LAD, and CTO of the LCX (Figure 1). We first treated the LAD with standard stenting (Figure 2). Computed tomography after successful revascularization of LAD revealed a short and mildly calcified CTO; and a stump was revealed after sending out the small branch (Figure 3(a)). Thereafter, we tried to treat the LCX-CTO. The middle LCX was occluded with a Rentrop grade 2 collateral flow from the posterolateral branch channel and the apical channel (Figure 3(b), Videos 1–2). However, interventional collateral channels were unclear.

We started PCI with the antegrade approach. We engaged an SPB 3.0, 8Fr (ASAHI Intecc, Nagoya, Japan) in the left coronary artery and progressed with the XT-R (ASAHI Intecc) supported by Corsair Pro (ASAHI Intecc) into the CTO stump. However, stiff wires and the parallel wire technique resulted in subintimal wiring (Figure 4). We chose to convert to the retrograde approach. Tip injection revealed that the apical channel was connected to the posterolateral branch (Figure 5(a)). The SUOH 03 (ASAHI Intecc) passed the channel and bidirectional angiography revealed the short CTO length (Figure 5(b)), and the Gaia 2nd (ASAHI Intecc) directly crossed the CTO lesion (Figure 5(c)). Intravascular ultrasound imaging confirmed that the retrograde wire was in the true lumen (Figure 5(d)). However, a Mizuki (KANEKA MEDIX, Osaka, Japan) microcatheter could not pass the CTO lesion despite wire trapping by balloon catheter in the middle of the LCX. Even after the progression of the Gaia 2nd directly into the guiding catheter, the microcatheter could not pass the CTO lesion. Attempts were made to instead use the new Caravel microcatheter (ASAHI Intecc), which is thinner and has a softer body; however, it could not pass the CTO lesion as well. Thus, we planned to catch the retrograde wire with a snaring catheter, but that did not work. Therefore, we performed the rendezvous technique that meant full insertion of the

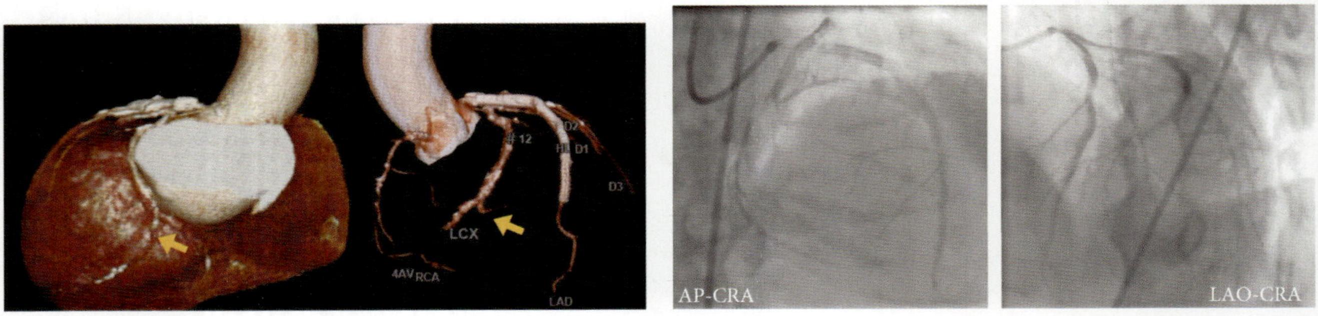

(a) (b)

FIGURE 3: (a) Computed tomography after successful revascularization of the left anterior descending artery; the short and mildly calcified chronic total occlusion of the left circumflex artery; a stump presents after sending out the small branch (yellow arrows). (b) The middle left circumflex artery is occluded with Rentrop grade 2 collateral flow from the posterolateral branch channel and the apical channel. AP: antero-posterior; CRA: cranial; LAO: left anterior oblique.

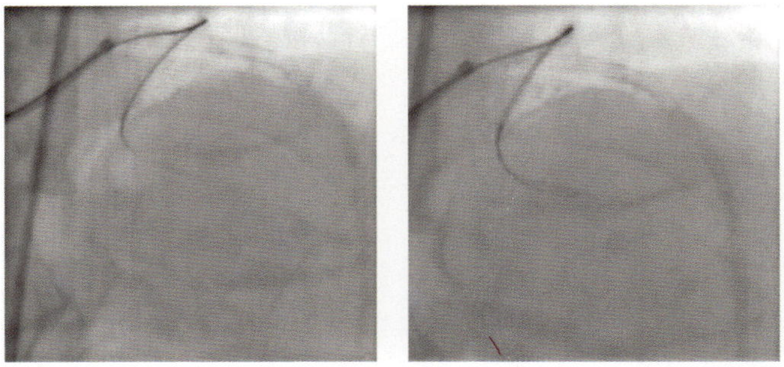

(a) (b)

FIGURE 4: The antegrade approach with tapered wire (a) and stiff wires using the parallel wire technique (b) results in subintimal wiring.

retrograde Gaia 2nd into the antegrade Corsair Pro (Figure 6(a), Video 3). The antegrade Corsair Pro could advance into the CTO, tracking on the retrograde guidewire, but could not pass through the CTO completely (Figure 6(b)). Then, we tried the chasing wire technique, pushing the antegrade wire and pulling the retrograde wire simultaneously (Figure 7, Video 4). We chose the SION black (ASAHI Intecc) polymer jacket wire as an antegrade wire expecting smooth tracking along the route made by the retrograde guidewire before reocclusion. These techniques resulted in antegrade CTO crossing. We subsequently dilated the CTO with a small balloon and deployed the drug-eluting stent as usual (Figure 8, Videos 5–6).

3. Discussion

The CTO-PCI was developed along with novel techniques and devices [6, 7]. In particular, the bidirectional approach led to dramatic improvements in CTO-PCI success rates [5]. If interventionists established the bidirectional approach, some strategies, such as the direct retrograde guidewire crossing, kissing-wire technique, controlled antegrade and retrograde subintimal tracking (CART) technique [17, 18], or reverse CART technique [19], can be considered. After the retrograde guidewire has crossed the CTO lesion, the wire externalization can primarily be attempted and the retrograde microcatheter is required to reach the antegrade guiding catheter. Bidirectional approach for CTO-PCI with a single guiding catheter limits procedural choices in this situation. In the double guiding-catheter system, if the retrograde microcatheter could not track on the retrograde guidewire similar to our case, then (1) using a new microcatheter, (2) applying a guide-extension catheter, (3) performing wire trapping in the guiding catheter, or (4) catching the wire by snare catheter can be considered. Option 1 failed. Option 2, which utilized a small-sized catheter (e.g., 6Fr guide-extension catheter for 7Fr guiding catheter), was feasible, and the gap allowed the retrograde guidewire to progress in the antegrade guiding catheter; however, this was not considered at that time. In addition, options 3 and 4 are complicated when conducted via the bidirectional approach using the ipsilateral collaterals with the single guiding catheter. One solution could be the wire rendezvous technique and the chasing wire technique.

The wire rendezvous technique was first reported by Kim et al. [20]. They reported that the antegrade and retrograde microcatheters were aligned in the same guiding catheter, and the antegrade guidewire advanced into the retrograde microcatheter and reached the distal CTO lumen. The difference in the current case was that the

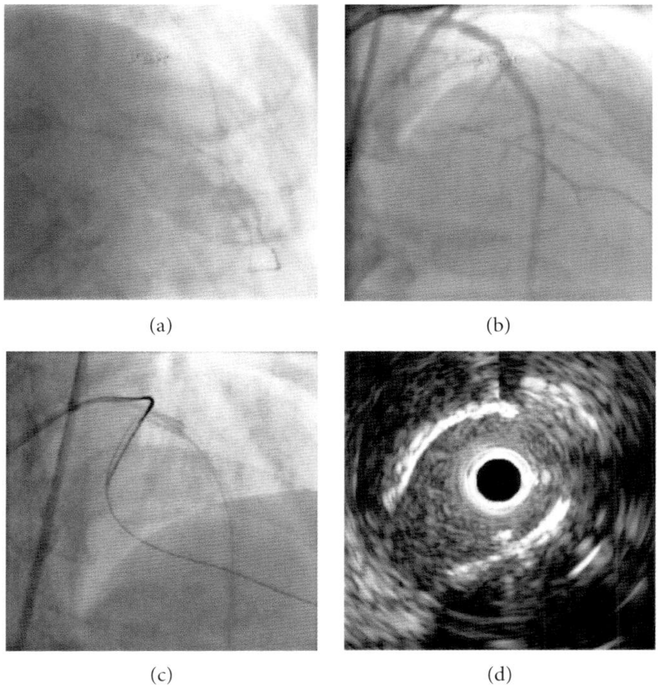

FIGURE 5: (a) Tip injection reveals the connection from the apical channel to the posterolateral branch. (b) The bidirectional angiography shows the short chronic total occlusion length. (c) The Gaia 2nd directly crosses the chronic total occlusion lesion. (d) The intravascular ultrasound imaging confirms that the retrograde wire is in the true lumen.

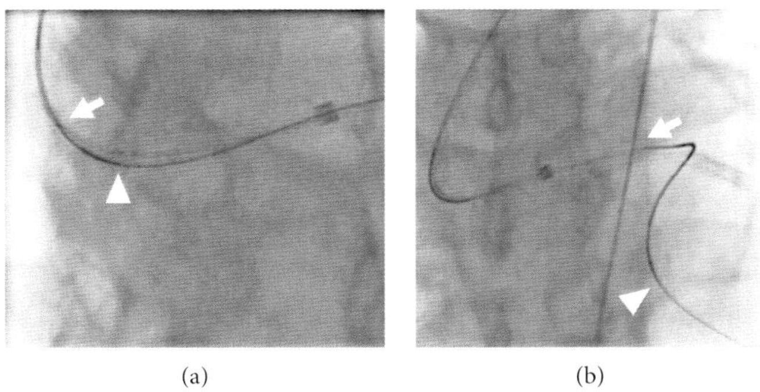

FIGURE 6: The wire rendezvous technique. (a) The insertion of the retrograde Gaia 2nd into the antegrade Corsair Pro. (b) The antegrade Corsair Pro advance in the chronic total occlusion, tracking on the retrograde guidewire, but cannot pass the chronic total occlusion completely. The arrowheads indicate the tip of the Corsair Pro. The arrows indicate the tip of the retrograde Gaia 2nd.

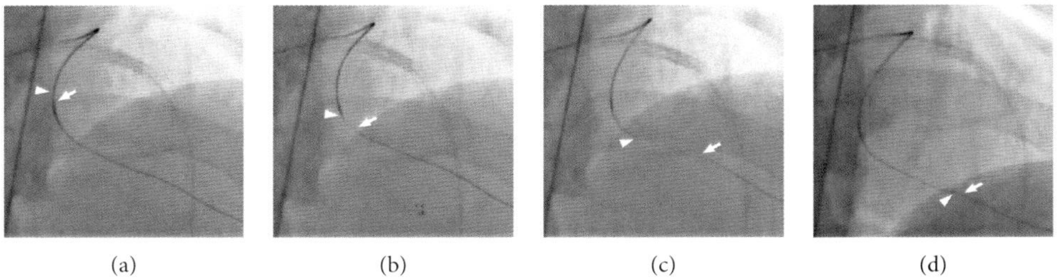

FIGURE 7: The chasing wire technique, pushing the antegrade guidewire and pulling the retrograde guidewire simultaneously. The arrowheads indicate the tip of the Corsair Pro. The arrows indicate the tip of the antegrade SION black. The arrows indicate the tip of the retrograde Gaia 2nd.

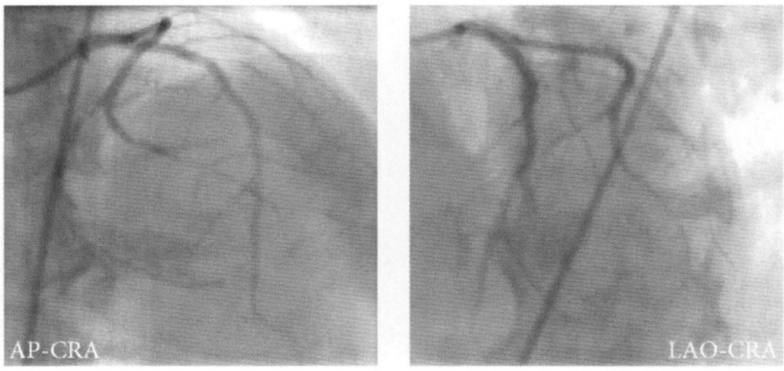

Figure 8: The final angiography. AP: antero-posterior; CRA: cranial; LAO: left anterior oblique.

retrograde microcatheter could not pass the CTO lesion. Therefore, we were required to perform the rendezvous technique inside the guiding catheter. There are recommendations regarding this approach. The rendezvous point should be at the greater curvature of the guiding catheter in the aortic sinus or aortic arch. Furthermore, inserting the guidewire near the tip of the microcatheter suppresses the microcatheter motion. In addition, several antegrade penetrations resulted in a large antegrade false lumen, which complicated securing the true lumen. Therefore, the antegrade microcatheter tracked on the retrograde guidewire, and the tip of that reached into the CTO entry, but not through the CTO lesion. This guaranteed that the antegrade guidewire was able to penetrate the true lumen from the CTO entry. Therefore, Corsair microcatheter could be suitable as the antegrade microcatheter.

To the best of our knowledge, the chasing wire technique has not been reported in the literature. The retrograde guidewire created a space with a width of 0.014 inches. Though this space might reocclude after wire retrieval, certain time lags could be expected. Therefore, we progressed the antegrade guidewire and pulled the retrograde guidewire simultaneously. The antegrade guidewire crossed the CTO through the space made by the retrograde guidewire. A polymer-coated wire, such as the SION black guidewire like our case, could be suitable as the antegrade wire because the surface of the CTO route might be narrow and rough. A tapered wire could also be appropriate in this situation, since the acute narrowing of the CTO route would occur after retrieving the retrograde guidewire.

Although the above techniques are technically feasible, they should be considered as last resort techniques because of the risk of rapid reocclusion. Since we easily succeeded in the direct retrograde guidewire crossing, recrossing seemed possible if needed. However, a very long CTO or a CTO requiring the CART technique can be riskier. In such cases, we should consider switching to the double guiding-catheter system by puncturing another access site.

4. Conclusion

Bidirectional approach for CTO-PCI using ipsilateral collaterals with single guiding catheter limits procedural choices. The wire rendezvous technique and the chasing wire technique might be possible solutions.

Abbreviations

CTO: Chronic total occlusion
LAD: Left anterior descending artery
LCX: Left circumflex artery
PCI: Percutaneous coronary artery
RCA: Right coronary artery.

Disclosure

This case was presented as an oral presentation in the Transcatheter Cardiovascular Therapeutics in Asia Pan-pacific (TCTAP) National Meeting 2018 (http://www.summit-tctap.com/2018/submission_case_accept.php), as the Winner for Case Competition of Complex PCI. In addition, the Journal of American College of Cardiology published only the abstract for this summit, which is available in https://www.sciencedirect.com/science/article/pii/S0735109718339019?via%3Dihub or http://www.onlinejacc.org/content/71/16_Supplement/S156.

References

[1] D. Joyal, J. Afilalo, and S. Rinfret, "Effectiveness of recanalization of chronic total occlusions: a systematic review and meta-analysis," *American Heart Journal*, vol. 160, no. 1, pp. 179–187, 2010.

[2] A. S. H. Cheng, J. B. Selvanayagam, M. Jerosch-Herold et al., "Percutaneous treatment of chronic total coronary occlusions improves regional hyperemic myocardial blood flow and contractility: insights from quantitative cardiovascular magnetic resonance imaging," *JACC: Cardiovascular Interventions*, vol. 1, no. 1, pp. 44–53, 2008.

[3] D. A. Jones, R. Weerackody, K. Rathod et al., "Successful recanalization of chronic total occlusions is associated with improved long-term survival," *JACC. Cardiovascular Interventions*, vol. 5, no. 4, pp. 380–388, 2012.

[4] S. George, J. Cockburn, T. C. Clayton et al., "Long-term follow-up of elective chronic total coronary occlusion angioplasty: analysis from the U.K. central cardiac audit database," *Journal of the American College of Cardiology*, vol. 64, no. 3, pp. 235–243, 2014.

[5] S. Rathore, O. Katoh, H. Matsuo et al., "Retrograde percutaneous recanalization of chronic total occlusion of the coronary arteries: procedural outcomes and predictors of success in contemporary practice," *Circulation. Cardiovascular Interventions*, vol. 2, no. 2, pp. 124–132, 2009.

[6] S. Rathore, H. Matsuo, M. Terashima et al., "Procedural and in-hospital outcomes after percutaneous coronary intervention for chronic total occlusions of coronary arteries 2002 to 2008: impact of novel guidewire techniques," *JACC: Cardiovascular Interventions*, vol. 2, no. 6, pp. 489–497, 2009.

[7] E. Tsuchikane, O. Katoh, M. Kimura, K. Nasu, Y. Kinoshita, and T. Suzuki, "The first clinical experience with a novel catheter for collateral channel tracking in retrograde approach for chronic coronary total occlusions," *JACC. Cardiovascular Interventions*, vol. 3, no. 2, pp. 165–171, 2010.

[8] S. Sumitsuji, K. Inoue, M. Ochiai, E. Tsuchikane, and F. Ikeno, "Fundamental wire technique and current standard strategy of percutaneous intervention for chronic total occlusion with histopathological insights," *JACC. Cardiovascular Interventions*, vol. 4, no. 9, pp. 941–951, 2011.

[9] A. Colombo, G. W. Mikhail, I. Michev et al., "Treating chronic total occlusions using subintimal tracking and reentry: the STAR technique," *Catheterization and Cardiovascular Interventions*, vol. 64, no. 4, pp. 407–411, 2005.

[10] M. Carlino, C. Godino, A. Latib, J. W. Moses, and A. Colombo, "Subintimal tracking and re-entry technique with contrast guidance: a safer approach," *Catheterization and Cardiovascular Interventions*, vol. 72, no. 6, pp. 790–796, 2008.

[11] E. S. Brilakis, W. B. Lombardi, and S. Banerjee, "Use of the Stingray guidewire and the Venture catheter for crossing flush coronary chronic total occlusions due to in-stent restenosis," *Catheterization and Cardiovascular Interventions*, vol. 76, no. 3, pp. 391–394, 2010.

[12] P. L. Whitlow, M. N. Burke, W. L. Lombardi et al., "Use of a novel crossing and re-entry system in coronary chronic total occlusions that have failed standard crossing techniques: results of the FAST-CTOs (facilitated antegrade steering technique in chronic total occlusions) trial," *JACC. Cardiovascular Interventions*, vol. 5, no. 4, pp. 393–401, 2012.

[13] L. Azzalini, P. Agostoni, S. Benincasa et al., "Retrograde chronic total occlusion percutaneous coronary intervention through ipsilateral collateral channels: a multicenter registry," *JACC: Cardiovascular Interventions*, vol. 10, no. 15, pp. 1489–1497, 2017.

[14] G. Christopoulos, R. V. Menon, D. Karmpaliotis et al., "The efficacy and safety of the "hybrid" approach to coronary chronic total occlusions: insights from a contemporary multicenter US registry and comparison with prior studies," *The Journal of Invasive Cardiology*, vol. 26, no. 9, pp. 427–432, 2014.

[15] C. P. Lin, J. H. Wang, W. L. Lee et al., "Mechanism and management of burr entrapment: a nightmare of interventional cardiologists," *Journal of Geriatric Cardiology*, vol. 10, no. 3, pp. 230–234, 2013.

[16] M. Koutouzis, G. Avdikos, G. Nikitas et al., ""Ping-pong" technique for treating a balloon uncrossable chronic total occlusion," *Cardiovascular Revascularization Medicine*, vol. 19, no. 1, pp. 117–119, 2018.

[17] J. F. Surmely, E. Tsuchikane, O. Katoh et al., "New concept for CTO recanalization using controlled antegrade and retrograde subintimal tracking: the CART technique," *The Journal of Invasive Cardiology*, vol. 18, no. 7, pp. 334–338, 2006.

[18] M. Kimura, O. Katoh, E. Tsuchikane et al., "The efficacy of a bilateral approach for treating lesions with chronic total occlusions the CART (controlled antegrade and retrograde subintimal tracking) registry," *JACC. Cardiovascular Interventions*, vol. 2, no. 11, pp. 1135–1141, 2009.

[19] D. Dash, "Retrograde coronary chronic total occlusion intervention using a novel reverse controlled antegrade and retrograde subintimal tracking," *Journal of Interventional Cardiology*, vol. 29, no. 1, pp. 70–74, 2016.

[20] M. H. Kim, L. H. Yu, and K. Mitsudo, "A new retrograde wiring technique for chronic total occlusion," *Catheterization and Cardiovascular Interventions*, vol. 75, no. 1, pp. 117–119, 2010.

A Novel Double Side Branch Protection Technique for a Left Main Trifurcation Lesion: Simultaneous Jailed Balloon and Jailed Corsair Technique

Masahito Munakata,[1] Yohei Numasawa,[2] Shiro Ishikawa,[1] and Takashi Koyama[1]

[1]*Department of Cardiology, Saitama Municipal Hospital, Saitama, Japan*
[2]*Department of Cardiology, Japanese Red Cross Ashikaga Hospital, Ashikaga, Japan*

Correspondence should be addressed to Yohei Numasawa; numasawa@cpnet.med.keio.ac.jp

Academic Editor: Markus Ferrari

Percutaneous coronary intervention for left main trifurcation disease is challenging. Although side branch protection techniques such as the jailed balloon technique and jailed Corsair technique are the established methods for treatment of coronary bifurcation lesions, little is known regarding the application and feasibility of these techniques for left main trifurcation disease. We herein describe a 72-year-old man with angina pectoris who was successfully treated with percutaneous coronary stent implantation for a left main trifurcation lesion. In this case, we performed a novel double side branch protection technique, the simultaneous jailed balloon and jailed Corsair technique, with a single 8 Fr guiding catheter. This is the first case report to highlight the feasibility and efficacy of combined use of the jailed balloon and jailed Corsair techniques during percutaneous coronary intervention for left main trifurcation disease.

1. Introduction

Percutaneous coronary intervention (PCI) for left main trifurcation disease remains one of the most technically challenging procedures for interventional cardiologists, even with the currently available drug-eluting stents (DESs). In general, provisional stenting using the jailed wire technique is considered the standard method for most coronary bifurcation lesions [1]. However, even when a protective guide wire is inserted into the side branch prior to main vessel stenting, there remains a risk of side branch occlusion after stent implantation due to plaque or carina shift [2, 3]. To overcome these difficulties associated with PCI for bifurcation lesions, the jailed balloon technique and jailed Corsair technique have been established [3–9]. Although these techniques are useful, PCI is more complex for coronary trifurcation than bifurcation lesions [10–13], and little is known regarding the application and feasibility of these side branch protection techniques for left main trifurcation disease. We herein describe a 72-year-old man with angina pectoris who was successfully treated with percutaneous coronary stent implantation for a left main trifurcation lesion using the simultaneous jailed balloon and jailed Corsair technique.

2. Case Presentation

A 72-year-old man presented to our hospital with a chief complaint of chest pain on exertion. He had multiple coronary risk factors including hypertension, dyslipidemia, and diabetes mellitus. Electrocardiography revealed no clear findings of ischemic ST-T changes or prior Q-wave myocardial infarction. Transthoracic echocardiography revealed an ejection fraction of 63.3% with mild left ventricular hypertrophy and no segmental wall motion abnormality. Coronary computed tomography angiography revealed a mixed plaque in the distal left main trifurcation with suspicion of significant stenosis. He was admitted to our hospital to undergo

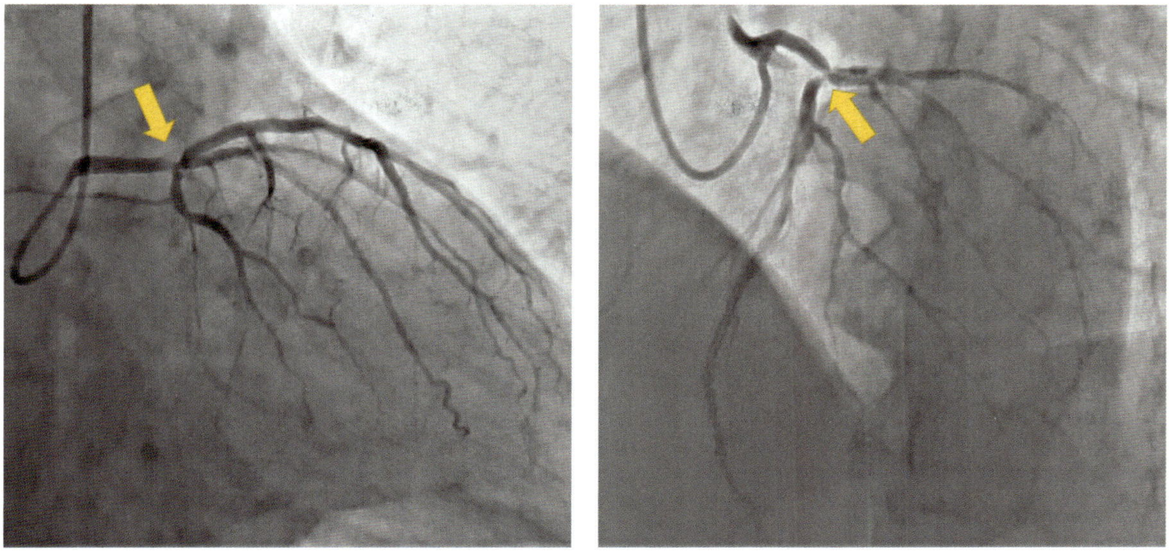

(a) (b)

Figure 1: Left coronary angiogram of the (a) right anterior oblique caudal view and (b) left anterior oblique cranial view revealed a significant distal left main trifurcation lesion (yellow arrows).

coronary angiography with a diagnosis of stable exertional angina pectoris.

Diagnostic coronary angiography revealed distal left main trifurcation disease including significant stenosis in the distal left main trunk (LMT), ostial left anterior descending artery (LAD), and ostial left circumflex artery (LCX) (modified Medina classification 1-1-1-0) (Figure 1) [11]. No significant stenosis was present in the right coronary artery. Because the SYNTAX score was calculated as 15 [14] and the patient refused a surgical approach, PCI using a DES was planned. Because both the LCX and intermediate branch were large vessels, it was essential to preserve the blood flow of these side branches after main vessel stenting. Therefore, we decided to perform PCI using the simultaneous jailed balloon and jailed Corsair technique for this left main trifurcation lesion.

After obtaining informed consent, PCI for the left main trifurcation lesion was performed. An 8 Fr AL 1.0 guiding catheter with a side hole (Hyperion; Asahi Intecc, Aichi, Japan) was engaged into the left coronary artery via the right femoral artery. A SION guide wire (Asahi Intecc) was initially inserted into the LAD. To protect the two large side branches, a Balance Middleweight Universal II guide wire (Abbott Vascular Japan, Tokyo, Japan) and a SION Blue guide wire (Asahi Intecc) with a Corsair Pro microcatheter (Asahi Intecc) were introduced into the intermediate branch and LCX, respectively (Figure 2(a)).

According to the angiographic and intravascular ultrasound images, we decided to perform direct crossover stenting from the LMT to LAD using the simultaneous jailed balloon and jailed Corsair technique. A DES (SYNERGY 3.0×16 mm; Boston Scientific, Natick, MA, USA) was advanced into the LAD, and a semicompliant balloon (canPass 2.5×15 mm; Japan Lifeline, Tokyo, Japan) was advanced into the intermediate branch. Subsequently, a Corsair Pro microcatheter was introduced into the LCX. The simultaneous jailed balloon and jailed Corsair technique was then performed. The side branch balloon in the intermediate branch was initially inflated at low pressure (3 atm) (Figure 2(b)). The main branch stent balloon in the LMT to LAD was then inflated three times at nominal pressure (11 atm), which simultaneously jailed the side branch semi-inflated balloon in the intermediate branch and the Corsair Pro microcatheter in the LCX (Figure 2(c)). When the jailed Corsair Pro microcatheter was removed with rotation of the shaft, only small friction was felt. Blood flow was preserved in both the intermediate branch and the LCX after main vessel stenting, and there were no signs of plaque or carina shift into the side branches (Figure 2(d)).

After reinsertion of a SION Black guide wire (Asahi Intecc) into the jailed intermediate branch via stent struts using a double-lumen catheter (Crusade K; Kaneka Medix, Osaka, Japan), kissing balloon inflation was performed with a 3.0×16 mm stent balloon in the LAD and a 2.5×15 mm canPass balloon in the intermediate branch (Figure 2(e)). Final kissing balloon angioplasty was then performed with a 3.0×16 mm stent balloon in the LAD and a 2.5×15 mm canPass balloon in the LCX (Figure 2(f)). A final coronary angiogram showed excellent results without any complications, including side branch narrowing or occlusion (Figure 3). The postprocedure course was uneventful, and no major complications including ischemic events, heart failure, or access-site complications were observed. The patient was discharged the day after the procedure, and his angina symptom completely disappeared after PCI.

Because left main trifurcation was anatomically crucial, an early follow-up coronary angiography was performed 2 weeks after the procedure. It showed excellent results and no findings of restenosis in both the main vessel and side branches. In addition, fractional flow reserve (FFR) was

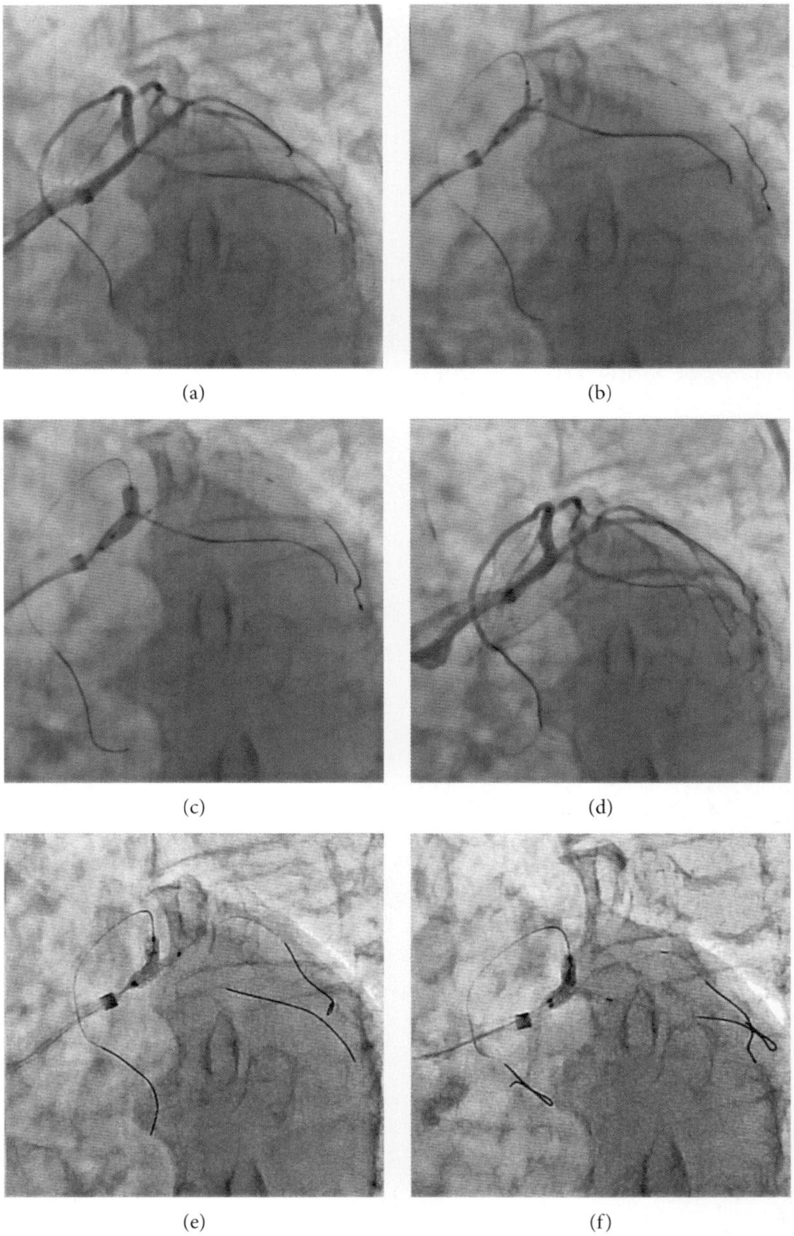

Figure 2: Stent implantation using the simultaneous jailed balloon and jailed Corsair technique. (a) Left coronary angiogram of the left anterior oblique caudal view before stent implantation. (b) The side branch balloon in the intermediate branch was initially inflated. (c) The main branch stent balloon was inflated, which jailed the side branch semi-inflated balloon in the intermediate branch and the Corsair Pro microcatheter in the left circumflex artery. (d) Blood flow was preserved in both side branches after stenting. (e, f) Final kissing balloon inflations were performed.

measured and there were no signs of significant ischemia in both distal LAD (FFR: 0.88) and LCX (FFR: 1.00).

3. Discussion

This case report highlights the feasibility and efficacy of the simultaneous jailed balloon and jailed Corsair technique with a single 8 Fr guiding catheter for the treatment of left main trifurcation disease. To the best of our knowledge, this is the first case report detailing successful percutaneous coronary stent implantation using this technique.

PCI for coronary bifurcation or trifurcation lesions, especially with left main trunk disease, remains challenging and is associated with a risk of side branch occlusion and a high rate of target lesion revascularization [11, 12]. The provisional stenting method using the jailed wire technique is generally recommended for most coronary bifurcation lesions [1]. However, side branch occlusion or side branch narrowing after main vessel stenting sometimes occurs because of

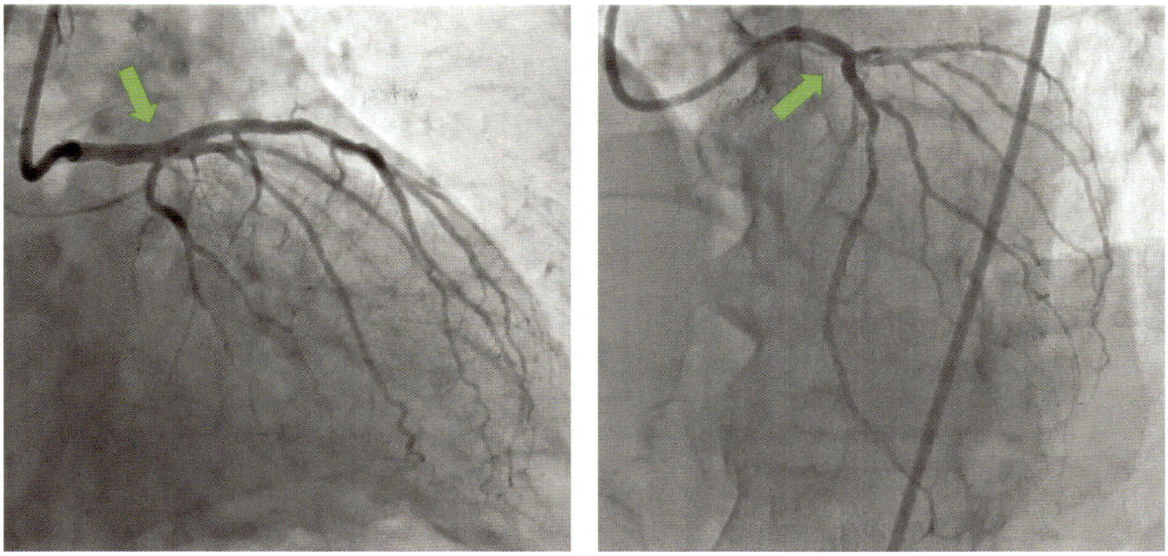

(a) (b)

FIGURE 3: Final coronary angiogram of the (a) right anterior oblique caudal view and (b) left anterior oblique cranial view showed excellent results without any complications including side branch narrowing or occlusion (green arrows).

plaque or carina shift, even when a protective guide wire is inserted into the side branch prior to stent implantation [2, 3]. Once the blood flow of the side branch is impaired, serious myocardial ischemia may develop along with chest pain and hemodynamic instability, even when the blood flow impairment is temporary [13]. Therefore, efforts to reduce the risk of temporary or chronic side branch occlusion during PCI are crucial. In addition, PCI is more complex for coronary trifurcation than for bifurcation lesions [10–13]. Although coronary artery bypass grafting surgery is generally recommended for patients with left main trifurcation disease, especially those with ostial plaque involvement of side branches, PCI may sometimes be required in selected patients with acute coronary syndrome at presentation and intolerance of or refusal to undergo a surgical approach mainly because of old age or systemic comorbidities [13].

To overcome difficulties associated with PCI for bifurcation lesions, the jailed balloon technique and jailed Corsair technique have been established [3–9]. The jailed semi-inflated balloon technique provides a high rate of procedural success and preservation of the side branch blood flow after main vessel stenting mainly because it prevents carina or plaque shift [5, 8]. However, this technique is associated with potential risks including jailed balloon entrapment, balloon rupture, and dissection of the side branch ostium by balloon inflation even with low pressure. Compared with the jailed balloon technique, the jailed Corsair technique is more suitable for protecting a small side branch, and the risk of dissection at the ostium of the side branch is lower [9]. In addition, because the shaft of the Corsair Pro microcatheter has both high strength and excellent lubricity due to its hydrophilic coating, the risk of device entrapment is minimal. The concept of the jailed Corsair technique is consistent with the "keep it open strategy" stated in the consensus document of the European Bifurcation Club [1]. Taking these advantages and disadvantages of the jailed balloon technique and jailed Corsair technique into account, the combined use of these two techniques for left main trifurcation disease may be reasonable. Because the intermediate branch was larger than the LCX in this case, we simultaneously performed the jailed balloon technique in the intermediate branch and the jailed Corsair technique in the LCX during main vessel stenting.

Our case report indicates that the basic treatment concepts for most coronary bifurcation lesions can be applied to trifurcation lesions including the jailed balloon and jailed Corsair technique. A provisional strategy with a single stent may also be a standard method, even in patients with left main trifurcation disease [11, 12], although the two side branches should be protected separately. In this situation, the simultaneous jailed balloon and jailed Corsair technique with a single 8 Fr guiding catheter is a useful alternative, as shown in this case report.

The simultaneous jailed balloon and jailed Corsair technique has some limitations. First, this technique requires an 8 Fr guiding catheter for simultaneous insertion of a stent delivery system, balloon catheter, and Corsair microcatheter. Therefore, this technique cannot be performed via the radial artery. Second, because the proximal marker of the side branch balloon should be located more proximal to the stent edge to prevent entrapment [6, 8], a long balloon with double radiopaque markers is necessary. Finally, the use of a semi-inflated balloon or Corsair microcatheter for side branch protection is off-label, and it may also be associated with an increase in the total procedural cost.

4. Conclusion

The simultaneous jailed balloon and jailed Corsair technique is a novel and effective double side branch protection technique for the treatment of left main trifurcation disease in selected patients. Further studies on this technique in larger populations are needed.

Acknowledgments

We thank Angela Morben, DVM, ELS, from Edanz Group (http://www.edanzediting.com/ac), for editing a draft of this manuscript.

References

[1] J. F. Lassen, F. Burzotta, A. P. Banning et al., "Percutaneous coronary intervention for the left main stem and other bifurcation lesions: 12th consensus document from the European Bifurcation Club," *EuroIntervention*, vol. 13, no. 13, pp. 1540–1553, 2018.

[2] J. Y. Hahn, W. J. Chun, J. H. Kim et al., "Predictors and outcomes of side branch occlusion after main vessel stenting in coronary bifurcation lesions: results from the COBIS II Registry (COronary BIfurcation Stenting)," *Journal of the American College of Cardiology*, vol. 62, no. 18, pp. 1654–1659, 2013.

[3] F. Burzotta and C. Trani, "Jailed balloon protection and rescue balloon jailing techniques set the field for safer bifurcation provisional stenting," *International Journal of Cardiology*, vol. 201, pp. 376-377, 2015.

[4] F. Burzotta, C. Trani, and G. Sianos, "Jailed balloon protection: a new technique to avoid acute side-branch occlusion during provisional stenting of bifurcated lesions. Bench test report and first clinical experience," *EuroIntervention*, vol. 5, no. 7, pp. 809–813, 2010.

[5] M. Cayli, T. Seker, M. Gur et al., "A novel-modified provisional bifurcation stenting technique: jailed semi-inflated balloon technique," *Journal of Interventional Cardiology*, vol. 28, no. 5, pp. 420–429, 2015.

[6] J. P. Depta, Y. Patel, J. S. Patel et al., "Long-term clinical outcomes with the use of a modified provisional jailed-balloon stenting technique for the treatment of nonleft main coronary bifurcation lesions," *Catheterization and Cardiovascular Interventions*, vol. 82, no. 5, pp. E637–E646, 2013.

[7] J. Singh, Y. Patel, J. P. Depta et al., "A modified provisional stenting approach to coronary bifurcation lesions: clinical application of the "jailed-balloon technique"," *Journal of Interventional Cardiology*, vol. 25, no. 3, pp. 289–296, 2012.

[8] Y. Numasawa, H. Hase, H. Yamazaki et al., "Three-dimensional optical frequency domain imaging of a true bifurcation lesion after stent implantation using the jailed semi-inflated balloon technique," *SAGE Open Medical Case Reports*, vol. 5, 2017.

[9] Y. Numasawa, K. Sakakura, K. Yamamoto et al., "A novel side branch protection technique in coronary stent implantation: jailed Corsair technique," *Cardiovascular Revascularization Medicine*, vol. 18, no. 4, pp. 295–298, 2017.

[10] U. Lopez-Pena, F. Garcia-Garcia, R. Robledo-Nolasco, E. Fernandez-Cesena, R. Borrego-Montoya, and N. Morales, "Distal left main trifurcation disease in a patient with porcelain aorta," *Cardiovascular Revascularization Medicine*, vol. 18, no. 5, pp. S27–S29, 2017.

[11] A. Ielasi, K. Takagi, A. Latib et al., "Long-term clinical outcomes following drug-eluting stent implantation for unprotected distal trifurcation left main disease: the Milan-New Tokyo (MITO) registry," *Catheterization and Cardiovascular Interventions*, vol. 83, no. 4, pp. 530–538, 2014.

[12] S. Kubo, K. Kadota, M. Sabbah et al., "Clinical and angiographic outcomes after drug-eluting stent implantation with triple-kissing-balloon technique for left main trifurcation lesion: comparison of single-stent and multi-stent procedures," *The Journal of Invasive Cardiology*, vol. 26, no. 11, pp. 571–578, 2014.

[13] L. Testa and F. Bedogni, "How should I treat a coronary "traffic jam"? A triple kissing balloon in distal left main trifurcation," *EuroIntervention*, vol. 6, no. 8, pp. 1011–1016, 2011.

[14] G. Sianos, M. A. Morel, A. P. Kappetein et al., "The SYNTAX score: an angiographic tool grading the complexity of coronary artery disease," *EuroIntervention*, vol. 1, no. 2, pp. 219–227, 2005.

Incidental Finding of the Anomalous Origin of Left Main Coronary Artery from Pulmonary Artery in an Adult Presenting with Arrhythmia-Induced Myocardial Ischemia

Shantanu Patil,[1] Mahek Shah,[2] Brijesh Patel,[2] Lohit Garg,[2] Larry Jacobs,[2] Nauman Islam,[2] and Matthew Martinez[2]

[1]*Department of Medicine, SSM Health St. Mary's Hospital, St. Louis, MO, USA*
[2]*Department of Cardiology, Lehigh Valley Hospital, Allentown, PA, USA*

Correspondence should be addressed to Shantanu Patil; shantanu115@gmail.com

Academic Editor: Ertugrul Ercan

Anomalous origin of the left main coronary artery from the pulmonary artery (ALCAPA) is a rare congenital coronary anomaly with high mortality. It is associated with cardiovascular complications and is usually diagnosed soon after birth. Those who survive into adulthood can present with signs of myocardial infarction, heart failure, mitral regurgitation, severe pulmonary hypertension, or sudden cardiac death. We present a 53-year-old female presenting with atrial fibrillation and found to have an incidental diagnosis of ALCAPA who refused surgical correction. We also review the epidemiology, diagnosis, age-based clinical presentations, and treatment options for ALCAPA.

1. Introduction

Coronary artery anomalies may be found in up to 1% of the general population [1]. Mostly, these anomalies are benign and can be found incidentally [2]. But certain coronary artery anomalies are associated with life-threatening cardiac complications including heart failure, ischemia, arrhythmias, and death. Anomalous origin of the left main coronary artery from pulmonary artery (ALCAPA), also known as Bland–White–Garland syndrome, is a rare congenital abnormality with high mortality. It causes a left to right shunt, thereby causing "coronary steal" and impaired myocardial perfusion. It is most commonly detected within the first one or two months of life. ALCAPA syndrome is one of the commonest causes of myocardial ischemia and infarction in children. If left untreated, up to 90% of patients with ALCAPA syndrome die within the first year of life [3]. Those who survive into adulthood can present with signs of myocardial infarction, heart failure, mitral regurgitation, severe pulmonary hypertension, or sudden cardiac death. In recent years, reports of adult patients with benign clinical presentation have been described. We present one such adult with undiagnosed ALCAPA syndrome presenting with atrial fibrillation accompanied by significant elevations in cardiac enzymes.

2. Case Description

A 53-year-old healthy female with known hypothyroidism being treated with thyroid hormone replacement presented to the emergency department with sudden-onset chest pain and palpitations. Her electrocardiogram revealed atrial fibrillation with a ventricular rate of 140 beats per minute. Cardiac auscultation revealed a continuous murmur at the left sternal border. She spontaneously converted to normal sinus rhythm with complete resolution of her chest pain. Her troponin I level was 17 ng/ml. EKG-gated multidetector cardiac computed tomographic angiography revealed the presence of a large anomalous left main coronary arising from the main pulmonary artery (Figure 1). The left anterior descending artery, diagonal branch, and left circumflex arteries arising from the left main were ectatic vessels with

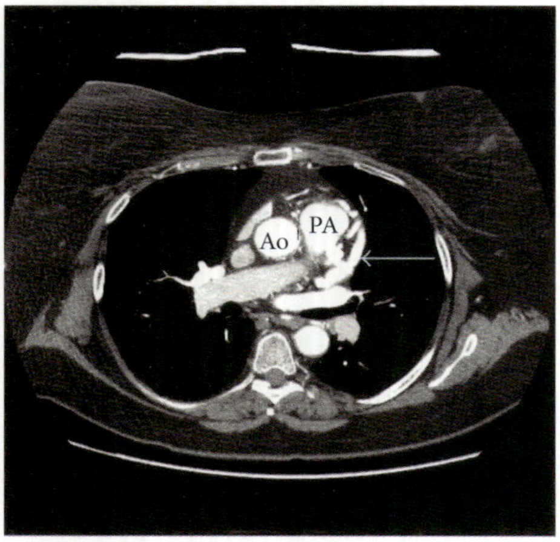

Figure 1: Axial view of multidetector cardiac CT angiogram shows the origin of the left main coronary artery (LMCA) from the main pulmonary artery (blue arrow).

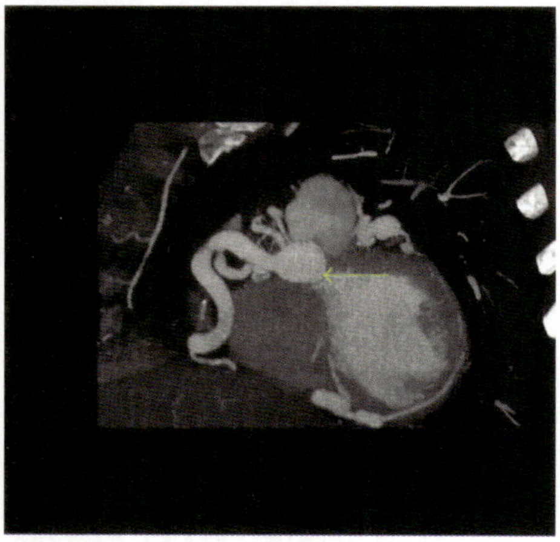

Figure 2: Sagittal view of multidetector cardiac CT angiogram shows an ectatic and dilated right coronary artery (RCA) (green arrow).

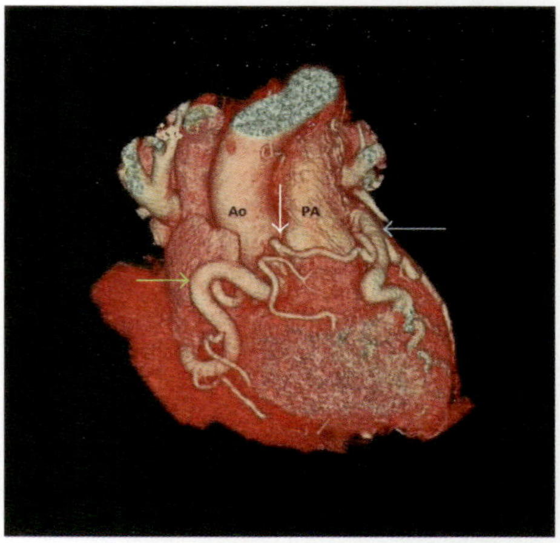

Figure 3: 3D reconstruction image of the heart in the right anterior oblique projection demonstrates severely dilated and tortuous RCA (green arrow) and dilated LMCA (blue arrow) along with large intercoronary collaterals (white arrow).

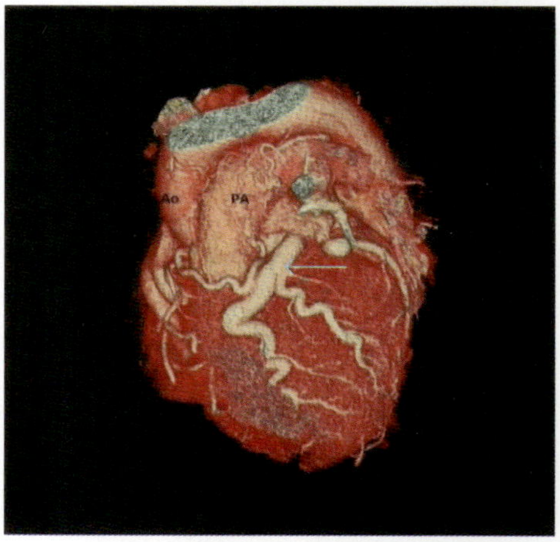

Figure 4: 3D reconstruction image of the heart in the left anterior oblique projection demonstrates the dilated LMCA and left anterior descending artery (blue arrow) coursing around the left side of the pulmonary artery.

extensive collateralization with a large ectatic right coronary artery arising from the right aortic coronary sinus (Figure 2). She remained asymptomatic, and her troponins normalized. Her atrial fibrillation was attributed to iatrogenic hyperthyroidism resulting from an excess in recommended doses for thyroid replacement therapy. The thyroid stimulating hormone level was noted to be low and reported at 0.05 mU/L.

A 2D echocardiogram revealed normal biventricular size and function with a left ventricular ejection fraction of 55%. Ventricular wall thickness was calculated to be normal in addition to normal left ventricular diastolic function and filling pressures. There were no advanced valvular abnormalities, and a mild degree of mitral and tricuspid regurgitation was present. There was evidence of markedly increased color Doppler signaling within the interventricular septum suggestive of high blood flow through septal collaterals (Figures 3 and 4). Coronary angiography showed evidence of retrograde blood flow in the left coronary system into the pulmonary trunk through collateral supply from the systemic side, secondary to relatively low right-sided pressures, and vascular resistance causing coronary steal (Video 1). Our patient was offered surgery for reimplantation of her left main into the aorta but she refused. Considering that her presentation of myocardial damage was secondary to a lack of oxygenated blood during increased demand at the time of tachycardia, a rhythm control strategy for the atrial fibrillation was adopted and the patient was discharged from the hospital on a reduced dose of thyroid replacement therapy with close follow-up.

3. Discussion

Krause first discovered anomalous origin of the left coronary artery from the pulmonary artery in the 1860s, which was later confirmed by Brooks in 1885 during a study on anatomical variations [4, 5]. However, the earliest clinical description was not until 1933 when Bland, White, and Garland observed a 3-month-infant with paroxysmal attacks of acute discomfort precipitated by exertion and associated with profound vasomotor collapse [6]. The EKG findings of this infant mimicked that of myocardial infarction in an adult. An autopsy showed anomalous origin of the left coronary artery arising from the pulmonary artery similar to that previously described by Krause and Brooks. Hence, it is also known as Bland–White–Garland syndrome.

Based on a Canadian heart registry, the incidence of ALCAPA is believed to be 1 per 300,000 live births [7]. ALCAPA occurs due to abnormal division of the conotruncus into the aorta and pulmonary artery or the persistence of the pulmonary buds together with involution of the aortic buds that form the coronary arteries during embryogenesis [8]. During the intrauterine period, the left coronary system has antegrade blood flow from the pulmonary artery, as pulmonary pressure is higher. As pulmonary resistance and oxygen content drops in the pulmonary arterial system during the neonate phase, the myocardium is perfused with blood with low oxygen content. Eventually, collaterals develop from the right coronary artery to supply the branches of the left coronary system, and the pressure in the left coronary system rises. This results in reversal of flow from the left coronary system to low pressure pulmonary system. The phenomenon is often regarded as "coronary steal." Depending on the extent of collaterals, the clinical spectrum can be divided in four types:

(1) *Infantile type*: in a review of postmortem cases, Kaunitz pointed out that closure of ductus arteriosus around 2 months of age was coincidental with development of symptoms [9]. Indeed, closure of ductus arteriosus decreases the oxygenated blood to the left coronary artery via the pulmonary artery. This leads to left ventricular ischemia. About 90% of cases present between 2 and 4 months, with signs of poor growth, tachypnea, profuse sweating, and angina-like episodes (usually occurring after nursing as the sudden onset of a distressed state with pallor). About 90% of those infants who are symptomatic and remain untreated die within first two years of life.

(2) *Asymptomatic adult type*: most adults with ALCAPA who survive infancy are found to have extensive collateralization and a dilated RCA. It is hypothesized that in infancy, the RCA supplies not only the posterior but also the lateral wall. These patients have continuous murmur due to collateral blood flow, or mild mitral regurgitation or incidental cardiomegaly on chest X-ray. While initial case reports showed a high percentage of patients present with sudden cardiac death, with recent advent of EKG-gated CT scans, cardiac MRIs, and easy accessibility of echo, higher numbers of asymptomatic and older individuals are being diagnosed in the last few years.

(3) *Symptomatic adult type*: these adults present with signs of angina due to increased flow from collaterals to the low-pressure pulmonary artery or coronary steal, which occurs during stress. These patients may also have moderate to severe mitral regurgitation. Mitral regurgitation occurs due to left ventricular dilatation or papillary muscle dysfunction [10].

(4) *Sudden cardiac death*: about 85% of adult cases have no previous cardiac symptoms. Histologic studies have shown substantial amount of viable but depressed contractile material and variable degree of fibrosis in myocardial tissue, which is believed to be a precursor to fatal ventricular tachyarrhythmias [11].

A comprehensive review of ECGs by Yau et al. showed Q waves in anterior leads in 50% of patients and left ventricular hypertrophy in up to 28% of all cases [12]. Using Doppler echocardiography, good visualization of the dilated RCA with retrograde flow into the left coronary artery and pulmonary artery along with septal collateralization is diagnostic in 90% of cases. Coronary angiography and cardiac CT scanning can be diagnostic when typical features of echocardiogram are not seen. Cardiac MRI has an advantage of finding scar tissue, areas of ischemia, and myocardial viability [13].

Surgery is the only definitive treatment. While ligation of the LCA at its origin was initially practiced, it was met with high incidence of late sudden cardiac deaths. In modern period, we found an adult case with primary use of the transcatheter closure device to occlude the LCA [14]. Establishing dual coronary supply using saphenous venous graft was found to be superior to ligation of LCA alone [15]. With advent of technology, direct reimplantation of the left coronary artery to the aorta has become very popular with good long-term results. Takeuchi procedure, introduced in 1979, involved the creation of an aortopulmonary window and intrapulmonary tunnel extending from the anomalous ostium to the window. This procedure is now unpopular due to late complications such obstruction of the baffle created between the anomalous coronary artery and supravalvular pulmonary stenosis in up to 33% of cases [16]. Normalization of cardiac function at rest is seen in all operative survivors in the first year itself, albeit exercise testing still may reveal subtle functional disability [17].

Majority of evidence suggests that mild to moderate MR corrects due to reverse LV modeling after the left coronary artery repair. Severe MR caused by irreversible myocardial necrotic damage or papillary muscle infarction needs concomitant repair to prevent long-term MR after alone ALCAPA repair [18]. Implantation of an ICD is usually reserved for patients who present with fatal ventricular arrhythmias. In a small cohort, no recurrence of ventricular arrhythmia was seen up to 10 years after ICD implantation [19].

4. Conclusion

ALCAPA is a rare but life-threatening disease. There should a strong clinical suspicion in young patients who present with unexplained cardiomegaly on imaging, continuous murmur on exam, or EKG findings of infarction without a history of ischemia. Due to lack of long-term data on medical therapy, surgical correction is the mainstay of therapy.

References

[1] T. Kristensen, K. F. Kofoed, S. Helqvist, M. Helvind, and L. Søndergaard, "Anomalous origin of the left coronary artery from the pulmonary artery (ALCAPA) presenting with ventricular fibrillation in an adult: a case report," *Journal of Cardiothoracic Surgery*, vol. 3, no. 1, p. 33, 2008.

[2] O. Yamanaka and R. E. Hobbs, "Coronary artery anomalies in 126,595 patients undergoing coronary arteriography," *Catheterization and Cardiovascular Diagnosis*, vol. 21, no. 1, pp. 28–40, 1990.

[3] H. Wesselhoeft, J. S. Fawcett, and A. L. Johnson, "Anomalous origin of the left coronary artery from the pulmonary trunk: its clinical spectrum, pathology, and pathophysiology, based on a review of 140 cases with seven further cases," *Circulation*, vol. 38, no. 2, pp. 403–425, 1968.

[4] W. Krause, "About the origin of accessory coronary artery from the pulmonary artery," *Ztschr Rat Med*, vol. 24, pp. 225–227, 1865.

[5] S. J. Brooks, "Two cases of an abnormal coronary artery of the heart arising from the pulmonary artery: with some remarks upon the effect of this anomaly in producing cirsoid dilatation of the vessels," *Journal of Anatomy and Physiology*, vol. 20, pp. 26–32, 1886.

[6] F. E. Bland, P. D. White, and J. Garland, "Congenital anomalies of the coronary arteries: report of an unusual case associated with cardiac hypertrophy," *American Heart Journal*, vol. 8, no. 6, pp. 787–801, 1933.

[7] J. D. Keith, "The anomalous origin of the left coronary artery from the pulmonary artery," *British Heart Journal*, vol. 21, no. 2, pp. 149–161, 1959.

[8] A. Dodge-Khatami, C. Mavroudis, and C. L. Backer, "Anomalous origin of the left coronary artery from the pulmonary artery: collective review from surgical therapy," *Annals of Thoracic Surgery*, vol. 74, no. 3, pp. 946–955, 2002.

[9] P. E. Kaunitz, "Origin of left coronary artery from the pulmonary artery: review of the literature and report of two cases," *American Heart Journal*, vol. 33, no. 2, pp. 182–206, 1947.

[10] G. Dahle, A. Fiane, and H. Lindberg, "ALCAPA, a possible reason for mitral insufficiency and heart failure in young patients," *Scandinavian Cardiovascular Journal*, vol. 41, no. 1, pp. 51–58, 2007.

[11] B. Shivalkar, M. Borgers, W. Daenen, M. Gewillig, and W. Flameng, "ALCAPA syndrome: an example of chronic myocardial hypoperfusion?," *Journal of the American College of Cardiology*, vol. 23, no. 3, pp. 772–778, 1994.

[12] J. M. Yau, R. Singh, E. J. Halpem, and D. Fischman, "Anomalous origin of the left coronary artery from the pulmonary artery in adults: a comprehensive review of 151 adult cases and a new diagnosis in a 53-year-old woman," *Clinical Cardiology*, vol. 34, no. 4, pp. 204–210, 2011.

[13] E. Pena, E. T. Nguyen, N. Merchant, and G. Dennis, "ALCAPA syndrome: not just a pediatric disease," *RadioGraphics*, vol. 29, no. 2, pp. 553–565, 2009.

[14] N. Collins, J. Colman, L. Benson, M. Hansen, N. Merchant, and E. Horlick, "Successful percutaneous treatment of anomalous left coronary artery from pulmonary artery," *International Journal of Cardiology*, vol. 122, no. 3, pp. e29–e31, 2007.

[15] C. L. Wilson, P. W. Dlabal, and S. A. McGuire, "Surgical treatment of anomalous left coronary artery from pulmonary artery: follow-up in teenagers and adults," *American Heart Journal*, vol. 98, no. 4, pp. 440–446, 1979.

[16] S. Takeuchi, H. Imamura, K. Katsumoto et al., "New surgical method for repair of anomalous left coronary artery from pulmonary artery," *Journal of Thoracic and Cardiovascular Surgery*, vol. 78, no. 1, pp. 7–11, 1979.

[17] T. Ojala, J. Salminen, J. M. Happonen et al., "Excellent functional result in children after correction of anomalous origin of left coronary artery from the pulmonary artery–a population-based complete follow-up study," *Interactive CardioVascular and Thoracic Surgery*, vol. 10, no. 1, pp. 70–75, 2010.

[18] P. A. Kazmierczak, K. Ostrowska, P. Dryzek, J. A. Moll, and J. J. Moll, "Repair of anomalous origin of the left coronary artery from the pulmonary artery in infants," *Interactive CardioVascular and Thoracic Surgery*, vol. 16, no. 6, pp. 797–801, 2013.

[19] P. Parizek, L. Haman, J. Harrer et al., "Bland–White–Garland syndrome in adults: sudden cardiac death as a first symptom and long-term follow-up after successful resuscitation and surgery," *Europace*, vol. 12, no. 9, pp. 1338–1340, 2010.

Persistent Hiccups as the Only Presenting Symptom of ST Elevation Myocardial Infarction

Nasreen Shaikh[1] **Rishi Raj**[1] **Srinivas Movva,**[1] **and Charles Mattina**[1,2]

[1]*Department of Internal Medicine, Monmouth Medical Center, 300 Second Avenue, Long Branch, NJ 07740, USA*
[2]*Department of Internal Medicine, Division of Cardiology, Monmouth Medical Center, 300 Second Avenue, Long Branch, NJ 07740, USA*

Correspondence should be addressed to Nasreen Shaikh; shaikh.drn@gmail.com

Academic Editor: Assad Movahed

Clinical manifestations of acute myocardial infarction can be more than just chest pain. Patients can present with dyspnea, fatigue, heart burn, diaphoresis, syncope, and abdominal pain to name a few. Our patient was a 74-year-old male with a past medical history of type 2 diabetes mellitus, hypertension, hyperlipidemia, and COPD due to chronic tobacco use, who presented with persistent hiccups for 4 days and no other complaints. Coincidently, he was found to have a diabetic foot ulcer with sepsis and acute kidney injury and hence was admitted to the hospital. A routine 12-lead EKG was done, and he was found to have an inferior wall ST elevation myocardial infarction. He underwent diagnostic catheterization which demonstrated 100% right coronary artery occlusion and a thallium viability study which confirmed nonviable myocardium; hence, he did not undergo percutaneous coronary intervention. Elderly patients who present with persistent hiccups should be investigated for an underlying cardiac etiology.

1. Introduction

This case report aims to spread awareness amongst the emergency department physicians and primary care physicians who often encounter patients with symptoms which seem trivial but have a grave underlying pathology. Persistent hiccups is one of them. Our case report highlights a patient who came in with similar complaints and was found to have an acute ST segment elevation myocardial infarction of the inferior wall. Persistent hiccups in the elderly with risk factors for coronary artery disease should be investigated further.

2. Presentation

A 74-year-old male with a past medical history of type 2 diabetes mellitus, hypertension, hyperlipidemia, and COPD from chronic tobacco use came with complaints of persistent hiccups for 4 days and no other complaints. Coincidently, he was noted to have a diabetic foot ulcer on the right great toe. On admission, the patient was afebrile with a blood pressure of 96/62 mm Hg and a heart rate of 72 beats per minute. Laboratory tests which included a complete blood count, comprehensive metabolic panel, and urinalysis were significant for a WBC count of $16\times10^3/\mu$L, creatinine of 1.29 mg/dL which was acute, and a lactic acid level of 2.3 mmol/L. The rest of the laboratory tests and chest X-ray were normal. Blood cultures were sent immediately and had no growth over the course of hospital stay. The admitting diagnosis was sepsis from a diabetic foot ulcer, and the patient was started on vancomycin and cefepime.

Blood cultures showed no growth, and on the basis of wound cultures showing methicillin-sensitive *Staphylococcus aureus*, doxycycline was substituted. A routine 12-lead EKG was performed on admission which showed ST elevation in inferior leads with Q waves and sinus rhythm with first-degree AV block (Figure 1) with troponin-I levels of 38.22 ng/dl, suggestive of a recent age indeterminate inferior

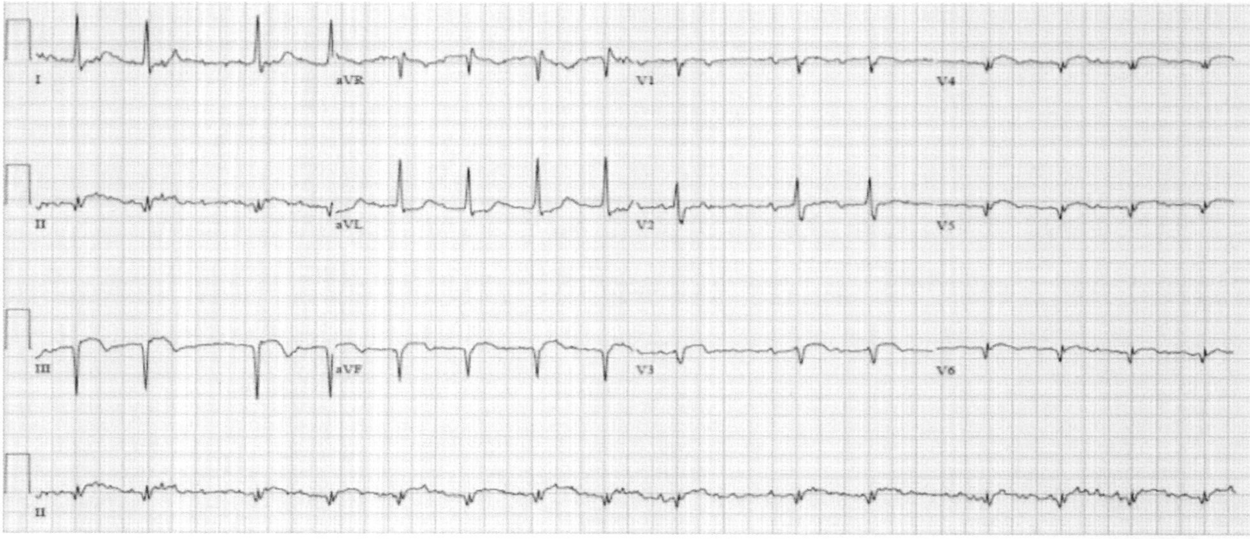

Figure 1: 12-lead EKG showing ST elevation and Q waves in leads II, III, and aVF and sinus rhythm with first-degree AV block.

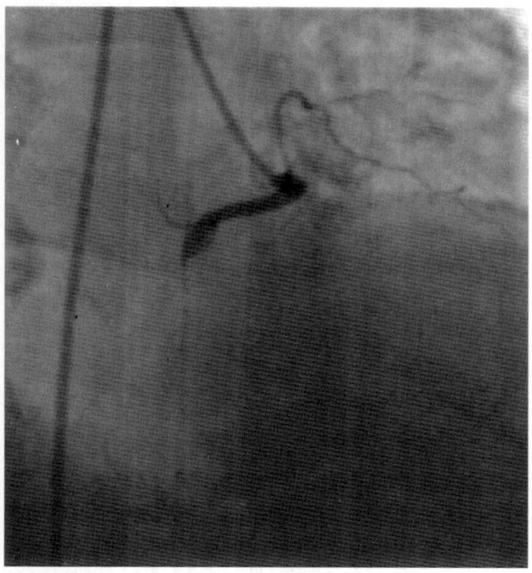

Figure 2: Coronary angiography showing 100% occlusion of the mid-right coronary artery.

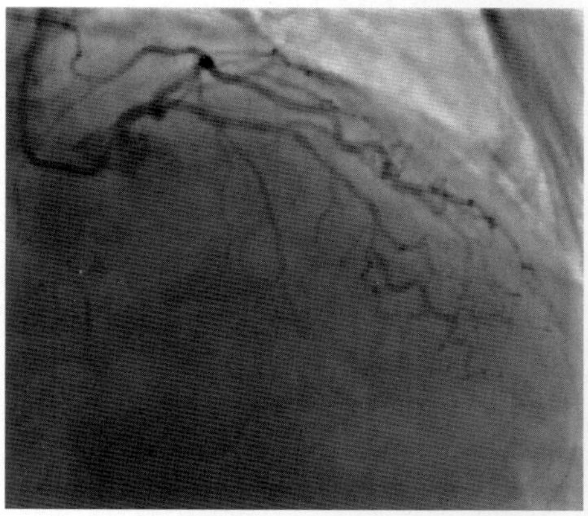

Figure 3: Coronary angiography showing 80% occlusion of the left anterior descending artery.

wall ST elevation myocardial infarction. He was given intravenous unfractionated heparin, aspirin, and ticagrelor. Lactic acid trended down within 4 hours. Hiccups resolved on day 2 of hospital stay, and troponins started to trend down within 6 hours of presentation. Echocardiogram showed LVEF of 30% with inferior wall akinesia. After the resolution of sepsis and acute kidney injury, diagnostic cardiac catheterization was performed which showed 100% mid-right coronary artery (RCA) occlusion (Figure 2), inferior wall akinesis, and 80% mid-left anterior descending (LAD) lesion (Figure 3), and ischemic cardiomyopathy was confirmed. A nuclear regadenoson stress test was performed which showed large inferoseptal wall defect with akinesia and surrounding anteroseptal wall hypokinesia (Figure 4). To rule out hibernating myocardium, a thallium viability scan was performed which showed a fixed inferoseptal and apical perfusion abnormality with no redistribution in 24-hour delayed imaging. As no viable tissue in the infarcted area was identified and there was no ischemic myocardium, medical therapy was recommended. The patient was discharged with an external cardiac defibrillator vest (LifeVest), and later on, he had an implantable cardiac defibrillator placed when there was no improvement in ejection fraction despite maximal medical therapy for secondary prevention of sudden cardiac death. The patient continues to do well on therapy and close follow-up.

3. Discussion

Our patient only complained of hiccups and displayed no other symptoms that would indicate myocardial ischemia. Although our patient did not have any other symptoms to suggest acute coronary syndrome, the patient did have multiple risk factors for coronary artery disease such as type 2 diabetes mellitus, hypertension, hyperlipidemia, and chronic smoking. "Anginal equivalent" is a term used for

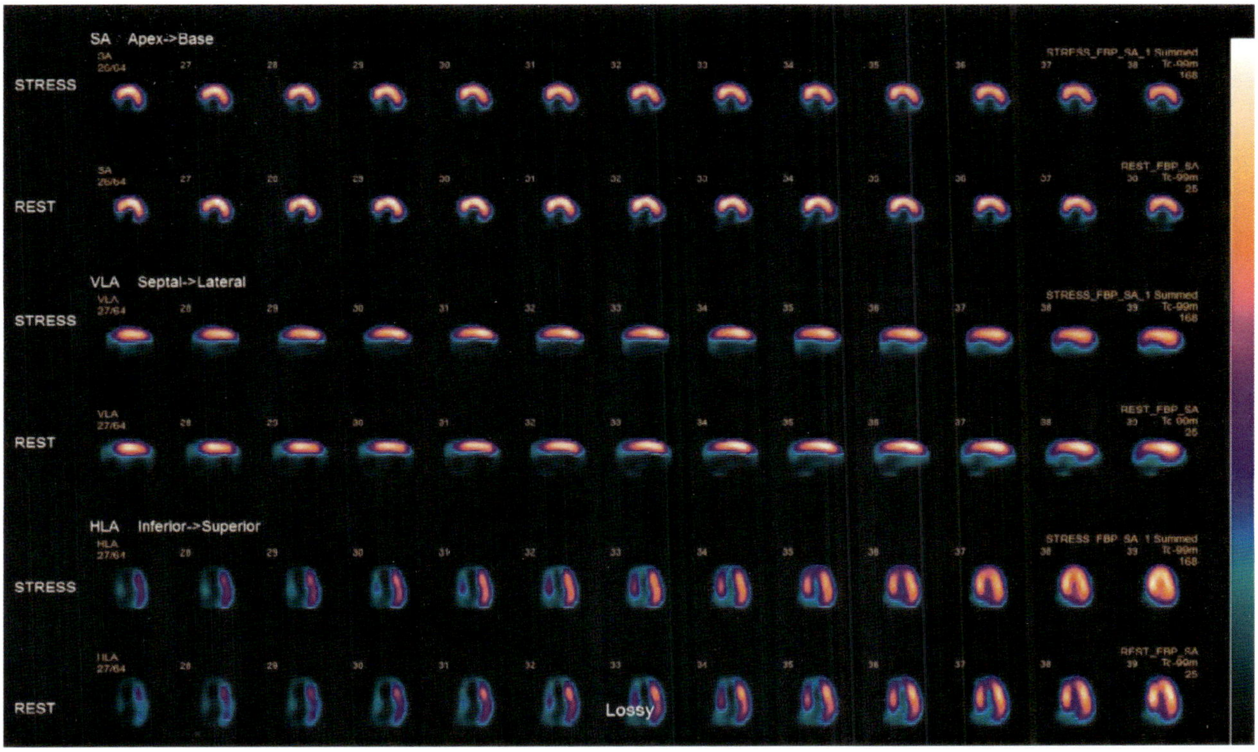

Figure 4: Nuclear regadenoson stress test showing inferoseptal wall defect.

symptoms of acute coronary syndrome other than chest pain and includes dyspnea, fatigue, heart burn, abdominal pain, nausea, and vomiting. Acute coronary syndrome in diabetics, elderly, and female patients may present with such anginal equivalents [1]. Our patient was an elderly diabetic male who presented with a sole complaint of persistent hiccups and was found to have ST elevation myocardial infarction. Their resolution as the patient entered the convalescent stage of their AMI suggests that it was not a coincidence. None of the guidelines mention persistent hiccups as an anginal equivalent.

Hiccups are defined as sudden onset of erratic diaphragmatic and intercostal muscle contraction, immediately followed by laryngeal closure leading to abrupt rush of air into the lungs eliciting a "hic" sound. Usually, they are self-limiting, but if episodes last >48 hours, they are defined as persistent hiccups [2]. The reflex arc of the hiccup has 3 components: the afferent limb composed of phrenic, vagus, and sympathetic nerves; a central processor in the midbrain; and the efferent limb composed of the phrenic nerve supplying the diaphragm and intercostal nerves supplying the intercostal muscle fibers [3]. Any irritants in the reflex pathway, such as physical, chemical, inflammatory, or neoplastic process, can trigger hiccups. Most commonly, persistent hiccups are caused by the nervous system disorder, either central (neoplastic and inflammatory) or peripheral by irritation of the phrenic nerve (goiter) or irritation of the vagus nerve (otolaryngologic diseases, meningitis, esophageal, stomach, and duodenal diseases, hepatitis, pancreatitis, and enteritis) [4].

This is the first case in literature in which ST segment elevation myocardial infarction presented with persistent hiccups as the sole presenting complaint. Myocardial ischemia has been reported to cause hiccups; however, there have been very few case reports in literature. Among the few reported cases, either hiccups was one of the associated symptoms in patients with myocardial ischemia or persistent hiccups presented as non-ST elevation myocardial infarction (NSTEMI). The earliest case report was in 1958, where a patient complained of dyspnea and orthopnea along with hiccups [5]. In 2 cases reported by Ikram et al. in 1971, patients developed intractable hiccups 2 to 3 days following acute inferoposterolateral and acute anterolateral MI, respectively [6]. Many other case reports cite hiccups as an associated symptom after admission for myocardial infarction [7, 8]. In a case reported by Davenport et al. in 2012, similar to our case, the patient presented with persistent hiccups without any other complaints; however, the patient was found to have inferior wall NSTEMI, and a subsequent cardiac catheterization revealed significant stenosis of the left circumflex and first obtuse marginal coronary arteries [9]. Zhang et al. reported a case of persistent hiccups with chest pain in a patient with cocaine-induced inferior wall STEMI with 99% occlusion of the mid-RCA and 80% stenosis of the LAD artery [4].

It is interesting to note that all the published literature about persistent hiccups and myocardial ischemia has identified the inferior wall of the myocardium to be affected. The inferior wall also known as the diaphragmatic surface of the heart lies in close proximity to the diaphragm. Irritation of phrenic nerves, which innervates the diaphragm, can be the cause of persistent hiccups in these patients. The other probable reason could be irritation of the vagus nerve supplying the pericardium [10].

Whether it is the inflammatory markers released from the infarcted inferior myocardium which irritate the diaphragm and trigger the hiccup reflex arc or it is the irritation of the vagus nerve directly remains to be elucidated [11]. In one of the case reports where both RCA and LAD were occluded, the symptoms of hiccups resolved after opening of only RCA even when LAD remained obstructed. This supports our observation of inferior wall MI causing hiccups [12]. This case reminds us of importance of having a high index of suspicion, especially in elderly diabetic patients where benign self-limiting condition like hiccups can be the only presenting symptoms of a serious underlying pathology like ST elevation myocardial infarction.

4. Conclusion

Whilst there are more common causes of acute onset persistent hiccups, if there are no other obvious causes, acute myocardial ischemia should be considered as a potential differential.

Authors' Contributions

Nasreen Shaikh was the primary resident taking care of the patient and wrote the case report. The case report was edited and finalized with the help of the senior resident Rishi Raj. Srinivas Movva was the primary attending of the patient and helped in gathering crucial information. Charles Mattina was the attending cardiologist who managed the patient, performed the coronary angiogram, and assisted in the preparation of the manuscript.

References

[1] A. Kumar and C. P. Cannon, "Acute coronary syndromes: diagnosis and management, part II," *Mayo Clinic Proceedings*, vol. 84, no. 11, pp. 1021–1036, 2009.

[2] F. Y. Chang and C. L. Lu, "Hiccup: mystery, nature and treatment," *Journal of Neurogastroenterology and Motility*, vol. 18, no. 2, pp. 123–130, 2012.

[3] D. E. Becker, "Nausea, vomiting, and hiccups: a review of mechanisms and treatment," *Anesthesia Progress*, vol. 57, no. 4, pp. 150–157, 2010.

[4] F. Zhang, N. D. Tongo, V. Hastings et al., "ST-segment elevation myocardial infarction with acute stent thrombosis presenting as intractable hiccups: an unusual case," *American Journal of Case Reports*, vol. 18, pp. 467–471, 2017.

[5] N. S. Gilbert, "Hiccups as sole presenting symptom of myocardial infarction," *Journal of the Florida Medical Association*, vol. 44, pp. 960–963, 1958.

[6] H. Ikram, R. T. Orchard, and S. E. Read, "Intractable hiccuping in acute myocardial infarction," *British Medical Journal*, vol. 2, no. 5760, p. 504, 1971.

[7] A. H. Douthwaite, "Intractable hiccuping in acute myocardial infarction," *British Medical Journal*, vol. 2, no. 5763, p. 709, 1971.

[8] N. G. Kounis, "Persistent hiccuping in acute myocardial infarction–report of a case," *Irish Medical Journal*, vol. 67, no. 24, pp. 644-645, 1974.

[9] J. Davenport, M. Duong, and R. Lanoix, "Hiccups as the only symptom of non-ST-segment elevation myocardial infarction," *American Journal of Emergency Medicine*, vol. 30, no. 1, pp. 266.e1–266.e2, 2012.

[10] D. Howes, "Hiccups: a new explanation for the mysterious reflex," *Bioessays*, vol. 34, no. 6, pp. 451–453, 2012.

[11] N. Sinha, R. C. Ahuja, R. K. Saran, and G. C. Jain, "Clinical correlates of acute right ventricular infarction in acute inferior myocardial infarction," *International Journal of Cardiology*, vol. 24, no. 1, pp. 55–61, 1989.

[12] W. Krysiak, S. Szabowski, M. Stepień, K. Krzywkowska, A. Krzywkowski, and P. Marciniak, "Hiccups as a myocardial ischemia symptom," *Polskie Archiwum Medycyny Wewnętrznej*, vol. 118, no. 3, pp. 148–151, 2008.

45

Coil Embolization of Coronary-Cameral Fistula Complicating Revascularization of Chronic Total Occlusion

Amy Mertens,[1] Pratik Dalal,[1] Michael Ashbrook,[1] and Ivan Hanson[1,2]

[1]*Department of Cardiovascular Medicine, Beaumont Health System, Royal Oak, MI, USA*
[2]*Oakland University William Beaumont School of Medicine, Royal Oak, MI, USA*

Correspondence should be addressed to Ivan Hanson; ivan.hanson@beaumont.org

Academic Editor: Ramazan Akdemir

Traumatic vessel perforation is a potential complication of chronic total occlusion (CTO) percutaneous coronary artery intervention (PCI). A rare consequence of this complication is a coronary-cameral fistula. The management of this condition is not well elucidated. Herein, we present such a case of symptomatic left anterior descending to the right ventricle (LAD-RV) fistula which was treated with coil embolization.

1. Introduction

Coronary artery chronic total occlusion (CTO) is present in 18–26% of all patients with coronary disease and in up to 50% of patients after coronary artery bypass grafting [1, 2]. These procedures are known to have higher complication rates compared to traditional PCI and require careful procedural planning and case selection for success. Potential complications include coronary perforation with or without tamponade due to equipment exit or stent overdilation, vessel thrombosis or occlusion, high radiation exposure leading to skin injury, vascular access complications, and contrast nephropathy [3]. Iatrogenic coronary artery fistulas are seen in only 0.25% of cases and typically involve coronary artery to coronary vein communication [4, 5]. We present a case of a left anterior descending (LAD) artery to the right ventricle (RV) fistula complicating a LAD CTO revascularization.

2. Case Presentation

A 71-year-old man with progressive angina was found to have severe stenosis in the circumflex artery and complex CTO of the left anterior descending artery (Figure 1, Supplementary Video 1). Coronary artery bypass surgery was offered to the patient but declined. He underwent uncomplicated stenting of the circumflex artery, followed by staged CTO recanalization of the LAD. A guidewire was passed relatively easily across the occlusion into the true lumen of the distal LAD beyond the bifurcation. Antegrade wiring of the diagonal artery was difficult. An epicardial collateral from the distal right coronary artery was used to access the diagonal branch retrograde, and this wire was steered into the antegrade guide catheter and externalized (Figure 2). Both the LAD and diagonal were dilated with 3.0 mm noncompliant balloons. The diagonal was stented into the proximal LAD, and the distal LAD was rewired. The distal LAD was dilated through the stent struts to allow passage of stents into the distal LAD (Culotte technique). The distal LAD was stented using four everolimus drug-eluting stents. The stents were postdilated with 3.0 mm noncompliant balloons in the diagonal and distal LAD and 4.0 mm noncompliant balloon in the proximal LAD. Within the distal-most stent in the distal LAD, the balloon had a persistent waist until an inflation pressure of 12 ATM. At that point, the balloon suddenly expanded. Angiography revealed contrast filling of the right ventricle (RV), with the appearance of one or two focal jets of contrast extravasation at the location of the rigid lesion in the distal LAD, consistent with iatrogenic LAD-RV fistula (Figure 3, Supplementary Video 2). Of note, the flow beyond the stents in the distal LAD was not seen, likely due to shunt flow and "coronary steal." The patient remained hemodynamically stable and

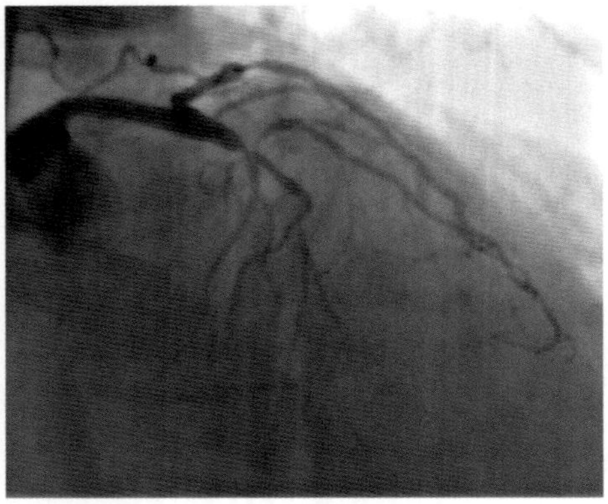

FIGURE 1: Left coronary angiography demonstrating severe stenosis of the left circumflex artery and CTO of the LAD.

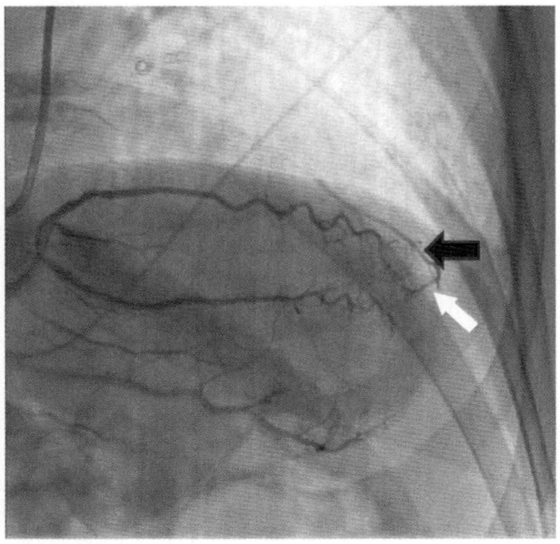

FIGURE 2: Epicardial vessel from the distal right coronary artery (white arrow) collateralizing the diagonal branch (black arrow).

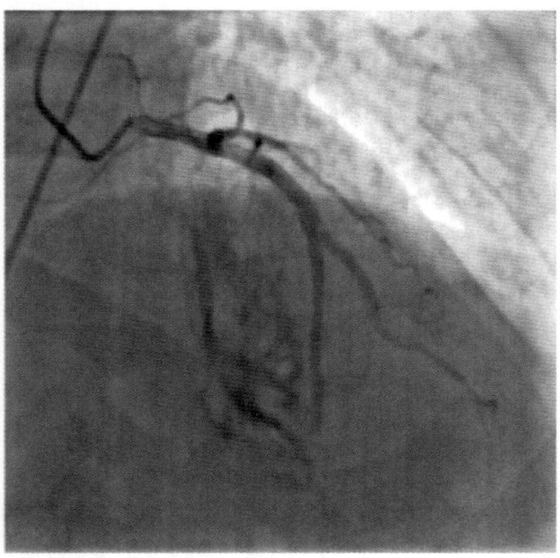

FIGURE 3: Angiography of the LAD demonstrating an iatrogenic LAD to RV fistula.

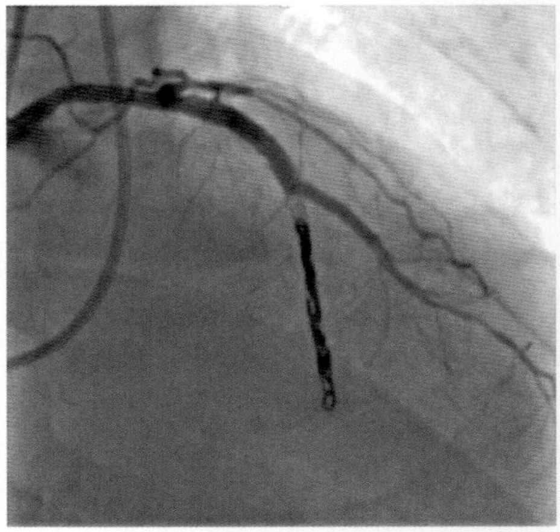

FIGURE 4: Angiography of the LAD showing successful coil embolization and complete cessation of flow into the RV.

was asymptomatic, and it was elected to manage the fistula conservatively. Serial echocardiograms revealed only trace pericardial effusion. He was discharged in stable condition.

Approximately three weeks after the CTO procedure, the patient was presented to the emergency department with chest pain and dyspnea. He described several episodes of "tearing" sensation in the chest. Blood pressure and heart rate were 123/69 mmHg and 64 beats per minute, respectively. A 12-lead ECG revealed inferior T wave inversion. Troponin I was elevated to 0.06 ng/mL. Urgent coronary angiography was performed, which revealed patent stents in the proximal LAD and diagonal branch. LAD-RV fistula appeared relatively unchanged compared to during the CTO procedure (Figure 3). The right coronary artery was normal and provided a very faint collateral to the apical LAD. Left ventriculography in the left anterior oblique projection revealed no evidence of a ventricular septal defect. The patient developed profound hypotension of unclear etiology during angiography. A right heart catheterization revealed normal filling pressures, normal cardiac output and ratio of pulmonic to systemic flow (Qp:Qs) 1.7. A transthoracic echocardiogram revealed preserved ejection fraction and normal left ventricular wall motion with turbulent flow signals at the LV and RV apex throughout the cardiac cycle (Supplementary Video 3). There was no pericardial effusion. The patient was transferred to the cardiac intensive care unit in stable condition.

Heart team evaluation was undertaken, and it was decided to perform coil embolization of the distal LAD. A standard 6 French left coronary guide catheter was used to advance a ProGreat (Terumo Medical Corp., Somerset, New Jersey) guidewire and 2.8 French catheter into the distal LAD. This was used to deploy two Ruby (Penumbra, Inc., Alameda, California) coils at the distal end of the stent.

There was still persistent shunt flow, so two Tornado (Cook Medical, Bloomington, Indiana) coils were subsequently deployed. Angiogram of the LAD confirmed complete cessation of flow into the distal LAD and absence of shunt flow (Figure 4, Supplementary Video 4). Hemodynamics postprocedure demonstrated a 20 mmHg increase in systolic blood pressure and normalization of Qp:Qs. A follow-up echocardiogram revealed the obliteration of apical shunt flow, normal left ventricular ejection fraction, and no left ventricular wall motion abnormalities. Creatine kinase eight-hour postprocedure was normal. The patient was discharged home in stable condition. At follow-up, one month later, the patient remained asymptomatic.

3. Discussion

To our knowledge, this is the first reported case of a traumatic LAD to RV fistula precipitated by CTO PCI that was successfully closed with percutaneous coil embolization. There have been 3 other reported cases of iatrogenic coronary artery fistulae in the literature, two of which were caused by RCA guidewire perforation and one secondary to LAD stent deployment [6, 7].

Development of LAD-RV fistula in this patient may have related to stent/balloon oversizing and rupture of the relatively small distal vessel. It is conceivable that the distal LAD had an intramyocardial course, which could explain why flow was preferentially tracked into RV, and not the pericardial space. The symptoms of chest pain, described as "tearing," along with low-level troponin release, may have been caused by the ongoing myocardial rupture. Although there was a significant shunting, there was no evidence of typical angina, which may have been expected if coronary steal had occurred [8].

Definitive management of symptomatic coronary-cameral fistula has not been well elucidated. Approaches may include conservative management, surgical ligation, prolonged balloon inflation, covered stents, and device embolization [9, 10].

The GRAFTMASTER (Abbott Vascular, Santa Clara, California) is a polytetrafluoroethylene- (PTFE-) covered stent that can be delivered into the coronary arteries via a 6 French guide catheter. The crimped profile of the device is 1.63–1.73 mm, making it difficult to deliver in tortuous or calcified/stented vessels. The smallest expanded stent diameter is 2.8 mm, so for smaller vessels, it is less useful. In addition, the GRAFTMASTER requires guidewire "purchase" beyond the site of deployment, but in the present case, distal intraluminal guidewire position could not be confirmed. Deployment of a covered stent has a potential advantage of maintaining distal flow in the vessel beyond the treatment site. If covered stent deployment is not possible, device embolization can be considered.

Coil embolization requires placement of a delivery catheter to the segment of interest, followed by advancement of coils, which are initially elongated and then conformed to their prespecified shape and volume once they are extruded. Ruby is a detachable coil, so it can be withdrawn or completely removed if needed. This type of coil was selected for initial delivery in the present case in order to achieve a precise position and avoid extension of the coil into the fistula tract or RV. Tornado is available in thickness as small as $0.018''$ and is coated with thrombogenic fronds to promote faster hemostasis. It is not detachable.

In the present case, distal LAD embolization resulted in complete occlusion of the stented segment beyond the large diagonal branch. It is important to note that embolization may not have been the preferred strategy if the perforation had occurred in a larger vessel or one supplying a large myocardial territory. The lack of a rise in cardiac biomarkers and the absence of left ventricular wall motion abnormalities suggested that the apical LAD and interventricular septum were adequately collateralized. Finally, the large diagonal branch, which was felt to be a more important vessel due to its large size and myocardial territory, was preserved.

4. Conclusion

Traumatic vessel perforation leading to LAD-RV fistula is a potential complication of CTO PCI and may lead to untoward symptoms and significant intracardiac shunting. A working knowledge of transcatheter closure techniques, including covered stents and device embolization, is mandatory for coronary interventionalists and CTO operators in particular.

References

[1] P. Fefer, M. L. Knudtson, A. N. Cheema et al., "Current perspectives on coronary chronic total occlusions: the Canadian Multicenter Chronic Total Occlusions Registry," *Journal of the American College of Cardiology*, vol. 59, no. 11, pp. 991–997, 2012.

[2] O. M. Jeroudi, M. E. Alomar, T. T. Michael et al., "Prevalence and management of coronary chronic total occlusions in a tertiary Veterans Affairs hospital," *Catheterization and Cardiovascular Interventions*, vol. 84, no. 4, pp. 637–643, 2014.

[3] P. Tajti and E. S. Brilakis, "Chronic total occlusion percutaneous coronary intervention: evidence and controversies," *Journal of the American Heart Association*, vol. 7, no. 2, article e006732, 2018.

[4] S. Banerjee and S. Patra, "Coronary–cameral fistula caused by guidewire trauma and resolved by coil embolization," *Texas Heart Institute Journal*, vol. 43, no. 4, pp. 338–340, 2016.

[5] Z. Elghoul and M. A. Leesar, "Iatrogenic fistula between the left anterior descending coronary artery and anterior interventricular vein following stenting," *The Journal of Invasive Cardiology*, vol. 19, no. 7, pp. E188–E191, 2007.

[6] P. Lipiec, J. Z. Peruga, M. Krzeminska-Pakula, J. Forys, J. Drozdz, and J. D. Kasprzak, "Right coronary artery-to-right ventricle fistula complicating percutaneous transluminal angioplasty: case report and review of the literature," *Journal of the American Society of Echocardiography*, vol. 17, no. 3, pp. 280–283, 2004.

[7] W. H. Chen, P. Y. Lee, and E. P. Wang, "Left anterior descending artery-to-right ventricle fistula and left ventricular free wall perforation after rotational atherectomy and stent implantation," *The Journal of Invasive Cardiology*, vol. 17, no. 8, pp. 450-451, 2005.

[8] S. A. M. Said and T. Van der Werf, "Dutch survey of coronary artery fistulas in adults: congenital solitary fistulas," *International Journal of Cardiology*, vol. 106, no. 3, pp. 323–332, 2006.

46

A Rare Presentation of Cardiac Tamponade from Metastatic Urothelial Carcinoma of the Bladder

Sowmya Palam, Ridhima Kapoor, and Jacquelyn Kulinski

Department of Internal Medicine, Medical College of Wisconsin, 9200 W. Wisconsin Ave., Suite 5100, Milwaukee, WI 53226, USA

Correspondence should be addressed to Sowmya Palam; spalam@mcw.edu

Academic Editor: Assad Movahed

A 62-year-old man presented with 2 weeks of progressive dyspnea and chest pain. He was previously diagnosed with high-grade invasive urothelial carcinoma (UC) of the bladder and underwent neoadjuvant chemotherapy followed by radical cystectomy 10 months earlier, resulting in pathologic complete remission. Clinical evaluation and echocardiographic imaging was consistent with a diagnosis of cardiac tamponade. Due to a history of malignancy, the patient was referred for a surgical pericardial window, to include biopsy of the pericardium. Pericardial fluid and pericardial biopsy specimens were consistent with metastatic UC. Cardiac tamponade due to metastatic UC is a rare presentation, and, to our knowledge, there have been only 5 cases reported in the English literature. We report a rare case of cardiac tamponade due to isolated pericardial metastases from high grade UC of the bladder and discuss the symptoms, treatment, and prognosis of this pathologic condition. We also present a brief review of previously published literature. Through this discussion, we would like to emphasize the (1) consideration of cardiac metastases in the differential diagnosis for patients with a history of UC presenting with cardiac or pulmonary symptoms and (2) improved diagnostics with pericardial biopsy and pericardiocentesis over pericardiocentesis alone.

1. Introduction

Bladder cancer is the ninth most common malignancy worldwide involving the urinary system. Urothelial carcinoma (UC) is the most prevalent histologic type in the United States and Western Europe and accounts for approximately 90% of bladder cancers [1, 2]. Common sites of metastasis of UC include regional and distant lymph nodes, liver, lung, and bone [3]. However, in rare cases, metastasis to the pericardium can also be seen. Approximately ten percent of autopsied cases of UC have shown cardiac metastasis [4]. However, in most cases, the metastases are clinically silent. We report a rare case of cardiac tamponade caused by metastatic UC of the bladder and discuss the patient's symptoms, management, and prognosis.

2. Case Presentation

A 62-year-old man presented with 2 weeks of progressive dyspnea and chest pain. He was previously diagnosed with high-grade invasive urothelial carcinoma (UC) of the bladder. He underwent neoadjuvant chemotherapy followed by radical cystectomy, resulting in complete pathologic remission. On examination, patient was afebrile with a heart rate of 136 bpm, blood pressure of 122/74 mm Hg, respiratory rate of 18 breaths/min, and O_2 saturation of 98% on room air. Heart sounds were muffled. Heart rhythm was irregularly irregular. Distention of the jugular veins was observed and Kussmaul's sign was present. Although pulsus paradoxus was not observed, other physical findings were extremely concerning for cardiac tamponade. Bibasilar crackles were present on lung auscultation. Laboratory data was remarkable for a creatinine of 1.42 (baseline of 1.08) and international normalized ratio (INR) of 3.6 (on warfarin for a history of pulmonary embolism). His complete blood counts and electrolytes were normal. His electrocardiogram revealed atrial fibrillation with a rapid ventricular rate (RVR) and electrical alternans. Chest radiograph showed enlargement of the cardiac silhouette.

Due to high clinical suspicion for cardiac tamponade, a bedside transthoracic echocardiogram (TTE) was obtained which showed a large pericardial effusion with diastolic

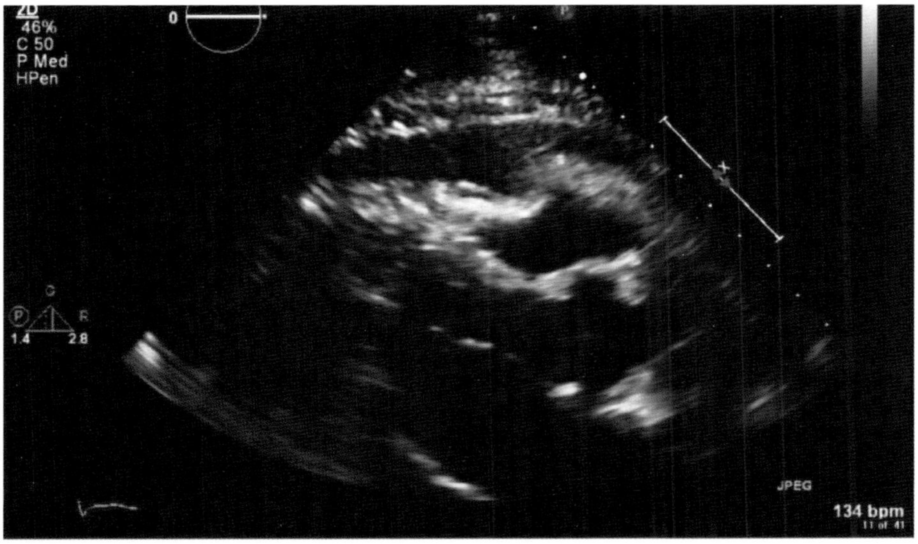

FIGURE 1: Transthoracic echocardiogram, parasternal long view, demonstrating large pericardial effusion and RV diastolic collapse.

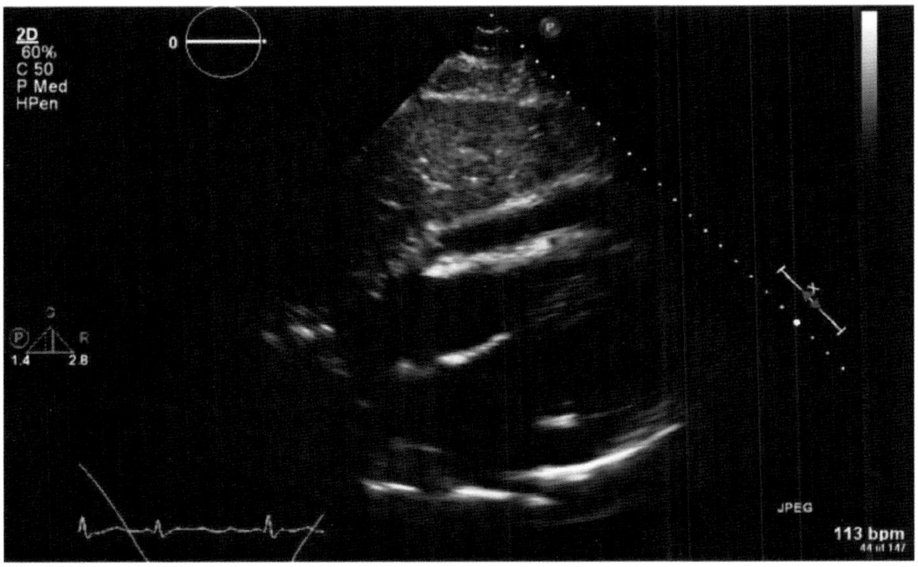

FIGURE 2: Transthoracic echocardiogram, subcostal view.

compression of the right ventricle, suggestive of cardiac tamponade, as well as mild left ventricular systolic dysfunction (see Figures 1 and 2). Patient's INR was reversed to <1.5 and he underwent emergent subxiphoid pericardial window with the removal of 700 ml of turbid, dark, bloody pericardial fluid. He had significant improvement in hemodynamics and respiratory distress. The pericardial fluid cytology and pericardial biopsy were both positive for malignancy, consistent with metastatic UC (see Figure 3).

One week after the pericardial window, the patient underwent a computerized tomography (CT) scan of the chest, abdomen, and pelvis which did not show evidence of metastatic disease elsewhere. Given the recurrence of UC with metastasis to the pericardium, he was started on atezolizumab. Subsequently, he was noted to have recurrent pericardial effusion suggesting failure of treatment (see Figure 4). He was then started on pemetrexed, a folate antimetabolite chemotherapy drug, for metastatic UC with plans to complete 6 cycles.

3. Discussion

Metastases to the heart typically occur late in the course of malignant disease. The incidence of cardiac metastasis, regardless of primary, has been estimated from 2.3% to 18.3% [5]. The pericardium is involved in about two thirds of all cardiac metastasis. Bussani et al. reported a large autopsy case series of 18,751 in-hospital deceased patients and found one or more malignant neoplasms in 7289 patients. The incidence of cardiac metastasis diagnosed postmortem was 9.1%

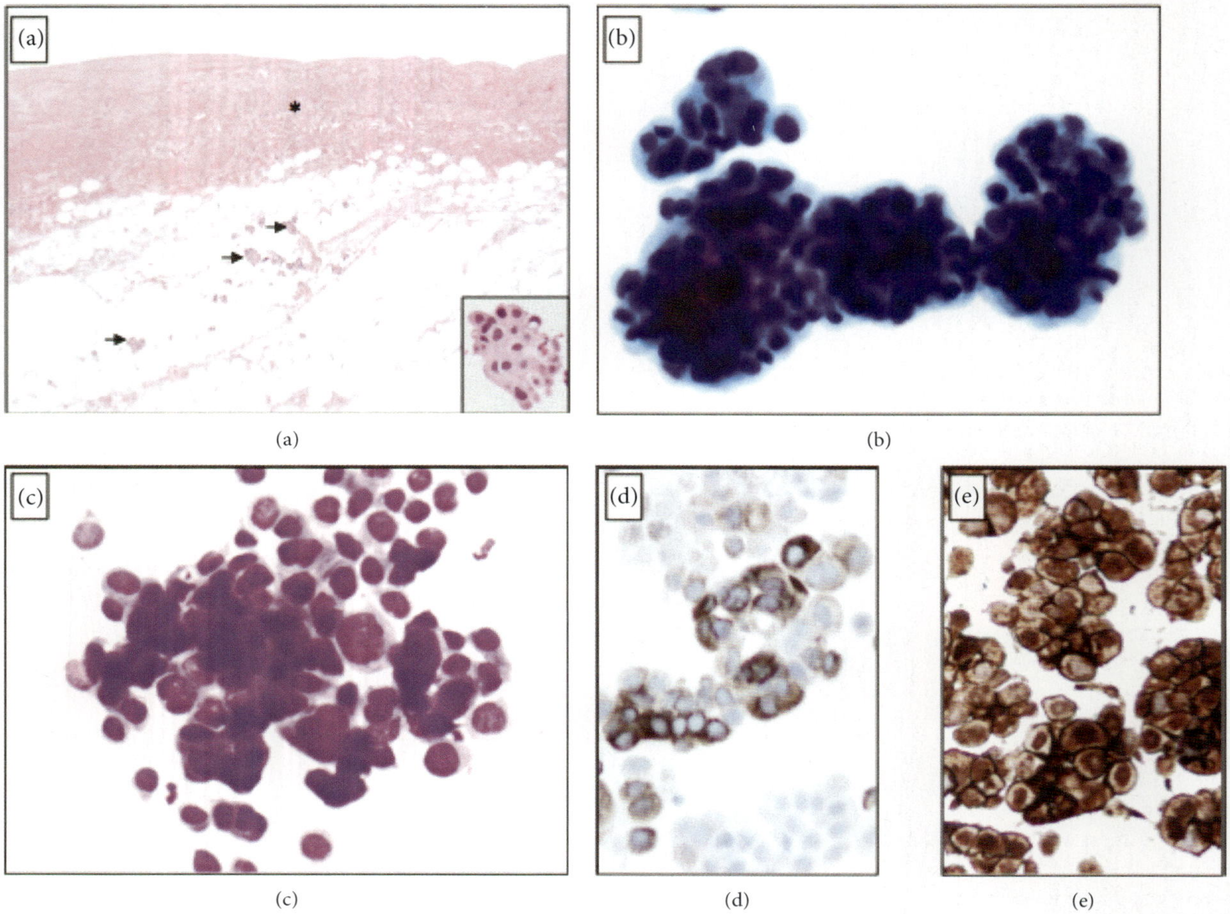

Figure 3: (a) H&E section shows thickening and fibrosis of the pericardium (asterisk) and scattered aggregates of metastatic urothelial carcinoma (black arrows). Insert: high power view of the malignant cells. The pericardial effusion demonstrates 3D clusters of large highly atypical malignant cells (b, Papanicolaou stain), variable in size and hyperchromatic with a high nuclear to cytoplasmic ratio (c, Diff-Quick stain). The malignant cells are immunoreactive for uroplakin and MOC-31 while negative for calretinin (not shown).

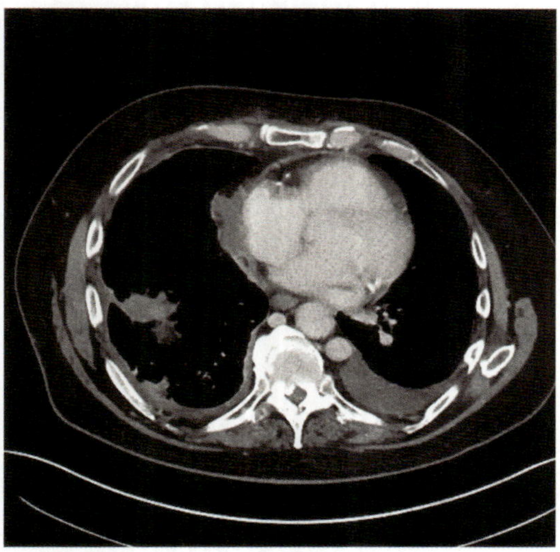

Figure 4: CT scan of the chest obtained one week after the pericardial window showing loculated pericardial fluid adjacent to the right atrium that is slightly higher in attenuation, suggestive of bloody or proteinaceous effusion.

and the tumors leading to the highest rates of cardiac metastasis were pleural mesothelioma (48.4%), melanoma (27.8%), lung adenocarcinoma (21%), undifferentiated carcinomas (19.5%), lung squamous cell carcinoma (18.2%), and breast carcinoma (15.5%). In contrast, only 3.9% of autopsied cases of UC revealed cardiac metastases.

To the best of our knowledge after a review of the literature, there have been only five cases of cardiac tamponade due to metastatic UC, with our case being the sixth [6–10]. In four of these cases, patients presented with symptoms of dyspnea, cough, fatigue, orthopnea, and chest pain [7–10]. In all cases, a chest radiograph showed the enlargement of the cardiac silhouette. An echocardiogram was utilized to evaluate the extent of pericardial effusion. Pericardiocentesis was performed for drainage and sent for cytology in all cases. However, in three of the cases, the pericardial fluid cytodiagnosis was equivocal and a pericardial biopsy was also obtained which led to the diagnosis of metastasis from UC [6, 8, 10]. In one case, the cytology was negative and no pericardial biopsy was performed; however, a large echogenic mass abutting the proximal free wall of the left ventricle and extending into the base of the pericardial cavity was noted [9]. In our case, pursuing a surgical approach for the pericardial window allowed us to obtain a pericardial biopsy in addition to pericardial fluid analysis in a patient with a prior history of malignancy. Both the pericardial fluid and pericardial biopsy showed malignant cells, which helped us establish the diagnosis of metastasis UC and guide appropriate management for the patient.

Of note, a minimum of 60 ml of pericardial fluid is necessary to ensure that benign diagnosis is truly benign and improves the likelihood of detecting malignancy with a sensitivity of 91.7%–92.1% [11, 12]. The false negative rates of cytology and biopsy range from 4% to 14.7% and 40% to 54.5%, respectively [13–15]. However, combining pericardial biopsy with pericardial effusion cytology further increases overall sensitivity for identifying malignancy by approximately 8% [9]. In this case, performing the surgical approach for the window allowed us to not only obtain a pericardial biopsy but also decompress the pericardial effusion and provide immediate restoration of improved hemodynamics and help prevent immediate recurrence of the pericardial effusion. Therefore, in patients with a history of malignancy, this approach should be considered.

Systemic chemotherapy is the standard approach for the initial treatment of patients with metastatic UC. However, the optimum management of UC with cardiac metastasis remains unclear at this time. In case of symptomatic cardiac metastases, the prognosis is extremely poor. Hattori et al., in their review of 14 reported cases in the literature found that most patients died within one year after diagnosis of symptomatic cardiac metastases from UC [7].

In patients with a history of malignancy who present with clinical, ECG, or CXR findings concerning pericardial effusion, one must consider a diagnosis of cardiac tamponade, particularly in a hemodynamically unstable patient. Cardiac metastasis should be on the differential diagnosis as an etiology. An echocardiogram may be performed for confirmation. However, if the patient is hemodynamically unstable, we recommend emergent pericardiocentesis, preferably with pericardial biopsy via surgical approach for accurate and early diagnosis of cardiac metastasis and for rapid relief of hemodynamic compromise. Treatment options for metastatic UC include systemic chemotherapy; however, prognosis of symptomatic cardiac metastasis from UC remains extremely poor.

References

[1] M. Ploeg, K. K. H. Aben, and L. A. Kiemeney, "The present and future burden of urinary bladder cancer in the world," *World Journal of Urology*, vol. 27, no. 3, pp. 289–293, 2009.

[2] N. E. Fleshner, H. W. Herr, A. K. Stewart, G. P. Murphy, C. Mettlin, and H. R. Menck, "The National Cancer Data Base report on bladder carcinoma," *Cancer*, vol. 78, no. 7, pp. 1505–1513, 1996.

[3] R. J. Babaian, D. E. Johnson, L. Llamas, and A. G. Ayala, "Metastases from transitional cell carcinoma of urinary bladder," *Urology*, vol. 16, no. 2, pp. 142–144, 1980.

[4] E. C. Klatt and D. R. Heitz, "Cardiac metastases," *Cancer*, vol. 65, no. 6, pp. 1456–1459, 1990.

[5] R. Bussani, F. De-Giorgio, A. Abbate, and F. Silvestri, "Cardiac metastases," *Journal of Clinical Pathology*, vol. 60, no. 1, pp. 27–34, 2007.

[6] R. Khan, W. Jehangir, S. Tulpule, M. Osman, S. Singh, and S. Sen, "Pericardial metastasis induced tamponade from urothelial carcinoma: a rare entity," *Case Reports in Medicine*, vol. 2016, Article ID 6162732, 3 pages, 2016.

[7] S. Hattori, A. Miyajima, T. Maeda et al., "Metastatic urothelial carcinoma to pericardia manifested by dyspnea from cardiac tamponade during systemic chemotherapy: case report and literature review," *Canadian Urological Association Journal*, vol. 6, no. 5, pp. E184–E188, 2012.

[8] S. J. Fabozzi, J. R. Newton Jr., R. P. Moriarty, and P. F. Schellhammer, "Malignant pericardial effusion as initial solitary site of metastasis from transitional cell carcinoma of the bladder," *Urology*, vol. 45, no. 2, pp. 320–322, 1995.

[9] N. Islam and M. Y. Ahmedani, "Renal carcinoma presenting as cardiac tamponade: a case report and review of literature," *International Journal of Cardiology*, vol. 64, no. 2, pp. 207–211, 1998.

[10] K. Spiliotopoulos, M. Argiriou, T. Argyrakos et al., "Solitary metastasis of urothelial carcinoma of the urinary bladder to the heart: an unusual clinical manifestation," *The Journal of Thoracic and Cardiovascular Surgery*, vol. 136, no. 5, pp. 1377–8, 1378.e1, 2008.

[11] L. M. Rooper, S. Z. Ali, and M. T. Olson, "A minimum volume of more than 60 ml is necessary for adequate cytologic diagnosis of malignant pericardial effusions," *American Journal of Clinical Pathology*, vol. 145, no. 1, pp. 101–106, 2016.

[12] J. Saab, R. S. Hoda, N. Narula et al., "Diagnostic yield of cytopathology in evaluating pericardial effusions: clinicopathologic analysis of 419 specimens," *Cancer Cytopathology*, vol. 125, no. 2, pp. 128–137, 2017.

[13] G. R. Corey, P. T. Campbell, P. van Trigt et al., "Etiology of large pericardial effusions," *The American Journal of Medicine*, vol. 95, no. 2, pp. 209–213, 1993.

[14] E. A. Dragoescu and L. Liu, "Pericardial fluid cytology: an analysis of 128 specimens over a 6-year period," *Cancer Cytopathology*, vol. 121, no. 5, pp. 242–251, 2013.

[15] H. M. Yazdi, S. I. Hajdu, and M. R. Melamed, "Cytopathology of pericardial effusions," *Acta Cytologica*, vol. 24, no. 5, pp. 401–412, 1980.

Staphylococcus aureus Myocarditis with Associated Left Ventricular Apical Thrombus

Michael McGee,[1] Emily Shiel,[2] Stephen Brienesse,[1,3] Stuart Murch,[1] Robert Pickles,[2,3] and James Leitch[1,3]

[1]*Cardiovascular Department, John Hunter Hospital, Lookout Road, New Lambton Heights, NSW 2305, Australia*
[2]*Infectious Diseases Department, John Hunter Hospital, Lookout Road, New Lambton Heights, NSW 2305, Australia*
[3]*Department of Medicine, University of Newcastle, Newcastle, NSW, Australia*

Correspondence should be addressed to Michael McGee; mcgee.michael.j@gmail.com

Academic Editor: Ertugrul Ercan

Staphylococcus aureus myocarditis is a rare diagnosis with a high mortality rate, usually seen in people who are immunocompromised. Here, we report a case of a 44-year-old man on methotrexate for rheumatoid arthritis who presented in septic shock and was diagnosed with *staphylococcus aureus* myocarditis. The myocarditis was associated with a left ventricular apical thrombus, with normal systolic function. The myocarditis and associated thrombus were characterised on transthoracic echocardiogram and subsequently on cardiac magnetic resonance imaging. Cardiac magnetic resonance (CMR) imaging showed oedema in the endomyocardium, consistent with acute myocarditis, associated with an apical mural thrombus. Repeat CMR 3 weeks following discharge from hospital showed marked improvement in endomyocardial oedema and complete resolution of the apical mural thrombus. He was treated with a 12-week course of antibiotics and anticoagulated with apixaban. The patient was successfully managed with intravenous antibiotics and anticoagulation with complete recovery.

1. Introduction

Staphylococcus aureus is widely reported to be the most common bacterial cause of myocarditis and usually occurs in the setting of bacteraemia and sepsis. Rarely, it occurs without associated infective endocarditis [1, 2]. Furthermore, difficulty in determining the diagnosis, prevalence, and aetiology of myocarditis is complicated by the infrequent use of endomyocardial biopsy (EMB), the diagnostic gold standard [2, 3].

Noninvasive imaging such as cardiac magnetic resonance (CMR) imaging has been shown to be reliable in the diagnosis and monitoring of disease progression in acute myocarditis [4, 5]. Despite the advances of noninvasive imaging, the sensitivity and specificity of CMR for acute myocarditis are reported at 81% and 71% and 63% and 40% in chronic myocarditis [6]. Ideally, CMR and EMB are both obtainable and are complimentary, overcoming limitations of either technique alone [4].

Here, we present a case of *Staphylococcus aureus* myocarditis with associated left ventricular apical thrombus.

2. Case History

A 44-year-old male was admitted to the intensive care unit (ICU) critically unwell with septic shock. On the day prior to admission, he had complained of lethargy, diffuse body aches, epigastric pain, nausea, and vomiting and had experienced rigors. He had a medical background significant for rheumatoid arthritis, treated with methotrexate 10 mg weekly for the last five years and had recently travelled to Fiji.

On arrival of paramedics, the patient was nonresponsive, febrile, and tachycardic, with an unrecordable blood pressure and mottled appearance of the skin. He was drowsy and confused on arrival to the emergency department and had prolonged capillary refill of five seconds, a lactate of 6.8. There was no clear focus of infection on examination, and cardiovascular examination was normal at this time. He was found

Table 1: Blood work on presentation to hospital and peak values.

	Presentation	Peak	Laboratory reference
White blood cell count	12.5	15.4	10^9/L 4–11
Neutrophils	8.2	12.7	10^9/L 2–8
Haemoglobin	162	162	g/L 130–180
Platelets	87	466	10^9/L 150–400
Bicarbonate	17	25	mmol/L 22–32
Urea	16.3	16.3	mmol/L 3.5–8
Creatinine	290	290	μmol/L 60–110
Bilirubin	69	69	μmol/L < 20
GGT	70	70	U/L 5–50
ALP	76	105	U/L 30–100
ALT	69	69	U/L < 50
AST	74	92	U/L < 45
C-reactive protein	339	348	mg/L < 5
HS troponin		139	Ng/L < 26

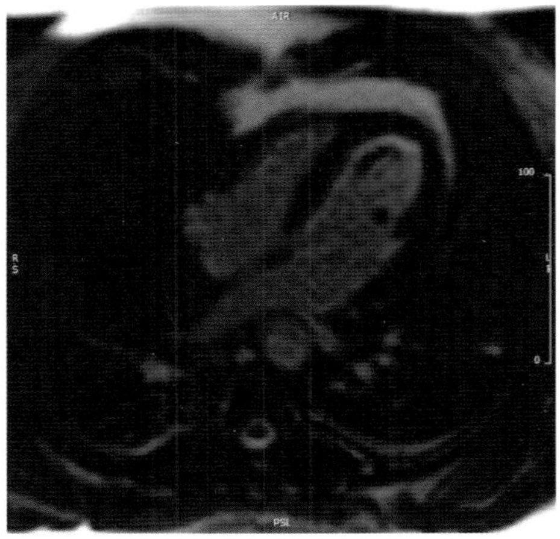

Figure 1: Cardiac magnetic resonance imaging 4-chamber-view post gadolinium injection revealing late gadolinium enhancement of the endomyocardium at the left ventricular apex.

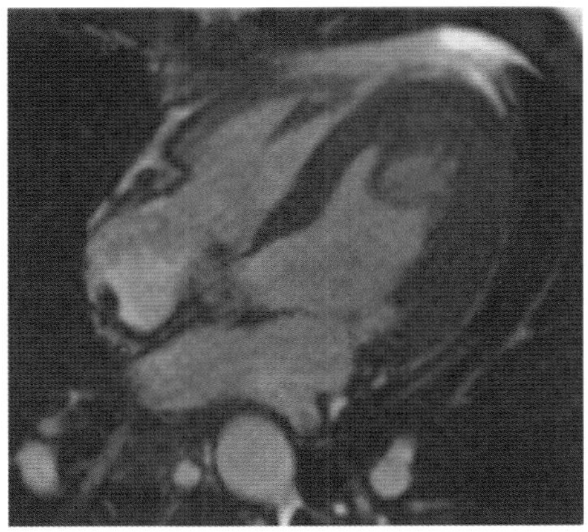

Figure 2: Cardiac magnetic resonance imaging 4-chamber view (still frame from a steady-state free precession (SSFP) cine sequence) with the left ventricular apical mass taken shortly after presentation.

to have an acute kidney injury, hepatic impairment, and coagulopathy, see Table 1. Blood cultures returned positive in 11 hours for methicillin-sensitive *Staphylococcus aureus*, and antibiotics were changed to intravenous (IV) flucloxacillin. He was culture positive for 48 hours.

His course was further complicated by development of left olecranon bursitis, treated by open drainage. The bursitis was culture negative but presumed septic. He also had several episodes of atypical chest pain. Electrocardiogram at the time of pain revealed sinus tachycardia, with lateral T wave inversion, and high-sensitivity troponin was elevated at 139 ng/L (NR < 26 ng/L). Transthoracic echocardiogram revealed normal left ventricular systolic function, with an echo-dense mass in the apex, no valvular abnormality, and mild left atrial dilatation. The patient proceeded to cardiac magnetic resonance (CMR) imaging which showed increased wall thickness in the mid to apical wall segments and high signal intensity in the mid to apical endocardium on short tau inversion recovery (STIR) imaging. There was late gadolinium enhancement in the same area, consistent with oedema in the apical endomyocardium (Figure 1). There was also a nonenhancing mass in the left ventricular apex consistent with thrombus and small bilateral pleural effusions (Figure 2).

Anticoagulation with therapeutic dose enoxaparin was commenced, which was subsequently changed to apixaban 5 mg twice daily prior to discharge.

A repeat echocardiogram was performed 10 days after the initial echocardiogram, which did not reveal any interval change. The patient was discharged with IV flucloxacillin to continue via a peripherally inserted central catheter (PICC) line and ongoing anticoagulation with apixaban. Repeat CMR was performed 3 weeks following discharge and revealed normal left ventricular cavity size, with mildly increased wall thickness in the mid to apical wall segments. Tissue characterisation was consistent with apical wall oedema, which had reduced significantly in size since the previous CMR, and complete resolution of the left ventricular apical mural thrombus and pleural effusions (Figure 3). He completed a 6-week course of IV flucloxacillin, followed by a 6-week course of oral dicloxacillin, and remained clinically well throughout this time.

3. Discussion

The majority of published cases of bacterial myocarditis are autopsy studies and predate the use of antibiotics [1]. Flaxman in 1943 described 17 cases of staphylococcal myocardial abscesses without endocarditis [7]. Sanders in 1963 reported nine similar cases [8]. A further seven cases of staphylococcal myocarditis have been reported, six of which died with diagnosis confirmed at autopsy [9–14]. One case had aortic valve insufficiency requiring valve replacement secondary to a massive intramyocardial abscess [15]. All cases developed septic shock as a result of staphylococcal bacteraemia, and one case died as a result of ventricular rupture [10]. Risk

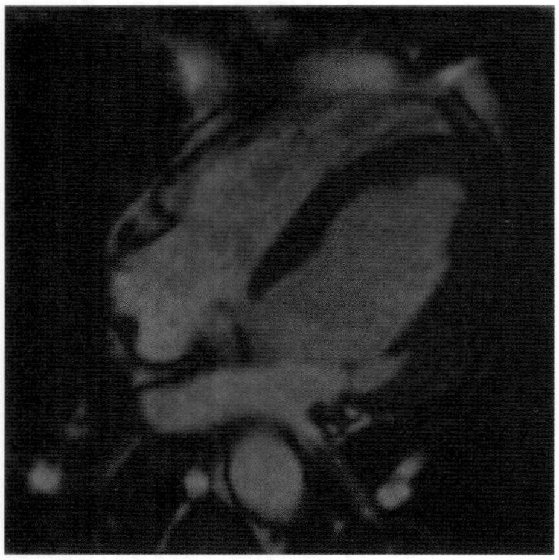

Figure 3: Cardiac magnetic resonance imaging 4-chamber view (still frame from a steady-state free precession (SSFP) cine sequence) taken 3 weeks after the previous study and on treatment (apixaban and antibiotics) demonstrating resolution of the apical mass.

factors for infection were identified in four cases including end-stage renal disease on haemodialysis [12], steroid-dependent Crohn's disease, and initiation of infliximab [15] and two cases with AIDS [13].

This case demonstrates two aspects of myocarditis that are unusual: firstly, isolated *staphylococcus aureus* myocarditis with no evidence of valvular involvement and secondly, left ventricular apical thrombus formation in a patient with normal left ventricle systolic function.

Isolated *staphylococcus aureus* myocarditis remains a rare condition. There have been case reports of both methicillin-sensitive and methicillin-resistant infections. As distinct from endocarditis and device infections, these cases of myocarditis are almost exclusively described in individuals who are immunocompromised.

Several conditions can present with thrombus or thrombus-like formation in the left ventricular apex, including dilated cardiomyopathy, Loeffler's endocarditis, myxoma, Chagas disease, and aneurysms. Factors that influence thrombus formation include blood stagnation, endothelial injury, and hypercoagulable states [16, 17].

In this case, the predominant force of Virchow's triad is likely endothelial injury and inflammation secondary to myocarditis. Echocardiography demonstrated the apical mass but was not able to define the thrombus or associated inflammation in the myocardium, whereas CMR was useful for tissue characterisation but not able to identify the aetiology.

Anticoagulation in cases of left ventricular thrombus, especially in the context of normal systolic function, has limited evidence but is used to reduce the risk of embolisation. Warfarin has historically been used due to familiarity and lack of evidence with direct acting oral anticoagulants (DOACs). Several cases of successful treatment with DOACs have been described [18], but to our knowledge, this is the first case of thrombus treatment with apixaban in the context of normal systolic function.

References

[1] F. Wasi and J. Shuter, "Primary bacterial infection of the myocardium," *Frontiers in Bioscience*, vol. 8, pp. s228–s231, 2003.

[2] A. L. P. Caforio, S. Pankuweit, E. Arbustini et al., "Current state of knowledge on aetiology, diagnosis, management, and therapy of myocarditis: a position statement of the European Society of Cardiology Working Group on Myocardial and Pericardial Diseases," *European Heart Journal*, vol. 34, no. 33, pp. 2636–2648, 2013.

[3] O. Leone, J. P. Veinot, A. Angelini et al., "2011 consensus statement on endomyocardial biopsy from the Association for European Cardiovascular Pathology and the Society for Cardiovascular Pathology," *Cardiovascular Pathology*, vol. 21, no. 4, pp. 245–274, 2012.

[4] H. Baccouche, H. Mahrholdt, G. Meinhardt et al., "Diagnostic synergy of non-invasive cardiovascular magnetic resonance and invasive endomyocardial biopsy in troponin-positive patients without coronary artery disease," *European Heart Journal*, vol. 30, no. 23, pp. 2869–2879, 2009.

[5] M. Gutberlet, B. Spors, T. Thoma et al., "Suspected chronic myocarditis at cardiac MR: diagnostic accuracy and association with immunohistologically detected inflammation and viral persistence," *Radiology*, vol. 246, no. 2, pp. 401–409, 2008.

[6] P. Lurz, I. Eitel, J. Adam et al., "Diagnostic performance of CMR imaging compared with EMB in patients with suspected myocarditis," *JACC: Cardiovascular Imaging*, vol. 5, no. 5, pp. 513–524, 2012.

[7] N. Flaxman, "Myocardial Abscess," *JAMA*, vol. 122, no. 12, pp. 804–806, 1943.

[8] V. Sanders, "Viral myocarditis," *American Heart Journal*, vol. 66, no. 5, pp. 707–713, 1963.

[9] A. K. Sikary, A. R. Mridha, and C. Behera, "Sudden death of a child due to pyogenic bacterial myocarditis," *Medico-Legal Journal*, vol. 85, no. 2, pp. 105–107, 2017.

[10] R. M. LeLeiko, D. J. Bower, and C. P. Larsen, "MRSA-associated bacterial myocarditis causing ruptured ventricle and tamponade," *Cardiology*, vol. 111, no. 3, pp. 188–190, 2008.

[11] Y. P. Lee, W. H. Hoi, and R. C. Wong, "A case of myopericarditis in a patient with methicillin-resistant Staphylococcus aureus community-acquired pneumonia," *Annals of the Academy of Medicine, Singapore*, vol. 37, no. 3, pp. 243–242, 2008.

[12] B. Khan, R. W. Strate, and R. Hellman, "*ASDIN Original Investigations*: Myocardial abscess and fatal cardiac arrhythmia in a hemodialysis patient with an arterio-venous fistula infection," *Seminars in Dialysis*, vol. 20, no. 5, pp. 452–454, 2007.

[13] P. Hofman, J. F. Michiels, E. Rosenthal et al., "Acute Staphylococcus aureus myocarditis in AIDS. 2 cases," *Archives des Maladies du Coeur et des Vaisseaux*, vol. 86, no. 12, pp. 1765–1768, 1993.

[14] P. Jariwala, A. Punjani, S. Mirza, B. Harikishan, and D. B. Madhawar, "Myocardial abscess secondary to staphylococcal septicemia: diagnosis with 3D echocardiography," *Indian Heart Journal*, vol. 65, no. 1, pp. 124-125, 2013.

[15] P. Reichardt, I. Dahnert, G. Tiller, and H. J. Hausler, "Possible activation of an intramyocardial inflammatory process (*Staphylococcus aureus*) after treatment with infliximab in a boy with Crohn disease," *European Journal of Pediatrics*, vol. 161, no. 5, pp. 281–283, 2002.

[16] R. Delewi, F. Zijlstra, and J. J. Piek, "Left ventricular thrombus formation after acute myocardial infarction," *Heart*, vol. 98, no. 23, pp. 1743–1749, 2012.

[17] S. Solheim, I. Seljeflot, K. Lunde et al., "Prothrombotic markers in patients with acute myocardial infarction and left ventricular thrombus formation treated with pci and dual antiplatelet therapy," *Thrombosis Journal*, vol. 11, no. 1, p. 1, 2013.

[18] Y. Mano, K. Koide, H. Sukegawa, M. Kodaira, and T. Ohki, "Successful resolution of a left ventricular thrombus with apixaban treatment following acute myocardial infarction," *Heart and Vessels*, vol. 31, no. 1, pp. 118–123, 2016.

Brugada Phenocopy Induced by Recreational Drug Use

Adedoyin Akinlonu,[1] Ranjit Suri,[2] Priyanka Yerragorla,[1] Persio D. López,[1] Tuoyo O. Mene-Afejuku,[1] Olatunde Ola,[1] Carissa Dumancas,[1] Jumana Chalabi,[1] Gerald Pekler,[3] Ferdinand Visco,[3] and Savi Mushiyev[3]

[1]*Department of Medicine, Health+Hospitals/Metropolitan, New York Medical College, Valhalla, NY, USA*
[2]*Cardiovascular Department, Arrhythmia Services Mount Sinai Health System Hospitals, Mount Sinai St. Luke's, New York, NY, USA*
[3]*Department of Medicine, Division of Cardiology, Health+Hospitals/Metropolitan, New York Medical College, Valhalla, NY, USA*

Correspondence should be addressed to Adedoyin Akinlonu; aakinlonu@gmail.com

Academic Editor: Man-Hong Jim

Recreational drugs are commonly abused in all age groups. Intoxication with these substances can induce silent but significant electrocardiographic signs which may lead to sudden death. In this case study, we present a 49-year-old male with no medical comorbidities who came to the emergency department requesting opioid detoxification. Toxicology screen was positive for cocaine, heroin, and cannabis. Initial electrocardiogram (EKG) showed features of a Brugada pattern in the right precordial leads, which resolved within one day into admission. This presentation is consistent with the recently recognized clinical entity known as Brugada phenocopy.

1. Introduction

The Brugada electrocardiographic pattern (BEP) is a coved-type, downsloping, ≥2 mm ST segment elevation with T-wave inversion among the right precordial leads V1-V2 (occasionally only in V1 and unusually also in V3) termed type 1 BEP, or a saddle-back convex ST segment elevation with variable T wave in V1, and positive or flat T wave in lead V2 (types 2 or 3 BEP) [1]. Initial guidelines required documented, polymorphic ventricular tachycardia or fibrillation, a family history of sudden cardiac death (≤45 years old), coved-type electrocardiograms in family members, syncope, or nocturnal agonal respiration in addition to the type 1 BEP for a diagnosis of Brugada syndrome (BrS) [2–4]. The latest guidelines, nonetheless, only require the documentation of type 1 BEP, either spontaneously or as a consequence of a provocative test with sodium channel blockers for a diagnosis of BrS [5].

2. Case Presentation

A 49-year-old Hispanic man presented to our institution requesting opioid detoxification. He had no specific clinical complaints, and the review of systems was negative. The patient's physical examination was unremarkable. Initial workup revealed normal complete blood count, electrolyte panel, and renal and hepatic function; a urine toxicology screen was positive for cocaine, opioid, and cannabinoid use.

An electrocardiogram obtained on admission (Figure 1(a)) revealed a Brugada pattern which was not present on previous studies. He was monitored on a telemetry unit, and a repeat electrocardiogram the morning after showed complete resolution of the Brugada-type abnormalities (Figure 1(b)). On targeted interrogation, he denied any syncopal episodes and he had not been informed of nocturnal breathing abnormalities by his partner; there had been no sudden, unexplained deaths in his family. The patient's parents were contacted, and their electrocardiograms were found to be normal. Since the patient's

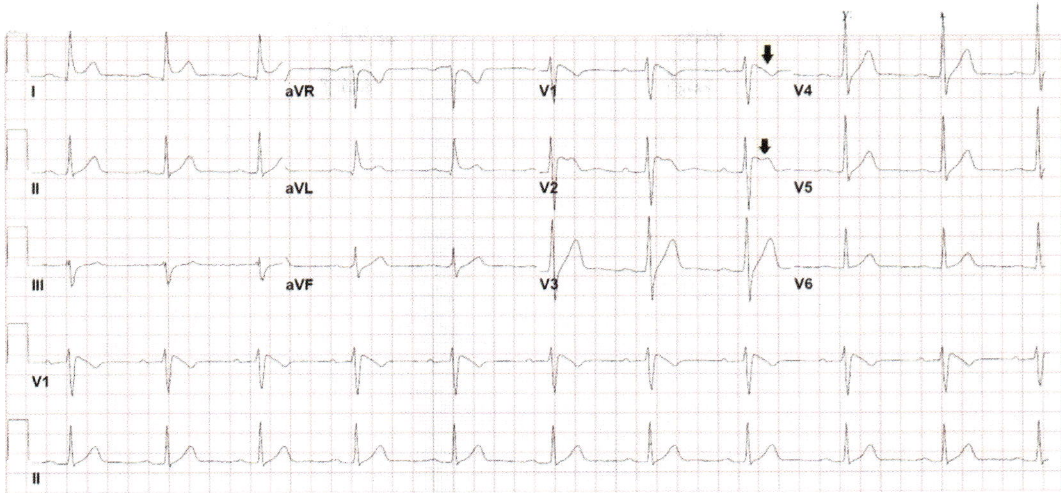

(a)

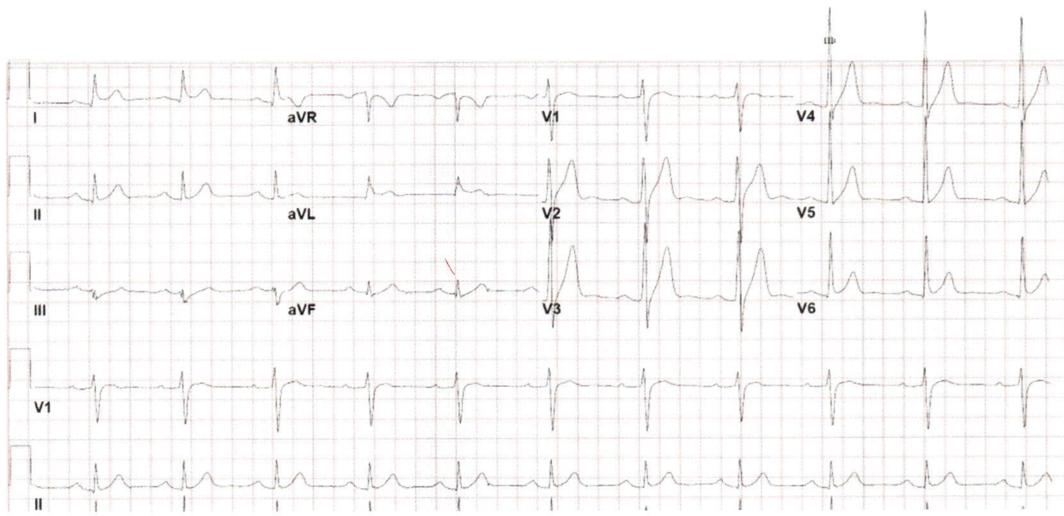

(b)

FIGURE 1: Electrocardiograms of the first admission revealing transient Brugada pattern (a, arrow) with complete resolution the following morning (b).

electrocardiogram was not completely normal, he was referred to an affiliated tertiary institution for provocative testing with sodium channel blockers; however, he did not follow-up. Multiple attempts to convince the patient to undergo further workup were unsuccessful. Five months later, he was readmitted to the observation unit of our institution for evaluation of cocaine-associated chest pain. The urine toxicology screen was again positive for cocaine, opioid, and cannabinoid use. His admission electrocardiogram revealed recurrence of the Brugada pattern (Figure 2(a)), which resolved after 24 hours (Figure 2(b)). Both a transthoracic echocardiogram and a stress myocardial perfusion scintigraphy were normal. Once more, he declined further workup. The patient was asymptomatic and hemodynamically stable at the time of hospital discharge.

3. Discussion

BrS is an autosomal dominant, low-penetrance disease caused by several different loss-of-function gene mutations that affect the $Na_v1.5$ sodium channel [6]. In addition, mutations causing loss of function of the calcium channel currents and a gain of function of potassium channel currents have also been associated with BrS [7]. These genetic abnormalities are thought to induce defective depolarization and/or early repolarization [8, 9], which lead to the clinical manifestations of BrS: life-threatening arrhythmias and sudden cardiac death.

Not all patients with BrS, however, become symptomatic [6], which has led to recommendations regarding risk stratification [7]. Moreover, BEP has been reported in association to several acute and persistent conditions: acute

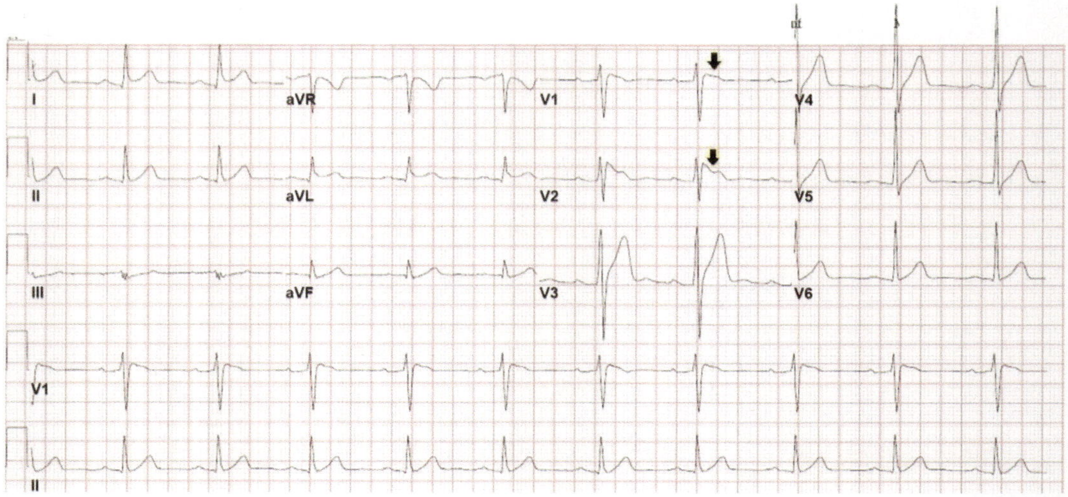

(a)

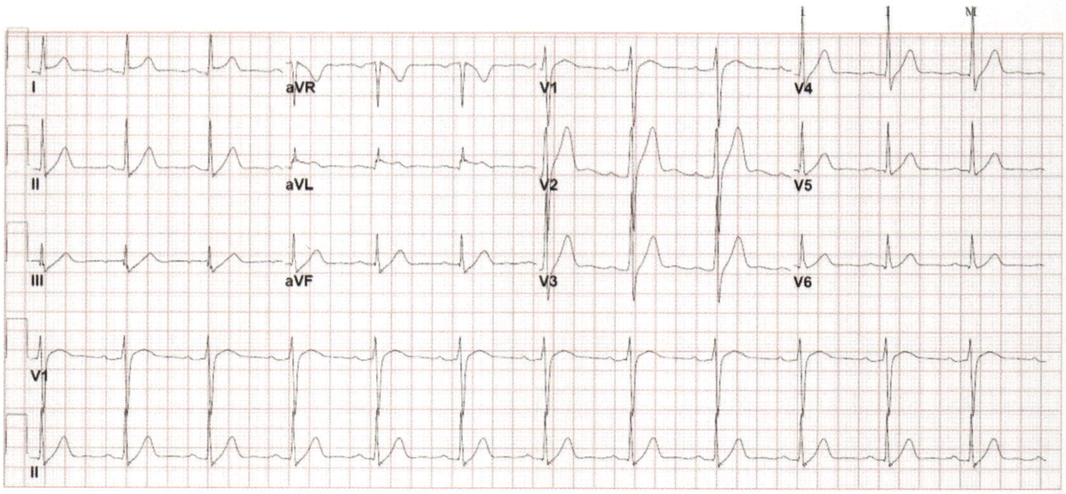

(b)

FIGURE 2: Electrocardiograms revealing recurrence of the Brugada pattern in the setting of recreational drug use (a, arrow) and complete resolution after approximately 24 hours without substance use (b).

coronary events, pericarditis, myocarditis, pulmonary embolism, metabolic disorders, electrolyte imbalances, dissecting aorta aneurysm, thiamine deficiency, electric shock, certain pharmacologic agents, left ventricular hypertrophy, athlete's heart, right bundle branch block, pectus excavatum, septal hypertrophy, arrhythmogenic right ventricular cardiomyopathy or dysplasia, autonomic nervous system abnormalities, Duchenne dystrophy, Friedreich's ataxia, mediastinal tumor, and Chagas disease [7, 10].

Recently, the term "Brugada phenocopy" (BrP) has been used to describe these cases, provided they fulfill the following criteria: there is an identifiable trigger, BEP resolves after removal of said trigger (when possible), and the results of a provocative test with sodium channel blockers are negative [10]. Patients with BrP would be classified morphologically according to the type of BEP and further qualified depending on whether all diagnostic criteria are met [10, 11]. The term is still controversial, as it has been argued that data regarding a genetic predisposition are lacking in almost all cases [7]. We believe it is a helpful descriptor to identify patients with a lower risk of developing the feared complications of BrS that would warrant invasive therapeutics.

Both cannabis and cocaine have been associated with BrP [12–14], possibly due to their activities on the cardiac voltage-gated sodium channel [14, 15]. The EKG changes seen with cannabis use are a result of its action as a partial agonist of the cardiac sodium channels, and arrhythmias can be induced if the action potential is shortened [12, 13, 15]. Cocaine, on the other hand, blocks sodium and potassium ion channels and also inhibits calcium entry into the cardiac myocytes thereby impairing action potential and altering the normal electrical activity of the heart [9, 16]. A synergistic effect is observed by coingestion of the above two drugs since cannabis increases the plasma concentration of cocaine [16]. Heroin has also been associated with BEP, though the exact cardiovascular mechanism remains to be described [16, 17]. A combination of the effects of these substances likely triggered the appearance of BEP in our patient. Unlike in symptomatic patients, individuals with drug-induced Brugada EKG pattern who are asymptomatic generally have good prognosis (i.e., there is a low risk of lethal arrhythmias), and the observed EKG changes is likely to be benign [9, 18]. Therefore, the need for provocative testing in these groups of patients might be unwarranted but reasonable to pursue when feasible with due considerations given to the risks and benefits [11, 18].

This presentation of highly suspected BrP in the setting of cocaine, cannabinoid, and heroin use continues to raise the alarm about the cardiovascular effects of these substances. Although the clinical implications of BrP remain to be elucidated, genetic testing may help in differentiating BrP from BrS and thus with managing these patients.

Authors' Contributions

All authors had access to the case and participated in the elaboration of this manuscript.

References

[1] A. Bayés de Luna, J. Brugada, A. Baranchuk et al., "Current electrocardiographic criteria for diagnosis of Brugada pattern: a consensus report," *Journal of Electrocardiology*, vol. 45, no. 5, pp. 433–442, 2012.

[2] C. Antzelevitch, P. Brugada, M. Borggrefe et al., "Brugada syndrome: report of the second consensus conference: endorsed by the Heart Rhythm Society and the European Heart Rhythm Association," *Circulation*, vol. 111, no. 5, pp. 659–670, 2005.

[3] A. A. Wilde, C. Antzelevitch, M. Borggrefe et al., "Proposed diagnostic criteria for the Brugada syndrome," *European Heart Journal*, vol. 23, no. 21, pp. 1648–1654, 2002.

[4] A. A. Wilde, C. Antzelevitch, M. Borggrefe et al., "Proposed diagnostic criteria for the Brugada syndrome: consensus report," *Circulation*, vol. 106, no. 19, pp. 2514–2519, 2002.

[5] S. G. Priori, A. A. Wilde, M. Horie et al., "Executive summary: HRS/EHRA/APHRS expert consensus statement on the diagnosis and management of patients with inherited primary arrhythmia syndromes," *EP Europace*, vol. 15, no. 10, pp. 1389–1406, 2013.

[6] A. Curcio, G. Santarpia, and C. Indolfi, "The Brugada syndrome–from gene to therapy," *Circulation Journal*, vol. 81, no. 3, pp. 290–297, 2017.

[7] C. Antzelevitch and B. Patocskai, "Brugada syndrome: clinical, genetic, molecular, cellular, and ionic aspects," *Current Problems in Cardiology*, vol. 41, no. 1, pp. 7–57, 2016.

[8] M. M. Refaat, M. Hotait, and M. Scheinman, "Brugada syndrome," *Cardiac Electrophysiology Clinics*, vol. 8, no. 1, pp. 239–245, 2016.

[9] Y. G. Yap, E. R. Behr, and A. J. Camm, "Drug-induced Brugada syndrome," *EP Europace*, vol. 11, no. 8, pp. 989–994, 2009.

[10] A. Baranchuk, T. Nguyen, M. H. Ryu et al., "Brugada phenocopy: new terminology and proposed classification," *Annals of Noninvasive Electrocardiology*, vol. 17, no. 4, pp. 299–314, 2012.

[11] B. Gottschalk, D. D. Anselm, and A. Baranchuk, "Brugada phenocopy: morphological classification and importance of provocative testing," *Annals of Noninvasive Electrocardiology*, vol. 19, no. 6, pp. 604-605, 2014.

[12] M. Daccarett, M. Freih, and C. Machado, "Acute cannabis intoxication mimicking Brugada-like ST segment abnormalities," *International Journal of Cardiology*, vol. 119, no. 2, pp. 235-236, 2007.

[13] J. V. Alonso, B. H. Teo, F. J. Pozo, M. A. Aguayo, and A. Sanchez, "Brugada electrocardiogram pattern induced by cannabis; is cannabis safe?," *American Journal of Emergency Medicine*, vol. 34, no. 8, pp. 1738e.1–1738e.4, 2016.

[14] R. B. Weiner, S. D. Weiner, and P. M. Yurchak, "Removing the mask," *American Journal of Medicine*, vol. 121, no. 2, pp. 113–116, 2008.

[15] S. Johnson and E. F. Domino, "Some cardiovascular effects of marihuana smoking in normal volunteers," *Clinical Pharmacology & Therapeutics*, vol. 12, no. 5, pp. 762–768, 1971.

[16] A. Ghuran and J. Nolan, "Recreational drug misuse: issues for the cardiologist," *Heart*, vol. 83, no. 6, pp. 627–633, 2000.

[17] M. Rambod, S. Elhanafi, and D. Mukherjee, "Brugada phenocopy in concomitant ethanol and heroin overdose," *Annals of Noninvasive Electrocardiology*, vol. 20, no. 1, pp. 87–90, 2015.

[18] M. Nishizaki, H. Sakurada, N. Yamawake, A. Ueda-Tatsumoto, and M. Hiraoka, "Low risk for arrhythmic events in asymptomatic patients with drug-induced type 1 ECG," *Circulation Journal*, vol. 74, no. 11, pp. 2464–2473, 2010.

Spontaneous Regression of Cardiac Rhabdomyoma Presenting as Severe Left Ventricular Inlet Obstruction in a Neonate with Tuberous Sclerosis

Eun Song Song, Kumi Jeong, Gun Kim, In Ji Hwang, Mi-Ji Lee, Hwa Jin Cho, and Young Kuk Cho

Department of Pediatrics, Chonnam National University Medical School, Chonnam National University Hospital, Gwangju, Republic of Korea

Correspondence should be addressed to Young Kuk Cho; youngcx@hanmail.net

Academic Editor: Assad Movahed

Cardiac rhabdomyoma can be subclinical or have a fatal presentation according to the onset age and involved site, size, and degree of invasion. Although most cardiac rhabdomyomas become smaller with time, emergency intervention is indicated when severe obstruction has occurred. In this report, we describe the spontaneous regression of a large cardiac rhabdomyoma (20.5 × 15.6 mm) presenting as severe left ventricular inlet obstruction in a neonate with tuberous sclerosis. Although a cardiac rhabdomyoma can be large enough to induce left ventricular inlet obstruction, conservative treatment without aggressive surgical intervention can be considered if the hemodynamic condition does not deteriorate.

1. Introduction

Rhabdomyoma is the most common cardiac tumor in infants and children and is reported in up to 50–64% of infants with tuberous sclerosis [1, 2]. Its expression ranges from subclinical to fatal presentation, according to the onset age and the site, size, and degree of invasion [3]. Although rhabdomyomas become smaller with time, when severe obstruction induces hemodynamic instability or a rhythm abnormality, emergency intervention is indicated [4–6]. Rhabdomyoma causing left ventricular (LV) inlet obstruction can necessitate an emergency operation [3, 7–10]. However, there is no recorded report of spontaneous resolution of a huge cardiac rhabdomyoma causing LV inlet obstruction. We report a case of spontaneous regression of a large symptomatic cardiac rhabdomyoma presenting as severe LV inlet obstruction, occupying 75–90% of the mitral valve (MV) annulus in a neonate with tuberous sclerosis.

2. Case Presentation

A male infant was born at 39 weeks of gestation by vaginal delivery to a healthy 35-year-old female. There was no family history of congenital heart disease or tuberous sclerosis. At 31 weeks of gestation, a fetal echocardiogram revealed a large, solitary LV mass and multiple right ventricular (RV) masses. The delivery was uneventful. The Apgar score was 10 at both 1 and 5 minutes. Birth weight of 3,450 g, length of 51.0 cm, and head circumference of 35.5 cm were normal. Transcutaneous oxygen saturation was 95% on room air, heart rate was 132 bpm, respiratory rate was 48/minute, arterial pressure was 62/38 mmHg, a grade 2/6 mid-diastolic rumbling murmur was heard at the left sternal border, and there were no skin lesions. Chest X-ray showed mild cardiomegaly with increased pulmonary vascular markings. Transcranial ultrasonography was normal.

Two-dimensional echocardiographic examination revealed a large solitary tumor measuring 20.5 × 15.6 mm and occupying 75–90% of the mitral annulus (Figures 1(a)–1(c)). This tumor was attached to the anterior leaflet of the MV, causing LV inlet obstruction. The peak velocity through the MV was 1.66 m/s (Figure 1(d)). Right atrial and RV dilatation and pressure overload secondary to pulmonary hypertension were observed (Figure 1(e)). The peak jet velocity through the regurgitant tricuspid valve was 4.13 m/s (Figure 1(f)). Mild mitral

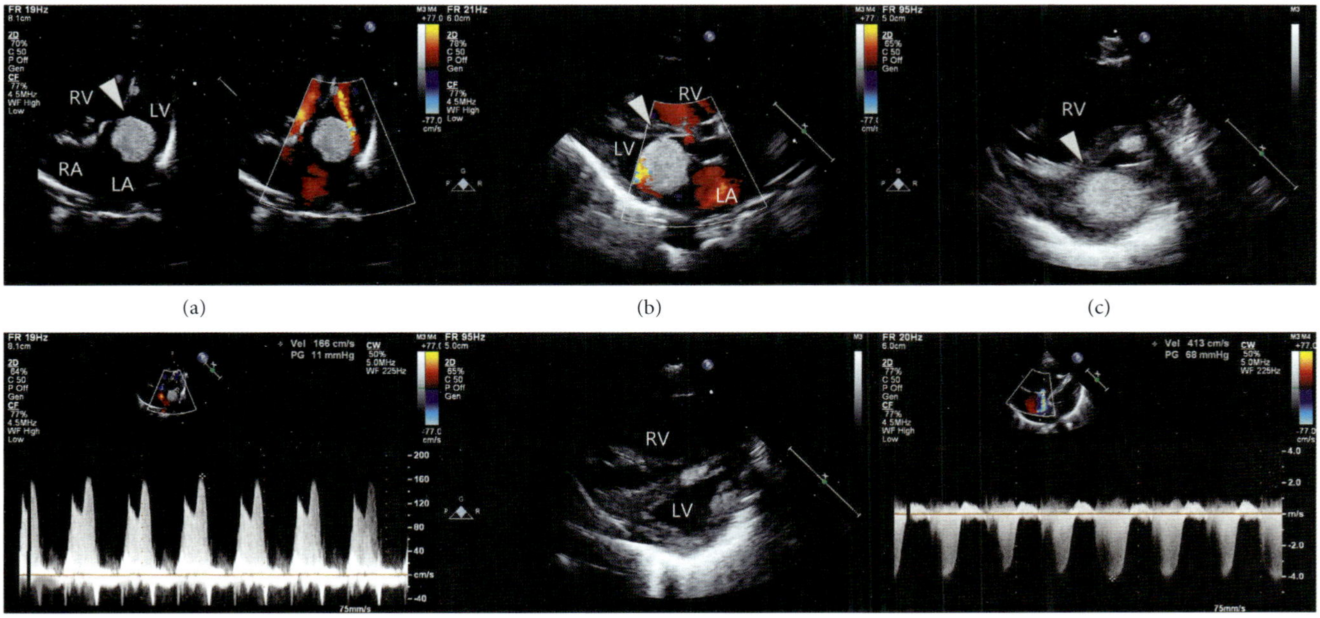

(a) (b) (c)

(d) (e) (f)

FIGURE 1: Two-dimensional echocardiography shows a large rhabdomyoma (arrowhead), 20.5 × 15.6 mm in diameter, occupying 75–90% of the mitral annulus, in addition to multiple small tubers in both ventricles and the left ventricular outflow tract after birth in apical 4-chamber (a), parasternal long-axis (b), and parasternal short-axis (c) views. Right atrial, right ventricular (RV), and left atrial dilatation were also observed. Pulse Doppler echocardiography showed a peak velocity through the mitral valve of 1.66 m/s (d). RV dilatation and pressure overload secondary to pulmonary hypertension were observed in a parasternal, end-diastolic short-axis view (e). The peak velocity through the tricuspid valve was 4.13 m/s (f).

regurgitation (MR), left atrial (LA) enlargement without LV dilatation, and multiple small tubers in both ventricles and the LV outflow tract were observed (Figures 1(a)–1(c)). LV ejection fraction was normal at 67.2%. Although the newborn had mild subcostal chest retractions, his vital signs were stable; therefore, inotropes and oxygen were not provided. At 5 h of age, paroxysmal supraventricular tachyarrhythmia at 240 bpm developed. Because intermittent supraventricular tachyarrhythmia with desaturation and irritability continued, repeated doses of adenosine were administered intravenously to restore sinus rhythm. Digoxin was started for long-term management and the tachyarrhythmia resolved. Genetic analysis was performed to detect mutations of tuberous sclerosis complex (*TSC*) 1 and 2 genes. *TSC1* mutation was absent, but a *TSC2* mutation (*c.5161–1G* > C) was detected. Ophthalmic examination revealed a jagged-edged, linear depigmented retina in the right eye. During the 14-day hospital stay, blood pressure was well maintained without inotropes, tachypnea improved, the frequency of breast-feeding increased, and weight gain was observed. Follow-up chest X-ray showed regression of cardiomegaly and pulmonary vascular markings. Follow-up echocardiography demonstrated decreased MR and pulmonary hypertension and normal systolic LV function. The infant was discharged with only digoxin to prevent arrhythmias.

At 40 days of age, symptoms and signs associated with LV inlet obstruction and tachyarrhythmia were absent. Echocardiography showed good LV function with decreased rhabdomyoma size (16.8 × 11.5 mm). At 3 months of age, a tonic-type seizure occurred and right frontal cortical tubers, multifocal white-matter lesions, and subependymal nodules were discovered on brain magnetic resonance imaging (Figures 2(a) and 2(b)). Vigabatrin as an antiepileptic drug was started. Depigmented skin lesions were also found that time on the right shoulder and chest.

At 6 months of age, echocardiography revealed a further decrease in rhabdomyoma size (13.8 × 12.1 mm); the lesion occupied a smaller portion (about 50%) of the mitral annulus (Figure 3(a)). Tricuspid regurgitation and pulmonary hypertension were improved. MR and LA dilatation were not observed. Digoxin was maintained up to 24 months of age. After discontinuation of medication, no further tachyarrhythmias occurred.

At 3 years of age, echocardiography showed a very small (6.5 × 2.3 mm), ellipse-shaped rhabdomyoma attached to the MV anterior leaflet without LV inlet obstruction (peak velocity = 0.76 m/s) (Figures 3(b) and 3(c)). At that time, fibroadenomas began to develop on the face. Convulsions were controlled by vigabatrin and topiramate. A developmental delay of about 18 months was apparent.

3. Discussion

Although cardiac rhabdomyomas are known to spontaneously regress in patients with tuberous sclerosis, many complications associated with tumor location and size are possible [1–3]. Some patients are very symptomatic, with signs of severe heart failure or valve dysfunction due to blood flow

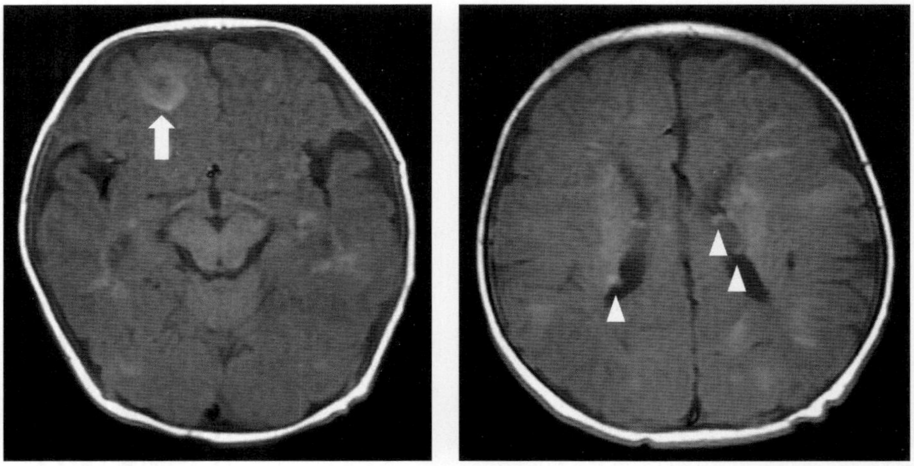

(a) (b)

Figure 2: At 3 months of age, T1-weighted magnetic resonance imaging showed a right frontal cortical tuber (arrow) (a) and high signal intensity lesions in both cerebral hemispheres, with multiple nodular lesions (arrowheads) along the lateral ventricular caudothalamic grooves (b).

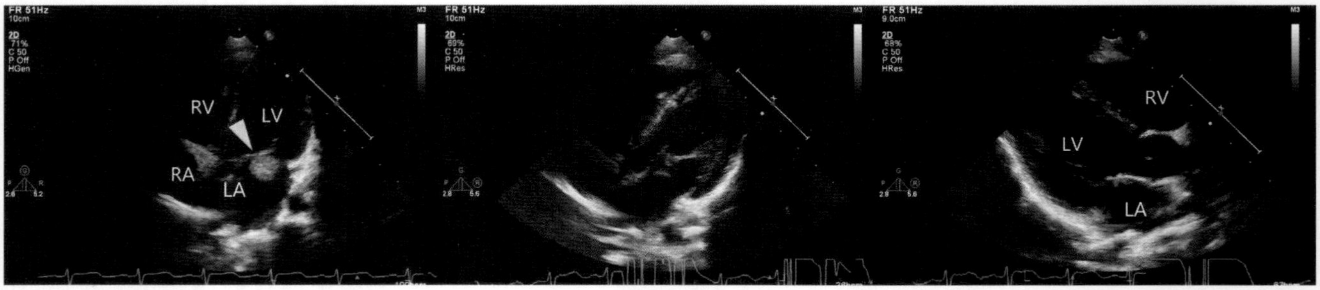

(a) (b) (c)

Figure 3: Two-dimensional follow-up echocardiography showed that rhabdomyoma size was significantly decreased at 6 months of age (a). At 3 years of age, a very small (6.5 × 2.3 mm), ellipse-shaped rhabdomyoma attached to the MV anterior leaflet without LV inlet obstruction (peak velocity = 0.76 m/sec) (b and c) was observed.

obstruction, and even univentricular physiology [7]. Only five case reports of hemodynamically significant LV inflow obstruction caused by cardiac rhabdomyoma have been published (Table 1). Four cases were associated with tuberous sclerosis [3, 7, 9, 11], and most were detected in infancy and the perinatal period. The other case involved a tumor detected in adulthood. Common initial symptoms were related to heart failure, including cyanosis and dyspnea with or without cardiomegaly [9]. Surgical resection of tumor was performed in four patients in whom the lesions were attached to the septum. A 1-day-old infant underwent atrial septostomy by cardiac catheterization due to hemodynamic instability.

In our case, a large rhabdomyoma (20.5 × 15.6 mm) occupied 75–90% of the LV inlet and caused obstruction, LA enlargement, and pulmonary hypertension. The patient did not undergo surgical intervention because he was hemodynamically stable. Since the rhabdomyoma was attached to the anterior leaflet of the MV, there was a risk of valve dysfunction after surgery. With increasing age, the LV inflow obstruction was attenuated by decreasing rhabdomyoma and increasing mitral annulus size. At 3 years of age, the rhabdomyoma had decreased to an ellipse-shaped mass 6.5 × 2.3 mm in size and showed no LV flow disturbance. Repeat echocardiography to confirm hemodynamic stability played a critical role in determining treatment. Many reports have emphasized the usefulness of echocardiography in the management of cardiac rhabdomyoma in neonates or children. Di Liang et al. [11] described serial echocardiographic evaluation of cardiac rhabdomyoma. Follow-up echocardiography revealed that of 22 tumors in 8 patients, 7 completely regressed, 7 partially regressed, and 8 remained stable. In addition, Batmaz et al. [12] reported a huge spherical rhabdomyoma originating from the MV in an asymptomatic patient with a murmur and experienced spontaneous regression with conservative treatment alone. In the present case, the neonate had an arrhythmia and evidence of congestive heart failure. Hemodynamic stability was confirmed accurately and continuously with echocardiography. Therefore, we provided conservative treatment.

TABLE 1: Clinical features of patients with significant LV inlet obstruction caused by cardiac rhabdomyoma.

Reference, year	Age at diagnosis	Initial presentation	Rhabdomyoma number	Rhabdomyoma treatment	Spontaneous rhabdomyoma regression	Genetic analysis	Tuberous sclerosis-associated sign	Outcome
Mair et al., 1977 [7]	1 day	Cyanosis Tachypnea Tachycardia Cardiomegaly Hepatomegaly	Multiple	Atrial septostomy	No	None	Cerebral hamartoma	Died
Muhler et al., 1994 [3]	5 weeks	Pulmonary edema	1	Tumor resection	No	None	None	Died
Dyamenahalli et al., 1998 [8]	1 day	Cyanosis Tachycardia	1	Tumor resection	No	None	Unknown	Alive
Abdel-Rahman et al., 2005 [9]	Prenatal	Cyanosis Cardiomegaly	3	Tumor resection	Unknown	None	Unknown	Alive
Ono et al., 2007 [10]	20 years	Dyspnea	Multiple	Tumor resection	No	None	None	Alive
This case	1 day	Tachypnea Tachycardia Cardiomegaly	Multiple	None	Yes	*TSC2*	Depigmented nevus Adenoma sebaceum Depigmented retina Developmental delay	Alive

TSC2: tuberous sclerosis 2.

4. Conclusion

Although a cardiac rhabdomyoma can be large enough to induce LV inlet obstruction, conservative treatment without aggressive surgical intervention can be considered if hemodynamic conditions do not deteriorate. In addition, repeated echocardiography may play a pivotal role in understanding hemodynamic status and establishing a treatment plan.

Disclosure

This case was presented at the poster session of the annual conference of Korean Pediatrics Society held in Seoul, South Korea, on Thursday, November 10, 2016.

Acknowledgments

This study was supported by a grant (NRF-2015R1D1A1A01059017) of the Basic Science Research Program through the National Research Foundation of Korea (NRF) funded by the Ministry of Education, Republic of Korea.

References

[1] W. Tworetzky, D. B. McElhinney, R. Margossian et al., "Association between cardiac tumors and tuberous sclerosis in the fetus and neonate," *American Journal of Cardiology*, vol. 92, no. 4, pp. 487–489, 2003.

[2] D. G. Holley, G. R. Martin, J. I. Brenner et al., "Diagnosis and management of fetal cardiac tumors: a multicenter experience and review of published reports," *Journal of the American College of Cardiology*, vol. 26, no. 2, pp. 516–520, 1995.

[3] E. G. Muhler, V. Turniski-Harder, W. Engelhardt, and G. von Bernuth, "Cardiac involvement in tuberous sclerosis," *British Heart Journal*, vol. 72, no. 6, pp. 584–590, 1994.

[4] T. Hishitani, K. Hoshino, K. Ogawa et al., "Rapid enlargement of cardiac rhabdomyoma during corticotropin therapy for infantile spasms," *Canadian Journal of Cardiology*, vol. 13, no. 1, pp. 72–74, 1997.

[5] C. M. Ikemba, B. W. Eidem, V. V. Dimas et al., "Fetal rhabdomyoma causing postnatal critical left ventricular outflow tract obstruction," *Annals of Thoracic Surgery*, vol. 80, no. 4, p. 1529, 2005.

[6] H. S. Chan, M. J. Sonley, C. A. Moes et al., "Primary and secondary tumors of childhood involving the heart, pericardium, and great vessels. A report of 75 cases and review of the literature," *Cancer*, vol. 56, no. 4, pp. 825–836, 1985.

[7] D. D. Mair, J. L. Titus, G. D. Davis, and D. G. Ritter, "Cardiac rhabdomyoma simulating mitral atresia," *Chest*, vol. 71, no. 1, pp. 102–105, 1977.

[8] U. Dyamenahalli, M. D. Black, C. Boutin et al., "Obstructive rhabdomyoma and univentricular physiology: a rare combination," *Annals of Thoracic Surgery*, vol. 65, no. 3, pp. 835–837, 1998.

[9] U. Abdel-Rahman, F. Ozaslan, A. Esmaeili, and A. Moritz, "A giant rhabdomyoma with left ventricular inflow occlusion and univentricular physiology," *Thoracic and Cardiovascular Surgeon*, vol. 53, no. 4, pp. 259-260, 2005.

[10] M. Ono, D. Boethig, E. Akin et al., "Coexistent cardiac rhabdomyoma with mitral valve anomaly in patients with tuberous sclerosis: a case report," *Thoracic and Cardiovascular Surgeon*, vol. 55, no. 2, pp. 120-121, 2007.

50

Severe Stenosis of an Anomalous Circumflex Artery Mimicking a Chronic Total Occlusion

George Mawardi and Anbukarasi Maran

Coronary CTO Program, Medical University of South Carolina, 30 Courtenay Street, MSC 592, Charleston, SC 29425, USA

Correspondence should be addressed to Anbukarasi Maran; maran@musc.edu

Academic Editor: Expedito E. Ribeiro

The prevalence of anomalous circumflex coronary arteries is rare. Identifying the presence of an anomalous coronary is quite easy when there is no severe stenosis. However, in the presence of severe stenosis, there is limited anterograde flow, which makes it challenging to visualize the course of the stenotic artery, and it can be assumed to be a chronic total occlusion (CTO). This case demonstrates how the anomalous circumflex artery with severe stenosis masqueraded as a CTO and the patient was treated medically for several years, despite continued symptoms. The retrograde filling of an anomalous circumflex has a specific angiographic pattern which should be recognized. This case is an excellent illustration of the said angiographic pattern.

1. Introduction

Coronary chronic total occlusion (CTO) can occur in up to 30% of patients with coronary artery disease. The foundation of CTO percutaneous intervention is understanding the coronary anatomy. This case report demonstrates the pitfalls of single catheter angiography in the presence of a coronary CTO. Because of the lack of understanding of the patient's coronary anatomy and failure to recognize the demonstrated specific angiographic pattern, the patient suffered with angina and did not receive appropriate treatment. Dual angiography is an essential initial step in patients undergoing CTO percutaneous coronary intervention (PCI) to define the anatomy completely. This case report illustrates how understanding the coronary anatomy with dual angiography completely changed the approach to intervention.

2. Case Presentation

The patient is a 65 year-old male with a past medical history significant for coronary artery disease (status post a drug-eluting stent to his right coronary artery in 2011, with occluded left circumflex), paroxysmal atrial fibrillation (status post ablation in 2015, rhythm controlled, on apixaban), abdominal aortic aneurysm (status post endovascular repair), diabetes mellitus (A1C of 6%), polymyalgia rheumatica on chronic prednisone, and colon cancer (status post resection), who was admitted to the General Medicine Service for lumbar 5-sacral 1 discitis. Cardiology was consulted for chest pain. The patient normally had stable angina pectoris but now had been experiencing unstable angina and nocturnal angina. His electrocardiogram at the time demonstrated sinus rhythm with anterolateral ST segment depressions and T wave inversions and isolated ST segment elevation in aVR. He was treated with sublingual nitroglycerin, after which the chest pain and electrocardiographic changes were resolved (EKG at rest showed sinus bradycardia, occasional premature atrial contractions (PAC), and upright T waves, with no ischemic changes).

About five months before the current episode, he had a nuclear stress test which demonstrated a small reversible perfusion defect of moderate severity in the basal, lateral region, consistent with mild ischemia. His ejection fraction was 53%.

His cardiac medications include carvedilol, aspirin, isosorbide, and lovastatin.

His physical exam was not remarkable for any physical exam findings.

His echocardiogram here showed normal ejection fraction, with inferior wall hypokinesis with a pseudonormal filling pattern.

A cardiac heart catheterization was recommended given the significant symptoms and significant electrocardiographic changes as part of his preoperative risk assessment.

The catheterization showed that the left main bifurcates into the left anterior descending (LAD) and a small left circumflex (LCx). There was also mild disease of the mid and distal left main.

The LAD wraps around the left ventricle apex, with diffuse mild-moderate disease. It gives off a large diagonal branch with mild diffuse disease (Figure 1).

The LCx was described as a small vessel with proximal occlusion at the takeoff of a large marginal branch that has mild diffuse disease (Figures 2(a) and 2(b)).

The right coronary artery (RCA) is a dominant vessel with a focal area of moderate eccentric disease in the mid vessel. Otherwise, it has mild diffuse disease. It gives off a large posterior descending artery (PDA) and posterolateral branch (PLB) that directly provide retrograde collateral supply to the distal atrioventricular (A-V) circumflex. The A-V circumflex turns at an acute angle away from the left main artery (Figure 3) (video file 1).

The patient underwent uncomplicated back surgery. He continued to have exertional angina (Canadian Cardiovascular Society (CCS) class III-IV) with substernal chest tightness and radiation to the shoulder with minimal activity and at rest at night. Symptoms were relieved by sublingual nitroglycerin. He was subsequently referred for hemodynamic assessment of the left main and left anterior descending with planned CTO PCI of the occluded circumflex.

During CTO PCI, initial dual angiogram demonstrated that the RCA collateral to the circumflex was in a different plane than the left main coronary artery (Figure 4).

This raised the suspicion that the circumflex artery was probably anomalous in origin (Figure 5).

Further probing of the right coronary cusp demonstrated an anomalous origin of the circumflex artery. The patient did not have CTO of the circumflex but instead had severe stenosis of his anomalous circumflex (Figure 6).

The patient was found to have an anomalous left circumflex artery, the most common coronary anomaly. Fractional flow reserve of the left main and the left anterior descending were 0.91 at rest and 0.82 at hyperaemia.

The patient underwent successful PCI of the anomalous circumflex with drug-eluting stents (Figure 7) (video file 1).

3. Follow-Up

The patient did not have CTO of the left circumflex artery as described in his cardiac catheterizations previously but instead had severe stenosis of his anomalous circumflex artery. Angiographic pattern recognition of an anomalous course of a coronary artery in the presence of severe stenosis/chronic total occlusion is of importance to avoid treatment delays. The patient was followed up in a cardiology clinic 4 weeks after the procedure. He was angina free and had stopped taking long-acting nitrates.

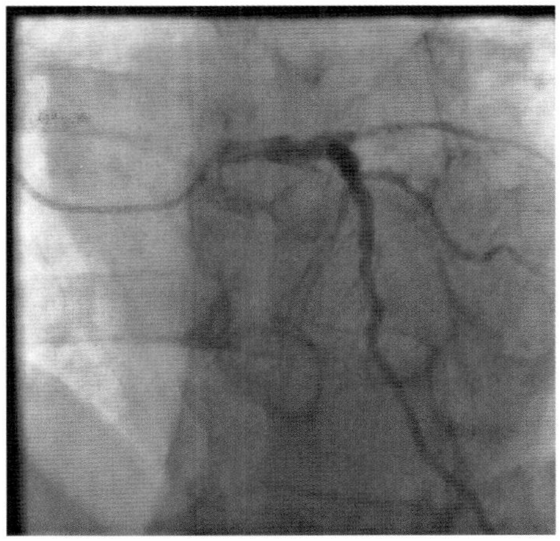

Figure 1: Diagnostic angiogram: left anterior oblique/cranial view demonstrating the LAD and diagonal branches.

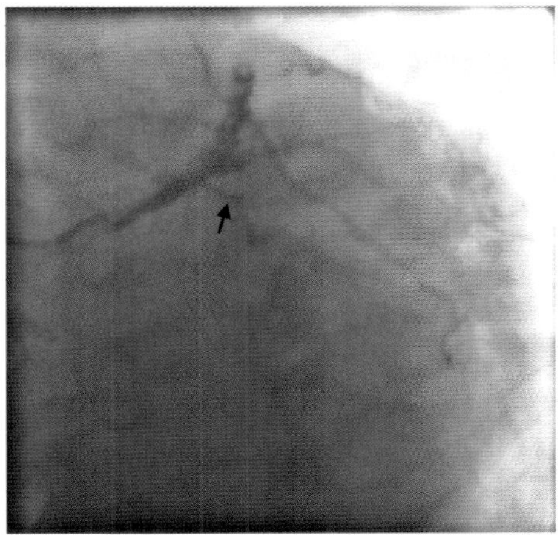

(a)

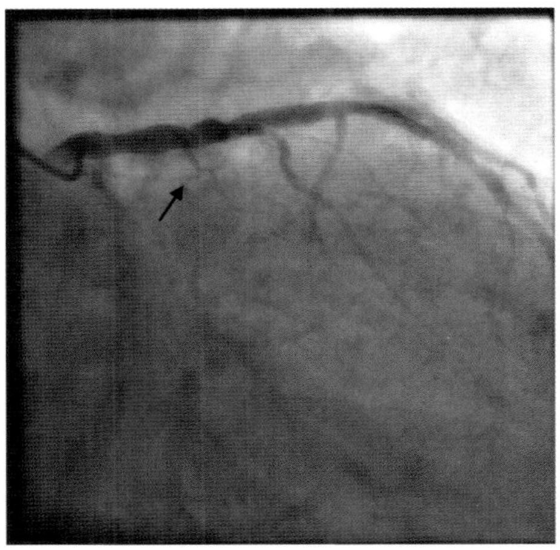

(b)

Figure 2: (a) Diagnostic angiogram in left anterior oblique/caudal view; (b) right anterior oblique/caudal view demonstrating the LAD ramus branch with moderate disease and diminutive circumflex branches (arrow).

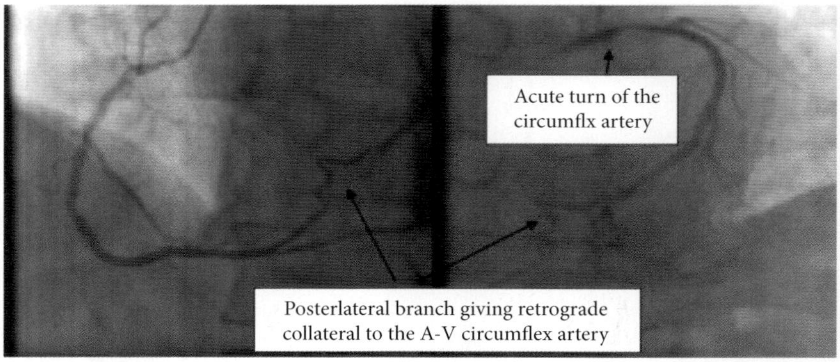

Figure 3: Right coronary artery with collaterals to the circumflex artery.

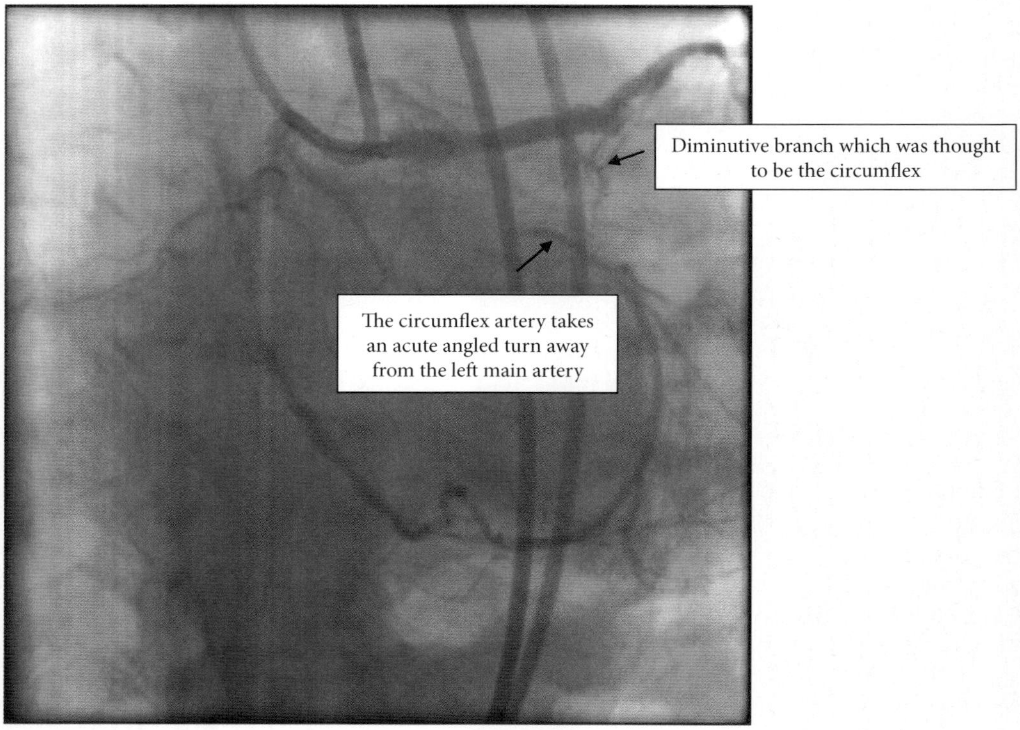

Figure 4: Dual angiogram demonstrating the different plane of origin of the circumflex artery.

4. Discussion

4.1. Anomalous Circumflex Artery. Coronary anomalies generally are reported to be present in about 0.2–1.3% in the population based on angiographic studies and about 0.3% based on autopsy studies [1, 2]. The most common anatomic variation is an anomalous left circumflex artery, present in about 0.7% of patients [1]. The circumflex invariably courses posterior to the aortic root. The artery can arise from a separate ostium within the right sinus or as a proximal branch of the right coronary artery. The arterial course to the aorta and pulmonary artery relationship has been associated with many serious conditions, including congestive heart failure, arrhythmias, myocardial infarction, and even sudden death [3–6]. This sudden death phenomena is thought to may be due to the fact that the vessel's tangential origin during demand can lead to ischemia and arrhythmias [7]. Retroaortic portion of the anomalous circumflex also predisposes patients to atherosclerotic disease [1]. In this case, there was severe stenosis in the anomalous circumflex artery which mimicked a CTO. Because of this, the patient was treated medically and suffered with angina for more than 6 years and did not receive appropriate treatment.

4.2. PCI for Chronic Total Occlusion. Even though the patient was referred for CTO PCI, he did not have a CTO. However, the systematic approach to CTO PCI helped in identifying the anomalous coronary anatomy. Chronic total occlusion interventions (CTO PCI) are increasing in frequency secondary to advances in techniques and development of the North American Hybrid Algorithm [8]. Despite the increase in CTO PCI, many non-CTO operators attempt

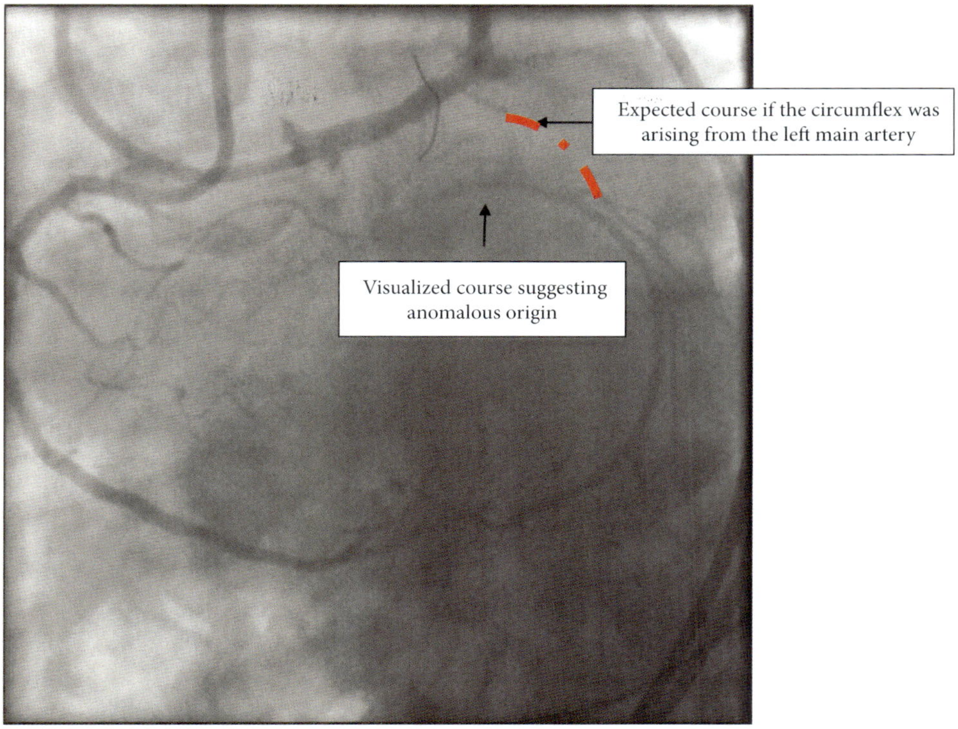

FIGURE 5: Dual angiogram demonstrating the course of the circumflex artery in a plane different from the left main artery—guide catheters in the right coronary artery and left main coronary artery in left anterior oblique/caudal view.

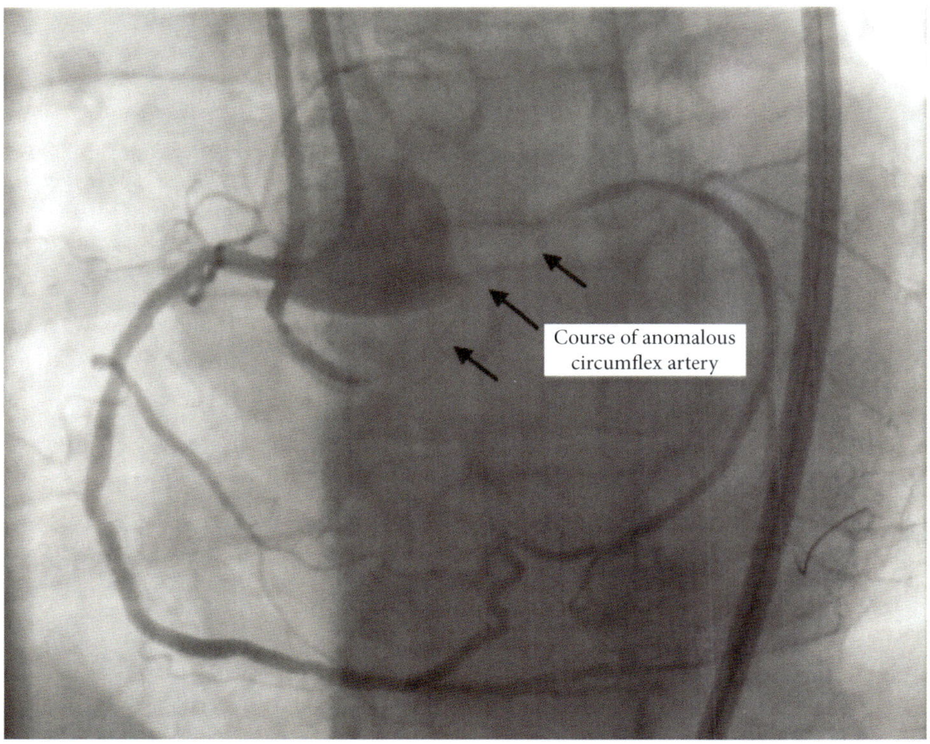

FIGURE 6: Dual angiogram with guide catheters in the right coronary artery and the anomalous origin of the circumflex artery.

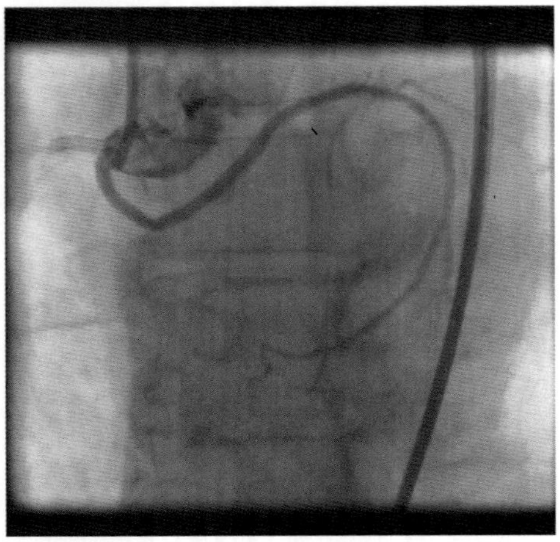

FIGURE 7: Final angiographic result after PCI of the anomalous circumflex artery.

the conventional wiring techniques, where a guide wire is attempted to be passed across the lesion without proper visualization of the distal vessel with dual angiogram. Conventional work horse wires with over-the-wire (OTW) balloons are usually used. This has been called the "Poke and Hope" technique. In some cases, this results in complete dissection and shut down of the vessel or wire perforation of the native vessel. In the case that we have described, if the "Poke and Hope" technique was to be used, it would have resulted in perforation of a small branch coming off the left anterior descending artery which was initially thought to be the diminutive left circumflex artery.

This case demonstrates the importance of dual angiography in clearly defining the coronary anatomy. Dual angiography remains the cornerstone for decision making on CTO PCI [9]. The angiogram of the right coronary artery with the right posterolateral branch giving collateral flow to the atrioventricular circumflex branch is the second most common collateral pattern for circumflex CTOs [10]; however, the turn taken by the A-V circumflex vessel is not the usual course. In the normal course of the circumflex artery, the artery runs towards the left main artery. In the case that we have described, the circumflex runs in a different plane from the left main artery, which should raise suspicion of an anomalous origin of the circumflex. Therefore, angiographic pattern recognition of this coronary angiogram is of extreme importance. If this angiographic pattern was recognized during his initial cardiac catheterization, the patient would have received appropriate treatment for his angina pectoris.

This case report serves to reiterate the unusual angiographic pattern of the anomalous circumflex artery in the presence of severe stenosis, which mimicked a chronic total occlusion. Furthermore, recognition of this angiographic pattern can facilitate further evaluation for the presence of an anomalous artery and PCI can be done in the same setting. Delays in patient care can be avoided.

References

[1] N. E. J. West, C. J. McKenna, O. Ormerod, J. C. Forfar, A. P. Banning, and K. M. Channon, "Percutaneous coronary intervention with stent deployment in anomalously-arising left circumflex coronary arteries," *Catheterization and Cardiovascular Interventions*, vol. 68, no. 6, pp. 882–890, 2006.

[2] O. Yamanaka and R. E. Hobbs, "Coronary artery anomalies in 126,595 patients undergoing coronary arteriography," *Catheterization and Cardiovascular Diagnosis*, vol. 21, no. 1, pp. 28–40, 1990.

[3] S. Yuksel, M. Meric, K. Soylu et al., "The primary anomalies of coronary artery origin and course: a coronary angiographic analysis of 16,573 patients," *Experimental & Clinical Cardiology*, vol. 18, no. 2, pp. 121–123, 2013.

[4] L. J. Zhang, G. F. Yang, W. Huang, C. S. Zhou, P. Chen, and G. M. Lu, "Incidence of anomalous origin of coronary artery in 1879 Chinese adults on dual-source CT angiography," *Netherlands Heart Journal*, vol. 18, no. 10, pp. 466–470, 2010.

[5] D. Andreini, S. Mushtaq, G. Pontone et al., "Additional clinical role of 64-slice multidetector computed tomography in the evaluation of coronary artery variants and anomalies," *International Journal of Cardiology*, vol. 145, no. 2, pp. 388–390, 2010.

[6] H. Liu, C. Zhu, Y. Guo, M. Zhang, and J. Li, "A rare case of complex anomalous origin of coronary arteries with severe atherosclerosis," *Chinese Medical Journal*, vol. 127, no. 24, pp. 4297-4298, 2014.

[7] A. T. Marler, J. A. Malik, and A. M. Slim, "Anomalous left main coronary artery: case series of different courses and literature review," *Case Reports in Vascular Medicine*, vol. 2013, Article ID 380952, 5 pages, 2013.

[8] W. M. Wilson, S. J. Walsh, A. T. Yan et al., "Hybrid approach improves success of chronic total occlusion angioplasty," *Heart*, vol. 102, no. 18, pp. 1486–1493, 2016.

[9] B. V. Rangan, A. Kotsia, G. Christopoulos et al., "The hybrid approach to intervention of chronic total occlusions," *Current Cardiology Reviews*, vol. 11, no. 4, pp. 299–304, 2015.

[10] M. B. McEntegart, A. A. Badar, F. A. Ahmad et al., "The collateral circulation of coronary chronic total occlusions," *EuroIntervention*, vol. 11, no. 14, pp. e1596–e1603, 2016.

Pheochromocytoma, "the Great Masquerader," Presenting as Severe Acute Decompensated Heart Failure in a Young Patient

Hans A. Reyes,[1] **Jason J. Paquin**,[2] **and David M. Harris**[1]

[1]*Division of Cardiovascular Health and Disease, University of Cincinnati College of Medicine, Cincinnati, OH, USA*
[2]*Division of Cardiology, Mercy Heart Institute, Cincinnati, OH, USA*

Correspondence should be addressed to Hans A. Reyes; hansreyesg@gmail.com

Academic Editor: Assad Movahed

A 22-year-old man presented to the hospital with progressive shortness of breath, chest discomfort, sinus tachycardia, and emesis. The echocardiogram demonstrated global hypokinesis with a left ventricle ejection fraction of 15–20%. The patient was treated for acute systolic heart failure decompensation with diuresis and afterload reduction. Unexpectedly, an abdominal computed tomography showed a left adrenal mass and subsequent serum/urine metanephrine tests suggested pheochromocytoma. Once the patient had stabilized, he underwent an uneventful adrenalectomy with histology results confirming the diagnosis of pheochromocytoma. After six months follow-up, he is currently doing well with close outpatient follow-up by cardiology.

1. Introduction

Pheochromocytoma, the "great masquerader," is a neoplasm of neuroectodermal chromaffin cells which produces excess catecholamines. The classical clinical triad is described with headaches, palpitations, and sweating. However, this tumor can be asymptomatic or present with a myriad of symptoms including headaches, anxiety attacks, hypertension, and in rare cases, multiorgan failure [1–3]. These symptoms are secondary to excess catecholamines. Once diagnosed, the medical management can be further challenging. Our patient initially presented with severe cardiomyopathy and decompensated heart failure which required optimization prior to adrenalectomy.

2. Case

A 22-year-old male presented to the emergency department (ED) complaining of shortness of breath and abdominal swelling that had progressed over the previous two months. His symptoms were associated with intermittent chest discomfort and palpitations. Upon developing increased nausea, emesis, and diarrhea, he presented to the ED. The patient reported a history of hypertension and intermittent severe headaches but stated he did not seek additional evaluation or treatment. He had no history of tobacco or recreational drugs but reported occasional alcohol consumption. Initial vital signs included blood pressure 110/70 mmHg, heart rate 114 bpm, respiratory rate 18 per minute, O_2 sat of 99% on room air, and temperature of 98°F. The physical exam was remarkable for a jaundiced patient in mild distress with jugular venous distention, tachycardia, and S3 gallop. Electrocardiogram confirmed sinus tachycardia with anterior ST depression. Laboratory data revealed the following: WBC 9800/μL, Hb/Hct 14.5/45 g/dL, normal electrolytes, BUN/Cr 13/0.8, hepatic function was remarkable for ALT 153 mg/dL and AST 85 mg/dL, total bilirubin 3.9 mg/dL, normal coagulation profile, and troponin I < 0.01 ng/mL. The chest X-ray was notable for an enlarged cardiopericardial silhouette and prominent central pulmonary vasculature. The echocardiogram revealed severe global hypokinesis with left ventricular ejection fraction (LVEF) of 15–20%, apical akinesis with an organized 2.2×1.4 cm fixed thrombus (Figure 1), and a right ventricular systolic pressure estimated at 55 mmHg. A

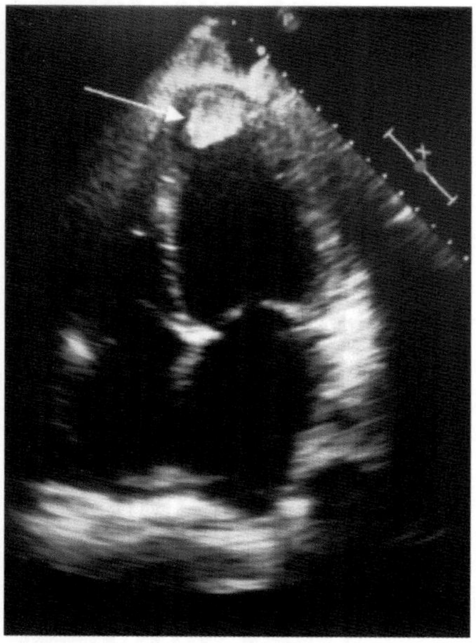

Figure 1: Echocardiogram: an apical four-chamber view showing a 2.2×1.4 cm left ventricular thrombus.

computed tomography (CT) pulmonary angiogram excluded pulmonary embolism but did show cardiomegaly and a right pleural effusion. An abdominal and pelvic CT with contrast was ordered due to gastrointestinal symptoms, and unexpectedly, it showed a 4×3 cm enhancing mass on the left adrenal gland (Figure 2).

The patient was admitted with a diagnosis of acute decompensated heart failure; the therapy included diuresis and afterload reduction with lisinopril, carvedilol as tolerated, and digoxin. Due to the suggestion of left ventricular thrombus by the echocardiogram, anticoagulation was initiated. A single-photon emission computed tomography (SPECT) stress test was done revealing severe global hypokinesis with regional variability, LVEF of 17%, and no evidence of ischemia. Incidentally, increased uptake associated with the left adrenal gland was noted. Plasma and 24-hour urine metanephrines were elevated at 11.8 nmol/L (normal value: 0–0.89 nmol/L) and 2223 μg/24 h (normal value: 0–400 μg/24 h), respectively, supporting the diagnosis of pheochromocytoma. Once heart failure condition was stabilized, carvedilol was switched to prazosin and metoprolol. The patient was transferred to a facility with cardiothoracic surgical support capabilities including left ventricular-assisted device and cardiac transplant prior to the planned adrenalectomy. Surgery was completed successfully with balloon pump backup and with histology results confirming the diagnosis of pheochromocytoma.

Subsequently, a cardiac magnetic resonance imaging (CMRI) performed two weeks after discharge showed moderate dilation of the left ventricle with a LVEF of 23%, diffuse hypokinesis, resolution of the intracavitary left ventricular thrombus, and a midventricular, midmyocardial linear stripe and inferior right midventricular insertion enhancement on the delayed gadolinium enhancement (DGE) (Figures 3(a) and 3(b)). Six months after adrenalectomy, the patient was able to return to work doing light activities four hours daily and his last echocardiogram showed an improved LVEF of 40%.

3. Discussion

Our case of a young male patient with a history of hypertension who presented with congestive heart failure highlights the importance of screening for secondary etiologies of hypertension in this population. While heart failure is uncommon in this population, the differential diagnosis includes viral myocarditis, drug-induced cardiomyopathy, familial cardiomyopathies, cardiac sarcoidosis, congenital heart disease, and, even rarer, ischemic cardiomyopathy.

Our patient had a history of hypertension for two years, was noncompliant, and was lost to follow-up. His acute presentation with heart failure was initially attributed to an uncontrolled hypertension. However, during the initial work-up, an abdominal CT showed a mass in the left adrenal gland with incidental radionuclide uptake during cardiac stress testing. Based on these findings, pheochromocytoma was suspected, which was subsequently confirmed by ancillary tests and pathology.

Pheochromocytoma, known as the "great masquerader," is a neoplasm of neuroectodermal chromaffin cells which produces excess catecholamines. Its annual incidence is approximately 0.8 per 100,000 person-years and probably occurs in less than 0.5 percent of patients with hypertension [1, 2]. Pheochromocytoma can be sporadic or familial; sporadic forms are usually diagnosed between the ages of 40 and 50, while the hereditary forms present in childhood or early adulthood [3]. This tumor has varied clinical manifestations ranging from an asymptomatic subclinical picture to symptoms such as headaches, palpitations, sweating, anxiety, emesis, hypertension, and, in rare cases, multiorgan failure [4–7]. All of these symptoms are secondary to excess catecholamines. Importantly, relatively large numbers of patients are not diagnosed during their lives or are diagnosed only after the occurrence of significant cardiovascular damages [4], as with our patient.

Although the majority of patients with pheochromocytoma have a normal or increased ventricular systolic function on echocardiography, the pattern of left ventricular dysfunction may be variable. Only around 10–20% of patients with pheochromocytoma present with catecholamine-induced cardiomyopathy [8, 9]. When catecholamine-induced cardiomyopathy is present, most of the cases demonstrate a stress-induced cardiomyopathy, Takotsubo syndrome [7, 10]. In those patients, an echocardiogram demonstrates transient left ventricular apical ballooning with midventricular dyskinesis that extends beyond the distribution of any single coronary artery. Unlike stress-induced cardiomyopathy, our patient's echocardiogram demonstrated global hypokinesis and not apical ballooning which was initially suspected to be a consequence of occult hypertension leading to a "burned-out" ventricle.

Pheochromocytomas have been associated with other various cardiovascular complications due to overwhelming catecholamine levels. The most common complications

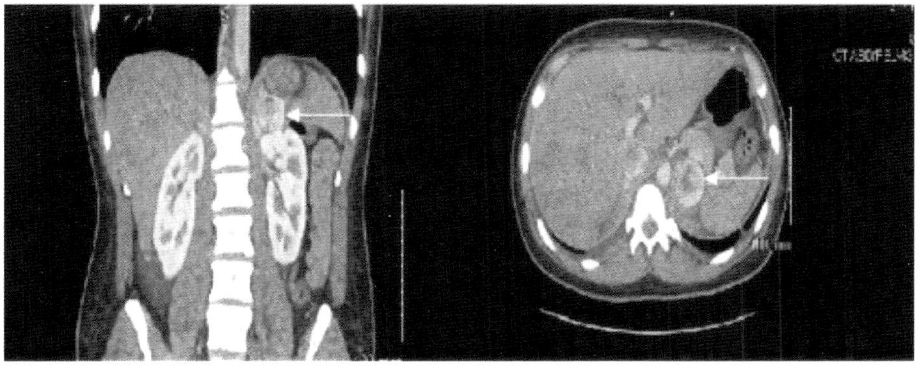

Figure 2: Abdomen/pelvic CT with contrast, coronal, and axial views showing the 4 × 3 cm left pheochromocytoma.

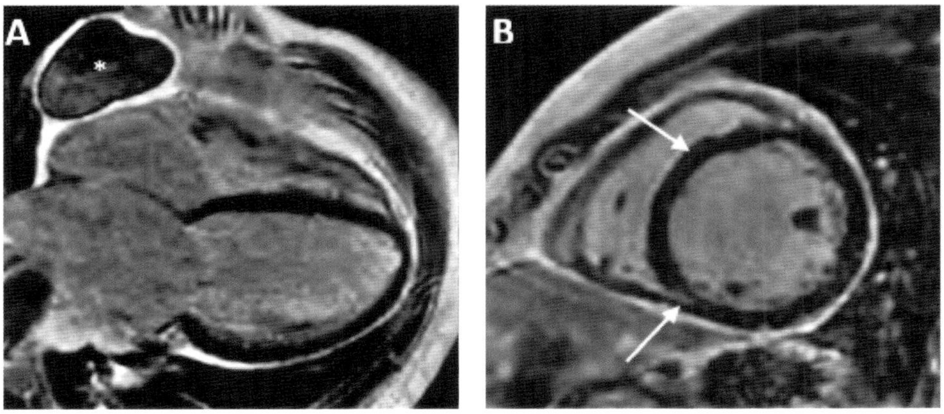

(a) (b)

Figure 3: (a) CMRI showing the resolution of the left ventricular thrombus and an incidental pericardial cyst (asterisk). (b) CMRI showing slight delayed gadolinium enhancement with a left midventricular, midmyocardial septal stripe (superior arrow) and also an inferior right midventricular insertion delayed gadolinium enhancement (inferior arrow).

include left ventricular hypertrophy, ischemic heart disease, disturbances in rhythm and conduction, malignant ventricular arrhythmias, and even shock [3, 5, 11]. The potentially fatal cardiovascular complications of these tumors are due to the potent effects of catecholamines, especially noradrenaline, the main transmitter released from sympathetic nerve terminals.

According to Batisse-Lignier et al. [7], which performed a systematic review in 145 cases with either acute or chronic pheochromocytoma-induced cardiomyopathy, the LVEF recovery after surgical resection of the tumor is higher in patients who presented with stress-induced cardiomyopathy than in others who presented with catecholamine-induced cardiomyopathies (64.9% versus 40.8%, $p = 0.005$). Even after a multivariate analysis, only stress-induced cardiomyopathy was associated with a better left ventricle recovery ($p = 0.03$).

The exact mechanism of cardiomyopathy in patients with pheochromocytoma remains unclear. However, there are some mechanisms that can explain the myocardial damage associated with catecholamines. These can cause a direct toxic effect on the myocardium through calcium overload due to altered sodium and calcium transporters, enhanced lipid mobility, free radical production, or increased sarcolemmal permeability [5, 10, 12]. In addition, myocardial damage may occur secondary to a decrease in myocardial oxygen supply combined with a sustained myocardial oxygen demand [12, 13]. Usually, catecholamines bind to beta1 and beta2-adrenergic receptors and produce positive inotropic and lusitropic effects. Nevertheless, in situations of increased stress with very high levels of catecholamines, beta1-adrenergic receptors' activation can induce apoptosis of the cardiac myocytes. Moreover, the binding of epinephrine to beta2-adrenergic receptors produces a negative inotropic effect [5, 10]. Thus, catecholamines also have a dose-dependent cardiotoxic effect.

Considering the previous mechanisms of cardiac injury, the myocardial damage produced in acute or chronic exposure to catecholamines could be different. Acute catecholamine exposure, such as in stress-induced cardiomyopathy, exposes the myocardial beta receptors to an enormous amount of catecholamines leading to a stunning of the left ventricle and slight histological apoptosis. On the other hand, in chronic adrenergic exposure, it is hypothesized that the heart gets gradually used to the surge of catecholamines with desensitization of adrenergic receptors [7]. Unlike acute exposure, long-standing catecholaminergic burden leads to structural myocardial alterations such as interstitial fibrosis, inflammation, and a subsequent dysfunction [10, 13]. This chronic exposure may explain the lower level of LVEF recovery in the catecholamine-induced cardiomyopathy subgroup described by Batisse-Lignier et al.

Previous reports have showed that pheochromocytoma-induced cardiomyopathy can be reversed with medical therapy first followed by a subsequent tumor extirpation [4, 6–9], as with our patient. The prognosis of catecholamine-induced cardiomyopathy depends on early diagnosis and prompt medical and surgical treatment. Once diagnosed, the medical management of these tumors prior to surgery may be challenging in the context of heart failure [14]. The usual therapy includes initial blockade of alpha-adrenergic receptors [8, 9]; beta-blockers are added after several days to ensure adequate alpha-adrenergic blockade. Beta blockers should never be administered without appropriate alpha blockade as this could worsen hypertensive episodes by exacerbating vasoconstriction while inhibiting vasodilation. Our patient had clear symptoms of decompensated heart failure on presentation, requiring reduction of both preload and afterload. Thus, we believe that the use of carvedilol, an alpha- and beta-adrenergic receptor blocker, was a rational and adequate option due to the possibility of pheochromocytoma. An alpha blocker is not a recommended treatment for heart failure, but its use in patients with pheochromocytoma is mandatory. Patients with pheochromocytoma may be intravascularly volume depleted, and diuretics should be administered with caution. However, in patients with catecholamine-induced cardiomyopathy, diuretic use is warranted. Regarding ancillary tests, interpretation of metanephrine levels in the context of established cardiomyopathy is also difficult as cardiac failure of any etiology generates an adrenergic response [14]. In this particular presentation of heart failure, where the culprit is an uncommon cause, multidisciplinary management is needed, including physiologically directed pharmacologic therapy which may deviate from guidelines given the need for alpha blockers and individualized care.

Our patient's CMRI showed minimal DGE consistent with mild myocardial fibrosis or scar, which was encouraging for left ventricular functional recovery. At six months follow-up, the patient is doing well, without significant symptoms, and has shown improvement of LVEF by echocardiogram. Given his young age at presentation with pheochromocytoma, he underwent genetic testing and is continuing to be followed by endocrinology.

With this case, we want to emphasize that the diagnosis of pheochromocytoma requires high clinical alertness due to its rare incidence and extremely variable clinical presentation and to highlight the relevance of considering pheochromocytoma in the differential diagnosis of unexplained cardiomyopathy in a young patient. We also want to stress the importance of routine follow-up in hypertensive patients as early diagnosis and appropriate treatment can significantly reduce morbidity and mortality in this group of patients. Finally, once diagnosed, it is essential to closely follow these patients to monitor the LVEF and provide optimal medical management for their cardiomyopathy.

References

[1] C. M. Beard, S. G. Sheps, L. T. Kurland, J. A. Carney, and J. T. Lie, "Occurrence of pheochromocytoma in Rochester, Minnesota, 1950 through 1979," *Mayo Clinic Proceedings*, vol. 58, no. 12, pp. 802–804, 1983.

[2] K. Pacak, W. M. Linehan, G. Eisenhofer, M. C. M. Walther, and D. S. Goldstein, "Recent advances in genetics, diagnosis, localization, and treatment of pheochromocytoma," *Annals of Internal Medicine*, vol. 134, no. 4, pp. 315–329, 2001.

[3] M. Satendra, C. de Jesus, A. L. Bordalo e Sá et al., "Reversible catecholamine-induced cardiomyopathy due to pheochromocytoma: case report," *Revista Portuguesa de Cardiologia (English Edition)*, vol. 33, no. 3, pp. 177.e1–177.e6, 2014.

[4] M. Mannelli, J. W. M. Lenders, K. Pacak, G. Parenti, and G. Eisenhofer, "Subclinical phaeochromocytoma," *Best Practice & Research Clinical Endocrinology & Metabolism*, vol. 26, no. 4, pp. 507–515, 2012.

[5] V. Agarwal, G. Kant, N. Hans, and F. H. Messerli, "Takotsubo-like cardiomyopathy in pheochromocytoma," *International Journal of Cardiology*, vol. 153, no. 3, pp. 241–248, 2011.

[6] T. Pereira-da-Silva, J. Abreu, R. Ramos et al., "Unexpected triggers for pheochromocytoma-induced recurrent heart failure," *International Archives of Medicine*, vol. 7, no. 1, p. 30, 2014.

[7] M. Batisse-Lignier, B. Pereira, P. Motreff et al., "Acute and chronic pheochromocytoma-induced cardiomyopathies," *Medicine*, vol. 94, no. 50, article e2198, 2015.

[8] J. H. Park, K. S. Kim, J. Y. Sul et al., "Prevalence and patterns of left ventricular dysfunction in patients with pheochromocytoma," *Journal of Cardiovascular Ultrasound*, vol. 19, no. 2, pp. 76–82, 2011.

[9] G. D. Sanna, G. Talanas, G. Fiore, A. Canu, and P. Terrosu, "Pheochromocytoma presenting as an acute coronary syndrome complicated by acute heart failure: the challenge of a great mimic," *Journal of the Saudi Heart Association*, vol. 28, no. 4, pp. 278–282, 2016.

[10] C. M. Mulla and P. E. Marik, "Pheochromocytoma presenting as acute decompensated heart failure reversed with medical therapy," *Case Reports*, vol. 2012, no. 1, article bcr2012006319, 2012.

[11] F. Galetta, F. Franzoni, G. Bernini et al., "Cardiovascular complications in patients with pheochromocytoma: a mini-review," *Biomedicine & Pharmacotherapy*, vol. 64, no. 7, pp. 505–509, 2010.

[12] A. Prejbisz, J. W. M. Lenders, G. Eisenhofer, and A. Januszewicz, "Cardiovascular manifestations of phaeochromocytoma," *Journal of Hypertension*, vol. 29, no. 11, pp. 2049–2060, 2011.

[13] M. De Lazzari, A. Cipriani, M. P. Marra et al., "Heart failure due to adrenergic myocardial toxicity from a pheochromocytoma," *Circulation: Heart Failure*, vol. 8, no. 3, pp. 646–648, 2015.

[14] Y. Mamoojee, M. Arham, W. Elsaify, and S. Nag, "Lesson of the month 2: catecholamine-induced cardiomyopathy - pitfalls in diagnosis and medical management," *Clinical Medicine*, vol. 16, no. 2, pp. 201–203, 2016.

52

Bisoprolol Transdermal Patch Is Effective for the Treatment of AF Tachycardia

Yoh Arita, Hajime Saeki, Miwa Miyoshi, and Shinji Hasegawa

Department of Cardiology, Japan Community Healthcare Organization (JCHO) Osaka Hospital, 4-2-78 Fukushima, Fukushima-ku, Osaka 553-0003, Japan

Correspondence should be addressed to Yoh Arita; arita-yo@osaka.jcho.go.jp

Academic Editor: Tayfun Sahin

Atrial fibrillation (AF) is an irregular and often rapid heart rate that can increase the risk of stroke, heart failure, and other heart-related complications. Its incidence increases with age and the presence of concomitant heart disease. We present the cases of a 93-year-old woman, an 82-year-old man, and an 87-year-old woman who developed AF tachycardia. This report highlights the use of a bisoprolol transdermal patch to treat AF tachycardia in 3 adult elderly patients. In this paper, we report an initial treatment strategy using a bisoprolol transdermal patch and show heart rate trends for 24 hours.

1. Introduction

Clinical atrial fibrillation (AF) is associated with increased rates of stroke, heart failure, mortality, hospitalization, and cognitive decline, much of which may present suddenly and constitute irretrievable harm [1, 2]. AF symptoms often include heart palpitations, shortness of breath, and weakness. Rate control is possible in the majority of patients with AF. Beta- (β-) blockers have been the most effective drugs [3]. However, swallowing tablets or capsules is sometimes difficult for elderly people because of dysphagia [4]. Moreover, aspiration pneumonia can be associated with dysphagia [5]. Bisoprolol is also available as a transdermal patch in Japan. Medication adherence is better with the use of a transdermal patch than with the use of tablets, particularly in elderly patients who might have difficulty with oral administration. In this paper, we report an initial treatment strategy for AF tachycardia using a bisoprolol transdermal patch in elderly patients.

2. Case Presentation

2.1. Case 1. This 93-year-old woman, a resident of a special elderly care nursing home, was referred to our hospital for the treatment of cellulitis. She related a history of treatment for hypertension and atrial fibrillation (AF). Upon arrival, her blood pressure (BP) was 119/83 mmHg and heart rate (HR) was 82 bpm. An electrocardiogram (ECG) demonstrated AF and a complete right bundle branch block (Figure 1(a)). During the treatment for cellulitis using antibiotics, she complained of dyspnea. Her HR increased to 140 bpm and her chest X-ray (CXR) showed pulmonary edema and congestion (Figure 1(b)). Echocardiography demonstrated preserved cardiac contractility with an ejection fraction (EF) of 60%, indicating heart failure with a preserved EF. She was administered furosemide (20 mg/day) to treat heart failure. In addition, a bisoprolol transdermal patch (2 mg) was applied to her chest. Her HR trends were significantly decreased within 8 hours and the control of HR continued for 24 hours (Figure 2). Eventually, her CXR and symptoms improved.

2.2. Case 2. An 82-year-old man was admitted to our hospital for the treatment of ileus. He related a history of treatment for persistent AF and hypertension. He was administered bisoprolol fumarate tablets (2.5 mg/day) for AF before admission. His HR on admission was 87 bpm. However, he could not take oral medicine because of fasting for treatment of ileus. After 3 days of fasting, he developed AF tachycardia and his HR increased to 150 bpm. Bisoprolol transdermal patch (4 mg) was applied to his chest. This dose was equal

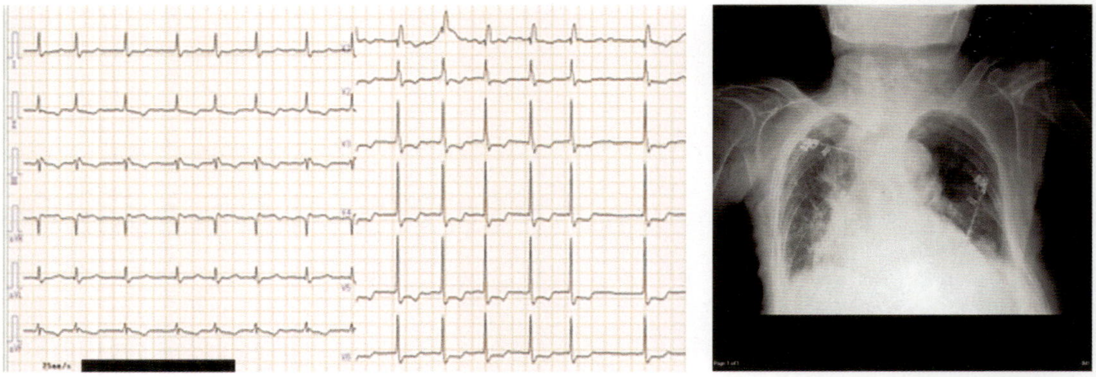

(a) (b)

Figure 1: (a) Electrocardiogram (ECG, case 1) findings upon admission. ECG showing atrial fibrillation (AF) and a complete right bundle branch block. (b) Chest X-ray (CXR) findings during AF tachycardia. CXR showing severe pulmonary edema and congestion.

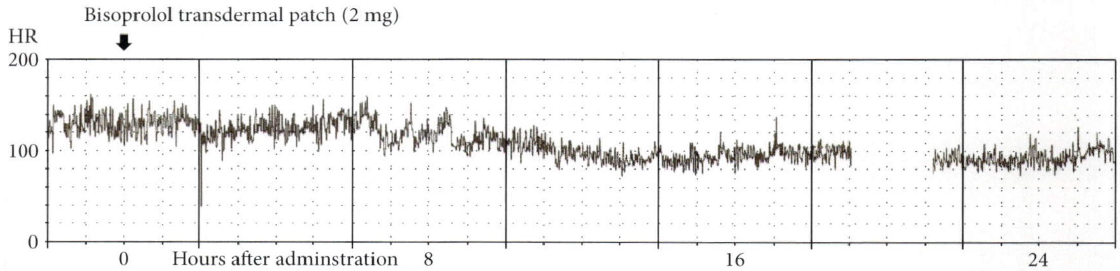

Figure 2: Patient (case 1) heart rate (HR) trends during treatment. The gap in the record is due to battery exhaustion.

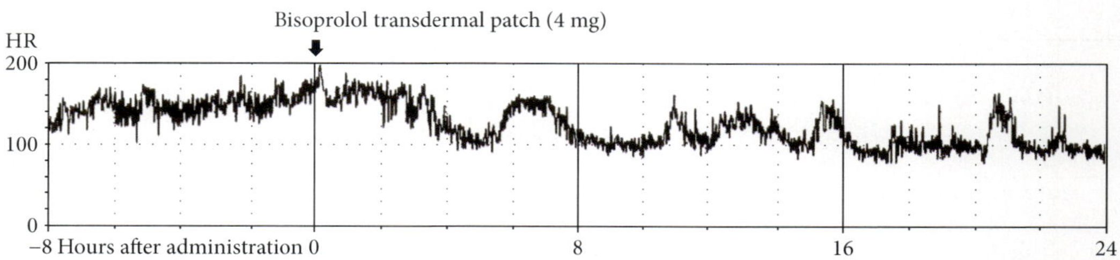

Figure 3: Patient (case 2) heart rate (HR) trends during treatment.

to a 2.5 mg bisoprolol fumarate tablet. His HR trends were significantly decreased after 8 hours of bisoprolol transdermal patch, and the frequency and duration of AF decreased until 24 hours after administration (Figure 3).

2.3. Case 3. An 87-year-old woman was referred to our hospital for treatment of AF with palpitation and dyspnea (Figure 4(a)). She related a history of treatment for hypertension and cerebral infarction but no history of heart failure and/or arrhythmia. Upon arrival, her BP was 102/54 mmHg and HR was 151 bpm. Her heart rhythm often spontaneously alternated between AF and sinus rhythm (Figure 4(b)). Echocardiography demonstrated preserved cardiac contractility with an EF of 64%, indicating heart failure with preserved EF. She was administered verapamil (5 mg) injection; however, there was no decrease in HR or frequency of rhythm alternation. Next, bisoprolol transdermal patch (4 mg) was applied to her chest. Her HR trends were significantly decreased after 6 hours on the bisoprolol transdermal patch and the frequency and duration of AF decreased until 24 hours after administration (Figure 5). Moreover, her symptoms were improved.

3. Discussion

AF is an irregular and often rapid heart rate that can increase the risk of stroke, heart failure, and other heart-related complications. Its incidence increases with age and the presence of concomitant heart disease [6]. Rate control in AF improves the quality of life, reduces morbidity, and decreases

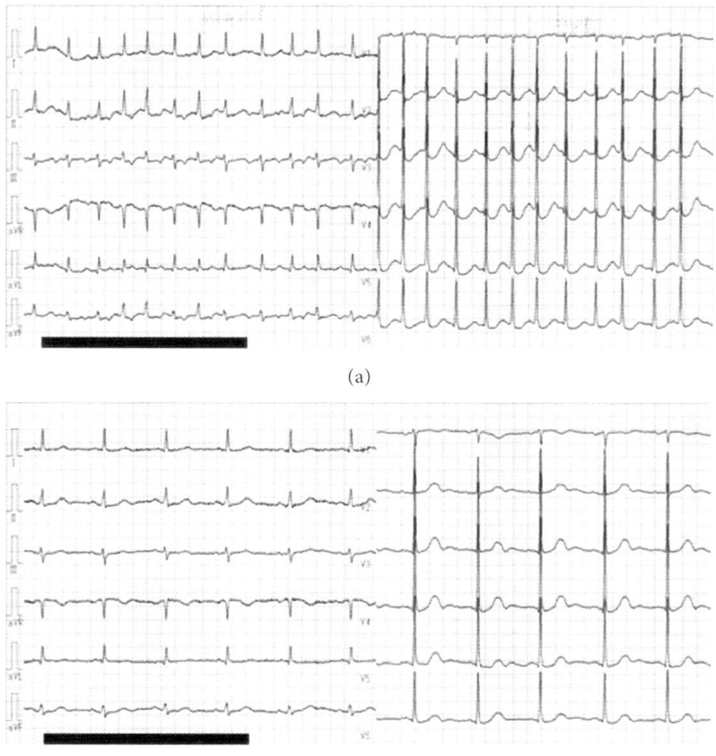

FIGURE 4: Electrocardiogram (ECG, case 3) findings upon admission. (a) ECG showing atrial fibrillation (AF). (b) ECG showing sinus rhythm (SR). The heart rhythm often spontaneously alternated between AF and SR.

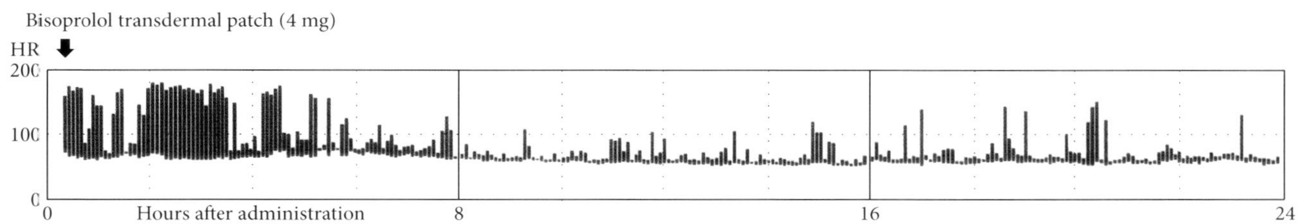

FIGURE 5: Patient (case 3) heart rate (HR) trends during treatment.

the potential for tachycardia-induced cardiomyopathy. Multiple agents, including β-blockers, nondihydropyridine calcium channel blockers, digoxin, and certain antiarrhythmic drugs, including amiodarone and sotalol, have been evaluated for efficacy in attaining rate control [1]. β-blockers are the most commonly used drugs to control the ventricular rate during AF [3]. β-blockers also have an antiarrhythmic effect due to the suppression of sympathetic activity [7]. By reducing sympathetic tone, conduction over the atrioventricular node is slowed and atrioventricular nodal refractoriness is increased.

Bisoprolol, also available as a transdermal patch in Japan, is indicated for the management of hypertension [8]. However, bisoprolol fumarate tablets are used for the management of patients with AF tachycardia [6]. Switching therapy from landiolol to bisoprolol transdermal patch is often performed in patients with AF tachycardia because the latter is relatively easy to manage [9–11]. A recent study reported efficacy and safety when switching from bisoprolol fumarate tablets to a bisoprolol transdermal patch at a dose conversion rate of 5 : 8 [12]. There are several benefits to using a transdermal patch instead of tablets. First, medication adherence is better because patients or caregivers can monitor medication through direct observation of the transdermal patch. Second, a transdermal patch can be used in patients for whom oral treatment is difficult, including those whose swallowing function has been impaired, those with gastrointestinal disease, and those who require tracheal intubation for an operation or pneumonia.

The current cases may provide physicians with an initial treatment strategy for the use of a bisoprolol transdermal patch for AF tachycardia patients and especially in elderly patients who are relatively difficult to treat with oral medication.

References

[1] C. T. January, L. S. Wann, J. S. Alpert et al., "2014 AHA/ACC/HRS guideline for the management of patients with atrial fibrillation: a report of the American College of Cardiology/American Heart Association Task Force on Practice Guidelines and the Heart Rhythm Society," *Journal of the American College of Cardiology*, vol. 64, no. 21, pp. e1–76, 2014.

[2] A. L. Waldo and A. J. Camm, "Atrial fibrillation: atrial high-rate events (AHRES): look and you will find-then what?," *Circulation*, vol. 136, no. 19, pp. 1795–1797, 2017.

[3] B. Olshansky, L. E. Rosenfeld, A. L. Warner et al., "The Atrial Fibrillation Follow-up Investigation of Rhythm Management (AFFIRM) study: approaches to control rate in atrial fibrillation," *Journal of the American College of Cardiology*, vol. 43, no. 7, pp. 1201–1208, 2004.

[4] P. Clave and R. Shaker, "Dysphagia: current reality and scope of the problem," *Nature Reviews Gastroenterology & Hepatology*, vol. 12, no. 5, pp. 259–270, 2015.

[5] S. Ebihara, H. Sekiya, M. Miyagi, T. Ebihara, and T. Okazaki, "Dysphagia, dystussia, and aspiration pneumonia in elderly people," *Journal of Thoracic Disease*, vol. 8, no. 3, pp. 632–639, 2016.

[6] E. N. Prystowsky, B. J. Padanilam, and R. I. Fogel, "Treatment of atrial fibrillation," *JAMA*, vol. 314, no. 3, pp. 278–288, 2015.

[7] H. Ishiguro, T. Ikeda, A. Abe et al., "Antiarrhythmic effect of bisoprolol, a highly selective β_1-blocker, in patients with paroxysmal atrial fibrillation," *International Heart Journal*, vol. 49, no. 3, pp. 281–293, 2008.

[8] H. Matsuoka, I. Kuwajima, K. Shimada, H. Mitamura, and T. Saruta, "Comparison of efficacy and safety between bisoprolol transdermal patch (TY-0201) and bisoprolol fumarate oral formulation in Japanese patients with grade I or II essential hypertension: randomized, double-blind, placebo-controlled study," *The Journal of Clinical Hypertension*, vol. 15, no. 11, pp. 806–814, 2013.

[9] K. Nakamura, R. Inokuchi, T. Hiruma, K. Tokunaga, K. Doi, and S. Nakajima, "Switching therapy from intravenous beta blocker to bisoprolol transdermal patch for atrial fibrillation tachycardia," *Journal of Anesthesia*, vol. 30, no. 5, pp. 891–894, 2016.

[10] S. Godo, Y. Kawazoe, H. Ozaki et al., "Switching therapy from intravenous landiolol to transdermal bisoprolol in a patient with thyroid storm complicated by decompensated heart failure and gastrointestinal dysfunction," *Internal Medicine*, vol. 56, no. 19, pp. 2603–2609, 2017.

[11] Y. Arita, T. Segawa, S. Yamamoto, and S. Hasegawa, "Landiolol is effective for the treatment of tachycardia-induced cardiogenic shock in patients during septic shock therapy," *BMJ Case Reports*, vol. 2017, 2017.

[12] S. I. Momomura, Y. Saito, Y. Yasumura et al., "Efficacy and safety of switching from oral bisoprolol to transdermal patch in Japanese patients with chronic heart failure," *Circulation Journal*, vol. 82, no. 1, pp. 141–147, 2017.

53

Treatment of an Unusual Occurrence of a Complex Left Subclavian Artery/Left Internal Mammary Artery Bifurcation Stenosis in the Setting of Coronary Subclavian Steal Syndrome and Ischemic Left Ventricular Systolic Dysfunction

Michael J. Martinelli[1] **and Michael B. Martinelli**[2]

[1]*St. Peter's Health Partners, 2 Palisades Drive, Albany, NY 12205, USA*
[2]*College of Biomedical Sciences, Thomas Jefferson University, Philadelphia, PA, USA*

Correspondence should be addressed to Michael J. Martinelli; michael.martinelli@sphp.com

Academic Editor: Ertugrul Ercan

This case will illustrate the clinical and unique technical challenges, not previously reported, in a patient with a history of progressive left ventricular (LV) systolic dysfunction, congestive heart failure (CHF), myocardial infarction (MI), and a complex bifurcation lesion of the left subclavian artery (SA) involving the left internal mammary artery (LIMA) in the setting of coronary subclavian steal syndrome (CSSS). The approach to this lesion is complicated by significant LIMA involvement requiring intervention directed toward both the SA and the LIMA in the presence of severe LV systolic dysfunction. This clinical scenario necessitates a careful technique, utilizing bifurcation methods similar to those used in coronary intervention.

1. Introduction

Coronary subclavian steal syndrome (CSSS), first described in 1974, is characterized by a stenotic proximal left subclavian artery (SA) causing reversal of flow in the LIMA resulting in a "steal" phenomenon [1]. This syndrome typically presents with angina during left upper extremity exertion. Less common manifestations include acute myocardial infarction (MI), ischemic cardiomyopathy, and ventricular arrhythmias [2, 3]. The case reported here demonstrates a lesion of the proximal SA, which could be expected to result in CSSS, but which atypically involves both the LIMA and the SA beyond the LIMA. This lesion morphology not only creates a steal phenomenon but further compromises LIMA flow to the LAD by inhibiting inflow to and outflow from the LIMA. This complex anatomy may further worsen the clinical severity beyond which is typically seen in CSSS alone. Both the lesion morphology and the severity of the clinical manifestations noted in this patient increase the risk and technical difficulty of the procedure.

2. Case

A 75-year-old Caucasian male was referred for evaluation with the following history: coronary artery bypass grafting (CABG) with left internal mammary artery (LIMA) to left anterior descending (LAD) and sequential saphenous vein grafting (SVG) to ramus, obtuse marginal, right posterolateral and right posterior descending arteries, repeat CABG two years later with revision of the SVG, severe peripheral arterial disease (PAD) with a history of left lower extremity surgical revascularization, right iliac artery occlusion, atherosclerotic carotid artery disease, and chronic kidney disease (CKD) Stage III. He had been hospitalized for the treatment of CHF and non-ST elevation myocardial infarction (NSTEMI) within the prior three months and continued to experience increasing angina and dyspnea on exertion (NYHA Class III), which was refractory to medications. He was noted to have had a decrease in LV ejection fraction by echocardiogram from 45% to 15% and underwent cardiac catheterization.

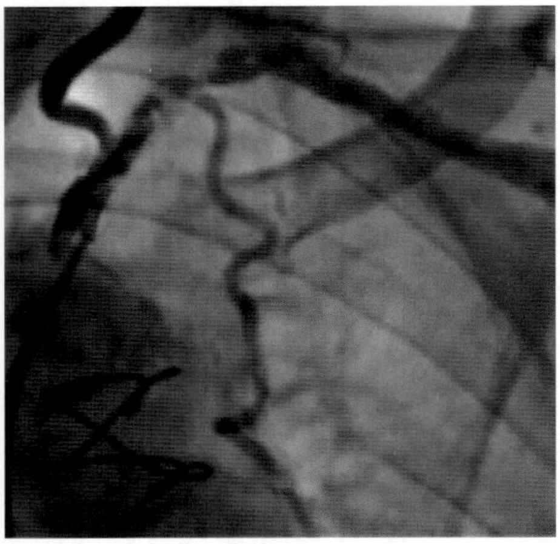

Figure 1: SA angiogram showing diffuse, severe atherosclerosis of the SA/LIMA bifurcation. SA, subclavian artery; LIMA, left internal mammary artery.

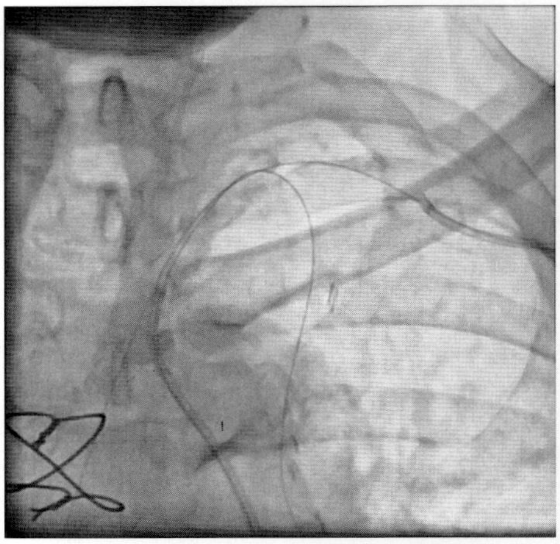

Figure 2: Retrograde wiring of the SA via the left radial artery and anterograde wiring of the LIMA via the left femoral artery. SA, subclavian artery; LIMA, left internal mammary artery.

Cardiac catheterization revealed a patent sequential SVG and severe disease of the body of the SA, distal to the left vertebral artery, and involving the LIMA (Figure 1). The lesion involved the LIMA and the SA, immediately both proximal and distal to the LIMA. Cardiac surgical consultation was obtained, and the patient was deemed a prohibitive risk for a third CABG. Vascular surgical treatment (subclavian-carotid transposition or bypass) was not an option as it would not address the compromised LIMA. Percutaneous therapy directed toward the SA/LIMA bifurcation was planned.

A 6 Fr FR 4.0 Medtronic Launcher coronary guide catheter was placed via the left femoral artery (LFA) into the proximal SA, and a 6-French IMA Medtronic Launcher coronary guide catheter was placed via the left radial artery (LRA) into the SA distal to the LIMA origin. Initial attempts to cross the diffusely calcific SA stenosis anterograde via the LFA, using multiple wire sizes and tips, were unsuccessful. A 0.018 Terumo Glidewire Advantage wire was then placed retrograde via the LRA across the SA stenosis and into the ascending aorta. A 0.014 Terumo Runthrough NS Hypercoat coronary guidewire was placed from the LFA into the LIMA (Figure 2). The SA was predilated via the LRA. A 5 mm × 28 mm balloon expandable stent (Multi-Link Ultra, Abbott Vascular) was then placed into the SA crossing the ostium of the LIMA, trapping the LIMA guidewire (Figure 3). This was followed by postdilatation of the stent with a 5 mm × 15 mm noncompliant balloon (NC Trek, Abbott Vascular). A second Terumo Runthrough NS Hypercoat coronary guidewire was then placed through the stent into the LIMA from the LFA, and the trapped guidewire was removed. Multiple unsuccessful attempts were made to pass a balloon through the stent struts into the LIMA from the LFA. Despite the use of small, low profile balloons and a guide extender (Guide Liner, Vascular Solutions), the LIMA could not be accessed from the LFA. At this point, the decision was made to change the angle of approach to the LIMA by attempting percutaneous intervention via the LRA.

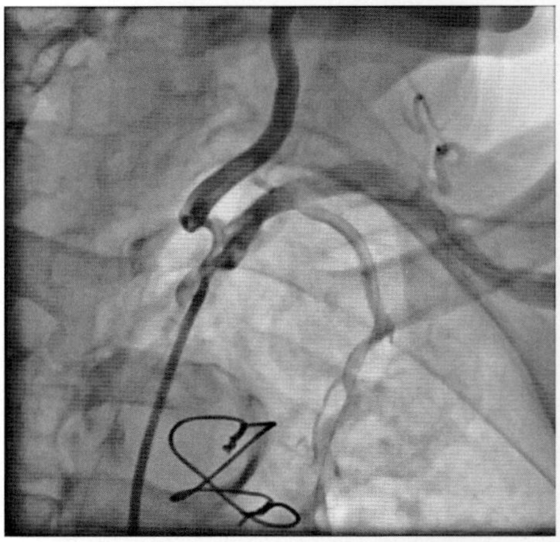

Figure 3: SA stented, trapping the LIMA wire. Persistent significant disease is noted in the proximal LIMA. SA, subclavian artery; LIMA, left internal mammary artery.

A 0.014 Terumo Runthrough NS Hypercoat coronary guidewire was then placed from the LRA through the stent struts into the LIMA. The coronary guidewire which had been placed into the LIMA from the LFA was removed. A 0.035 Terumo Glidewire Advantage wire was then placed from the LFA into the SA.

The stent struts were then dilated via the LRA, and a 3 mm × 12 mm drug-eluting stent (Xience Alpine, Abbott Vascular) was easily passed through. A 5 mm × 15 mm noncompliant balloon (NC Trek, Abbott Vascular) was then placed into the SA stent via the LFA, and a small portion of the LIMA stent was pulled back into the SA stent in order to perform "T and small Protrusion" or TAP stenting [4] of the SA/LIMA bifurcation (Figure 4). A final kissing balloon angioplasty was accomplished, and post-op angiography demonstrated a patent SA/LIMA bifurcation (Figure 5).

The patient was symptom free with improved LV ejection fraction to 30% by echocardiography at 6 months.

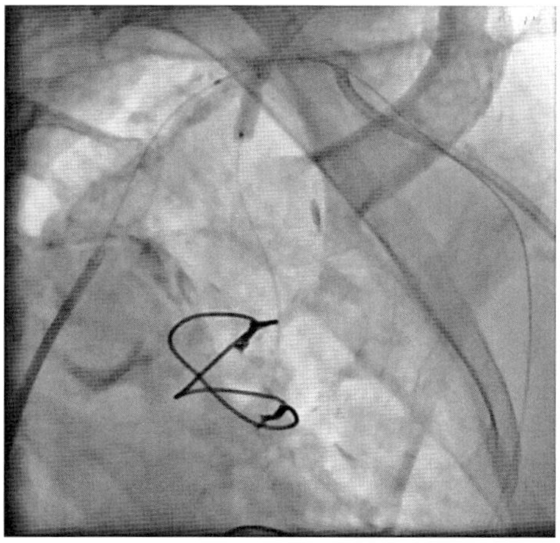

FIGURE 4: The DES is deployed in the LIMA with a balloon placed in the SA. The balloon will be inflated following stent deployment prior to concluding with final kissing angioplasty. DES, drug-eluting stent; LIMA, left internal mammary artery; SA, subclavian artery.

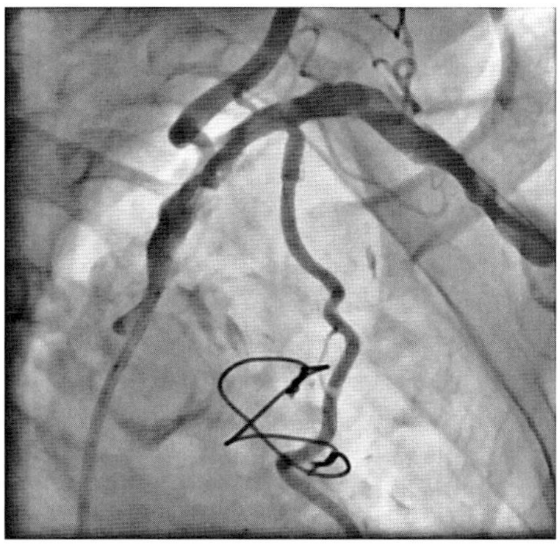

FIGURE 5: Final angiogram demonstrating a patent SA/LIMA bifurcation. SA, subclavian artery; LIMA, left internal mammary artery.

3. Discussion

Subclavian artery stenosis (SAS) is found in up to 18% of patients with PAD [5]. Proximal left SAS was found to occur in 11.8% of patients with both PAD and coronary artery disease requiring CABG [2, 6]. In patients who have undergone CABG with LIMA, the estimated incidence of CSSS is between 0.2% and 6.8% [2, 7]. Based on data from 98 case reports, the most common manifestation of CSSS is stable/unstable angina (88.6%), MI (11.4%), and CHF or worsening LV systolic dysfunction (13.2%) [8].

Endovascular treatment of SAS has evolved into first-line therapy. Balloon expandable stents have been associated with low periprocedural complication rates. In addition, ten-year patency and event-free survival appear comparable to surgical treatment of SAS [2, 9].

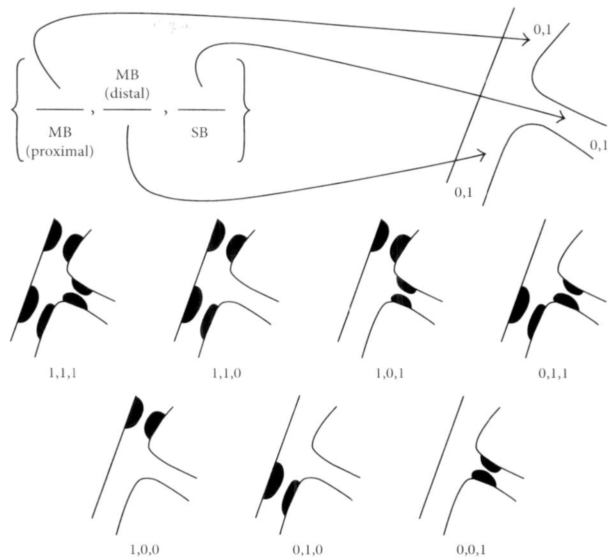

FIGURE 6: The Medina classification of coronary bifurcation lesions [11].

The case described is anatomically unique due to the presence of extensive atherosclerosis of the subclavian/LIMA bifurcation resulting in severe ischemia leading to progressive LV systolic dysfunction and congestive heart failure. This complex bifurcation anatomy creates not only substrate for CSSS but compromises inflow to and outflow from the LIMA, likely compounding the severity of the LAD territory ischemia causing significant cardiac compromise [10].

The lesion was classified as a Medina 1,1,1 bifurcation type (Figure 6) using the Medina classification for coronary bifurcations [11]. In this case, the SA was considered the main branch (MB) and the LIMA the side branch (SB), and the procedure was planned accordingly.

Accessing the lesion from both the proximal and distal SA (MB) provided a unique approach to bifurcation stenting, which is not available in the coronary tree. The decision to utilize a two-stent technique was based on the large size of the SB (LIMA) with disease extending greater than 5 mm from the carina into the SB [12]. The "T and small protrusion" or TAP technique was the chosen bifurcation technique [4]. The "crush" bifurcation technique has been reported in SA/vertebral artery bifurcation stenoses [13]; however, the technically less demanding TAP technique was chosen based on lesion complexity and difficult lesion access [4]. Also, the near ninety-degree angle of the bifurcation favors the TAP technique [12]. It should be noted that despite the high-risk nature of the intervention, mechanical support was not utilized. This patient had significant bilateral lower extremity PAD, including a totally occluded right iliac artery making the use of support devices problematic. This case illustrates a severe clinical manifestation of CSSS and LIMA compromise secondary to a complex bifurcation stenosis. As demonstrated, with careful planning and the meticulous use of bifurcation techniques adapted from the coronary experience, a procedure of this nature can be performed safely and with an excellent outcome.

Acknowledgments

The authors thank Eric S. Roccario, MD, Chief, Cardiac Catheterization Laboratory, St. Peter's Hospital, Albany, NY, and Harold G. Card, MD, St. Peter's Health Partners Medical Associates, Saratoga Springs, NY.

References

[1] P. T. Harjola and M. Valle, "The importance of aortic arch or subclavian angiography before coronary reconstruction," *Chest*, vol. 66, no. 4, pp. 436–438, 1974.

[2] B. Cua, N. Mamdani, D. Halpin, S. Jhamnani, S. Jayasuriya, and C. Mena-Hurtado, "Review of coronary subclavian steal syndrome," *Journal of Cardiology*, vol. 70, no. 5, pp. 432–437, 2017.

[3] T. J. Takach, G. J. Reul, J. M. Duncan et al., "Myocardial thievery: the coronary-subclavian steal syndrome," *Annals of Thoracic Surgery*, vol. 80, no. 2, pp. 564–569, 2005.

[4] F. Burzotta, V. Dzavik, M. Ferenc, C. Trani, and G. Stankovic, "Technical aspects of the T and small protrusion (TAP) technique," *EuroIntervention*, vol. 11, pp. V91–V95, 2015.

[5] G. R. Gutierrez, P. Mahrer, V. Ahraronian, P. Mansukhani, and J. Bruss, "Prevalence of subclavian artery stenosis in patients with peripheral vascular disease," *Angiology*, vol. 52, no. 3, pp. 189–194, 2001.

[6] J. A. English, E. S. Carell, S. A. Guidera, and H. F. Tripp, "Angiographic prevalence and clinical predictors of left subclavian stenosis in patients undergoing diagnostic cardiac catheterization," *Catheterization and Cardiovascular Interventions*, vol. 54, no. 1, pp. 8–11, 2001.

[7] J. F. Iglesias, S. Degrauwe, P. Monney et al., "Coronary subclavian steal syndrome and acute anterior myocardial infarction: a new treatment dilemma in the era of primary percutaneous coronary intervention," *Circulation*, vol. 132, pp. 70-71, 2015.

[8] M. Sintek, E. Coverstone, and J. Singh, "Coronary subclavian steal syndrome," *Current Opinion in Cardiology*, vol. 29, no. 6, pp. 506–513, 2014.

[9] E. Ballotta, G. Da Giau, E. Abbruzzese, E. Mion, R. Manara, and C. Baracchini, "Subclavian carotid transposition for symptomatic subclavian artery stenosis or occlusion. A comparison with the endovascular procedure," *International Angiology*, vol. 21, no. 2, pp. 138–144, 2002.

[10] A. Alcocer, G. Castillo, J. M. Rivera-Capello, V. Gonzalez, and E. Meaney, "Anterograde flow compromise of a patent left internal mammary artery graft from a proximal subclavian stenosis. Myocardial ischemia not driven by the coronary subclavian steal mechanism," *Archivos de Cardiología de México*, vol. 82, no. 2, pp. 135–138, 2012.

[11] A. Medina, J. S. de Lezo, and M. Pan, "A new classification of coronary bifurcation lesions," *Revista Española de Cardiología*, vol. 59, no. 2, p. 183, 2006.

[12] D. Hildick-Smith, J. F. Lassen, R. Albiero et al., "Consensus from the 5th European bifurcation club meeting," *EuroIntervention*, vol. 6, no. 1, pp. 34–38, 2010.

[13] A. Roguin and I. A. Alhaddad, "Crush stenting of bifurcational left subclavian-vertebral artery stenosis," *Catheterization and Cardiovascular Interventions*, vol. 62, no. 3, pp. 393–395, 2004.

Transcatheter Aortic Valve Replacement Incidentalomas: A Multimodality Imaging Case of Giant Right Coronary Aneurysm

Jamal Janjua,[1] Esosa G. Odigie-Okon,[2] Premnauth Rabindranauth,[3] Richard J. Wittchow,[4] and Aiman Riaz[1]

[1]*Department of Internal Medicine, Gundersen Health System, La Crosse, WI 54601, USA*
[2]*Department of Cardiology, Gundersen Health System, La Crosse, WI 54601, USA*
[3]*Department of Cardiothoracic Surgery, Gundersen Health System, La Crosse, WI 54601, USA*
[4]*Department of Pathology, Gundersen Health System, La Crosse, WI 54601, USA*

Correspondence should be addressed to Jamal Janjua; jamaljanjua@gmail.com

Academic Editor: Ertugrul Ercan

Giant coronary artery aneurysms (CAAs) are defined as having a diameter of greater than 2 cm. We report a case of an 82-year-old male with severe aortic stenosis incidentally diagnosed with giant right coronary artery aneurysm (gRCAA) while undergoing evaluation for transcather aortic valve replacement (TAVR). It was causing a mass effect on the right cardiac chambers but was otherwise asymptomatic. Our patient was successfully treated with surgical excision of aneurysm with concomitant coronary artery bypass grafting (CABG) and surgical aortic valve replacement (SAVR). The patient remained stable at discharge and on serial follow-ups for two years. In conclusion, due to the associated complication and increased risk of mortality with giant coronary aneurysms, we recommend surgical approach instead of medical management alone. We also call for evidence-based recommendations and guidelines for management of TAVR incidentalomas.

1. Introduction

Transcatheter aortic valve replacement (TAVR) has been proven to be a safe and effective minimally invasive procedure for aortic stenosis and has been shown to reduce mortality among high-risk patients with aortic valve stenosis irrespective of their candidacy for surgical replacement, typically octogenarians and nonagenarians [1]. As a result of patients' advanced age, incidentalomas ranging from intracardiac thrombi, extracardiac malignancies and congenital heart diseases are frequently encountered and alter the surgical plan. Coronary artery aneurysm (CAA) is a rare entity typically diagnosed incidentally through imaging studies or at postmortem. Giant coronary artery aneurysms (gCAAs) are even rarer and are defined as having a diameter more than 2 cm. It can be broadly classified into congenital or acquired (e.g., iatrogenic, atherosclerosis, and infectious). We present a multimodality imaging case of a giant right coronary artery aneurysm (gRCAA) found incidentally during workup for aortic valve replacement and outline the unique challenge it presented in this setting.

2. Case Report

An 82-year-old male with symptomatic severe aortic stenosis, permanent atrial fibrillation, ascending aorta enlargement, and obstructive sleep apnea, was referred to our institution. Retrospectively, a transthoracic echocardiogram (TTE) performed 4 years prior had demonstrated an echolucent mass external to the heart located in the right atrioventricular junction causing mass effect on the right atrium and ventricle (Figure 1); however, it was not investigated further. Computed tomography angiogram (CTA) of the aorta was performed in consideration for TAVR based

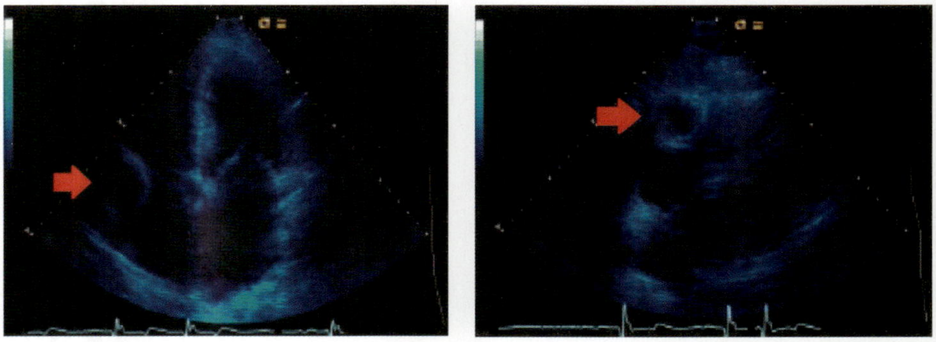

(a) (b)

Figure 1: (a, b) 2D Echocardiogram showing echolucent mass in the right AV groove with mass effect. AV: atrioventricular.

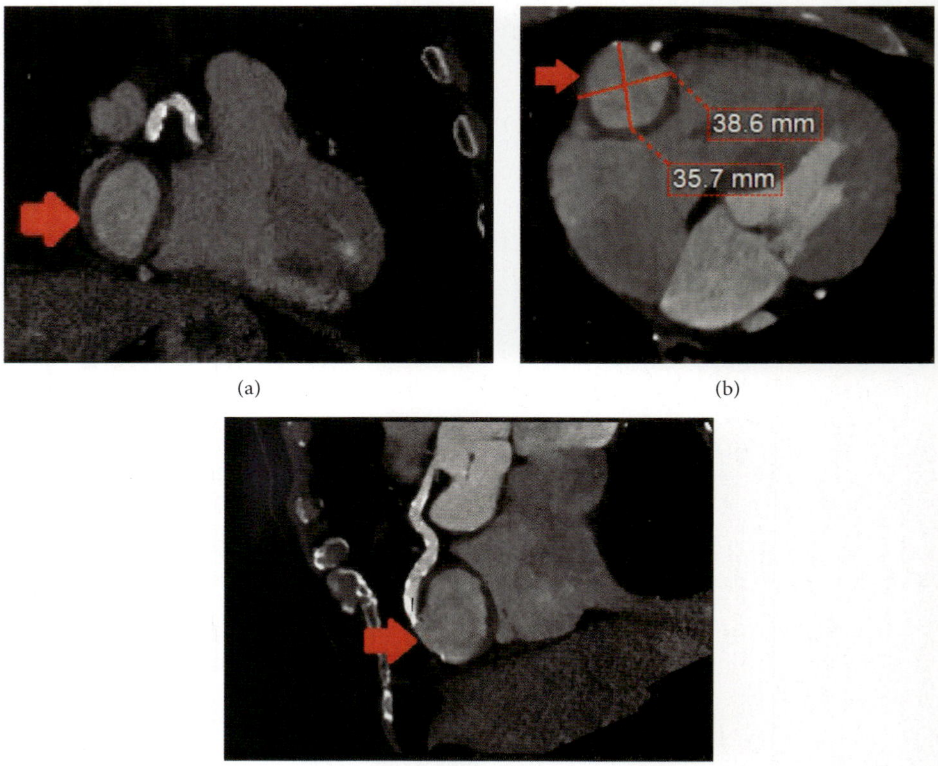

(a) (b)

(c)

Figure 2: CT coronary angiogram. Thrombosed RCA aneurysm in coronal (a) and axial (b) view in right AV groove. (c) Curved multiplanar reformatted image displaying full length of the RCA. AV: atrioventricular; RCA: right coronary artery.

on his high-risk status as well as patient not wanting to undergo surgical aortic valve replacement (SAVR) for personal reasons. It showed a large encapsulated spherical mass with wall thickening in the right atrioventricular groove measuring 38.6 mm by 47.4 mm, continuous with the right coronary artery in the mid-occluded mid-right coronary artery (RCA) segment, findings consistent with a thrombosed gRCAA (Figures 2(a)–2(c)). Coronary angiography confirmed a totally occluded RCA with a mid-RCA dilation that demonstrated contrast swirling in the aneurysm (Figures 3(a) and 3(b)). The left coronary arterial system was without significant disease. The heart team including the cardiologists and cardiothoracic surgeons agreed that TAVR does not address his gRCAA, which could potentially be fixed by coiling, but this would likely lead to complications from the aneurysm including an RCA infarction, fistula, or other fatal complication intraoperatively. As such, he underwent a surgical aortic valve replacement with a 27 mm Sorin Solo Smart tissue valve, coronary artery bypass grafting was done using a saphenous vein graft to the distal posterior descending artery with end to side to acute marginal anastomosis, the gRCAA was excised and repaired with over sew of proximal and distal coronary artery (Figures 4(a)–4(c)) with a left atrial appendage amputation

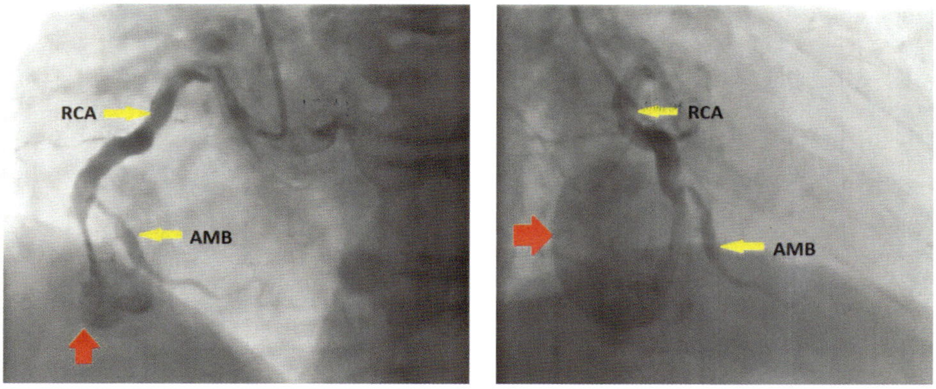

(a) (b)

FIGURE 3: (a, b) Invasive coronary angiogram showing thrombosed RCA aneurysm with contrast and no distal flow. AMB: acute marginal branch; RCA: right coronary artery.

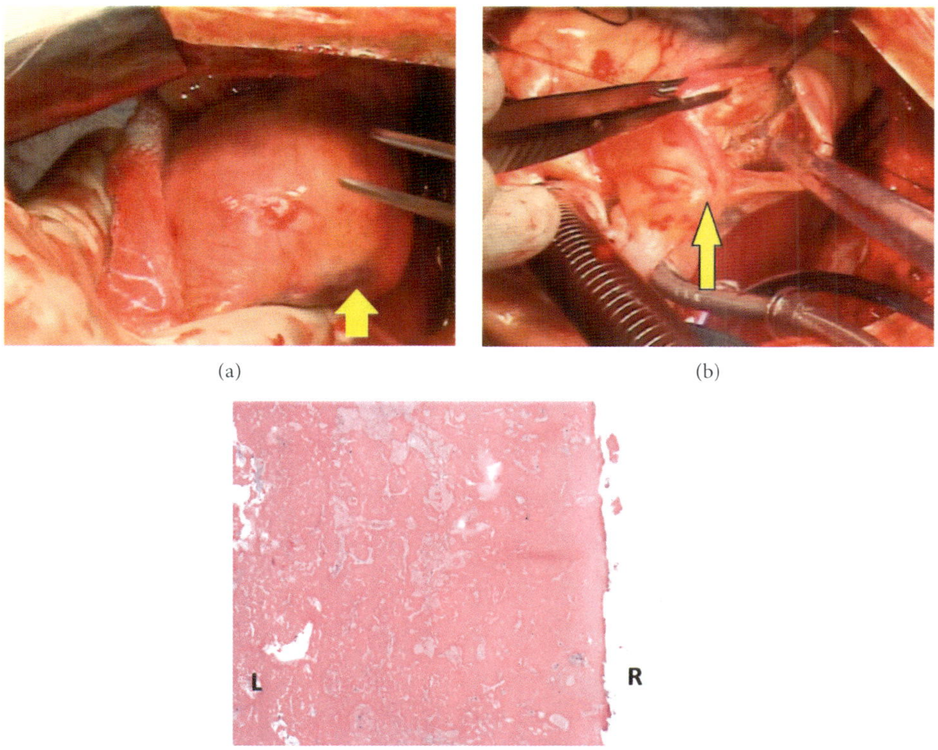

(a) (b)

(c)

FIGURE 4: Intraoperative surgeons' view of the RCA aneurysm intact (a) and excised (b). (c) Photomicrographs of the fibrin thrombus removed from the RCA aneurysm taken at 40x magnification. Shown is the more mature portion of the thrombus on the right side composed of dense, laminated fibrin, while the luminal side (left) has more recent thrombus deposition composed of blood/platelets alternating with fibrin bands (lines of Zahn). RCA: right coronary artery.

for his atrial fibrillation. Postoperative course was uneventful, and he was discharged home in a stable condition.

3. Discussion

Coronary artery aneurysm is defined as dilation of greater than 1.5 times than the reference vessel. It is rare with incidence of 0.02–0.04% in the general population [2]. Increased incidence, however, is reported in patients undergoing diagnostic procedures like angiography, ranging from 1.1 to 4.9% [3]. It usually involves the right coronary artery. In a study by Keyser et al., right-sided gCAA was found in 89% of the cases [4]. One of the most common childhood conditions associated with CAAs is Kawasaki disease, but it can also be found in connective tissue diseases (e.g., Marfan's and Ehlers-Danlos syndrome), infections (e.g., syphilis), inflammation (e.g., polyarthritis nodosa and systemic lupus erythematosus), and iatrogenic causes (like coronary angiography and stenting). The most common acquired cause of CAA is atherosclerosis as suggested in studies by Makris et al. [5] and Hartnell et al. [6] in as early as 1976 and 1985, respectively. The dreaded complications include rupture of CAA [2], thrombosis, embolization and myocardial infarction [7], congestive heart failure, and fistulous connections [8] among others.

Management remains controversial. Recommended surgical treatment involves resection of aneurysm with or without coronary bypass graft [2]. Other options include patch repair, coil embolization, and stents [9]. More recently, percutaneous techniques have been used as well [10]. Dai et al. reported a case of gRCAA which was successfully treated percutaneously with multiple overlapping stents [11]. Conservative management includes statins and antiplatelet agents or anticoagulation due to the fear of thrombus formation and distal embolization [12] although evidence is still lacking. In our patient, no evidence for vasculitis, infection or connective tissue disease was found. CT angiogram demonstrated significant calcific atherosclerotic coronary artery disease allowing us to positively confirm atherosclerosis as the most likely etiology.

Since our patient had aneurysm that remained asymptomatic for the past 4 years, one approach could have been to manage it conservatively. It was supported by the data from coronary artery surgery study (CASS) registry which followed patients throughout the 1980s, and no aneurysmal ruptures were found [13]. However, the authors of this paper propose the individualization of treatment based on patient-related factors and preferences. In our case, the patient required aortic valve replacement and had significant coronary artery disease in addition to the mass effect caused by the gCAA, so it made sense to address it at time of valve repair. An isolated, asymptomatic gCAA without valvular stenosis requiring intervention would have steered us in the direction of medical management alone.

4. Conclusion

Giant coronary aneurysm is a rare entity. However, the probability of encountering it in geriatric cardiology clinical practice is likely to increase with rising rates of percutaneous cardiac interventions like TAVR. With the increasing expansion of TAVR over SAVR to intermediate risk and possibly low-risk patients in the near future, percutaneous options for management of these pathologies will be of paramount importance to justify the eventual cost of TAVR over SAVR for these patients with otherwise limited life expectancies. In addition, knowledge of the various etiologies, associated complications, and treatment options of these incidentalomas are paramount. Optimal management option of GCA is still controversial, but we recommend surgical excision especially if aneurysm is causing a mass effect as seen in our patient. Most incidentalomas found during TAVR evaluation may be benign but can also represent lesions requiring therapeutic interventions that would otherwise not be necessary based on the patient's life expectancy, thus leading to more expensive medical costs. The specific relevance and implications of the pathologies will vary for the interventional cardiologist as well as the cardiothoracic surgeon. There is therefore a growing need for evidence-based recommendations and guidelines for management of TAVR incidentalomas.

References

[1] M. B. Leon, C. R. Smith, M. J. Mack et al., "Transcatheter or surgical aortic-valve replacement in intermediate-risk patients," *New England Journal of Medicine*, vol. 374, pp. 1609–1620, 2016.

[2] D. Li, Q. Wu, L. Sun et al., "Surgical treatment of giant coronary artery aneurysm," *Journal of Thoracic and Cardiovascular Surgery*, vol. 130, no. 3, pp. 817–821, 2005.

[3] A. S. Daoud, D. Pankin, H. Tulgan, and R. A. Florentin, "Aneurysms of the coronary artery. Report of ten cases and review of literature," *American Journal of Cardiology*, vol. 11, no. 2, pp. 228–237, 1963.

[4] A. Keyser, M. K. Hilker, O. Husser, C. Diez, and C. Schmid, "Giant coronary aneurysms exceeding 5 cm in size," *Interactive CardioVascular and Thoracic Surgery*, vol. 15, no. 1, pp. 33–36, 2012.

[5] J. E. Markis, C. D. Joffe, P. F. Cohn, D. J. Feen, M. V. Herman, and R. Gorlin, "Clinical significance of coronary arterial ectasia," *American Journal of Cardiology*, vol. 37, no. 2, pp. 217–222, 1976.

[6] G. G. Hartnell, B. M. Parnell, and R. B. Pridie, "Coronary artery ectasia. Its prevalence and clinical significance in 4993 patients," *British Heart Journal*, vol. 54, no. 4, pp. 392–395, 1985.

[7] S. Suzuki, S. Ichimiya, M. Kanashiro, H. Okamoto, H. Ishii, and T. Murohara, "Acute thrombotic occlusion of a giant right coronary artery aneurysm," *Journal of Cardiac Surgery*, vol. 30, no. 5, pp. 436-437, 2015.

[8] H. Morita, H. Ozawa, S. Yamazaki et al., "A case of giant coronary artery aneurysm with fistulous connection to the pulmonary artery: a case report and review of the literature," *Internal Medicine*, vol. 51, no. 11, pp. 1361–1366, 2012.

[9] R. A. Aqel, G. J. Zoghbi, and A. Iskandrian, "Spontaneous coronary artery dissection, aneurysms, and pseudoaneurysms: a review," *Echocardiography*, vol. 21, no. 2, pp. 175–182, 2004.

[10] M. A. Peterson, L. H. Monsein, G. Dangas, R. Mehran, and M. B. Leon, "Percutaneous transcatheter management of giant coronary aneurysms," *Circulation*, vol. 100, pp. e8–e11, 1999.

[11] H. Dai, X. Guang, L. Jiang, Q. Xue, and W. Zhang, "Overlapping-stent intervention treatment of a giant right coronary artery pseudoaneurysm," *JACC: Cardiovascular Interventions*, vol. 8, no. 15, pp. e255–e256, 2015.

[12] P. Banerjee, T. Houghton, M. Walters, and G. C. Kaye, "Giant right coronary artery aneurysm presenting as a mediastinal mass," *Heart*, vol. 90, no. 9, p. e50, 2004.

[13] T. Robertson and L. Fisher, "Prognostic significance of coronary artery aneurysm and ectasia in the coronary artery surgery study (CASS) registry," *Progress in Clinical and Biological Research*, vol. 250, pp. 325–339, 1987.

Transcatheter Coil Embolization of Single Coronary Artery Fistula Using the Occlusion Test

Shin Takahashi,[1] **Yurie Takizawa**,[1] **Satoshi Nakano**,[1] **Junichi Koizumi**,[2] **and Kotaro Oyama**[1]

[1]*Department of Pediatrics, School of Medicine, Iwate Medical University, Morioka, Japan*
[2]*Department of Cardiovascular Surgery, School of Medicine, Iwate Medical University, Morioka, Japan*

Correspondence should be addressed to Shin Takahashi; shint@iwate-med.ac.jp

Academic Editor: Kuan-Rau Chiou

The case of a patient in whom hemodynamic and electrocardiographic studies using the occlusion test for coronary artery fistulas (CAF) were safely performed prior to catheter embolization is reported. A 1-year-old girl had a separate right coronary artery arising from a left single coronary artery that formed a significant coronary artery fistula to the right ventricle. Coronary steal by the large coronary artery fistula narrowed the left coronary artery. The right coronary artery branches could not be clearly identified due to an overlap with the fistula. Due to the long porous CAF, embolic procedures could cause serious complications. We confirmed the safety by performing an occlusion test of the CAF's proximal blood vessels. Following total occlusion of the CAF for 10 minutes, pulmonary arterial pressure and aortic blood pressure were not significantly changed. No bradycardia, atrioventricular block, or ST changes were observed. Coil embolization treatment was performed safely. For patients with long distal CAF complicated with a single coronary artery, myocardial ischemia and conduction system disorders can be identified by performing the occlusion test before embolization.

1. Introduction

Coronary artery fistula (CAF) has congenital and acquired coronary artery abnormalities. This abnormality accounts for 0.27–0.4% of all congenital cardiac defects. Congenital single coronary artery comprises about 0.04% of congenital cardiac anomalies [1]. In addition, CAF complicated with single coronary artery is rare. Myocardial ischemia due to coronary steal is an extremely difficult problem, and its presence can be an indication for treatment. Acute complications associated with embolization of CAF include myocardial ischemia and conduction system disorders [2]. A case of significant CAF is presented in a heart with normal structure. A hemodynamic study involving an occlusion test of the fistula's proximal vessel prior to catheter embolization was performed, and the patient safely underwent catheter treatment.

2. Case Presentation

The parents of the following patient have given their consent for the publication of this report.

2.1. Case. A 1-year-old girl presented with continuous heart murmur. Chest radiography showed slight cardiomegaly (cardiothoracic ratio, 55%). Electrocardiogram showed sinus rhythm and no ST changes. Echocardiography showed a dilated left main coronary trunk artery (LMT) and a right coronary artery (RCA) entering a right ventricular fistula. Coronary computed tomography angiography (CTA) with three-dimensional volume rendering revealed the thick and torsional RCA originating from the left anterior descending coronary artery (LAD), with fistulous communication to the right ventricle via a large vessel (Figure 1(a)). In cardiac catheterization, the Qp/Qs was 2.6. The CAF was a "beaded

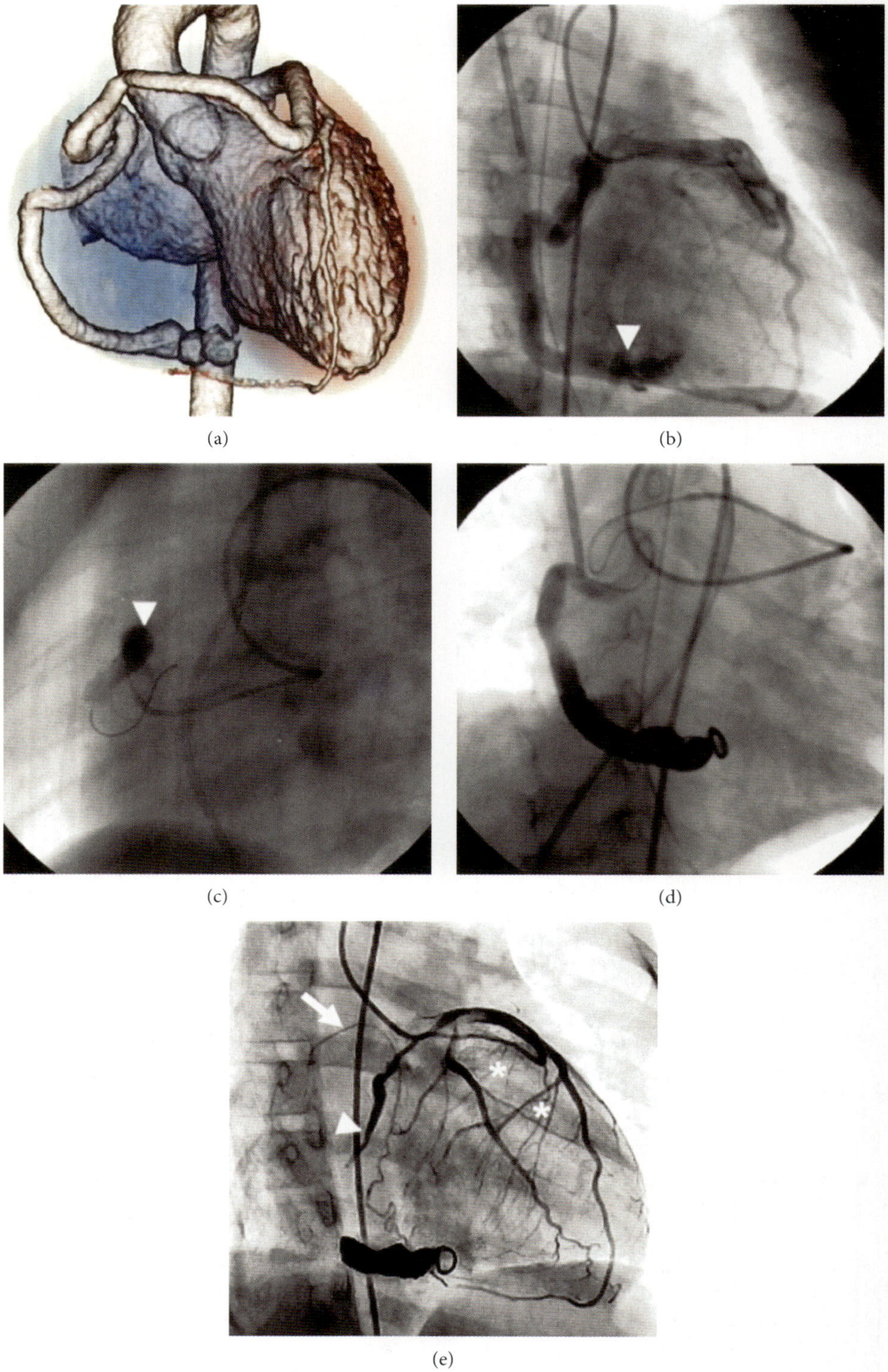

FIGURE 1: (a) 320-row coronary CTA. The single coronary artery view shows the anterior course of the separate right coronary artery coming off the LAD. This is the anterior view. (b) Selective coronary angiography of the LMT shows the LAD and the LCX with weak contrast effects and a CAF with "multiple caliber change" of the RCA to the right ventricle (arrowhead). (c) Occlusion test on the proximal site of CAF using an occlusion balloon (arrowhead). (d) Engaged microcatheter in the distal RCA and embolization using a detachable coil. (e) One year after coil embolization, selective LMT coronary angiography clearly distinguishes the contrast effect of the LAD and LCX, the sinus node branch branching from LCX (white arrow), and right ventricular branches from the proximal side of the RCA (asterisks). The proximal end of the coil-embolized CAF formed a thrombus and occluded (arrowhead). CAF: coronary artery fistula; CTA: computed tomography angiography; LAD: left anterior descending coronary artery; LCX: left circumflex coronary artery; LMT: left main coronary trunk artery; RCA: right coronary artery.

and caliber change" form. Coronary angiography could not distinguish the RCA's peripheral branches (Figure 1(b)). The sinus node branch, right ventricular branches, and acute marginal branch from the RCA could not be clearly identified. Additionally, neither the atrioventricular nor the posterior descending branch on the peripheral site could be identified due to an overlap with the fistula. Collateral vessels from the LCA to the same site also could not be identified. Because of the long porous CAF, there was a concern about the embolism disrupting peripheral branch blood flow. We tried the occlusion test on the proximal vessel of the CAF. Using the PercuSurge GuardWire™ system (Medtronic, Santa Rosa, CA, USA), an occlusion test was performed in the proximal site of the RCA using a 6 mm balloon (Figure 1(c)). Following total occlusion for 10 minutes, the pulmonary arterial pressure (systolic/diastolic/mean) changed from 19/10/15 to 18/10/14 mmHg and the aortic blood pressure changed from 109/49/64 to 109/57/66 mmHg, both of which had no significant changes. In addition, no bradycardia, atrioventricular block, or ST changes were observed on electrocardiogram. Coil embolization was performed with GDC™ Detachable Coils (Boston Scientific, Fremont, CA, USA) (Figure 1(d)). Because of the long porous CAF, the target vessel was an embolus of a long lumen. However, the embolic area did not cross the balloon occlusion site. Coil embolization treatment techniques were safely performed.

After this procedure, anticoagulation therapy was continued. In cardiac catheter examination one year after coil embolization, the contrast effect of the LAD and left circumflex coronary artery (LCX) increased, and each coronary branch was easy to distinguish. The residual shunt from the CAF did not have a contrast effect. The proximal end of the coil-embolized CAF formed a thrombus and occluded. However, there existed right ventricular branches from the proximal side of the RCA. The sinus node branch revealed branching from the LCX. The collateral vessels from the developed septal branch, LAD, and sinus node branch supplemented the peripheral areas of the RCA (Figure 1(e)). The patient's hemodynamics are now stable, and she is in good health.

3. Discussion

Up to 57% of patients with a CAF also have another congenital cardiovascular anomaly [3]. In patients with coronary fistulas, a coronary artery "steal" phenomenon can result in coronary blood preferentially passing through the fistula instead of the more distal myocardial capillaries. Angina has been reported in many patients with large fistulas and may be aggravated by distal coronary artery disease. In comparing CAF symptoms between adults and children, children more often have abnormal murmur and associated defects and rarely have CAF aneurysms and coronary artery disease. Symptoms are more likely to develop with advancing age, although treating asymptomatic CAF patients still poses management difficulties [4].

CAF are classified as distal or proximal. The proximal type arises near the origin of the coronary artery. A short proximal segment of the feeding coronary artery may be dilated, but the distal end of the original coronary artery is thin. The original coronary branches responsible for blood flow steal are hard to identify. The distal type of CAF originates near the distal end of a branch coronary artery. The feeding coronary artery proximal to a distal fistula gives rise to coronary branches that supply the myocardium [5]. This case was a right distal CAF, in which the left coronary branches responsible for blood flow steal could not be identified.

Therapies to close congenital CAF during childhood have been recommended to avoid complications such as myocardial ischemia, congestive heart failure, endocarditis, and aneurysmal dilatation [2]. Whether to treat CAF surgically or by percutaneous intervention in childhood is controversial. Of the acute complications following coil embolization, the most important are myocardial ischemia and conduction system disorders. Early complications have been reported to include transient ST-T wave changes, transient arrhythmias, distal coronary spasm, and fistula dissection [6]. In addition, there are many variations of the origin and course of coronary arteries in congenital heart disease, making percutaneous coronary intervention technically difficult. Asymptomatic children with large CAF who underwent therapeutic intervention have been reported [7]. Catheter techniques are difficult or impossible in a small percentage of patients, particularly younger pediatric cases, due to extreme vessel tortuosity and inability to deliver a catheter far enough distally [8]. The single coronary artery seen in this case is especially rare, making percutaneous coronary intervention technically difficult.

A balloon occlusion test before coil embolization of a CAF is necessary to avoid complications, particularly when many coronary branches cannot be distinguished clearly in small pediatric patients [9].

4. Conclusion

In patients with CAF, the coronary artery branches sometimes cannot be identified due to the presence of blood flow steal. In such cases, myocardial ischemia and conduction system disorders can be identified by performing the occlusion test before embolization.

References

[1] K. R. Shyam Sunder, K. G. Balakrishnan, J. A. Tharakan et al., "Coronary artery fistula in children and adults: a review of 25 cases with long-term observations," *International Journal of Cardiology*, vol. 58, no. 1, pp. 47–53, 1997.

[2] C. Mavroudis, C. L. Backer, A. P. Rocchini, A. J. Muster, and M. Gevitz, "Coronary artery fistulas in infants and children: a surgical review and discussion of coil embolization," *The Annals of Thoracic Surgery*, vol. 63, no. 5, pp. 1235–1242, 1997.

[3] N. Collins, R. Mehta, L. Benson, and E. Horlick, "Percutaneous coronary artery fistula closure in adults: technical and procedural aspects," *Catheterization and Cardiovascular Interventions*, vol. 69, no. 6, pp. 872–880, 2007.

[4] H. S. Singh, C. Nagy, A. W. Wan, M. D. Osten, L. N. Benson, and E. M. Horlick, "Complex interventions in the adult with

congenital heart disease: percutaneous solutions for venous baffles, coronary artery fistulas, and ruptured sinus of Valsalva aneurysms," *Interventional Cardiology Clinics*, vol. 2, no. 1, pp. 153–172, 2013.

[5] S. T. Gowda, L. A. Latson, S. Kutty, and L. R. Prieto, "Intermediate to long-term outcome following congenital coronary artery fistulae closure with focus on thrombus formation," *The American Journal of Cardiology*, vol. 107, no. 2, pp. 302–308, 2011.

[6] L. R. Armsby, J. F. Keane, M. C. Sherwood, J. M. Forbess, S. B. Perry, and J. E. Lock, "Management of coronary artery fistulae: patient selection and results of transcatheter closure," *Journal of the American College of Cardiology*, vol. 39, no. 6, pp. 1026–1032, 2002.

[7] K.-S. Hsieh, T.-C. Huang, and C.-L. Lee, "Coronary artery fistulas in neonates, infants, and children: clinical findings and outcome," *Pediatric Cardiology*, vol. 23, no. 4, pp. 415–419, 2002.

[8] L. A. Latson, "Coronary artery fistulas: how to manage them," *Catheterization and Cardiovascular Interventions*, vol. 70, no. 1, pp. 111–118, 2007.

[9] G. C. Kung, P. Moore, D. B. McElhinney, and D. F. Teitel, "Retrograde transcatheter coil embolization of congenital coronary artery fistulas in infants and young children," *Pediatric Cardiology*, vol. 24, no. 5, pp. 448–453, 2003.

56

Postural Tachycardia Syndrome and Vasovagal Syncope: A Hidden Case of Obstructive Cardiomyopathy without Severe Septal Hypertrophy

Kenneth A. Mayuga,[1] Natalie Ho,[1] Robert W. Shields Jr.,[2] Paul Cremer,[1] and L. Leonardo Rodriguez[1]

[1]*Department of Cardiovascular Medicine, Heart and Vascular Institute, Cleveland Clinic, Cleveland, OH, USA*
[2]*Neurological Institute, Cleveland Clinic, Cleveland, OH, USA*

Correspondence should be addressed to Kenneth A. Mayuga; mayugak@ccf.org

Academic Editor: Hajime Kataoka

A 36-year-old female with symptoms of orthostatic intolerance and syncope was diagnosed with vasovagal syncope on a tilt table test and with postural tachycardia syndrome (POTS) after a repeat tilt table test. However, an echocardiogram at our institution revealed obstructive cardiomyopathy without severe septal hypertrophy, with a striking increase in left ventricular outflow tract gradient from 7 mmHg at rest to 75 mmHg during Valsalva, with a septal thickness of only 1.3 cm. Cardiac MRI showed an apically displaced multiheaded posteromedial papillary muscle with suggestion of aberrant chordal attachments to the anterior mitral leaflet contributing to systolic anterior motion of the mitral valve. She underwent surgery with reorientation of the posterior medial papillary muscle head, resection of the tethering secondary chordae to the A1 segment of the mitral valve, chordal shortening and tacking of the chordae to the A1 and A2 segments of the mitral valve, and gentle septal myectomy. After surgery, she had significant improvement in her prior symptoms. To our knowledge, this is the first reported case of obstructive cardiomyopathy without severe septal hypertrophy with abnormalities in papillary muscle and chordal attachment, in a patient diagnosed with vasovagal syncope and POTS.

1. Introduction

Postural tachycardia syndrome (POTS) is a clinical syndrome characterized by frequent symptoms that occur with standing, an increase in heart rate of 30 bpm when moving from a recumbent to a standing position, and the absence of orthostatic hypotension [1]. Vasovagal syncope is defined as syncope that usually occurs with upright posture held for more than 30 seconds, features diaphoresis, warmth, nausea, and pallor, and is associated with hypotension and relative bradycardia [1]. Obstructive cardiomyopathy without severe septal hypertrophy (OCM), such as from papillary muscle abnormalities or abnormal chordal attachment, can lead to a decrease in cardiac output due to obstruction in the left ventricular outflow tract. To our knowledge, OCM from papillary muscle abnormalities and abnormal chordal attachment has not previously been reported in a patient diagnosed with POTS as well as vasovagal syncope.

2. Case Presentation

A 36-year-old female was referred to our institution for evaluation of symptoms of orthostatic intolerance. Consent was obtained from the patient to publish this as a case report, with documentation of verbal consent in the electronic medical record. She reported symptoms including dizziness, palpitations, nausea, and a warm sensation while upright that improved with assuming a recumbent posture. She also reported symptoms during exertion, documented as light-headedness and feeling of her heart racing when physically active, as well as a decreased tolerance to walking. Her symptoms occurred a few times per week up to several times per day and were worse during the beginning of her menstrual cycle. Her symptoms significantly improved with wearing compression stockings. She also reported two episodes of loss of consciousness. With the first episode, she was lying on the couch then sat up and felt nauseated, and then she stood up and had an abrupt loss of consciousness. With the second episode, she was walking in the kitchen, had a brief prodrome of not feeling well, and then had an abrupt loss of consciousness. She had evaluations at an outside institution with a Holter monitor showing episodes of sinus tachycardia, an echocardiogram that was reportedly normal, and a tilt table test reporting a vasovagal reaction following the administration of nitroglycerin. She reported that her father had multiple episodes of syncope but never sought medical treatment; she did not report any family history of POTS.

She underwent further evaluations at our institution. A passive 70-degree head up tilt table test showed a postural increase in heart rate from 74 to 114 bpm at the end of the tilt, with some blood pressure oscillations but overall stable blood pressures (from 115/70 mmHg supine to 118/82 mmHg at the end of tilt) while eliciting her typical symptoms of nausea, warmth, a spinning sensation, and feeling like she would lose consciousness. She requested the test to be stopped early at 36 minutes out of a 45-minute protocol due to her symptoms. Of note, she was taking fludrocortisone 0.1 mg daily at the time of the head up tilt table test. She was diagnosed initially with POTS due to her clinical features and tilt table test results. She underwent blood volume and hemodynamic testing. Blood volume measured using a I-131-HSA-tagged human serum albumin technique with a Daxor BVA-100 system (Daxor Corporation, NY, USA) showed normal plasma volume at −2.8% from ideal (gender matched, weight, and height). Hemodynamic testing to assess circulatory kinetics was done using 99 m Technetium-RBC radionuclide imaging [2]. At 45-degree head up position, the heart rate increased by 18 bpm, cardiopulmonary volume fraction decreased by 34% (a marked decrease), cardiac index decreased from 2.6 L/min/m^2 to 1.777 L/min/m^2, stroke volume decreased from 79 ml to 50 ml, total peripheral resistance increased from 40 to 61 μm^2, and mean pulmonary transit time was rapid at 6.8 seconds. Plasma metanephrine and normetanephrine levels were checked and were within normal limits. An evaluation of autonomic function was done. Quantitative sudomotor axon reflex testing showed normal values at the right forearm, proximal leg, distal leg, and foot. The heart rate and blood pressure responses to Valsalva showed a normal Valsalva ratio of 1.47 and normal blood pressure responses in phase II and phase IV. An exercise treadmill test done as part of the evaluation for cardiac rehabilitation showed fair functional capacity at 8.6 METS, an increase in heart rate to 99% of maximal predicted heart rate, stable blood pressures, and no arrhythmias.

A resting echocardiogram repeated at our institution showed a normal EF of 71%, mild septal left ventricular hypertrophy measuring 1.3 cm, with a prominent posterior papillary muscle. At rest, there was chordal systolic anterior motion (SAM) of the mitral valve with trivial mitral regurgitation, and a left ventricular outflow tract (LVOT) gradient of only 7 mmHg. After Valsalva maneuver, the LVOT gradient increased strikingly to 75 mmHg (Figure 1) with a further increase to 81 mmHg after administration of amyl nitrite. A subsequent cardiac MRI demonstrated an apically displaced, multiheaded posteromedial papillary muscle. There was a suggestion that the more anteriorly displaced head of the posteromedial papillary muscle had aberrant chordal attachments to the anterior mitral valve leaflet that contributed to the SAM (Figure 2). There was mild hypertrophy of the anteroseptum (measuring 1.3 cm) with a normal left ventricular mass index of 57 gm/m^2 (normal 48–77 gm/m^2) and no delayed enhancement to suggest interstitial fibrosis. A subsequent transesophageal echocardiogram (TEE) demonstrated the mobile anteriorly displaced posterior papillary muscle with SAM (Figure 3).

After consultations with specialists in structural heart disease and cardiothoracic surgery, the patient ultimately underwent cardiac surgery consisting of very gentle septal myectomy focusing more midventricular at the basilar septum, reorientation of the posterior medial papillary muscle head, resection of the tethering secondary chordae to the A1 segment of the mitral valve, and chordal shortening and tacking of the chordae to the A1 and A2 segments of the mitral valve. During her several post-op visits with Cardiology and Cardiothoracic Surgery, she reported a significant improvement in her prior orthostatic symptoms and no longer reported syncope.

3. Discussion

Obstructive cardiomyopathy without severe septal hypertrophy, for example, from papillary muscle abnormalities or abnormal chordal attachment, is not as recognized as the more widely known hypertrophic obstructive cardiomyopathy with severe septal hypertrophy (HOCM) but can also lead to symptoms due to left ventricular outflow obstruction and decreased cardiac output. In the case presented, the patient underwent typical evaluations for a patient with orthostatic symptoms, syncope, and POTS, with expected findings on the initial evaluations, including a tilt table test. Typically, echocardiograms are done while the patient is at rest and without provocative maneuvers such as Valsalva or amyl nitrite unless a resting LVOT gradient is seen. Therefore, entities such as OCM can be readily underdiagnosed. The repeat echocardiogram at our institution disclosed no significant LVOT gradient at rest, but it did reveal a prominent posterior papillary muscle and mild septal hypertrophy. Valsalva maneuver demonstrated significant obstruction across the LVOT, with similar findings after administration of amyl nitrite, a vasodilator agent. The patient also underwent additional cardiac imaging with TEE and MRI that demonstrated the apically displaced, multiheaded posteromedial papillary muscle with SAM. Initial treatment with a beta-blocker can be considered to slow the heart rate and enhance left ventricular filling, but in some cases surgical correction is considered, as in this case. The diagnosis and treatment of obstructive cardiomyopathy without severe hypertrophy (≤1.8 cm) has recently been reported from our institution [3]. On multivariate analysis, the

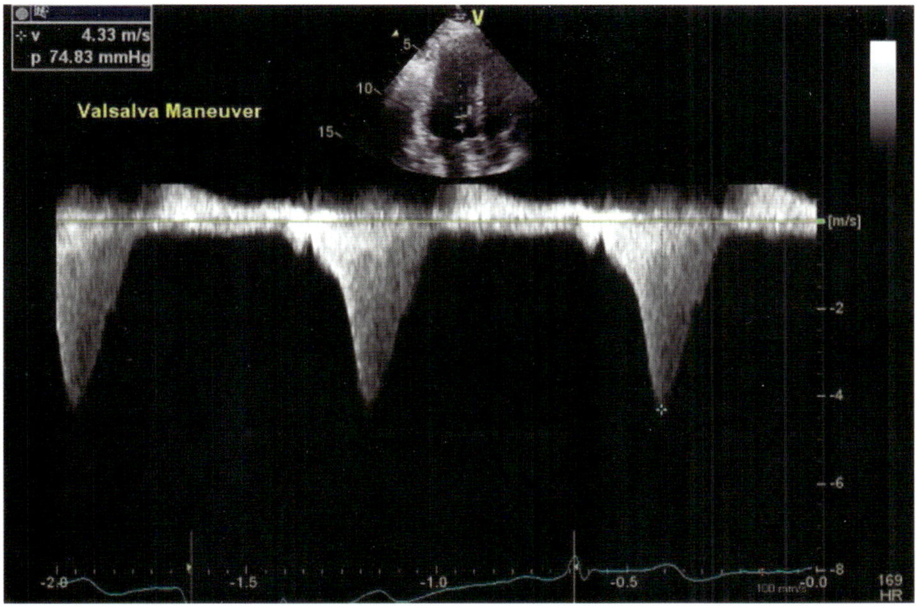

Figure 1: Echocardiogram showing 75 mmHg gradient in the left ventricular outflow tract with Valsalva.

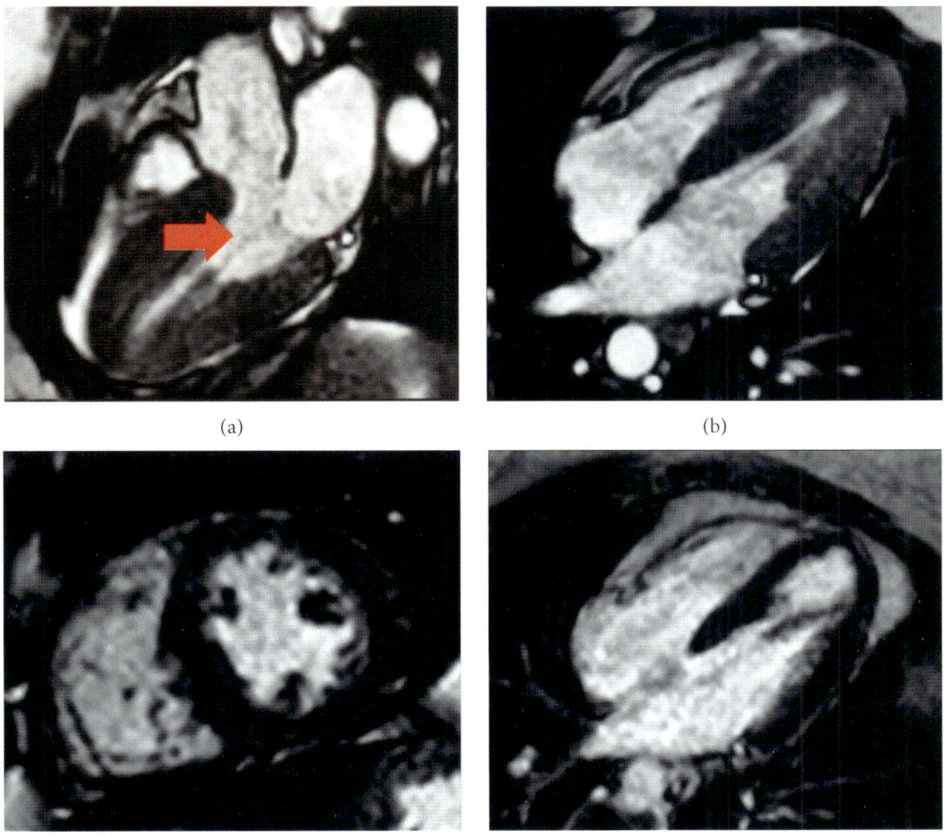

(a) (b)

(c) (d)

Figure 2: Cardiac MRI showing multiple heads of the posteromedial papillary muscle in the three chamber view (a), four chamber view (b), and short axis view (c), with a suggestion of an abnormal chordal attachment to the anterior mitral valve leaflet (red arrow). Delayed gadolinium imaging (d) showing no increased signal.

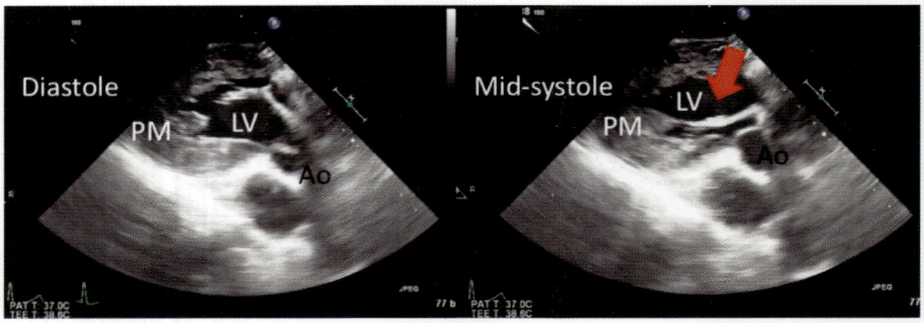

(a) (b)

Figure 3: Long axis of the LV from a deep transgastric view using transesophageal echocardiography. LV = left ventricle, PM = posterior papillary muscle, and Ao = aorta. During midsystole, there is anterior motion of the apically displaced posterior papillary muscle (red arrow).

predictors of maximal LVOT gradient included bifid papillary muscle mobility and abnormal chordal attachment to the base of the anterior mitral leaflet. In terms of management, it is important to differentiate patients with OCM as opposed to HOCM. As opposed to the surgical treatment of HOCM, which involves myectomy to relieve obstruction, performing myectomy in patients with OCM may not effectively relieve the obstruction. Patel et al. [3] showed that >50% of the patients with OCM required a non-myectomy approach to optimally relieve LV outflow tract obstruction, such as with papillary muscle reorientation. Newer techniques such as this have an added benefit of decreasing the need for mitral valve replacement for these patients.

In this case, given the venous pooling found on hemodynamic testing, a decrease in venous return to the heart with upright posture can provoke or worsen an LVOT gradient, resulting in reduced cardiac output, and subsequently causing symptoms. The hemodynamic testing indeed showed a decrease in the cardiac index when the patient was tilted to 45 degrees, even with an increase in the heart rate, due to a decrease in stroke volume. This may help explain the significant benefit that this patient derived from wearing lower extremity compression stockings with the limiting of venous pooling. Overall, this case illustrates the importance of maintaining a high degree of suspicion when assessing for cardiac etiologies, including considering the use of provocative maneuvers or multimodality cardiac imaging, in patients with otherwise presumed typical POTS and vasovagal syncope. To our knowledge, this is the first reported case of obstructive cardiomyopathy without severe septal hypertrophy with abnormalities in papillary muscle and chordal attachment, in a patient diagnosed with POTS and vasovagal syncope.

Abbreviations

POTS: Postural tachycardia syndrome
OCM: Obstructive cardiomyopathy without severe septal hypertrophy
HOCM: Hypertrophic obstructive cardiomyopathy
SAM: Systolic anterior motion
LVOT: Left ventricular outflow tract.

References

[1] R. S. Sheldon, B. P. Grubb II, B. Olshansky et al., "2015 heart rhythm society expert consensus statement on the diagnosis and treatment of postural tachycardia syndrome, inappropriate sinus tachycardia, and vasovagal syncope," *Heart Rhythm*, vol. 12, no. 6, pp. e41–e63, 2015.

[2] K. A. Mayuga, K. B. Butters, and F. Fouad-Tarazi, "Early versus late postural tachycardia: a re-evaluation of a syndrome," *Clinical Autonomic Research*, vol. 18, no. 3, pp. 155–157, 2008.

[3] P. Patel, A. Dhillon, Z. B. Popovic et al., "Left ventricular outflow tract obstruction in hypertrophic cardiomyopathy patients without severe septal hypertrophy: implications of mitral valve and papillary muscle abnormalities assessed using cardiac magnetic resonance and echocardiography," *Circulation: Cardiovascular Imaging*, vol. 8, p. e003132, 2015.

Inverted Yoga and Near Syncope: An Unusual Diagnosis of Right Ventricular Myxoma

Wadie David, Narmeen Rehman, Robby Singh, and Shukri David

Providence Hospital, Southfield, MI, USA

Correspondence should be addressed to Robby Singh; robby9697@gmail.com

Academic Editor: Assad Movahed

Primary cardiac tumors are extremely rare and are difficult to diagnose. Although usually benign in nature, myxomas require surgical resection due to their increased risk of embolic and cardiac complications, with the timing of resection dependent on the presentation and size of the tumor. However, if diagnosed early, patients with primary benign cardiac tumors have excellent prognosis following surgery. Therefore, a high index of suspicion and a wide differential diagnosis are very important in detecting rare conditions that can affect otherwise healthy individuals. We present an uncommon case of a right ventricular myxoma that was discovered when the patient was performing inverted yoga and experienced a near syncopal episode. Patient subsequently underwent an echocardiographic evaluation and was found to have a right ventricular myxoma that was excised. Although recurrence is rare, it is important for physicians to remain vigilant and continue careful and consistent follow-up for patients with a history of a cardiac myxoma.

1. Introduction

Primary cardiac tumors are very rare with an incidence rate of between 0.0017 and. 19% reported on autopsies of unselected patients and most are benign [1]. The vast majority, roughly 70–80%, are found in the left atrium and 10–20% in the right atrium [2]. Right ventricular myxomas are rarer still, with an incidence of only 2–4% [3]. Patients are typically asymptomatic and the malignancies are discovered either incidentally or when embolization or myocardial infiltration has occurred, which may lead to a rapid demise. We herein describe an extremely rare case of a right ventricular myxoma with an unusual clinical presentation.

2. Case Presentation

A 51-year-old previously healthy and physically active woman presented as an outpatient with complaints of lightheadedness and dizziness. In addition to her activities of daily living, the patient plays competitive tennis without any limitations or symptoms. Recently, while doing aerial yoga, she felt lightheaded and experienced a presyncopal episode, specifically while hanging upside down and performing hand stands. On physical exam, vital signs were normal and the exam was unremarkable except for the cardiac exam. The precordium was quiet with no displacement of the point of maximal impulse. There was a grade III/VI systolic murmur at the left sternal border and the electrocardiogram revealed a left bundle branch block. Subsequently, a transthoracic echocardiogram was performed and revealed a mass in the right ventricle attached to the posterior wall and prolapsing into the right ventricular outflow tract (RVOT) in systole (Figure 1).

Next, a transesophageal echocardiogram was performed to better characterize the mass, which measured 2.6 cm × 4.1 cm and was mobile and prolapsed into the RVOT during systole resulting in a mild dynamic obstruction (Figure 2(a)). Color Doppler revealed turbulent flow in the RVOT and pressure gradient measurements revealed a gradient of 26 mmHg across the RVOT while the patient was heavily sedated and in a supine position (Figure 2(b)).

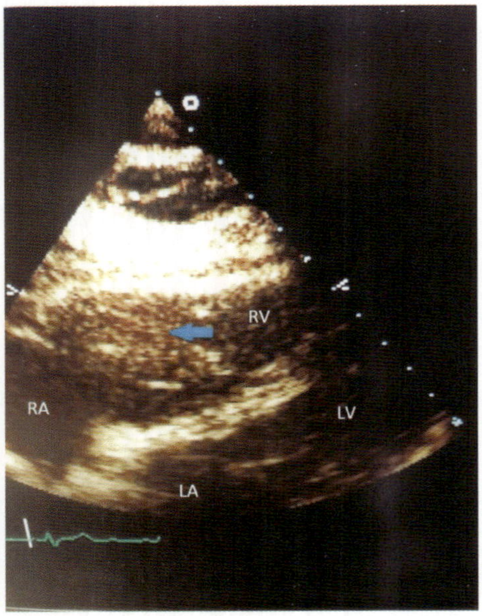

(a)

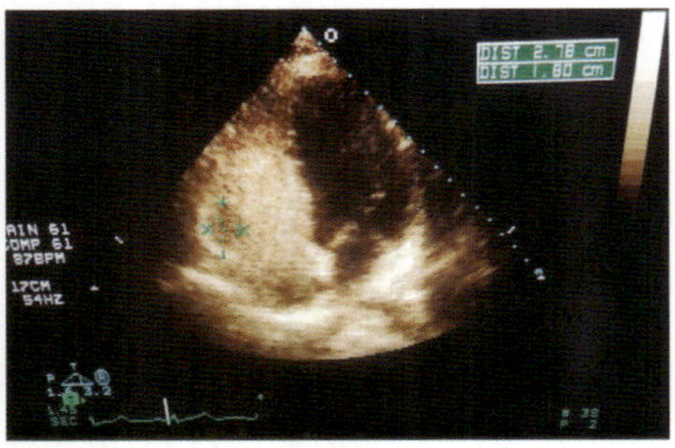

(b)

Figure 1: (a) Transthoracic echocardiogram with right ventricular myxoma (arrow). (b) Transthoracic echocardiogram with agitated saline revealing a right ventricular myxoma measuring 2.78 cm × 1.8 cm.

We suspect that with aerial yoga, and the resulting upside-down suspension, the gradient would be higher. Therefore, the obstruction would be enhanced, resulting in decreased cardiac output and cerebral hypoperfusion, which could explain the presenting symptoms of lightheadedness and dizziness. The patient was referred to cardiothoracic surgery for further evaluation and underwent a cardiac catheterization prior to thoracotomy which also showed evidence of a RV mass (Figure 3). A thoracotomy with excision of the mass was performed (Figure 4), and pathological examination revealed the mass as a myxoma (Figure 5). The patient had an uneventful recovery and was discharged home. She has been continued to follow up regularly two years postresection of the myxoma and continues to do well. She continues to experience no limitations in performing her activities of daily living nor while playing competitive tennis or performing aerial yoga. Repeat echocardiogram two years postresection did not reveal any evidence of recurrence of the myxoma (Figures 6(a) and 6(b)).

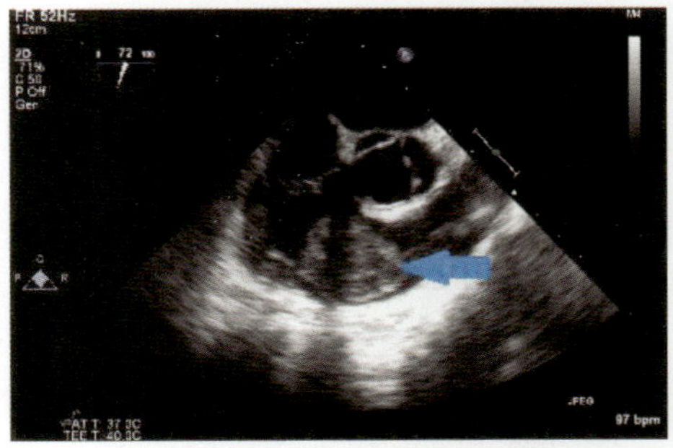

(a)

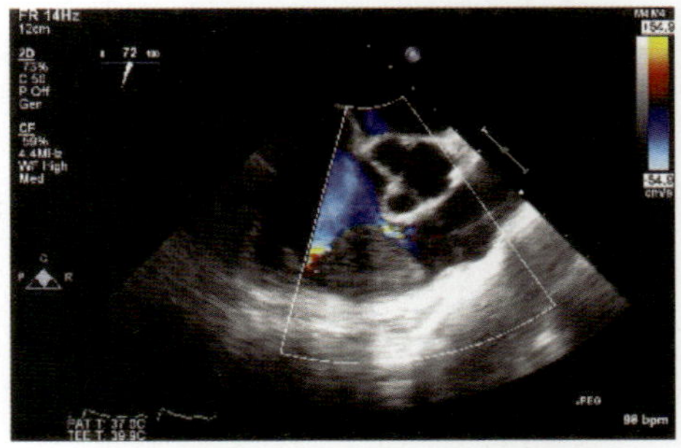

(b)

Figure 2: (a) RV myxoma on TEE (arrow). (b) Color flow around RV myoxoma on TEE.

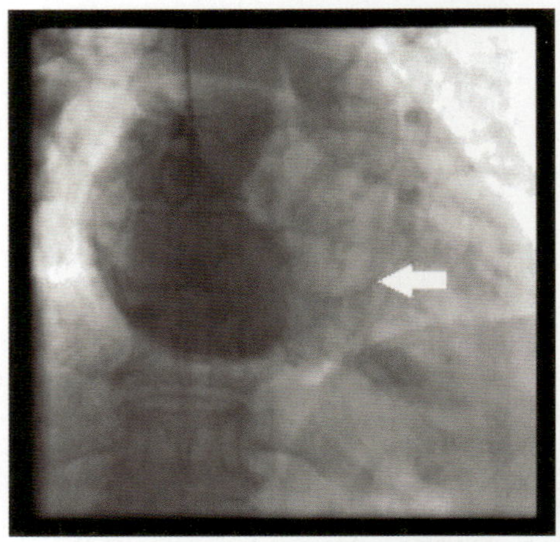

Figure 3: RV mass appreciated on cardiac catheterization.

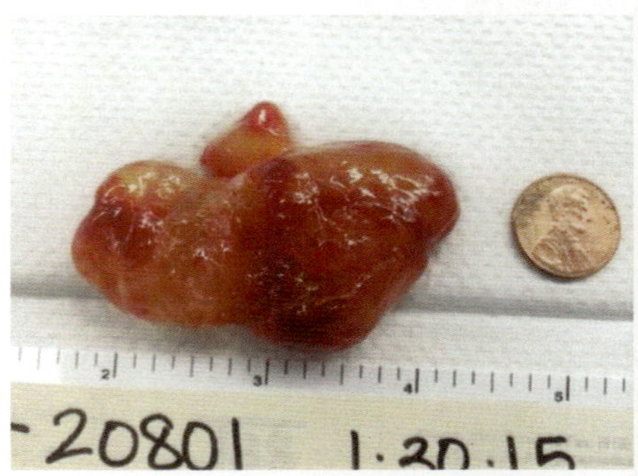

Figure 4: RV myxoma excised.

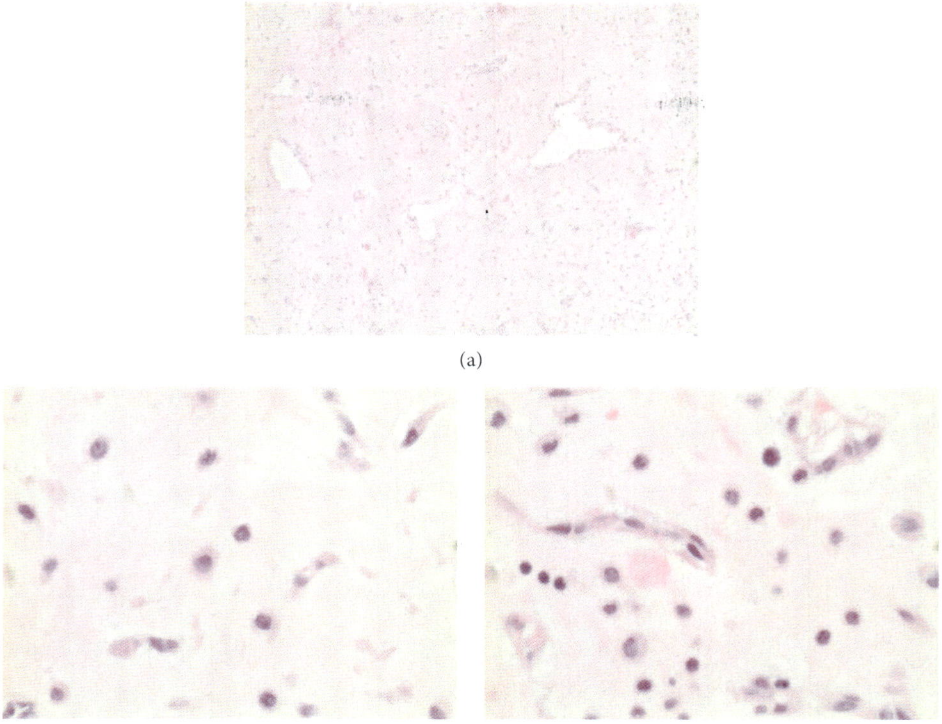

(a)

(b) (c)

FIGURE 5: The tumor is comprised of spindled or stellate cells with eosinophilic cytoplasm and uniform, round nuclei with inconspicuous nucleoli in a background of myxoid stroma. Chronic inflammatory cells including hemosiderin-laden macrophages are also present. The cellularity is variable; however, no foci of increased cellularity marked nuclear pleomorphism or increased mitotic activity seen.

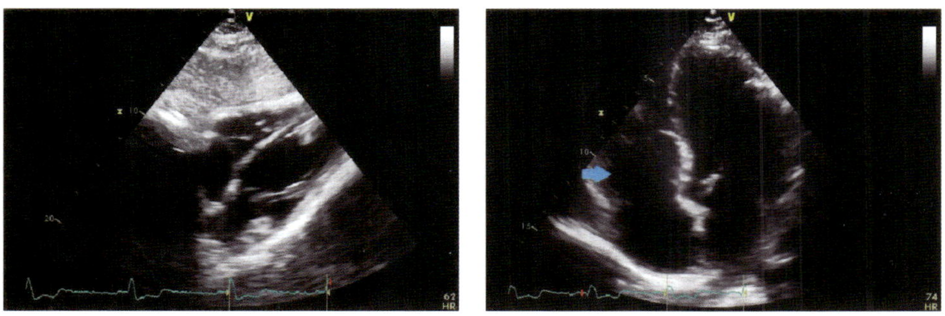

(a) (b)

FIGURE 6: (a) Subcostal view on transthoracic echocardiogram two years postprocedure without evidence of recurrence of RV myxoma. (b) Apical view from the same study (arrow: right ventricle).

3. Discussion

The majority of myxomas are found in the left atrium and symptoms are typically seen when tumor growth interferes with normal cardiac function [4]. Up to 12–15% of cardiac myxomas are asymptomatic and discovered incidentally or during postmortem examination. The majority present with a combination of symptoms such as obstruction of blood flow to the neighboring chamber, thromboembolic events, hemodynamic changes, conduction disease, and otherwise nonspecific symptoms. Obstruction of blood flow can lead to impaired atrial filling, heart failure, chronic passive congestion of the lungs, and dyspnea. Obstruction can also lead to hemodynamic changes caused by systemic emboli, particularly in right-sided lesions which can propagate to the pulmonary arteries and result in obstruction or left-sided lesions causing cerebral emboli. Additionally, depending on the location of the tumor, growth can disrupt nodal or septal conduction tissue leading to heart arrhythmia and sudden cardiac death [4].

Mitral valve stenosis and regurgitation may be seen in patients with mobile left atrial tumors. On physical exam, one can also listen for a "tumor plop," an acoustic diastolic sound that is caused by the presence of a mobile myxoma inside the atrial chamber. This is typically seen in 15% of patients and occurs when the tumor comes to rest over the mitral annulus. These tumors interfere with valve coaptation and can often be recognized by the astute clinician which may lead to further workup.

One unique characteristic of myxomas is its ability to mimic systemic autoimmune diseases. Myxomas have the capacity to secrete interleukin 6 and 8 (IL-6 and IL-8), especially IL-6, which is a pleiotropic cytokine that increases B cell differentiation and leads to increased synthesis of polyclonal immunoglobulins [4]. In addition, it is a strong hepatocyte-stimulating factor, which induces the release of acute-phase proteins [4]. IL-6 is also implicated in increased tumor growth and tumor recurrence. Theses cytokines also lead to nonspecific symptoms which are seen in about 80–85% of cases such as fatigue, lethargy, weakness, erythema, weight loss, and decreased appetite [4].

In addition, depending on the size of the tumor, many patients can present with chromic hemolytic anemia and thrombocytopenia [4]. These conditions are caused by abnormal blood flow leading to damaged RBCs as they pass over the tumor surface [4]. Diagnosis of these tumors is typically made by echocardiography which is highly sensitive and can differentiate cardiac tumors from other cardiac masses such as vegetation and thrombi [4].

While many patients present with multiple symptoms, these tumors may also be asymptomatic, making them especially difficult to diagnose. If gone undiagnosed and untreated, these can result in severe cardiac complications due to obstruction of blood flow and potential disruption of nodal conduction tissue. In our case, a right ventricular myxoma, among the rarest forms of cardiac malignancy, manifested with RVOT obstruction leading to syncope, though the outcome could have been more disastrous had the obstruction been more prolonged. For this reason, it is essential that the diagnosis is made early, and although most cases require surgical resection, recovery is often rapid. While recurrence is rare, it is important to have careful and consistent follow-up with patients who have a history of a cardiac myxoma.

References

[1] K. Reynen, "Cardiac myxomas," *The New England Journal of Medicine*, vol. 333, no. 24, pp. 1610–1617, 1995.

[2] T. Ermek, N. Aybek, W.-m. Zhang et al., "A rare case of biventricular myxoma," *Journal of Cardiothoracic Surgery*, vol. 12, no. 1, p. 17, 2017.

[3] A. B. Crummy jun and F. A. Hipona, "The radiographic aspects of right ventricular myxoma," *British Journal of Radiology*, vol. 37, no. 438, pp. 468–471, 1964.

[4] P. Singhal, A. Luk, V. Rao, and J. Butany, "Molecular basis of cardiac myxomas," *International Journal of Molecular Sciences*, vol. 15, no. 1, pp. 1315–1337, 2014.

Anomalous Left Main Coronary Artery Arising from the Right Sinus of Valsalva in a Young Man Presenting with Recurrent Syncope and Myocardial Infarction

Koroush Khalighi,[1,2] Munish Sharma ,[3] Amit Toor,[3] Rubinder S. Toor,[2,4] and Gary Costacurta[2]

[1]*EP Lab, Easton Hospital, Drexel University, Easton, PA, USA*
[2]*Department of Cardiology, Easton Cardiovascular Associates, Easton, PA, USA*
[3]*Department of Internal Medicine, Easton Hospital, Easton, PA, USA*
[4]*Department of Public Health, Milken Institute School of Public Health, George Washington University, Washington, DC, USA*

Correspondence should be addressed to Munish Sharma; munishintmed@gmail.com

Academic Editor: Expedito E. Ribeiro

A 19-year-old man with the left main coronary artery (LMCA) arising from the right sinus of Valsalva presented with recurrent episodes of syncope and myocardial infarction (MI). Anomalous aortic origin of a coronary artery (AAOCA) is an uncommon but extremely important differential diagnosis that should not be missed in patients presenting with syncope, MI, ventricular arrhythmias, or cardiac arrest. A definitive diagnosis with coronary angiography and prompt surgical intervention is imperative in such symptomatic patients.

1. Introduction

Left main coronary artery (LMCA) or left anterior descending coronary artery (LAD) arising from the right sinus of Valsalva or right coronary artery (RCA) is referred to as an anomalous aortic origin of a coronary artery (AAOCA). The subsequent course is mostly between the aorta and the pulmonary artery on its way to the left ventricle, which could compress the vessel and may give rise to fatal outcomes like myocardial ischemia, ventricular arrhythmias, and sudden cardiac death [1, 2]. This is an uncommon case of LMCA arising from the right sinus of Valsalva in a 19-year-old man with recurrent episodes of syncope due to myocardial ischemia and infarction.

2. Case Description

A 19-year-old African American man was brought to the emergency department (ED) by emergency medical services (EMS) after an episode of syncope earlier on the day of admission while playing basketball at his college. This occurred suddenly and was associated with a transient episode of lightheadedness, diaphoresis, and blurred vision. This was followed by lost consciousness for less than 10 seconds, with spontaneous recovery as witnessed by his friends on the sidelines. There was not any involuntary movement of the body, urinary or bowel incontinence, or postictal confusion as per the witnesses. After regaining consciousness, there was a complaint of nonradiating, substernal, burning chest pain with a "6 out of 10" intensity, which lasted approximately 20–30 minutes and was relieved with a nitroglycerin sublingual pill given by EMS. On arrival to the ED, the patient was asymptomatic. Blood pressure was 103/67 mmHg, heart rate 85 bpm and regular, afebrile oxygen saturation > 95% on room air, and respiratory rate 12 per minute. Physical examination findings revealed a supple neck with no jugular venous distention; no carotid bruits were audible. Cardiovascular examination

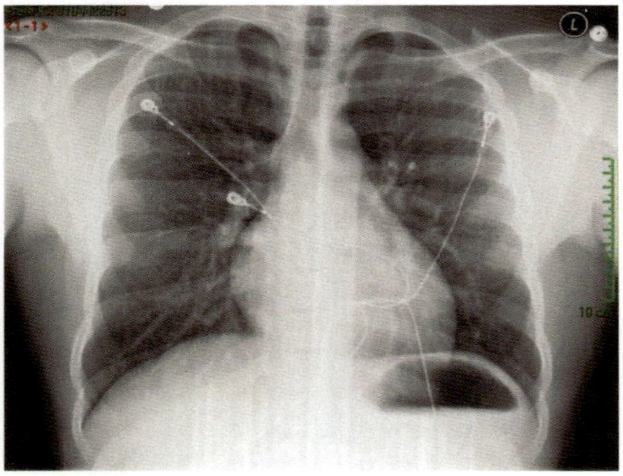

FIGURE 1: Chest X-ray did not reveal any significant radiographic abnormalities.

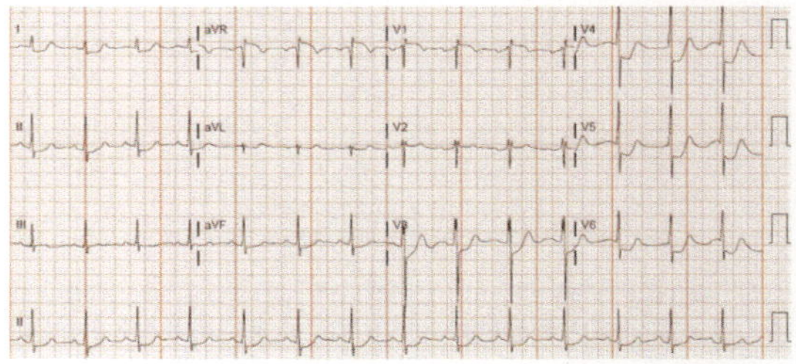

FIGURE 2: Admission EKG showed a rhythm of sinus origin at a rate of 80 BPM, with normal axis and 2-3 mm horizontal dawn sloping with ST segment depression in anterolateral leads.

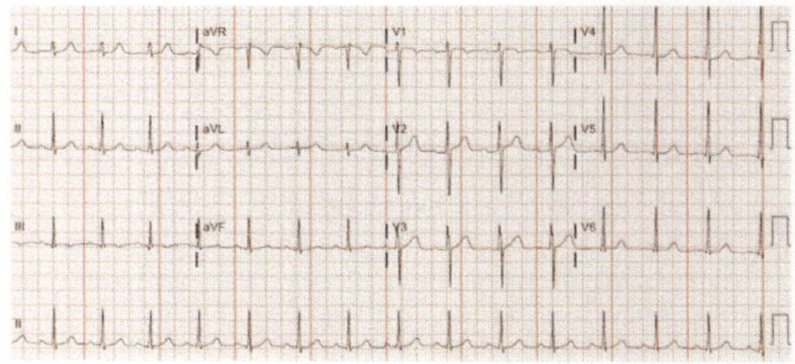

FIGURE 3: EKG 2 hours after admission showed a rhythm of sinus origin at a rate of 95 BPM, with normal axis and with reversal of ST-T wave changes present on admission.

revealed a regular heart rhythm with normal S1 and S2 and no significant audible murmurs, parasternal heave, or thrill. The lungs were clear to auscultation bilaterally. There was no pitting pedal edema, and all peripheral pulses were palpable. The abdomen was soft and nondistended; no focal neurological deficits were evident.

History was positive for two similar events in the past. The first episode occurred approximately 10 years ago in Nigeria while playing soccer, and another event occurred a year ago year while running a block to catch a bus. Medical attention was not sought on both occasions. Family history was negative for similar syncopal attacks, sudden cardiac arrest, or arrhythmias. Social history was positive for drinking heavy amounts of Vodka with friends occasionally on the weekends along with marijuana but negative for cigarette smoking or other illicit drug use.

Initial laboratory values in the ED showed hemoglobin of 12.3 gm %, serum creatinine of 1.4 mg/dl (normal reference range 0.50 to 1.20 mg/dl) and BUN of 24 mg/dl, elevated initial troponin I of 0.23 ng/ml (normal reference range 0.00 to 0.07 ng/ml), total creatinine kinase level of 585 units/liter (normal reference range: 49 to 397 U/l), and urine with 11–20 hyaline casts. Thyroid stimulating hormone, serum potassium, and serum magnesium were within normal limits. His chest X-ray did not reveal any acute cardiopulmonary process (Figure 1). His initial electrocardiogram (EKG) revealed significant 4 mm to 5 mm ST depression in the anterolateral leads but otherwise unremarkable (Figure 2). A repeat EKG done within 2 hours of the initial presentation showed reversal of ST depression (Figure 3). A repeat troponin done in 6 hours revealed staggering troponin I of 53.30 ng/ml. Immediate bedside echocardiogram showed a nondilated left ventricular cavity with normal LV wall thickness and a mildly diminished LV ejection fraction at 45–50% (Figure 4). In the emergency room, immediate treatment with 325 mg of Aspirin and therapeutic Lovenox (1 mg/kg) was given. Overnight, periodic 5–7-beat runs of nonsustained ventricular tachycardia on the cardiac monitor occurred. Cardiac tomography (CT) angiography of the heart revealed a common trunk for the right and left coronary arteries arising from the right coronary cusp. The right coronary artery had a normal course. The LMCA traveled posteriorly between the ascending aorta and pulmonary outflow tract before resuming its normal course.

The LMCA narrowed in its midportion as it passed between these two structures (Figures 5(a) and 5(b)). These findings were confirmed by cardiac catheterization which showed an anomalous origin of the LMCA, originating from the right sinus of Valsalva (Figures 6(a) and 6(b)). The LMCA narrowed in its midportion with over 60–70% luminal stenosis due to a stricture present between the ascending aorta and the left ventricular outflow track. Afterwards, medical stabilization was achieved and a transfer to a tertiary care center was carried out.

Upon arrival at the tertiary care center, a procedure was performed involving the unroofing of the anomalous aortic origin of the left main coronary artery, including retro pulmonary unroofing by a congenital cardiothoracic surgeon. Recovery was satisfactory after the surgery, and postoperative complications did not occur.

3. Discussion

The overall incidence of the abnormal aortic origin of the coronary arteries is estimated to be approximately 0.64% of births [3]. The most common anomaly is the origin of the left circumflex artery from the right sinus of Valsalva, followed by the origin of a single coronary artery from the left sinus of Valsalva, origin of both the right and the left coronary arteries from the right sinus of Valsalva, and the LAD originating from the right sinus of Valsalva. The prevalence of the RCA arising from the left sinus of Valsalva is approximately 0.17% while the rarest anomaly is the left coronary

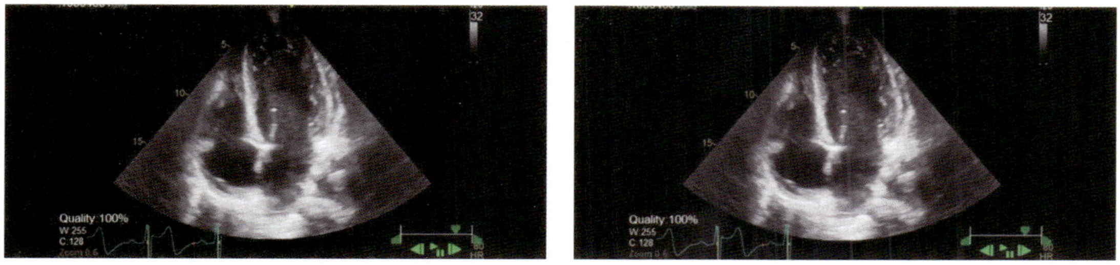

(a) (b)

FIGURE 4: Two-dimensional transthoracic echocardiogram showing normal sized cardiac chambers. Diastole phase (b) and systole phase (a).

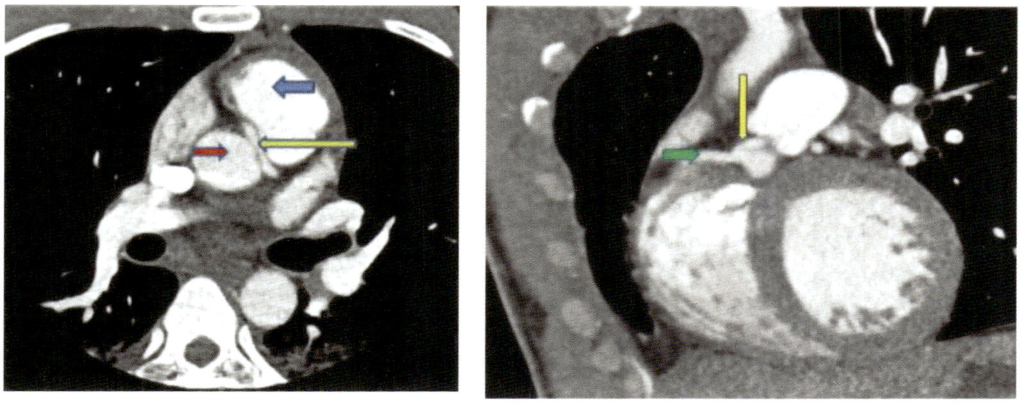

(a) (b)

FIGURE 5: (a) Anomalous LMCA course (yellow arrow) between the aorta (red arrow) and the pulmonary outflow track (blue arrow) showing narrowing. (b) Oblique view demonstrating the common origin of the right (green arrow) and the left coronary arteries (yellow arrow).

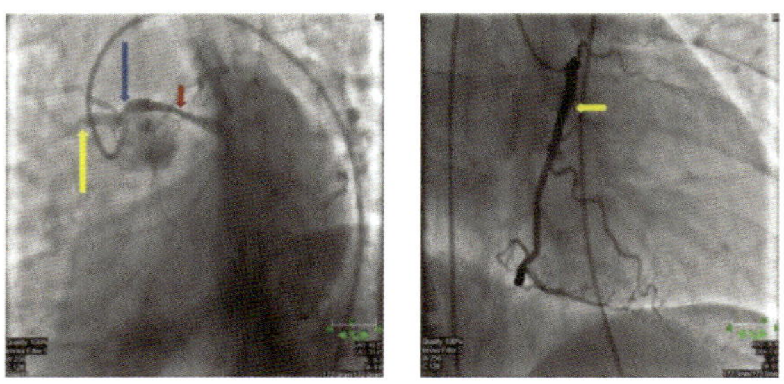

(a) (b)

FIGURE 6: (a) demonstrates the anomalous origin of the left main coronary artery (blue arrow) along with stenosis of the left main coronary (red arrow). (b) demonstrates the course of the RCA (yellow arrows).

artery arising from the right sinus of Valsalva and its prevalence is around 0.047% [4]. There are four major variations in the course taken by the LMCA after its origin from the right sinus of Valsalva, in relation to the aorta and the pulmonary trunk, on its way to the left ventricle. The LMCA can have a septal course beginning at the right ventricular infundibulum; it can have an anterior course, a retroaortic course, or an interarterial course between the aorta and the main pulmonary artery [5, 6].

The clinical presentation in AAOCA is commonly anginal chest pain or syncope that occurs mostly with exercise or other strenuous activities. In young athletes and military recruits, the first clinical presentation may unfortunately be sudden cardiac death [7]. In a registry of sudden cardiac death in 286 athletes, the anomalous coronary artery arising from the opposite sinus of Valsalva was the second most common cause of death (13%) besides hypertrophic cardiomyopathy [8]. Though the incidence of sudden cardiac death in patients with AAOCA is low overall, it is still comparatively higher for patients with AAOCA of the left coronary artery than with AAOCA of the RCA, especially in the absence of symptoms [9].

The pathophysiology behind syncope, myocardial ischemia, and sudden cardiac death has been postulated to be the compression of the anomalous coronary artery between the aorta and the pulmonary artery on its way to the left ventricle [1, 2, 10]. The intramural course and acute angle of take-off may predispose the affected artery to the obstruction of blood flow [11]. It has been proposed that there is an expansion of the aortic root and pulmonary trunk during exercise or strenuous physical activities which worsens the preexisting angulation of the coronary artery and thus reduces the diameter of the lumen in the proximal portion of the coronary artery [1]. The 19-year-old man might have had recurrent episodes of syncope and myocardial infarction on admission due to the compression of the interarterial portion of the LMCA between the aorta and the main pulmonary artery during strenuous physical activities.

Diagnosis is mainly based on the high index of clinical suspicion for the anomalous origin of the coronary artery. Coronary magnetic resonance angiography (CMRA) and coronary computed tomographic angiography (CCTA) are important noninvasive diagnostic tools that are being increasingly used to detect such cases. Several smaller studies have proven the efficacy of CMRA and CCTA [12, 13]. Coronary angiography is the gold standard for the diagnosis and evaluation of the origin and the course of anomalous coronary arteries and is particularly important when the noninvasive test fails to yield definitive results [14]. In patients with symptoms arising from ventricular tachyarrhythmia or myocardial infarction, surgical intervention is indicated, particularly in cases of the origin of the left coronary artery from the right sinus of Valsalva. The surgical intervention can consist of coronary artery bypass grafting (CABG) or unroofing (marsupialization) of the coronary artery that prevents further compression of the artery in its interarterial course [15]. For patients without any intramural course, the "hinge twist" procedure has been described [16]. Pulmonary artery translocation and intracoronary stents to prevent vessel compression are a few other alternative surgical procedures that have been described so far [17]. Benefits of surgical treatment in asymptomatic individuals with AAOCA have not been well established.

4. Conclusion

The left coronary artery arising from the right sinus of Valsalva is not a frequently encountered congenital coronary artery anomaly. In younger patients presenting with symptoms of syncope, myocardial ischemia, or ventricular arrhythmias, a high index of clinical suspicion is required. This man received a diagnosis at the age of 19 years despite having prior symptoms. A future fatal outcome may have occurred if anomalous coronary artery disease was not detected and treated promptly. Definitive diagnosis with coronary angiography and prompt surgical intervention is imperative in such symptomatic patients. Data regarding outcomes of surgical intervention in asymptomatic patients are still lacking. Noninvasive tests such as echocardiography and computed tomography angiography can aid in diagnosis and are becoming increasingly popular.

References

[1] J. M. Peñalver, R. S. Mosca, D. Weitz, and C. K. L. Phoon, "Anomalous aortic origin of coronary arteries from the opposite sinus: a critical appraisal of risk," *BMC Cardiovascular Disorders*, vol. 12, no. 1, pp. 83–83, 2012.

[2] S. M. Dogan, M. Gursurer, M. Aydin, H. Gocer, M. Cabuk, and A. Dursun, "Myocardial ischemia caused by a coronary anomaly left anterior descending coronary artery arising from right sinus of Valsalva," *International Journal of Cardiology*, vol. 112, no. 3, pp. e57–e59, 2006.

[3] D. Kimbiris, A. S. Iskandrian, B. L. Segal, and C. E. Bemis, "Anomalous aortic origin of coronary arteries," *Circulation*, vol. 58, no. 4, pp. 606–615, 1978.

[4] O. Yamanaka and R. E. Hobbs, "Coronary artery anomalies in 126,595 patients undergoing coronary arteriography," *Catheterization and Cardiovascular Diagnosis*, vol. 21, no. 1, pp. 28–40, 1990.

[5] P. K. Verma and D. Singh Bisht, "Anomalous origin of left main coronary artery from right sinus of Valsalva: a case report," *Angiology: Open Access*, vol. 3, no. 4, 2015.

[6] A. T. Marler, J. A. Malik, and A. M. Slim, "Anomalous left main coronary artery: case series of different courses and literature review," *Case Reports in Vascular Medicine*, vol. 2013, Article ID 380952, 5 pages, 2013.

[7] C. Basso, B. J. Maron, D. Corrado, and G. Thiene, "Clinical profile of congenital coronary artery anomalies with origin from the wrong aortic sinus leading to sudden death in young competitive athletes," *Journal of the American College of Cardiology*, vol. 35, no. 6, pp. 1493–1501, 2000.

[8] B. J. Maron, K. P. Carney, H. M. Lever et al., "Relationship of race to sudden cardiac death in competitive athletes with hypertrophic cardiomyopathy," *Journal of the American College of Cardiology*, vol. 41, no. 6, pp. 974–980, 2003.

[9] W. M. Gersony, "Management of anomalous coronary artery from the contralateral coronary sinus," *Journal of the American College of Cardiology*, vol. 50, no. 21, pp. 2083-2084, 2007.

[10] L. S. Cohen and L. D. Shaw, "Fatal myocardial infarction in an 11 year old boy associated with a unique coronary artery anomaly," *The American Journal of Cardiology*, vol. 19, no. 3, pp. 420–423, 1967.

[11] E. C. Lorenz, F. Mookadam, M. Mookadam, S. Moustafa, and K. J. Zehr, "A systematic overview of anomalous coronary anatomy and an examination of the association with sudden cardiac death," *Reviews in Cardiovascular Medicine*, vol. 7, no. 4, pp. 205–213, 2006.

[12] M. V. McConnell, P. Ganz, A. P. Selwyn, W. Li, R. R. Edelman, and W. J. Manning, "Identification of anomalous coronary arteries and their anatomic course by magnetic resonance coronary angiography," *Circulation*, vol. 92, no. 11, pp. 3158–3162, 1995.

[13] J. Datta, C. S. White, R. C. Gilkeson et al., "Anomalous coronary arteries in adults: depiction at multi-detector row CT angiography," *Radiology*, vol. 235, no. 3, pp. 812–818, 2005.

[14] T. P. Graham Jr., D. J. Driscoll, W. M. Gersony, J. W. Newburger, A. Rocchini, and J. A. Towbin, "Task force 2: congenital heart disease," *Journal of The American College of Cardiology*, vol. 45, no. 8, pp. 1326–1333, 2005.

[15] R. L. Romp, J. R. Herlong, C. K. Landolfo et al., "Outcome of unroofing procedure for repair of anomalous aortic origin of left or right coronary artery," *The Annals of Thoracic Surgery*, vol. 76, no. 2, pp. 589–596, 2003.

[16] L. Lopez, L. Mercer-Rosa, E. M. Zahn, N. R. Altman, R. Dubois, and R. P. Burke, "The "hinge-twist" technique for anomalous origin of the left coronary artery," *The Annals of Thoracic Surgery*, vol. 82, no. 2, pp. e19–e21, 2006.

[17] R. Gulati, V. M. Reddy, C. Culbertson et al., "Surgical management of coronary artery arising from the wrong coronary sinus, using standard and novel approaches," *The Journal of Thoracic and Cardiovascular Surgery*, vol. 134, no. 5, pp. 1171–1178.e5, 2007.

Acute Pericarditis Occurring Three Days after Intravesical Instillation of Mitomycin C after Transurethral Bladder Tumor Resection in a 64-Year-Old Woman

Vineet Meghrajani,[1] Arsalan Hashmi,[1] Shuo Cheng Lin,[1] Zvi Plawes,[2] and Shelly Brejt[2]

[1]*Department of Internal Medicine, Maimonides Medical Center, 4802 10th Avenue, Brooklyn, NY 11219, USA*
[2]*Department of Cardiology, Maimonides Medical Center, 4802 10th Avenue, Brooklyn, NY 11219, USA*

Correspondence should be addressed to Vineet Meghrajani; vineetmeghrajani@gmail.com

Academic Editor: Tayfun Sahin

We present a 64-year-old woman who developed symptoms of acute pericarditis three days after undergoing intravesical instillation of mitomycin C following transurethral bladder tumor resection. Mitomycin C is a chemotherapeutic agent which acts by alkylation of DNA and is known to be cardiotoxic when systemically administered. Despite classic pericarditis symptoms, the patient underwent an urgent coronary angiogram due to elevated cardiac troponin I level, EKG changes, and wall motion abnormalities on her echocardiogram. During her angiogram, it was found that she had multiple stenotic coronary artery lesions, with no acute total coronary occlusions, and percutaneous coronary intervention (PCI) was done with placement of a single drug-eluting stent for a 95% stenotic lesion in the left anterior descending artery. The patient was discharged after an uneventful hospitalization on dual antiplatelet therapy with aspirin and prasugrel, and colchicine for pericarditis. It is likely that the patient's presentation was the result of a perimyocardial inflammatory process secondary to intravesically administered mitomycin C, rather than an acute coronary syndrome. While the pathophysiological basis of cardiotoxicity of systemically administered mitomycin C is well documented, more studies are needed to determine whether intravesical MMC may cause cardiotoxicity.

1. Introduction

Acute pericarditis refers to inflammation of the pericardial sac—a tough double-layered fibroserous sac which covers the heart. Pericarditis has multiple causes, including infections, autoimmune diseases, metabolic disorders, neoplasms, trauma, radiation, and drugs [1–3], and its clinical manifestations typically include sharp and pleuritic chest pain that is improved by sitting up and leaning forward, a pericardial friction rub, EKG changes of new widespread ST elevations and PR depressions, and pericardial effusion [4]. Pericarditis is frequently self-limiting, and nonsteroidal anti-inflammatory agents remain the first-line treatment for uncomplicated cases [5]. We have here presented the case of a 64-year-old woman who developed acute pericarditis three days after intravesical instillation of mitomycin C chemotherapy after transurethral resection of bladder tumor (TURBT).

2. Case Presentation

A 64-year-old postmenopausal woman presented to the emergency department at 10 am in the morning with chest pain and shortness of breath of approximately 12 hours duration. Her medical history included right breast invasive ductal carcinoma with bilateral mastectomies in 2015, recently diagnosed bladder cancer with TURBT and intravesical mitomycin C instillation three days prior to current presentation, type 2 diabetes mellitus, hypertension, obstructive sleep apnea, chronic obstructive pulmonary disease, and prothrombin G20210A mutation. She had quit smoking 5 years ago, prior to that she had smoked 2 packs per day for 45 years. She was asymptomatic until about 10 pm the night before presentation, when she developed shortness of breath and sharp pleuritic chest pain while she was lying in bed. The patient reported that her chest pain was

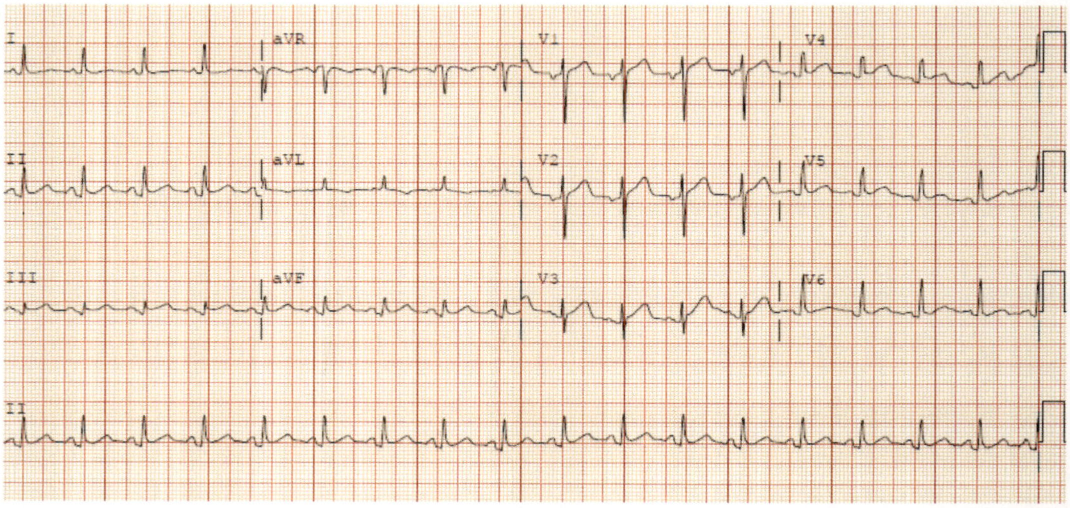

FIGURE 1: 12-lead electrocardiogram obtained on arrival of the patient to the emergency department 3 days after undergoing TURBT with intravesical mitomycin C instillation showing diffuse concave ST elevations with PR depressions in all leads, except in aVR which showed ST depression and PR elevation.

located in the substernal region, radiating to the back, aggravated by deep breaths and by lying down, and alleviated by sitting up and leaning forward. She said that she had taken some ibuprofen which had reduced the intensity of pain. She did endorse that she was also experiencing a less prominent pressure like sensation in addition to the sharp pleuritic type of pain. She denied fevers, chills, cough, diaphoresis, palpitations, dizziness, abdominal pain, heartburn, nausea or vomiting, flu-like symptoms, recent illnesses, or any history of chest pain in the past. Her family history was significant for her brother having an episode of myocardial infarction at age 55.

On detailed inquiry of the patient's history of bladder cancer, the patient reported that she was diagnosed in 2012 after undergoing cystoscopy for an episode of gross hematuria and was found to have a low-grade bladder cancer. She underwent transurethral bladder tumor resection and 1 cycle of intravesical BCG treatment in 2012 and was asymptomatic after that with regular follow-up with urology. On a surveillance cystoscopy performed by the patient's urologist in December 2016, a lesion was seen in the bladder, for which a biopsy was subsequently done which showed papillary hyperplasia and inflammation with no cancer. For this recurrence, the patient was planned for a cystoscopic transurethral bladder tumor resection and instillation of 40 mg of mitomycin C in the bladder, which she underwent three days before her current hospital presentation. The patient was intubated during this procedure which was uneventful, and was subsequently extubated without difficulty.

The patient's oral temperature on presentation was 98.0 F, heart rate of 107/min, respiratory rate of 25/min, and blood pressure of 152/63 mmHg (right arm, supine position). On examination, the patient was in no acute distress and appeared comfortable, although was complaining of having mild chest pain, alleviated by leaning forward. Her laboratory data were as follows: cardiac troponins on the day of presentation, 0.57 ng/ml at 12:30 pm; D-dimer, 257 ng/ml; and white blood cell count, 12.2 K/ml with 67.3% neutrophils. 12-lead electrocardiogram (Figure 1) showed diffuse concave ST elevations with PR depressions in all leads, except in aVR which showed ST depression and PR elevation.

The patient was treated with aspirin 325 mg orally and nebulized albuterol. An echocardiogram was performed which showed normal left ventricular ejection fraction of 61–65%, mid and apical inferior wall motion abnormality, mild to moderate left ventricular diastolic dysfunction, and trivial pericardial effusion. Although the patient's clinical presentation and electrocardiogram findings were consistent with pericarditis, an urgent coronary angiogram was planned due to the possibility of the patient having an acute coronary syndrome, considering her continuing chest pain, elevated cardiac troponin level, echocardiogram findings of mid and apical inferior wall motion abnormality, and the presence of multiple risk factors of ischemic heart disease. The coronary angiogram, performed through right radial artery access, showed a normal left main stem artery, proximal left anterior descending luminal irregularities, a 95% stenotic focal lesion of the mid left anterior descending artery, 40% stenosis of distal left circumflex artery, 30% stenosis of the ostial right coronary artery, 40% stenosis of proximal right coronary artery, 50% stenosis of mid right coronary artery, and 99% stenosis of right posterior descending artery. Left ventricular diastolic pressure was recorded to be 24 mmHg. A single 2.5×20 mm synergy monorail drug-eluting stent was placed in the stenosed segment of the mid left anterior descending artery. The patient received 60 mg of prasugrel orally during the procedure, a bolus dose of intravenous tirofiban followed by a maintenance dose intravenous tirofiban drip, and was admitted to the telemetry floor. Dual antiplatelet therapy with aspirin 81 mg daily and prasugrel 10 mg daily was initiated, and the patient was also started on colchicine 0.6 mg every 12 hours for pericarditis. The remainder of the hospitalization was uneventful, and the patient was discharged on the third hospital day, with a plan for a staged percutaneous coronary

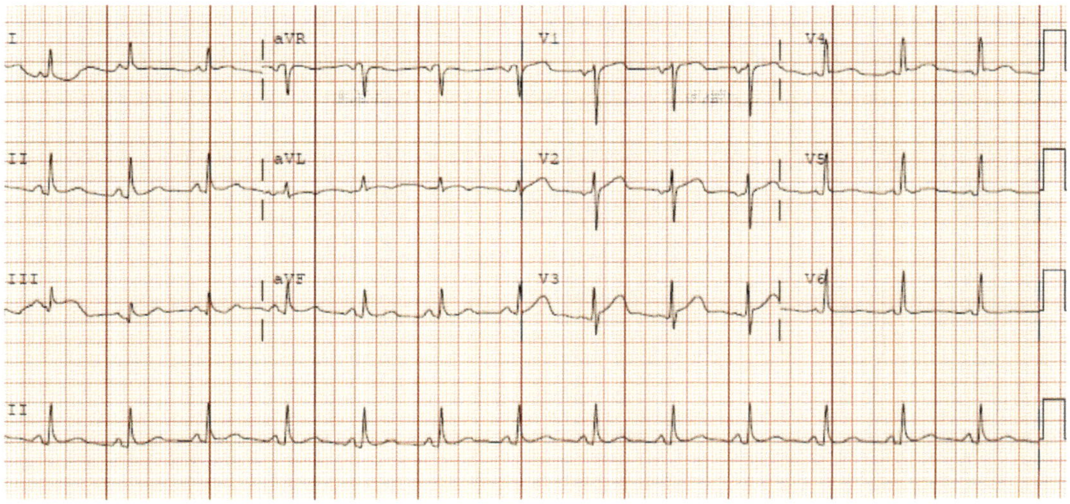

FIGURE 2: 12-lead electrocardiogram obtained 15 hours after presentation showing persistence of the ST elevations with PR depressions in all leads, except in aVR which showed ST depression and PR elevation.

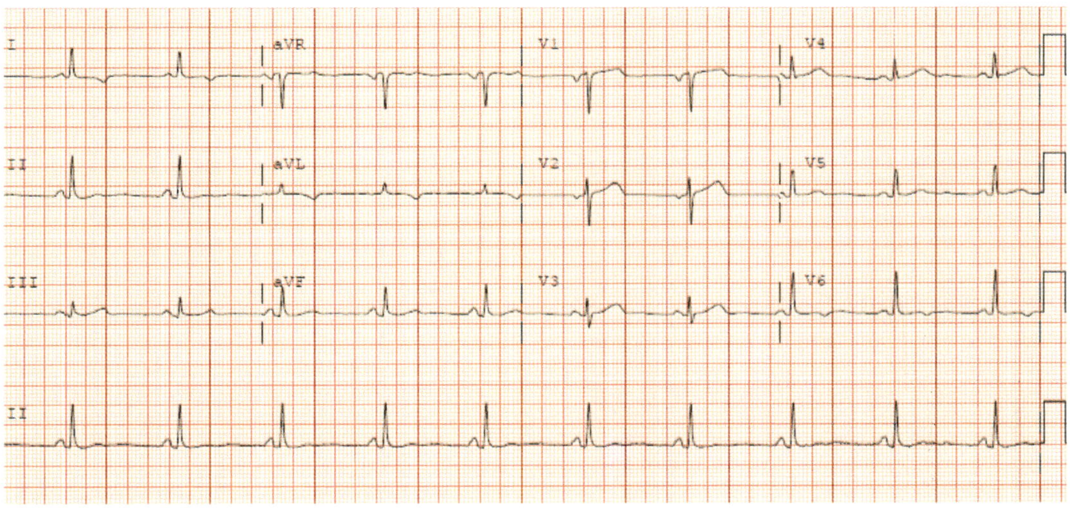

FIGURE 3: 12-lead electrocardiogram obtained 3 weeks after hospital discharge showing return of PR and ST segments to baseline.

intervention for the 99% stenotic lesion in the right posterior descending artery in a few weeks.

3. Discussion

The term "perimyocarditis" is used for cases of acute pericarditis that also demonstrate myocardial inflammation—it may be associated with increases in serum biomarkers of myocardial injury such as cardiac troponin I or T [6] and echocardiographic findings of diffuse/localized LV wall motion abnormalities [7, 8]. In clinical practice, it may be difficult to differentiate between perimyocarditis and ST elevation myocardial infarction due to EKG findings of ST elevation and cardiac biomarker elevation seen in both conditions [9, 10].

The patient's clinical presentation and EKG were strongly suggestive of pericarditis. Her chest pain was pleuritic and positional, with relief in a seated position and with ibuprofen—pointing more towards pericarditis than myocardial ischemia [1, 2]. The initial EKG obtained on presentation showed diffuse concave ST elevations with PR depressions in all leads, except in aVR which showed ST depression and PR elevation—a finding that is consistent with pericarditis [1, 2, 4]. Also, the distribution of the ST elevations on the EKG was more diffuse than what would be expected from her distal coronary lesions.

Due to her multiple risk factors—smoking, obesity, family history of early coronary artery disease, and a mildly elevated initial cardiac troponin I level of 0.57 ng/ml, an urgent echocardiogram was performed which showed wall motion abnormalities in the mid and apical inferior wall and trivial pericardial effusion. Coronary angiography performed subsequently showed a 95% focal stenotic lesion in the mid left anterior descending artery (LAD) and 99% lesion in the right posterior descending artery, with no acute total coronary occlusions. Since the patient had continued to

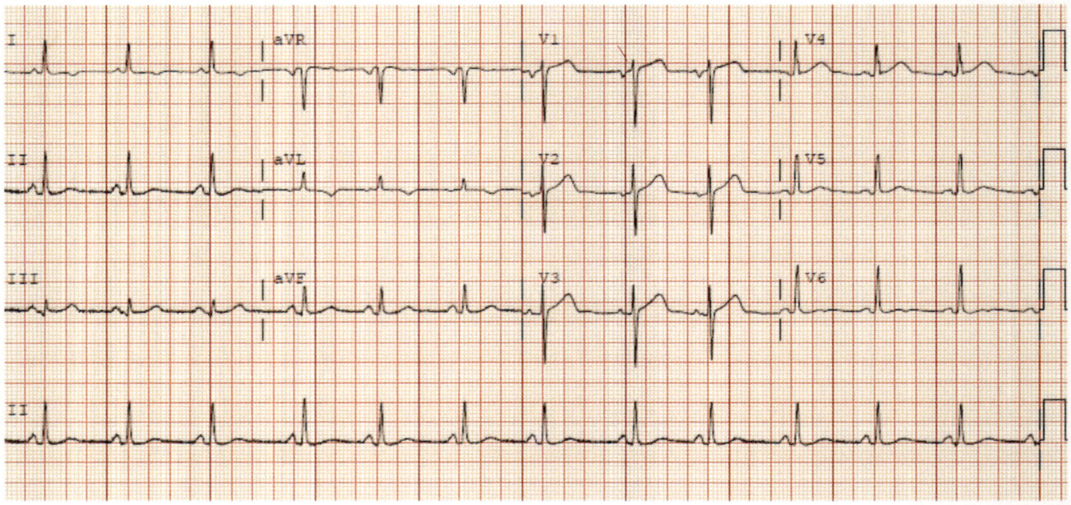

Figure 4: 12-lead electrocardiogram obtained one week prior to the patient undergoing TURBT with intravesical mitomycin C instillation showing normal PR and ST segments in all leads.

complain of chest pain through her presentation—which may have been worsened due the tachycardia caused by pericardial pain combined with the stenotic lesion in the LAD resulting in a possible ischemic component to the pain (similar to an exercise stress test)—and considering the apical wall motion abnormality seen on the echocardiogram, a decision was made to proceed with percutaneous coronary intervention (PCI) with placement of a drug-eluting stent for the LAD stenosis. However, based on the pathophysiology of coronary artery disease leading to acute coronary syndromes, the underlying pathology in most cases of acute myocardial infarction is an acute intraluminal coronary thrombus formation within an epicardial coronary artery leading to total or near-total acute coronary occlusion, something which our patient did not have [11]. A repeat troponin I level which resulted after angiography was 0.54 ng/ml at 5:30 pm (a downtrend from the earlier level of 0.57 ng/ml at 12:30 pm). Given her 12 hours of continuous chest pain, this is a particularly low troponin I level if acute coronary syndrome was her primary issue [12].

An EKG obtained 15 hours after intervention (Figure 2) showed neither the resolution of the ST elevation nor the evolution of pathological Q waves, either of which should have occurred if ischemia was the reason for her EKG findings [13]. A follow-up EKG performed 3 weeks after hospital discharge (Figure 3) shows complete resolution of the EKG findings and was essentially unchanged when compared to her EKG performed 1 week prior to the TURBT (Figure 4). This is consistent with resolution of her pericarditis.

Mitomycin C is the most commonly used intravesical chemotherapeutic agent [14] and has an established role in intravesical administration following resection of low-risk non-muscle-invasive bladder cancer [15]. It exerts its biological effects by alkylation of cellular nucleophiles, including DNA, after undergoing enzymatic bioreduction into a bis-electrophilic intermediate [16]. A study was done to determine the systemic absorption of intravesical mitomycin C (MMC) in which fourteen patients with primary or recurrent non-muscle-invasive bladder cancer (NMIBC) underwent single early intravesical instillation of MMC (40 mg in 50 mL distilled water) immediately after TURBT. The results showed that maximal MMC plasma concentrations were reached 40 minutes after instillation with a highest plasma peak of 49.25 ng/ml. In the first samples, at 20 minutes after instillation, the plasma concentration of MMC was significantly correlated with the extent of TURBT ($P = 0.026$) [17].

Side effects following intravesical administration of mitomycin C include myelosuppression [18], a self-limited chemical cystitis that rarely progresses to the shrunken contracted bladder [19], and a rash primarily involving the palms, soles, and genitalia, which is thought to be a manifestation of a hypersensitivity reaction [20]. While systemically administered mitomycin C has been known to be associated with dose-dependent cardiotoxicity, especially when combined with or given following doxorubicin [21], the association of cardiotoxicity with intravesically administered mitomycin C has not been studied. A study was done in 2013 which analyzed data retrospectively from 3 academic tertiary referral centers between 2000 and 2010, in which 47 patients (median age 70, range 32–85; 36 males and 11 females) who previously failed a median of 2 intravesical treatments, subsequently received 6 weekly treatments with sequential intravesical gemcitabine (1 g) and mitomycin C (40 mg) chemotherapy for non-muscle-invasive bladder cancer (NMIBC). Among the patients who developed complications as a result of the study, 1 patient was reported to have developed pericarditis shortly after the last treatment that was attributed to mitomycin C exposure [22].

4. Conclusion

The possibility of cardiotoxicity in the form of perimyocarditis occurring in association with intravesical mitomycin C instillation following TURBT has not been studied and with no documented case reports in existing literature and only one instance of pericarditis attributed to intravesical MMC instillation in a retrospective analysis [16]. While the pathophysiological basis of cardiotoxicity of systemically administered mitomycin C is well documented [14], more studies are needed to determine whether intravesical MMC may cause cardiotoxicity.

References

[1] M. LeWinter, "Clinical practice. Acute pericarditis," *New England Journal of Medicine*, vol. 371, no. 25, pp. 2410–2416, 2014.

[2] M. Imazio and F. Gaita, "Diagnosis and treatment of pericarditis," *Heart*, vol. 101, no. 14, pp. 1159–1168, 2015.

[3] M. Imazio, "Contemporary management of pericardial diseases," *Current Opinion in Cardiology*, vol. 27, no. 3, pp. 308–317, 2012.

[4] M. Imazio, F. Gaita, and M. LeWinter, "Evaluation and treatment of pericarditis: a systematic review," *Journal of the American Medical Association*, vol. 314, no. 14, pp. 1498–1506, 2015.

[5] R. W. Troughton, C. R. Asher, and A. L. Klein, "Pericarditis," *The Lancet*, vol. 363, no. 9410, pp. 717–727, 2004.

[6] M. Imazio, B. Demichelis, E. Cecchi et al., "Cardiac troponin I in acute pericarditis," *Journal of the American College of Cardiology*, vol. 42, no. 12, pp. 2144–2148, 2003.

[7] M. S. Nieminen, J. Heikkilä, and J. Karjalainen, "Echocardiography in acute infectious myocarditis: relation to clinical and electrocardiographic findings," *American Journal of Cardiology*, vol. 53, no. 9, pp. 1331–1337, 1984.

[8] B. Pinamonti, E. Alberti, A. Cigalotto et al., "Echocardiographic findings in myocarditis," *American Journal of Cardiology*, vol. 62, no. 4, pp. 285–291, 1988.

[9] J. B. Jayroe, D. H. Spodick, K. Nikus et al., "Differentiating ST elevation myocardial infarction and nonischemic causes of ST elevation by analyzing the presenting electrocardiogram," *American Journal of Cardiology*, vol. 103, no. 3, pp. 301–306, 2009.

[10] A. Deshpande and Y. Birnbaum, "ST-segment elevation: distinguishing ST elevation myocardial infarction from ST elevation secondary to nonischemic etiologies," *World Journal of Cardiology*, vol. 6, no. 10, pp. 1067–1079, 2014.

[11] J. A. Ambrose and M. Singh, "Pathophysiology of coronary artery disease leading to acute coronary syndromes," *F1000Prime Reports*, vol. 7, p. 8, 2015.

[12] M. C. Kontos, R. Shah, L. M. Fritz et al., "Implication of different cardiac troponin I levels for clinical outcomes and prognosis of acute chest pain patients," *Journal of the American College of Cardiology*, vol. 43, no. 6, pp. 958–965, 2004.

[13] F. Morris and W. J. Brady, "ABC of clinical electrocardiography: acute myocardial infarction—part I," *British Medical Journal*, vol. 324, no. 7341, pp. 831–834, 2002.

[14] S. Porten, M. Leapman, and K. Greene, "Intravesical chemotherapy in non-muscle-invasive bladder cancer," *Indian Journal of Urology*, vol. 31, no. 4, pp. 297–303, 2015.

[15] S. Shariat, D. Chade, P. Karakiewicz, D. Scherr, and G. Dalbagni, "Update on intravesical agents for non-muscle-invasive bladder cancer," *Immunotherapy*, vol. 2, no. 3, pp. 381–392, 2010.

[16] M. Paz, X. Zhang, J. Lu, and A. Holmgren, "A new mechanism of action for the anticancer drug mitomycin C: mechanism-based inhibition of thioredoxin reductase," *Chemical Research in Toxicology*, vol. 25, no. 7, pp. 1502–1511, 2012.

[17] M. Maffezzini, F. Campodonico, E. E. Manuputty et al., "Systemic absorption and pharmacokinetics of single-dose early intravesical mitomycin C after transurethral resection of non-muscle-invasive bladder cancer," *Urology*, vol. 82, no. 2, pp. 400–404, 2013.

[18] J. B. Thrasher and E. D. Crawford, "Complications of intravesical chemotherapy," *Urologic Clinics of North America*, vol. 19, no. 3, pp. 529–539, 1992.

[19] A. Böhle, D. Jocham, and P. R. Bock, "Intravesical bacillus Calmette-Guerin versus mitomycin C for superficial bladder cancer: a formal meta-analysis of comparative studies on recurrence and toxicity," *Journal of Urology*, vol. 169, no. 1, pp. 90–95, 2003.

[20] G. B. Colver, J. A. Inglis, E. McVittie, M. J. Spencer, D. A. Tolley, and J. A. Hunter, "Dermatitis due to intravesical mitomycin C: a delayed-type hypersensitivity reaction?," *British Journal of Dermatology*, vol. 122, no. 2, pp. 217–224, 1990.

[21] J. Verweij, A. J. Funke-Küpper, G. J. Teule, and H. M. Pinedo, "A prospective study on the dose dependency of cardiotoxicity induced by mitomycin C," *Medical Oncology and Tumor Pharmacotherapy*, vol. 5, no. 3, pp. 159–163, 1988.

[22] A. Lightfoot, B. Breyer, H. Rosevear, B. Erickson, B. Konety, and M. O'Donnell, "Multi-institutional analysis of sequential intravesical gemcitabine and mitomycin C chemotherapy for non–muscle invasive bladder cancer," *Urologic Oncology*, vol. 32, no. 1, pp. 35.e15–35.e19, 2014.

Delayed Development of Coronary Ostial Stenosis following Surgical Aortic Valve Replacement: A Case Report of Unusual Presentation

Doosup Shin,[1] **Kevin Huang**,[1] **Igor Sunjic**,[2] **Michael Berlowitz**,[2] **and Xavier Prida**[2]

[1]*Department of Internal Medicine, University of South Florida Morsani College of Medicine, Tampa, FL, USA*
[2]*Department of Cardiovascular Sciences, University of South Florida Morsani College of Medicine, Tampa, FL, USA*

Correspondence should be addressed to Xavier Prida; xavierprida@health.usf.edu

Academic Editor: Gianluca Di Bella

Coronary ostial stenosis is a rare but potentially life-threatening complication that occurs in 1%–5% of patients who undergo surgical aortic valve replacement (SAVR). Symptoms typically appear within the first 6 months and almost always within a year after SAVR. We report an unusually delayed presentation of non-ST segment elevation myocardial infarction due to coronary ostial stenosis 22 months after SAVR. A 71-year-old woman underwent uncomplicated SAVR with a bioprosthetic valve in August 2015 for severe aortic stenosis. A preoperative coronary angiogram demonstrated widely patent left and right coronary arteries. In June 2017, the patient presented to the hospital with chest pain. An electrocardiogram demonstrated 1 mm ST segment depression in the anterolateral leads, and serum troponin I level was elevated to 2.3 ng/ml. Diagnostic coronary angiography revealed severe ostial stenosis (99%) of the right coronary artery. A bare-metal stent was successfully placed with an excellent angiographic result, and the patient was asymptomatic at 4 months of follow-up after the procedure. As seen in our case, coronary ostial stenosis should be considered in the differential diagnosis of chest pain or arrhythmia in patients presenting with a history of SAVR, even if the procedure was performed more than 1 year prior to presentation.

1. Introduction

Coronary ostial stenosis is a rare but potentially life-threatening complication associated with surgical aortic valve replacement (SAVR). It has been reported to occur in 1%–5% of all patients who undergo the procedure [1–5]. Coronary ostial stenosis can present with diverse clinical symptoms ranging from angina to acute coronary syndrome (ACS) and even sudden cardiac death [4]. These symptoms typically appear within the first 6 months after SAVR and have rarely been identified beyond 1 year after surgery. We report an unusually delayed clinical presentation that developed 22 months after SAVR.

2. Case Presentation

The patient is a 71-year-old woman with a past medical history of hypertension, hyperlipidemia, type 2 diabetes mellitus, and severe aortic stenosis who underwent SAVR in August 2015. A preoperative coronary angiogram revealed normal coronary arteries without evidence of ostial obstruction. SAVR was successfully performed using a 23 mm diameter Magna bioprosthetic valve. During the surgery, antegrade cardioplegia was first administered to achieve electromechanical arrest. From this point, a dose of cold blood retrograde cardioplegia was administered to the coronary sinus every 15 minutes. The patient had an uncomplicated postoperative course and had returned to her usual lifestyle. A postoperative echocardiogram demonstrated a normal ejection fraction and a normally functioning bioprosthetic aortic valve with a mean gradient of 8–10 mmHg across the valve. The patient had been compliant with medications, including aspirin, statin, and beta-blocker. In June 2017, the patient presented with pressure-like exertional chest pain. An electrocardiogram demonstrated 1 mm ST segment depression in leads I, aVL, V2, and V3 (Figure 1). Laboratory investigations

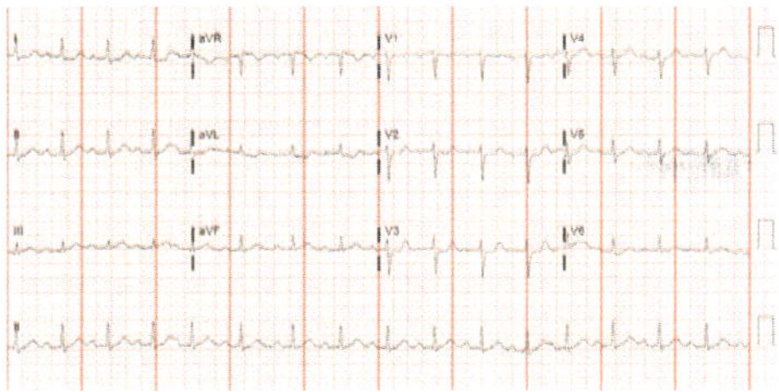

Figure 1: Electrocardiogram on admission demonstrates 1 mm ST segment depression in leads I, aVL, V2, and V3.

revealed elevation of the serum troponin I level to 2.3 ng/ml (normal value: less than 0.032 ng/ml). Guideline-directed medical therapy for non-ST elevation myocardial infarction (NSTEMI) was begun, and the patient was assigned to an invasive strategy. Diagnostic coronary angiography demonstrated isolated severe ostial stenosis (99%) of the right coronary artery with significant catheter pressure waveform dampening but no evidence of thrombus (Figure 2). It showed dramatically tapered appearance from what appeared to be normal arterial segment to a critical ostial stenosis. The lesion was less likely a catheter-induced spasm because (1) there was no direct catheter engagement or deep intubation of the vessel and (2) it persisted despite bolus administration of intracoronary nitroglycerin as well as continuous intravenous infusion of nitroglycerin prior to and during the procedure. Intravascular ultrasound (IVUS) could not be considered due to severity of the stenosis. The lesion was successfully treated using balloon dilations and a single 4.5 mm × 13 mm bare-metal stent (BMS) with excellent angiographic result (Figure 3). The patient was discharged from the hospital the next day without acute complications and was asymptomatic at 4 months of follow-up after the percutaneous coronary intervention (PCI).

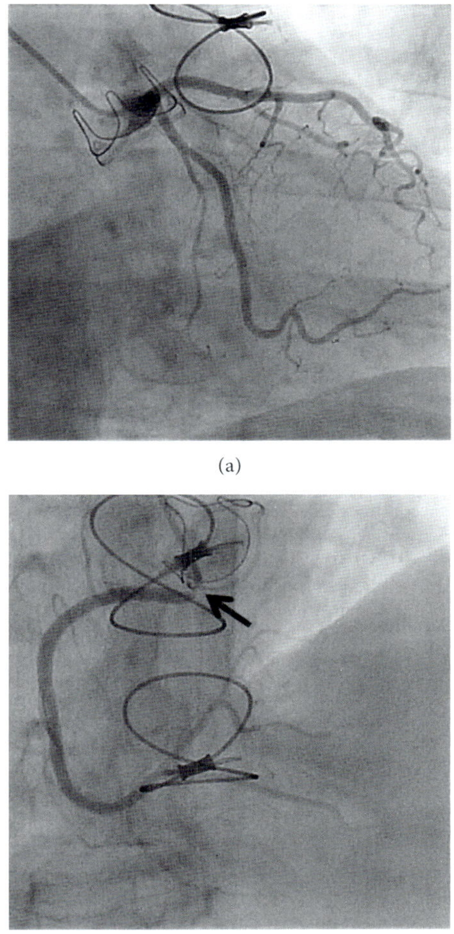

Figure 2: Diagnostic coronary angiogram shows (a) widely patent left coronary arteries and (b) severe ostial stenosis of the right coronary artery (arrow).

3. Discussion

In 1967, Roberts and Morrow first described coronary ostial stenosis as a complication of SAVR [6]. It has been reported as a rare but potentially lethal complication following SAVR. Its prevalence has been reported in 1%–5% of patients who undergo SAVR [1–5]. Coronary ostial stenosis secondary to SAVR more commonly affects the left main coronary artery (LMCA) but also affects the right coronary artery [5]. Clinical syndromes include stable angina, ACS, ventricular arrhythmia, congestive heart failure, and sudden cardiac death [4]. These clinical syndromes typically occur within the first 6 months after SAVR. Rarely has coronary ostial stenosis been identified in a patient more than one year after SAVR. To our knowledge, only one study has reported such a case [3]. Our patient represents one of the latest clinical presentations of coronary ostial stenosis occurred 22 months following SAVR.

Several different underlying mechanisms have been suggested to explain the development of this disease entity. In most cases, it has been attributed to the use of ostial cannulation for antegrade cardioplegia during surgery, which can cause a mechanical injury to the coronary ostium resulting in hyperplastic reaction and stenosis [5, 7, 8]. Furthermore,

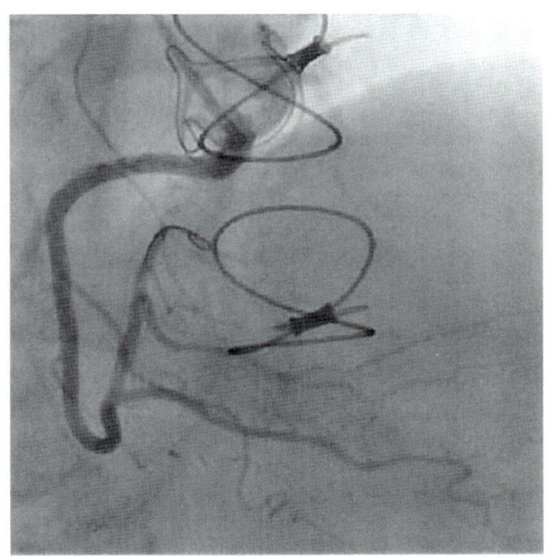

Figure 3: Postprocedure coronary angiogram shows successful revascularization of the right coronary artery with stent placement.

infusion pressure of the cardioplegic solution administered through the cannulation catheter may also contribute to this mechanical injury [9]. However, coronary ostial stenosis can develop after SAVR even without cannulation [10], and brief cannulation times with intermittent infusion of antegrade cardioplegic solution did not eliminate the risk [4, 11]. Similarly, in our case, only a dose of antegrade cardioplegia was given to achieve initial electromechanical arrest, and then, retrograde cardioplegia was used throughout the surgery. Therefore, other mechanisms might also play a role in the development of coronary ostial stenosis after SAVR. First, turbulent flow around the prosthetic valve can cause intimal thickening and fibrous proliferation near the aortic root resulting in ostial stenosis [4–7, 10, 11]. Second, an immunological reaction to the bioprosthetic aortic valve can be another possible mechanism [12, 13]. One study supported this immunological hypothesis by using IVUS which demonstrated a massive extravascular fibrosis and its extrinsic compression around the ostium of the coronary artery causing severe ostial stenosis after SAVR [13].

Revascularization alternatives for ostial coronary artery stenosis following SAVR include coronary artery bypass graft and PCI. Availability/selection of appropriate management strategies for ostial coronary artery stenosis, particularly unprotected LMCA disease, remains a controversial subject. With technological advancement, PCI and stent placement can successfully treat coronary ostial stenosis with good early and late outcomes [5, 7, 12, 14–17]. This approach was applied in our patient with good short-term outcomes. We chose the BMS over the drug-eluting stent (DES) due to its good radial strength and tightness of the lesion in the setting of a large vessel diameter. This anatomic consideration should be balanced with the risk of restenosis, especially in the aorto-coronary ostial lesions. At the same time, the patient's characteristics and the risk of bleeding should also be considered when selecting the type of stent, as DES placement would require longer dual-antiplatelet therapy [16].

In our case, further characterization of the ostial lesion by using prestenting IVUS was not possible because the IVUS catheter could not be negotiated through the critical narrowing of the lesion. Furthermore, the length of the procedure and the patient's disquiet did not allow us to extend the procedure for poststenting IVUS. Although IVUS could not be done in our case, it should be considered in future cases to better understand possible underlying mechanism and optimize stenting.

4. Conclusion

Although coronary ostial stenosis typically occurs within the first 6 months after SAVR, we describe its identification in association with NSTEMI 22 months after the surgery. Therefore, coronary ostial stenosis should be considered in the differential diagnosis of chest pain or arrhythmia in patients presenting with a history of SAVR, even if the procedure was performed more than 1 year prior to presentation. Also, we should continue to have a higher index of suspicion in these patients for ACS even after sufficient time has passed.

References

[1] J. D. Yates, M. M. Kirsh, T. M. Sodeman, J. A. Walton Jr., and J. F. Brymer, "Coronary ostial stenosis: a complication of aortic valve replacement," *Circulation*, vol. 49, no. 3, pp. 530–534, 1974.

[2] G. K. Sethi, S. M. Scott, and T. Takaro, "Iatrogenic coronary artery stenosis following aortic valve replacement," *Journal of Thoracic and Cardiovascular Surgery*, vol. 77, no. 5, pp. 760–767, 1979.

[3] D. G. Pennington, B. Dincer, H. Bashiti et al., "Coronary artery stenosis following aortic valve replacement and intermittent intracoronary cardioplegia," *The Annals of Thoracic Surgery*, vol. 33, no. 6, pp. 576–584, 1982.

[4] J. B. Pillai, T. M. Pillay, and J. Ahmad, "Coronary ostial stenosis after aortic valve replacement, revisited," *The Annals of Thoracic Surgery*, vol. 78, no. 6, pp. 2169–2171, 2004.

[5] A. G. Ziakas, F. I. Economou, N. A. Charokopos et al., "Coronary ostial stenosis after aortic valve replacement: successful treatment of 2 patients with drug-eluting stents," *Texas Heart Institute Journal*, vol. 37, no. 4, pp. 465–468, 2010.

[6] W. C. Roberts and A. G. Morrow, "Late postoperative pathological findings after cardiac valve replacement," *Circulation*, vol. 35, no. 4S1, pp. I48–I62, 1967.

[7] A. Funada, S. Mizuno, K. Ohsato et al., "Three cases of iatrogenic coronary ostial stenosis after aortic valve replacement," *Circulation Journal*, vol. 70, no. 10, pp. 1312–1317, 2006.

[8] A. S. Trimble, W. G. Bigelow, E. D. Wigle, and M. D. Silver, "Coronary ostial stenosis: a late complication of coronary perfusion in open-heart surgery," *Journal of Thoracic and Cardiovascular Surgery*, vol. 57, no. 6, pp. 792–795, 1969.

[9] E. Turillazzi, G. Di Giammarco, M. Neri, S. Bello, I. Riezzo, and V. Fineschi, "Coronary ostia obstruction after replacement of aortic valve prosthesis," *Diagnostic Pathology*, vol. 6, no. 1, p. 72, 2011.

[10] S. Rath, D. A. Goor, Y. Har-Zahav, A. Buttler, and Z. Ziskind, "Coronary ostial stenosis after aortic valve replacement without coronary cannulation," *American Journal of Cardiology*, vol. 61, no. 13, pp. 1156-1157, 1988.

[11] T. L. Force, D. S. Raabe Jr., L. H. Coffin, and J. D. DeMeules, "Coronary ostial stenosis following aortic valve replacement without continuous coronary perfusion," *Journal of Thoracic and Cardiovascular Surgery*, vol. 80, no. 4, pp. 637–641, 1980.

[12] M. Tsukiji, T. Akasaka, N. Wada et al., "Bilateral coronary ostial stenosis after aortic valve replacement with freestyle stentless bioprosthesis: a case report," *Journal of Cardiology*, vol. 44, pp. 207–213, 2004.

[13] S. W. Han, H. J. Kim, S. Kim, and K. H. Ryu, "Coronary ostial stenosis after aortic valvuloplasty (comprehensive aortic root and valve repair)," *European Journal of Cardio-Thoracic Surgery*, vol. 35, no. 6, pp. 1099–1101, 2009.

[14] M. A. Khan, F. Prati, and M. El-Omar, "Iatrogenic coronary ostial stenosis of left main stem following aortic valve replacement: visualization with optical coherence tomography," *Cardiovascular Revascularization Medicine*, vol. 14, no. 5, pp. 299–301, 2013.

[15] V. Marti, J. M. Auge, J. Garcia Picart, P. Guiteras, M. Ballester, and D. Obrador, "Percutaneous transluminal coronary angioplasty as alternative treatment to coronary artery bypass surgery in iatrogenic stenosis of the left main coronary artery," *Journal of Interventional Cardiology*, vol. 8, no. 3, pp. 229–231, 1995.

61

Successful Treatment of an Infant with Left Ventricular Noncompaction Presenting with Fatal Ventricular Arrhythmia Treated with Cardiac Resynchronization Therapy and an Implantable Cardioverter Defibrillator

Masato Kimura, Kengo Kawano, Hisao Yaoita, and Shigeo Kure

Department of Pediatrics, Tohoku University Graduate School of Medicine, 1-1 Seiryo-machi, Aoba-ku, Sendai, Miyagi 980-8574, Japan

Correspondence should be addressed to Masato Kimura; mkimura774@med.tohoku.ac.jp

Academic Editor: Tayfun Sahin

We herein report the successful treatment of a 4-year-old girl with left ventricular noncompaction (LVNC) who presented with incessant ventricular fibrillation at 5 months of age. An implantable cardioverter defibrillator (ICD) was implanted, and dual chamber (DDD) pacing was initiated at 7 months of age. At her 10-month follow-up, her left ventricular ejection fraction (LVEF) had decreased from 45% to 20% with mechanical dyssynchrony. After upgrading to cardiac resynchronization therapy (CRT), the LVEF improved to 50%. The usefulness of CRT in pediatric LVNC has not been fully elucidated. However, our case suggests that CRT therapy may be an effective option for LVNC-induced cardiac dysfunction.

1. Introduction

Left ventricular noncompaction (LVNC) is a rare congenital cardiomyopathy with a clinical presentation that ranges from no symptoms to sudden cardiac death due to fatal arrhythmia or heart failure. The onset of fatal ventricular arrhythmia under 1 year of age is a risk factor for cardiac death and an indication for heart transplantation [1]. LVNC is characterized by prominent left ventricular (LV) trabeculations and deep intertrabecular recesses, which are assumed to be the result of failure or abnormality of the myocardial compaction process during the prenatal period [2]. However, Jensen et al. recently hypothesized that hypertrabeculation may not be a failure of myocardial compaction, but rather an aberration of mammalian cardiogenesis [3]. Cardiac resynchronization therapy (CRT) for heart failure in pediatric congenital heart disease is an emerging option [4, 5]; however, few reports on CRT in pediatric LVNC patients are available [6].

2. Case Report

A 6-month-old girl was transferred to our university hospital presenting with incessant ventricular fibrillation (VF) after rewarming therapy for cerebral hypothermia. There was no family history of cardiovascular or neurologic disease. Her development until the event was normal, and at 5 months after birth, she went into cardiopulmonary arrest. During cardiopulmonary resuscitation by emergency medical services, VF was detected using an automated external defibrillator. Sinus rhythm was restored by defibrillation shock. Cerebral hypothermia treatment for 4 days was initiated at a tertiary emergency city hospital. After rewarming, VF occurred again and incessantly repeated without stimulation. She was moved to our university hospital, and her electrocardiogram (ECG) showed polymorphic ventricular tachycardia and VF (Figure 1(a)). After administration of various antiarrhythmic drugs and sedatives, the fatal arrhythmia finally stopped (Figure 1(b)). Laboratory blood

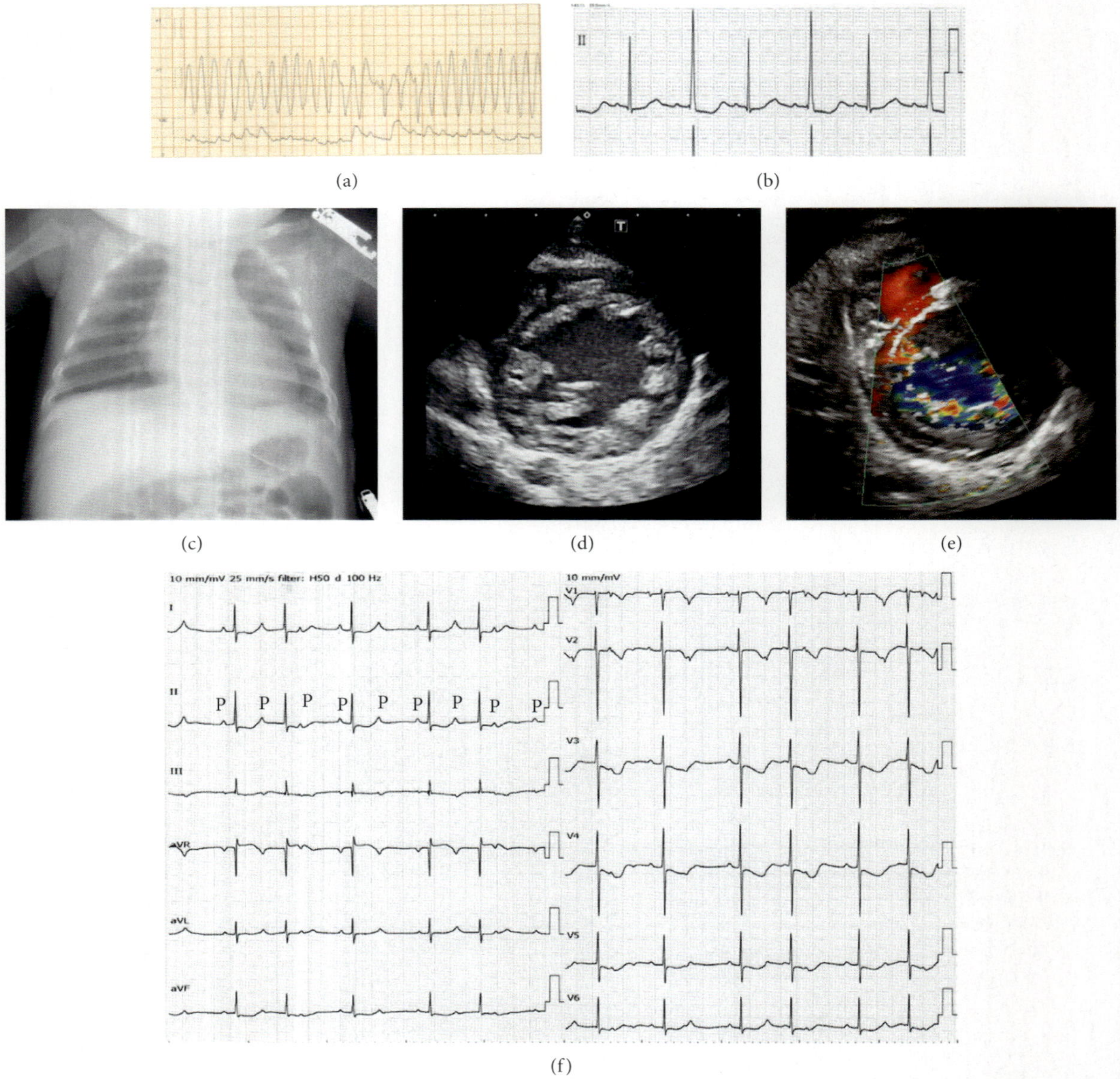

Figure 1: Electrocardiogram (ECG) and arterial blood pressure monitoring on admission (a). (Top panel) ECG shows polymorphic ventricular tachycardia, with a rate of approximately 300 bpm. (Bottom panel) arterial blood pressure monitoring. (b) Lead II of the ECG after polymorphic ventricular tachycardia was stopped. The heart rate (HR) was 79 bpm, PR interval was 160 msec, and QTc interval was 510 msec with alternate T waves. (c) Chest X-ray on admission showing a cardiothoracic ratio of 52%. Transthoracic echocardiography on admission. (d) Transthoracic echocardiography shows left ventricular noncompaction on the parasternal short axis view, with a ratio of noncompacted to compacted area at end-systole > 2. (e) Color Doppler imaging reveals communication between myocardial recesses and the left ventricular cavity. (f) The 12-lead ECG before implantable cardioverter defibrillator (ICD) implantation, showing 2 : 1 atrioventricular block. The HR was 76 bpm, PR interval was 170 msec, and QTc interval was 462 msec. P indicates the P wave in lead II.

tests did not indicate myocarditis or metabolic disease. A chest X-ray revealed no cardiomegaly with a cardiothoracic ratio (CTR) of 52% (Figure 1(c)). Transthoracic echocardiography confirmed global LV hypokinesis with an ejection fraction (EF) of 30%. B-mode analysis revealed a two-layer structure with a compacted thin epicardial band and a thick, noncompacted endocardial layer with prominent trabeculae and deep intertrabecular recesses at the LV apical and lateral walls. In the end-systolic phase, the ratio of noncompacted to compacted layers was 2.8. Color Doppler imaging revealed blood filling the recesses from the ventricular cavity (Figures 1(d) and 1(e)).

For secondary prevention, an implantable cardioverter defibrillator (ICD) (Protecta™ XT DR; Medtronic, Minneapolis, MN, USA) was implanted in the patient's left upper abdominal quadrant, and dual chamber (DDD) pacing was started due to 2 : 1 atrioventricular (AV) block (Figure 1(f)), which might have been induced by administration of amiodarone and beta-blocker (at 7 months of age; height 68 cm, weight 5.6 kg) (Figure 2(a)). The shock lead was run

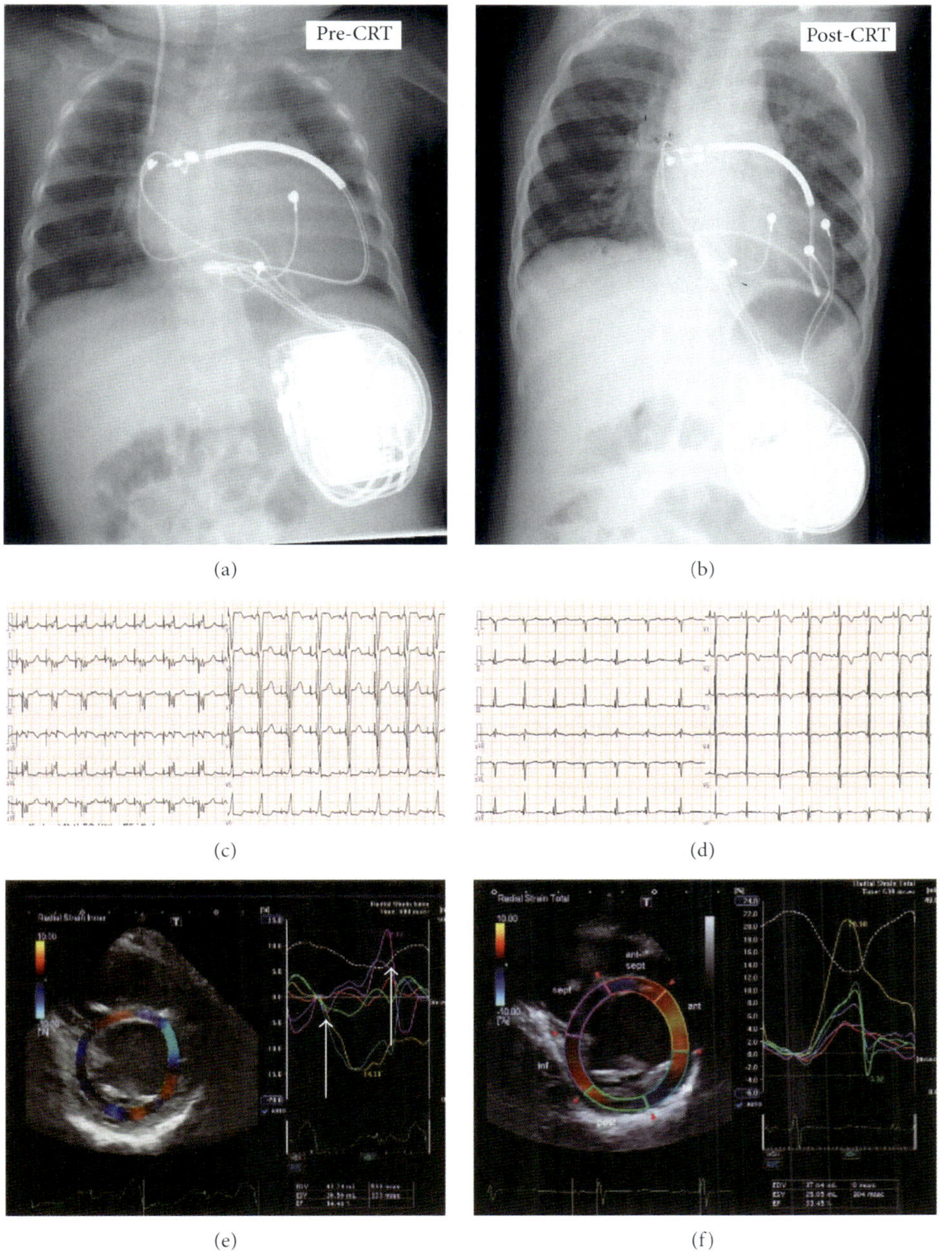

Figure 2: Chest X-rays pre- and postcardiac resynchronization therapy (CRT). (a) The defibrillator was placed into the left upper abdomen, and the shock lead was fixed at the level of the superior vena cava. The right ventricular (RV) epicardial lead was placed at the RV free wall. (b) The left ventricular (LV) lead was placed at the LV lateral wall. The 12-lead ECG pre- and post-CRT. Before CRT (c), the QRS duration was 114 msec. After CRT (d), the QRS duration was shortened to 80 msec. Speckle-tracking radial dyssynchrony pre- and post-CRT (Artida™; Toshiba Medical Systems, Tokyo, Japan). Pre-CRT (e), dyssynchrony is shown as a time difference (arrow) between time to peak strain in the anterior wall (yellow) and septum peak strain (purple) (dual chamber (DDD) 90–150 bpm with an atrioventricular (AV) delay of 130 msec). Post-CRT (C-II), dyssynchrony disappeared (DDD 80–160 bpm, with an AV delay of 120 msec and a LV-RV delay of 0 msec).

outside of the epicardium and fixed at the level of the superior vena cava. At discharge, the left ventricular ejection fraction (LVEF) was 45% and the brain natriuretic peptide (BNP) level was 96 pg/ml. At her 10-month follow-up, the LVEF decreased to 20% and the patient's mitral regurgitation had deteriorated severely. Moreover, mechanical dyssynchrony was observed on strain echocardiography (Figure 2(e)), and the patient's BNP levels increased to 1,300 pg/ml. After ICD implantation, appropriate discharge of the ICD occurred only once when she had developed acute gastroenteritis with ventricular tachycardia. ICD right ventricular (RV) pacing was upgraded to biventricular pacing with a cardiac resynchronization therapy defibrillator (CRTD) (Viva™ XT; Medtronic, NJ, USA) (height 72 cm, weight 8.5 kg). After this upgrade, her LV function gradually improved, with an LVEF of 50% without mechanical dyssynchrony and mild mitral regurgitation (Figure 2(f)). The BNP level decreased to 26 pg/ml, and the CTR was 53% (Figure 2(b)). Over a 3-year follow-up period, the patient's course was uneventful and she was maintained on bisoprolol (0.3 mg/kg), enalapril (0.25 mg/kg), aspirin, and diuretics. The extent and location of abnormal LV trabeculation did not change during this period. Her developmental delays improved, with exercise, social, and vocal capacities being at the 2-, 3-, and 3-year-old levels, respectively.

Whole exome sequencing revealed a nonsense mutation in exon 7 of the *DTNA* gene (C601T). While the patient's mother also had the same mutation in the *DTNA* gene, echocardiogram revealed that the mother's heart was morphologically and functionally normal. The patient's father did not have a mutation of the *DTNA* gene. The *DTNA* gene of the patient's older sister was not investigated because of her normal echocardiogram with no medical history.

3. Discussion

We herein report the successful treatment of a 4-year-old girl who presented with incessant VF and LVNC at 5 months of age. After RV pacing, her cardiac function deteriorated and LVEF decreased; however, CRT corrected her mechanical dyssynchrony, which subsequently improved cardiac function.

LVNC was first described pathologically by Grant in 1926 [7] and has been defined as a genetic cardiomyopathy by the American Heart Association since 2006 [8]. It is a rare disorder that is believed to develop due to cessation of the refinement of ventricular muscles between the 5th and 8th week of gestational age [2]. However, Jansen et al. recently hypothesized that hypertrabeculation is not a failure of myocardial compaction, but rather an aberration of mammalian cardiogenesis [3]. They proposed that the evolutionary and developmental models of normal and hypertrabeculated hearts and trabeculations in LVNC are not similar to the trabeculations of embryos or ectotherms, viewed in the light of histological and magnetic resonance imaging (MRI) findings.

The clinical presentation of LVNC ranges from no symptoms to sudden cardiac death due to fatal arrhythmia or heart failure. Brescia et al. investigated the long-term prognosis of 242 pediatric LVNC patients and reported that the mortality rate was 12.8%, the sudden cardiac death rate was 6.2%, and 5.4% of patients received a heart transplant [1]. The risk of death was strongly associated with cardiac dysfunction and ventricular arrhythmias for <1 year. LVNC is a genetically heterogeneous disorder, and gene mutations, which encode sarcomeric, cytoskeletal, and nuclear membrane proteins, are identified in only half of all reported cases [2]. In 2001, Ichida et al. reported a family with LVNC and a *DTNA* missense mutation in exon 4 (C362T) [9]. Whole exome sequencing in our patient revealed a nonsense mutation in exon 7 of the *DTNA* gene (C601T). Interestingly, our patient's mother also had the same mutation; however, her heart was morphologically normal. These differences may be due to incomplete penetrance of the *DTNA* gene in our case and/or the dominant negative effects of the missense mutation in exon 4. To the best of our knowledge, a *DTNA* gene mutation associated with LVNC was observed in only one family, and the function of the *DTNA* gene in LVNC has not been fully elucidated. No specific treatment has been established for LVNC, and ICD implantation is performed as a preventive measure for lethal ventricular arrhythmia. In a previous study, Kobza et al. reported that ICD implantation was effective as a primary and secondary preventive measure for sudden cardiac death in LVNC patients (30 patients; mean age 48 ± 14 years) [10]. Moreover, ICD with cardiac resynchronization improved LVEF from $22 \pm 5\%$ before implantation to $37 \pm 15\%$ after implantation, with a mean follow-up of 18 ± 11 months (six patients; mean age 58 ± 17 years). These studies were conducted in adult populations. However, implantation of ICD in pediatric patients is associated with several limitations. Indeed, the size of the devices and lead implantation result in placement difficulties of these therapeutic devices in pediatric patients. In our case, it seems that RV (DDD) pacing using an ICD caused LV function deterioration due to mechanical dyssynchrony. Cardiac function dramatically improved after introducing biventricular pacing using CRTD. It is known that in a certain proportion of pediatric patients with RV pacing, LV failure may develop. Indeed, Roman et al. demonstrated that epicardial RV free wall pacing is a risk factor for pacing-induced heart failure [11]. Moreover, due to their small heart size, selecting pacing lead positions is very difficult in infants. RV pacing-induced LV dysfunction responds well to biventricular pacing therapy [4]. Currently, there are no prospective randomized controlled trials evaluating pediatric CRT, and device therapy has become an emerging option for treating heart failure in pediatric heart disease [5]. Most reports in the medical literature concerning the use of CRT in pediatric patients are case reports that focus on the efficacy of CRT in treating severe heart failure. Only two large studies on the use of CRT in pediatric patients with dilated cardiomyopathy (DCM) have been published. Dubin et al. [12] reported their findings in 16 patients, while Cecchin et al. [13] included 10 patients with DCM in their study. No mortality was reported in these studies; however, additional reports of similar cases are needed to determine standard guidelines concerning the use of CRT in pediatric patients. The usefulness of CRT in pediatric LVNC remains to be fully elucidated. Our case suggests that CRT therapy could be an effective option for LVNC-induced cardiac dysfunction.

The present case provides important insights into the midterm effects of biventricular pacing and CRTD implantation for infantile LVNC. It is necessary to consider pediatric body size with respect to device and lead implantation. CRTD treatment is useful for the management of infantile LVNC with mechanical dyssynchrony and may improve prognosis.

References

[1] S. T. Brescia, J. W. Rossano, R. Pignatelli et al., "Mortality and sudden death in pediatric left ventricular noncompaction in a tertiary referral center," *Circulation*, vol. 127, no. 22, pp. 2202–2208, 2013.

[2] E. Oechslin and R. Jenni, "Left ventricular non-compaction revisited: a distinct phenotype with genetic heterogeneity?," *European Heart Journal*, vol. 32, no. 12, pp. 1446–1456, 2011.

[3] B. Jansen, P. Agger, B. A. de Boer et al., "The hypertrabeclated (noncompacted) left ventricle is different from the ventricle of embryos and ectothermic vertebrates," *Biochimica et Biophysica Acta*, vol. 1863, no. 7, pp. 1696–1706, 2016.

[4] J. Janousek and R. A. Gebauer, "Cardiac resynchronization therapy in pediatric and congenital heart disease," *PACE*, vol. 31, pp. S21–S23, 2008.

[5] K. S. Motonaga and A. M. Dubin, "Cardiac resynchronization therapy for pediatric patients with heart failure and congenital heart disease: a reappraisal of results," *Circulation*, vol. 129, no. 18, pp. 1879–1891, 2014.

[6] K. Saito, K. Ibuki, N. Yoshimura et al., "Successful cardiac resynchronization therapy in a 3-year-old girl with isolated left ventricular non-compaction and narrow QRS complex: a case report," *Circulation Journal*, vol. 73, pp. 2173–2177, 2009.

[7] R. T. Grant, "An unusual anomaly of the coronary vessels in the malformed heart of a child," *Heart*, vol. 13, pp. 273–283, 1926.

[8] B. J. Maron, J. A. Towbin, G. Thiene et al., "Contemporary definitions and classification of the cardiomyopathies," *Circulation*, vol. 113, no. 14, pp. 1807–1816, 2006.

[9] F. Ichida, S. Tsubata, K. R. Bowles et al., "Novel gene mutations in patients with left ventricular noncompaction or Barth syndrome," *Circulation*, vol. 103, no. 9, pp. 1256–1263, 2001.

[10] R. Kobza, J. Steffel, P. Erne et al., "Implantable cardioverter-defibrillator and cardiac resynchronization therapy in patients with left ventricular noncompaction," *Heart Rhythm*, vol. 7, no. 11, pp. 1545–1549, 2010.

[11] R. A. Gebauer, V. Tomek, A. Salameh et al., "Predictors of left ventricular remodelling and failure in right ventricular pacing in the young," *European Heart Journal*, vol. 30, no. 9, pp. 1097–1104, 2009.

[12] A. M. Dubin, J. Janousek, E. Rhee et al., "Resynchronization therapy in pediatric and congenital heart disease patients. An international multicenter study," *Journal of the American College of Cardiology*, vol. 46, pp. 2277–2283, 2005.

[13] F. Cecchin, P. A. Frangini, D. W. Brown et al., "Cardiac resynchronization therapy (and multisite pacing) in pediatrics and congenital heart disease: five years experience in a single institution," *Journal of Cardiovascular Electrophysiology*, vol. 20, no. 1, pp. 58–65, 2009.

Permissions

All chapters in this book were first published in CRC, by Hindawi Publishing Corporation; hereby published with permission under the Creative Commons Attribution License or equivalent. Every chapter published in this book has been scrutinized by our experts. Their significance has been extensively debated. The topics covered herein carry significant findings which will fuel the growth of the discipline. They may even be implemented as practical applications or may be referred to as a beginning point for another development.

The contributors of this book come from diverse backgrounds, making this book a truly international effort. This book will bring forth new frontiers with its revolutionizing research information and detailed analysis of the nascent developments around the world.

We would like to thank all the contributing authors for lending their expertise to make the book truly unique. They have played a crucial role in the development of this book. Without their invaluable contributions this book wouldn't have been possible. They have made vital efforts to compile up to date information on the varied aspects of this subject to make this book a valuable addition to the collection of many professionals and students.

This book was conceptualized with the vision of imparting up-to-date information and advanced data in this field. To ensure the same, a matchless editorial board was set up. Every individual on the board went through rigorous rounds of assessment to prove their worth. After which they invested a large part of their time researching and compiling the most relevant data for our readers.

The editorial board has been involved in producing this book since its inception. They have spent rigorous hours researching and exploring the diverse topics which have resulted in the successful publishing of this book. They have passed on their knowledge of decades through this book. To expedite this challenging task, the publisher supported the team at every step. A small team of assistant editors was also appointed to further simplify the editing procedure and attain best results for the readers.

Apart from the editorial board, the designing team has also invested a significant amount of their time in understanding the subject and creating the most relevant covers. They scrutinized every image to scout for the most suitable representation of the subject and create an appropriate cover for the book.

The publishing team has been an ardent support to the editorial, designing and production team. Their endless efforts to recruit the best for this project, has resulted in the accomplishment of this book. They are a veteran in the field of academics and their pool of knowledge is as vast as their experience in printing. Their expertise and guidance has proved useful at every step. Their uncompromising quality standards have made this book an exceptional effort. Their encouragement from time to time has been an inspiration for everyone.

The publisher and the editorial board hope that this book will prove to be a valuable piece of knowledge for researchers, students, practitioners and scholars across the globe.

List of Contributors

Zakaria Hindi and Rami Batarseh
Internal Medicine Department, Texas Tech University Health Sciences Center, Permian Basin, Odessa, TX, USA

Yousef Hindi
Cardiology Department, University of Texas Health Science Center at San Antonio, San Antonio, TX, USA

Furqan Khattak, Muhammad Khalid, Sathvika Gaddam, Vijay Ramu and Vipul Brahmbhatt
East Tennessee State University, Johnson City, TN, USA

Mohamad Kabach, Abdulah Alrifai, Lawrence Lovitz, Mark Rothenberg, Cristiano Faber and Marcos Nores
JFK Medical Center, University of Miami School of Medicine, Atlantis, FL, USA

Ahmed S. Yassin, Ahmed Subahi and Hossam Abubakar
Department of Internal Medicine, Wayne State University/Detroit Medical Center, Detroit, MI, USA

Ahmed Rashed and Mohamed Shokr
Division of Cardiovascular Medicine, Department of Internal Medicine, Wayne State University/Detroit Medical Center, Detroit, MI, USA

Makoto Nishimori, Tomoyuki Honjo, Kenji Kaihotsu, Naohiko Sone, Masanori Iwahashi, Sachiko Yoshikawa and Junichi Imanishi
Division of Cardiology, Department of Internal Medicine, Shinko Hospital, Kobe, Japan

Kazuhiko Nakayama
Division of Cardiovascular Medicine, Department of Internal Medicine, Kobe University Graduate School of Medicine, Kobe, Japan

Noriaki Emoto
Department of Clinical Pharmacy, Kobe Pharmaceutical University, Kobe, Japan

Khurram Butt, Ranjeet Kumar, Jason D'Souza, Joseph Limback, Rajesh Shah and Jeremy Burt
Florida Hospital, Orlando, USA

Daria Yunina, Dikshya Sharma and Hossam Amin
Department of Medicine, Maimonides Medical Center, Brooklyn, NY, USA

Richard Fazio and Yuriy Tsirlin
Division of Gastroenterology, Department of Medicine, Maimonides Medical Center, Brooklyn, NY, USA

Vijay Shetty
Department of Cardiology, Department of Medicine, Maimonides Medical Center, Brooklyn, NY, USA
Department of Medicine, SUNY Downstate School of Medicine, Brooklyn, NY, USA

Brunna Priscylla Amèrico Carvalho
Cardiology and Cardiovascular Surgery Department, São Josè do Rio Preto Medical School, São Josè do Rio Preto, SP, Brazil

Marcio Antônio Dos Santos, Wilson Pedro Guimarães Neto, Júlio Cèsar Queiroz De França, Mârcio Rogèrio de Souza Braite, Rodrigo Bottura De Araújo and Isabella Gomes Carvalho
Hemodynamic and Interventional Cardiology Service, Hospital de Base, São Josè do Rio Preto, SP, Brazil

Moacir Fernandes de Godoy
Cardiology and Cardiovascular Surgery Department, São Josè do Rio Preto Medical School, São Josè do Rio Preto, SP, Brazil
Hemodynamic and Interventional Cardiology Service, Hospital de Base, São Josè do Rio Preto, SP, Brazil

Sijan Basnet and Rashmi Dhital
Department of Medicine, Reading Hospital, 420 S Fifth Avenue, West Reading, PA 19611, USA

Priya Rajagopalan
Jefferson Medical College, 1025 Walnut Street, Philadelphia, PA 19107, USA

Biswaraj Tharu
Maharajgunj Medical Campus, Tribhuvan University, Kathmandu, Nepal

Yehia Saleh
Michigan State University, East Lansing, MI, USA
Faculty of Medicine, Alexandria University, Alexandria, Egypt

Basma Hammad
Faculty of Medicine, Alexandria University, Alexandria, Egypt
Massachusetts General Hospital and Harvard Medical School, Boston, MA, USA

Abdallah Almaghraby, Ola Abdelkarim, Hoda Shehata, Mahmoud Hammad, Bassem Ramadan, Mohamed Elshafei, Eman Elsharkawy, Mohamed Ayman Abdel-hay and Mohamed Seleem
Faculty of Medicine, Alexandria University, Alexandria, Egypt

Mahmoud Abdelnaby
Massachusetts General Hospital and Harvard Medical School, Boston, MA, USA

Oreoluwa Oladiran, Jared Segal and Salik Nazir
Reading Hospital, Tower Health System, Reading, PA, USA

Ifeanyi Nwosu
Benenden Hospitals Trust, Kent, UK

Sammy San Myint Aung, Kyaw Kyaw and Chanwit Roongsritong
Institute for Heart and Vascular Health, Renown Regional Medical Center, 1500 E 2nd St No. 302, Reno, NV 89502, USA

Htun Latt
Department of Internal Medicine, School of Medicine, University of Nevada-Reno, 1155 Mill St No.W11, Reno, NV 89502, USA

E. Fry, J. Urbanczyk, J. Price, R. Digiovanni, M. Jepson and D. Gantt
Baylor Scott and White Medical Center, Temple, TX, USA

Kristína Mikuš-Kuracinová, Pavel Babál and Eliška Kubíková
Department of Pathology and Institute of Anatomy, Comenius University Faculty of Medicine Bratislava, Sasinkova 4, 81372 Bratislava, Slovakia

Pradyumna Agasthi, Hemalatha Narayanasamy and Dan Sorajja
Department of Cardiovascular Diseases, Mayo Clinic, Arizona 85259, USA

James Slack
Department of Cardio-Oncology, Mayo Clinic, Arizona 85259, USA
Department of Internal Medicine, Mayo Clinic, Arizona 85259, USA

Farouk Mookadam
Department of Cardiovascular Diseases, Mayo Clinic, Arizona 85259, USA
Department of Cardio-Oncology, Mayo Clinic, Arizona 85259, USA

Adam Hafeez and Alexandra Halalau
Internal Medicine Department, Beaumont Hospital, Royal Oak, MI, USA
Oakland University William Beaumont School of Medicine, Rochester, MI, USA

Jonathan Sen, Michael Mok and Mark Perrin
University Hospital Geelong, Barwon Health, Geelong, VIC 3220, Australia

Miguel López Hidalgo
Interventional Cardiology Unit, Hospital Metropolitano Del Norte, Valencia, Venezuela

Risshi D. Rampersad
Caribbean Heart Care, Medcorp Ltd., St Clair Medical Centre, Port of Spain, Trinidad and Tobago

Peter J. Kennel
Department of Medicine, Weill Cornell Medicine, New York, NY, USA

Melvin Parasram
Department of Neurology, Weill Cornell Medicine, New York, NY, USA

Diane Zisa and Samuel Chung
Samuel Freedman, Katherine Knorr and Timothy Donahoe

Daniel Lu, Steven M. Markowitz and Hadi Halazun
Department of Cardiology, Weill Cornell Medicine, New York, NY, USA

Abdalla Ibrahim, Eoghan Meagher, Alexander Fraser and Thomas J. Kiernan
Cardiology Department, University Hospital Limerick, St. Nessan's Road, Dooradoyle, Limerick, Ireland
Rheumatology Department, University Hospital Limerick, St Nessan's Road, Dooradoyle, Limerick, Ireland

Manabu Ogita, Satoru Suwa, Taketo Sonoda and Shuta Tsuboi
Department of Cardiology, Juntendo University Shizuoka Hospital, Izunokuni, Japan

Katsumi Miyauchi and Hiroyuki Daida
Department of Cardiovascular Medicine, Juntendo University Graduate School of Medicine, Tokyo, Japan

Serena Sert Kim Khoo and Yin Khet Fung
Endocrinology Unit, Queen Elizabeth Hospital II, Kota Kinabalu, Sabah, Malaysia

Chong Mow Chu
Cardiology Department, Queen Elizabeth Hospital II, Kota Kinabalu, Sabah, Malaysia

K. Selthofer-Relatic
Department for Cardiovascular Disease, Osijek University Hospital, J. Huttlera 4, 31000 Osijek, Croatia
Department for Internal Medicine, Faculty of Medicine Osijek, Josip Juraj Strossmayer University of Osijek, Cara Hadrijana 10E, 31000 Osijek, Croatia

Haiyan Yang and Xiaojuan Ji
Department of Cardiology, Children's Hospital of Chongqing Medical University, Chongqing 400014, China
Ministry of Education Key Laboratory of Child Development and Disorders, Chongqing Key Laboratory of Child Infection and
Immunity, China International Science and Technology Cooperation Base of Child Development and Critical Disorders, Chongqing 400014, China

Jinqing Li
Department of Radiology, 324th Hospital of the PLA, Chongqing 400020, China

Bruno da Silva Matte, Gustavo Neves de Araujo, Felipe Homem Valle and Ana Maria Rocha Krepsky
Hospital de Clínicas de Porto Alegre, Federal University of Rio Grande do Sul, Porto Alegre, RS, Brazil

James J. Glazier, Amir Kaki and Theodore L. Schreiber
Detroit Medical Center Heart Hospital, Wayne State University, Detroit, MI, USA

Adam Hafeez, Dillon Karmo and Adrian Mercado-Alamo
Internal Medicine Department, Beaumont Hospital, Royal Oak, MI, USA
Oakland University William Beaumont School of Medicine, Rochester, MI, USA

Alexandra Halalau
Oakland University William Beaumont School of Medicine, Rochester, MI, USA
General Internal Medicine Division, Beaumont Hospital, Royal Oak, MI, USA

Sebhat Erqou
Department of Medicine, Alpert Medical School of Brown University, Providence, RI, USA
Department of Medicine, Providence VA Medical Center, Providence, RI, USA

Robert L. Kormos, Norman C. Wang, Dennis M. McNamara and Raveen Bazaz
Heart and Vascular Institute, University of Pittsburgh Medical Center, Pittsburgh, PA, USA

Evelyn Fennelly, Marcus Lee, Faisal Sharif and Darren Mylotte
Department of Cardiology, University Hospital Galway, Galway, Ireland

Mark Da Costa
Department of Cardiothoracic Surgery, University Hospital Galway, Galway, Ireland

Sherif Sultan
Department of Vascular Surgery, University Hospital Galway, Galway, Ireland

Ruben Jansen, Brigitte Bathgate and Jan-Erik Guelker
Department of Cardiology, Heartcentre Niederrhein, Helios Clinic Krefeld, Krefeld, Germany
Institute for Heart and Circulation Research, University of Cologne, Cologne, Germany

Alexander Bufe
Department of Cardiology, Heartcentre Niederrhein, Helios Clinic Krefeld, Krefeld, Germany
Institute for Heart and Circulation Research, University of Cologne, Cologne, Germany
University of Witten/Herdecke, Witten, Germany

Yae Min Park, Mi Sook Cha, Hanul Choi, Woong Chol Kang, Seung Hwan Han, In Suck Choi and Eak Kyun Shin
Cardiology Division, Department of Internal Medicine, Gachon University Gil Medical Center, Incheon, Republic of Korea

Young-Hoon Kim
Cardiology Division, Department of Internal Medicine, Korea University Anam Hospital, Seoul, Republic of Korea

Yu Yamada, Tomoko Ishizu and Hidekazu Tsuneoka
Department of Cardiology, Faculty of Medicine, University of Tsukuba, Ibaraki, Japan

Yutaka Eki
Department of Cardiology, Hitachi General Hospital, Ibaraki, Japan

Hitoshi Horigome
Department of Pediatrics, University of Tsukuba, Ibaraki, Japan

Gregor Leibundgut and Florian Riede
Department of Cardiology, Medizinische Universitätsklinik, Kantonsspital Baselland, Rheinstrasse 26, 4410 Liestal, Switzerland

Christian Degen
Departement of Internal Medicine, Medizinische Universitätsklinik, Kantonsspital Baselland, Rheinstrasse 26, 4410 Liestal, Switzerland

Dileep Unnikrishnan, Radhika Annam, Aasems Jacob, Braghadheeswar Thyagarajan and Peter Farrugia
Department of Internal Medicine, Monmouth Medical Center, Long Branch, NJ, USA

Nathaniel R. Smilowitz, Muhamed Saric, Michael J. Attubato and James N. Slater
Division of Cardiology, Department of Medicine, NYU School of Medicine, NYU Langone Health, New York, NY, USA

Raymond Pranata
Faculty of Medicine, Universitas Pelita Harapan, Tangerang, Banten, Indonesia
Tabanan General Hospital, Tabanan, Bali, Indonesia

Ian Huang
Faculty of Medicine, Universitas Pelita Harapan, Tangerang, Banten, Indonesia

Vito Damay
Faculty of Medicine, Universitas Pelita Harapan, Tangerang, Banten, Indonesia
Siloam Hospitals Lippo Village, Tangerang, Banten, Indonesia

Christina S. Chen-Milhone
Department of Internal Medicine and Pediatrics, University of Illinois College of Medicine at Peoria, Peoria, IL, USA

Kalyan Chakravarthy Potu and Sudhir Mungee
Department of Cardiology, University of Illinois College of Medicine at Peoria, Peoria, IL, USA

Francesco Summaria, Gregory A. Sgueglia, Fabrizio D'Errico, Antonella De Santis, Fabiana Piccioni, Gaetano Gioffr`e, and Achille Gaspardone
Department of Cardiology, San Eugenio Hospital, Rome, Italy

Karan Wats, Abhinav Saxena and Bilal Malik
Department of Cardiology, Maimonides Medical Center, 4802 10th Avenue, Brooklyn, New York 11219, USA

Ivan D. Hanson, Pratik K. Dalal, Brian M. Renard and George S. Hanzel
Department of Cardiovascular Medicine, Beaumont Health System, Royal Oak, MI, USA

Alessandro Vivacqua
Department of Cardiovascular Surgery, Beaumont Health System, Royal Oak, MI, USA

Keisuke Nakabayashi, Daisuke Sunaga, Nobuhito Kaneko, Akihiro Matsui, Kazuhiko Tanaka, Hiroshi Ando and Minoru Shimizu
Kasukabe Chuo General Hospital, Heart Center, Saitama, Japan

Yohei Numasawa
Department of Cardiology, Japanese Red Cross Ashikaga Hospital, Ashikaga, Japan

Masahito Munakata, Shiro Ishikawa and Takashi Koyama
Department of Cardiology, Saitama Municipal Hospital, Saitama, Japan

Shantanu Patil
Department of Medicine, SSM Health St. Mary's Hospital, St. Louis, MO, USA

Mahek Shah, Brijesh Patel, Lohit Garg, Larry Jacobs, Nauman Islam and Matthew Martinez
Department of Cardiology, Lehigh Valley Hospital, Allentown, PA, USA

Nasreen Shaikh, Rishi Raj and Srinivas Movva
Department of Internal Medicine, Monmouth Medical Center, 300 Second Avenue, Long Branch, NJ 07740, USA

Charles Mattina
Department of Internal Medicine, Monmouth Medical Center, 300 Second Avenue, Long Branch, NJ 07740, USA
Department of Internal Medicine, Division of Cardiology, Monmouth Medical Center, 300 Second Avenue, Long Branch,
NJ 07740, USA

Amy Mertens, Pratik Dalal and Michael Ashbrook
Department of Cardiovascular Medicine, Beaumont Health System, Royal Oak, MI, USA

Ivan Hanson
Department of Cardiovascular Medicine, Beaumont Health System, Royal Oak, MI, USA
Oakland University William Beaumont School of Medicine, Royal Oak, MI, USA

Sowmya Palam, Ridhima Kapoor and Jacquelyn Kulinski
Department of Internal Medicine, Medical College of Wisconsin, 9200 W. Wisconsin Ave., Suite 5100, Milwaukee, WI 53226, USA

Michael McGee
Cardiovascular Department, John Hunter Hospital, Lookout Road, New Lambton Heights, NSW 2305, Australia

Emily Shiel
Infectious Diseases Department, John Hunter Hospital, Lookout Road, New Lambton Heights, NSW 2305, Australia

Stephen Brienesse and James Leitch
Cardiovascular Department, John Hunter Hospital, Lookout Road, New Lambton Heights, NSW 2305, Australia
Department of Medicine, University of Newcastle, Newcastle, NSW, Australia

Stuart Murch
Cardiovascular Department, John Hunter Hospital, Lookout Road, New Lambton Heights, NSW 2305, Australia

Robert Pickles
Infectious Diseases Department, John Hunter Hospital, Lookout Road, New Lambton Heights, NSW 2305, Australia
Department of Medicine, University of Newcastle, Newcastle, NSW, Australia

Adedoyin Akinlonu
Department of Medicine, Health+Hospitals/Metropolitan, New York Medical College, Valhalla, NY, USA

Ranjit Suri
Cardiovascular Department, Arrhythmia Services Mount Sinai Health System Hospitals, Mount Sinai St. Luke's, New York, NY, USA

Priyanka Yerragorla, Persio D. López, Tuoyo O. Mene-Afejuku, Olatunde Ola, Carissa Dumancas and Jumana Chalabi
Department of Medicine, Health+Hospitals/Metropolitan, New York Medical College, Valhalla, NY, USA

Gerald Pekler, Ferdinand Visco and Savi Mushiyev
Department of Medicine, Division of Cardiology, Health+Hospitals/Metropolitan, New York Medical College, Valhalla, NY, USA

Eun Song Song, Kumi Jeong, Gun Kim, In Ji Hwang, Mi-Ji Lee, Hwa Jin Cho and Young Kuk Cho
Department of Pediatrics, Chonnam National University Medical School, Chonnam National University Hospital, Gwangju, Republic of Korea

George Mawardi and Anbukarasi Maran
Coronary CTO Program, Medical University of South Carolina, 30 Courtenay Street, MSC 592, Charleston, SC 29425, USA

Hans A. Reyes and David M. Harris
Division of Cardiovascular Health and Disease, University of Cincinnati College of Medicine, Cincinnati, OH, USA

Jason J. Paquin
Division of Cardiology, Mercy Heart Institute, Cincinnati, OH, USA

Yoh Arita, Hajime Saeki, Miwa Miyoshi and Shinji Hasegawa
Department of Cardiology, Japan Community Healthcare Organization (JCHO) Osaka Hospital, 4-2-78 Fukushima, Fukushima-ku, Osaka 553-0003, Japan

Michael J. Martinelli
St. Peter's Health Partners, 2 Palisades Drive, Albany, NY 12205, USA

Michael B. Martinelli
College of Biomedical Sciences and omas Jefferson University, Philadelphia, PA, USA

Jamal Janjua, 1 and Aiman Riaz1
Department of Internal Medicine, Gundersen Health System, La Crosse, WI 54601, USA

Esosa G. Odigie-Okon
Department of Cardiology, Gundersen Health System, La Crosse, WI 54601, USA

Premnauth Rabindranauth
Department of Cardiothoracic Surgery, Gundersen Health System, La Crosse, WI 54601, USA

Richard J. Wittchow
Department of Pathology, Gundersen Health System, La Crosse, WI 54601, USA

Shin Takahashi, Yurie Takizawa, Satoshi Nakano and Kotaro Oyama
Department of Pediatrics, School of Medicine, Iwate Medical University, Morioka, Japan

Junichi Koizumi
Department of Cardiovascular Surgery, School of Medicine, Iwate Medical University, Morioka, Japan

Kenneth A. Mayuga, Natalie Ho, Paul Cremer and L. Leonardo Rodriguez
Department of Cardiovascular Medicine, Heart and Vascular Institute, Cleveland Clinic, Cleveland, OH, USA

Robert W. Shields Jr.
Neurological Institute, Cleveland Clinic, Cleveland, OH,

Wadie David, Narmeen Rehman, Robby Singh and Shukri David
Providence Hospital, Southfield, MI, USA

Koroush Khalighi
EP Lab, Easton Hospital, Drexel University, Easton, PA, USA
Department of Cardiology, Easton Cardiovascular Associates, Easton, PA, USA

Munish Sharma and Amit Toor
Department of Internal Medicine, Easton Hospital, Easton, PA, USA

Gary Costacurta
Department of Cardiology, Easton Cardiovascular Associates, Easton, PA, USA

Rubinder S. Toor
Department of Cardiology, Easton Cardiovascular Associates, Easton, PA, USA
Department of Public Health, Milken Institute School of Public Health, George Washington University, Washington, DC, USA

Vineet Meghrajani, Arsalan Hashmi and Shuo Cheng Lin
Department of Internal Medicine, Maimonides Medical Center, 4802 10th Avenue, Brooklyn, NY 11219, USA

Zvi Plawes and Shelly Brejt
Department of Cardiology, Maimonides Medical Center, 4802 10th Avenue, Brooklyn, NY 11219, USA

Doosup Shin, Kevin Huang and Igor Sunjic
Department of Internal Medicine, University of South Florida Morsani College of Medicine, Tampa, FL, USA

Michael Berlowitz and Xavier Prida
Department of Cardiovascular Sciences, University of South Florida Morsani College of Medicine, Tampa, FL, USA

Masato Kimura, Kengo Kawano, Hisao Yaoita and Shigeo Kure
Department of Pediatrics, Tohoku University Graduate School of Medicine, 1-1 Seiryo-machi, Aoba-ku, Sendai, Miyagi 980-8574, Japan

Index